Neurosurgical Issues in Otolaryngology

Principles and Practice of Collaboration

Neurosurgical Issues in Otolaryngology
Principles and Practice of Collaboration

Editors

Moisés A. Arriaga, M.D., F.A.C.S.
Pittsburgh Ear Associates
Director
The Hearing and Balance Center
Allegheny General Hospital
Pittsburgh, Pennsylvania

J. Diaz Day, M.D.
Director of Neurological Surgery
House Ear Clinic
Los Angeles, California

Illustrator

Eugene New

LIPPINCOTT WILLIAMS & WILKINS
A **Wolters Kluwer** Company
Philadelphia • Baltimore • New York • London
Buenos Aires • Hong Kong • Sydney • Tokyo

Acquisitions Editor: Danette Knopp
Developmental Editor: Maureen Iannuzzi
Production Editor: Thomas Boyce
Manufacturing Manager: Kevin Watt
Cover Designer: QT Design
Compositor: Maryland Composition, Inc.
Printer: Edwards Brothers

227 East Washington Square
Philadelphia, PA 19106-3780 USA
LWW.com

Printed in the United States of America

Library of Congress Cataloging-in-Publication Data

Neurosurgical issues in otolaryngology: principles and practice of collaboration / editors, Moises A. Arriaga, J. Diaz Day.
p. cm.
Includes bibliographical references and index.
ISBN 0-7817-1579-2
1. Otolaryngology. 2. Nervous system—Surgery. I. Arriaga, Moises A. II. Day, J. Diaz (John Diaz)
[DNLM: 1. Neurosurgery. 2. Neurosurgical Procedures.
3. Otorhinolaryngologic Surgical Procedures. WL 368 N4958 1999]
RF46.5.N48 1999
617.5′1059—dc21
DNLM/DLC
for Library of Congress 99-23052
CIP

---

10 9 8 7 6 5 4 3 2 1

My family continues to provide motivation and joy.
Rosemary's patience, encouragement, and love are essential.
Rebecca, Moi, and Toby provide focus and the spark of spontaneity.
My parents continue to provide a perspective to me of what is truly important in life.

—MAA

Contents

Contributing Authors

Adnan A. Abla, M.Sc., M.D., F.A.C.S.
Department of Neurosurgery
Allegheny General Hospital
420 East North Avenue
Pittsburgh, Pennsylvania 15212

Felipe C. Albuquerque
Department of Neurosurgery
University of Southern California
1200 North State Street, Suite 5046
Los Angeles, California 90033

Arun P. Amar, M.D.
Department of Neurosurgery
University of Southern California
1200 North State Street, Suite 5046
Los Angeles, California 90033

Michael L. J. Apuzzo, M.D.
Department of Neurosurgery
University of Southern California
1200 North State Street, Suite 5046
Los Angeles, California 90033

Moisés A. Arriaga, M.D.
The Hearing and Balance Center
Allegheny General Hospital
320 East North Avenue
Pittsburgh, Pennsylvania 15212

Julian E. Bailes, M.D.
400 Celebration Place
Suite A290
Celebration, Florida 34747

Ghassan K. Bejjani, M.D.
Department of Neurosurgery
Allegheny University Hospitals
420 East North Avenue, Suite 302
Pittsburgh, Pennsylvania 15212

Philip A. Bird, M.B., Ch.B., F.R.A.C.S.
Department of Otolaryngology–Head and Neck Surgery
Christchurch Hospital
Riccarton Avenue
Christchurch, New Zealand

Derald E. Brackmann, M.D.
House Ear Clinic
2100 West Third Street
Los Angeles, California 90057

Hilary A. Brodie, M.D.
Department of Otolaryngology
University of California Davis Medical Center
2500 Stockton Boulevard
Sacramento, California 95817

Ricardo L. Carrau, M.D.
Department of Otolaryngology
University of Pittsburgh Medical Center
200 Lothrop Street
Pittsburgh, Pennsylvania 15213

Scott E. Celin, M.D.
University of Pittsburgh School of Medicine
Allegheny University of the Health Sciences
420 East North Avenue, Suite 302
Pittsburgh, Pennsylvania 15212

James P. Chandler, M.D.
Department of Neurological Surgery
Northwestern University Medical School
233 East Erie Street, Suite 614
Chicago, Illinois 60611

Douglas A. Chen, M.D.
Department of Surgery and Neurosurgery
Allegheny General Hospital
420 East North Avenue
Pittsburgh, Pennsylvania 15212

In Sup Choi, M.D.
Interventional Neuroradiology
Lahey Clinic Medical Center
41 Mall Road, Room 6W31
Burlington, Massachusetts 01805

Joseph D. Ciacci, M.D.
Department of Neurological Surgery
The Johns Hopkins Hospital
Baltimore, Maryland 21229

William D. Clark, M.D.
Department of Otolaryngology
Wilford Hall Air Force Medical Center
Lackland AFB
Department of Otolaryngology
University of Texas Health Science Center at San Antonio
59 MDW/MKCE
2200 Bergquist Drive, Suite 1
Lackland AFB, Texas 78236

Peter D. Costantino, M.D., F.A.C.S.
Department of Otolaryngology
Mount Sinai Medical Center
One Gustave Levy Place
New York, New York 10029

C. Phillip Daspit, M.D.
Department of Neurosurgery
The Barrow Neurological Institute
Mercy Healthcare Arizona
350 West Thomas Road
Phoenix, Arizona 85013-4496

Bolivia T. Davis, M.D.
Department of Radiology
Georgetown University Medical Center
3800 Reservoir Road, NW
Washington, D.C. 20007

J. Diaz Day, M.D.
Department of Neurological Surgery
House Ear Clinic
2100 West Third Street
Los Angeles, California 90057

Michael J. Fucci, M.D.
3487 Broadway
Fort Myers, Florida 33901

Takanori Fukushima, M.D.
Carolina Skull Base Surgery Center
Carolina Neuroscience and Ear Research Institute
3404 Wake Forest Road, Suite 303
Raleigh/Durham, North Carolina 27609

Michael W. Gorum, M.D.
Chief, Neurosurgery
Columbus Regional Medical Center
710 Center Street
Columbus, Georgia 31902

Regis W. Haid, M.D.
Department of Neurosurgery
Emory University School of Medicine
1365-B Clifton Road, NE
Atlanta, Georgia 30322

Richard E. Hayden, M.D.
Department of Otolaryngology
Allegheny University of the Health Sciences
Hahnemann Campus
2 Logan Square, Suite 1800
Philadelphia, Pennsylvania 19103

William E. Hitselberger, M.D.
2222 Ocean View, Suite 119
Los Angeles, California 90057

Annelle V. Hodges, Ph.D.
Department of Otolaryngology (D-48)
University of Miami School of Medicine
P.O. Box 016960
Miami, Florida 33101

Ivo P. Janecka, M.D., F.A.C.S.
Longwood Skull Base Program
Harvard Medical School
300 Longwood Avenue/HU-152
Boston, Massachusetts 02115

Hae-Dong Jho, M.D.
Department of Neurological Surgery
University of Pittsburgh Medical Center
203 Lothrop Street
Pittsburgh, Pennsylvania 15213

D. Kyle Kim, M.D., Ph.D.
Department of Neurosurgery
Allegheny General Hospital
420 East North Avenue, Suite 408
Pittsburgh, Pennsylvania 15212

Paul A. Lobaugh, Ph.D.
Allegheny Neuro-Monitors, Inc.
Neuromonitoring Services
Allegheny General Hospital
1321 Sandusky Street
Pittsburgh, Pennsylvania 15212

Joseph C. Maroon, M.D.
Department of Neurosurgery
Allegheny General Hospital
420 East North Avenue, Suite 302
Pittsburgh, Pennsylvania 15212

David Masel, M.D.
2600 North Oregon, Suite 800
El Paso, Texas 79902

Max Medary, M.D.
Department of Neuroscience
Celebration Hospital
400 Celebration Place, Suite A290
Celebration, Florida 34747

Anil Nanda, M.D.
Department of Neurosurgery
Louisiana State University Medical Center
1501 Kings Highway, P.O. Box 33932
Shreveport, Louisiana 71130-3932

Daniel W. Nuss, M.D., F.A.C.S.
Department of Otolaryngology–Head and Neck Surgery
Louisiana State University Medical Center
2020 Gravier Street, Suite A
New Orleans, Louisiana 70112-2234

Randall A. Ow, M.D.
Chief, Otolaryngology–Head and Neck Surgery
3rd Medical Group/SGOSL
5955 Zeamer Street
Elmendorf AFB, Alaska 99506

Ozcan Ozdamar, Ph.D.
Department of Biomedical Engineering
University of Miami
P.O. Box 248294
Coral Gables, Florida 33124

Zbigniew Petrovich, M.D.
Department of Radiation Oncology
University of Southern California
School of Medicine
1441 Eastlake Avenue, G34
Los Angeles, California 90033

Robert C. Platenberg, M.D.
Director of Diagnostic Services
MedTel International Corporation
1430 Spring Hill Road, Suite 500
McLean, Virginia 22102

Matthew R. Quigley, M.D.
Department of Neurosurgery
Allegheny General Hospital
320 East North Avenue
Pittsburgh, Pennsylvania 15212

Peter L. Rigby, M.D.
Department of Otolaryngology
Louisiana State University Medical Center
2020 Gravier Street, Suite A
New Orleans, Louisiana 70112-2234

Raimund Rueger, M.D.
Department of Otolaryngology
Allegheny General Hospital
320 East North Avenue
Pittsburgh, Pennsylvania 15212

Karl D. Schultz, Jr., M.D.
Department of Neurosurgery
Emory University School of Medicine
1365-B Clifton Road, NE
Atlanta, Georgia 30322

Gary W. Schurman, M.S.
Allegheny Neuro-Monitors, Inc.
Neuromonitoring Services
Allegheny General Hospital
1321 Sandusky Street
Pittsburgh, Pennsylvania 15212

Laligam N. Sekhar, M.D.
Department of Neurosurgery
Center for Cranial Base Surgery
George Washington University Medical Center
2150 Pennsylvania Avenue, NW
ACC #7-149
Washington, D.C. 20037

Robert F. Spetzler, M.D.
Department of Neurological Surgery
Barrow Neurological Institute
Mercy Healthcare Arizona
350 West Thomas Road
Phoenix, Arizona 85013-4496

Scott E. Strome, M.D.
Department of Otolaryngology–Head and Neck Surgery
Mayo Clinic
200 First Street SW
Rochester, Minnesota 55905-0002

Charles A. Syms III, M.D., M.B.A., F.A.C.S.
Ear Medical Group
Texas Neuroscience Institute
4410 Medical Drive, Suite 550
San Antonio, Texas 78229

Jarturon Tantivatana, M.D.
Department of Radiology
Faculty of Medicine
Chulalongkorn University
Bangkok 10330, Thailand

Lokesh S. Tantuwaya, M.D.
Alllegheny University Hospitals
420 East North Avenue, Suite 302
Pittsburgh, Pennsylvania 15212

Fred F. Telischi, M.E.E., M.D., F.A.C.S.
Department of Otolaryngology and Neurological Surgery
University of Miami School of Medicine
1666 NW Tenth Avenue
Miami, Florida 33136

A. Giancarlo Vishteh, M.D.
Division of Neurological Surgery
The Barrow Neurological Institute
Mercy Healthcare Arizona
350 West Thomas Road
Phoenix, Arizona 85013-4496

Jack Wilberger, M.D., F.A.C.S.
Department of Neurosurgery
Allegheny General Hospital
420 East North Avenue, Suite 302
Pittsburgh, Pennsylvania 15212

Joe B. Wiseman, M.D.
Department of Otolaryngology–Head and Neck Surgery
Wilford Hall Medical Center
Brooke Army Medical Center
59 MDW/MKCE
2200 Berquist Drive, Suite 1
Lackland AFB, Texas 78236-5300

Matthew E. Wolpoe
Department of Otolaryngology
Mount Sinai Medical Center
One Gustave Levy Place
New York, New York 10029

Donald C. Wright, M.D.
Department of Neurosurgery
George Washington University Medical Center
2150 Pennsylvania Avenue, NW
ACC #7-420
Washington, D.C. 20037

Esther L. Wylen, M.D.
Department of Ophthalmology
Alton Ochsner Medical Foundation Clinics
1516 Jefferson Highway
New Orleans, Louisiana 70121

Cheng Yu, Ph.D.
Department of Radiation Oncology
University of Southern California
1441 Eastlake Avenue
Los Angeles, California 90033-0804

Preface

The overlap between neurosurgery and otolaryngology is no longer a battle line for "turf wars." Instead, this overlap has become fertile ground for collaboration. Patient outcomes are certainly enhanced when there are coordinated efforts on behalf of the patient, utilizing the expertise of both specialties when surgical lesions involve areas or problems with which both otolaryngologists and neurosurgeons are familiar.

Despite this increased spirit of cooperation, neurosurgery and otolaryngology are distinct fields with different backgrounds. The motivation of this textbook is to bridge that difference in backgrounds. Otolaryngologists need familiarity with neurosurgical concerns about brain physiology, vascular management, and neural preservation to truly offer collaborative help in exposure and tissue management. Likewise, appropriate management of the middle ear, eustachian tube, otic capsule, paranasal sinuses, and nasal anatomy is crucial for successful functional outcomes in cases in which the neurosurgical interests are primarily with the deeper neurological structures.

This textbook is geared toward otolaryngologists who perform collaborative procedures with neurosurgeons and neurosurgeons who perform collaborative procedures with otolaryngologists–head and neck surgeons. We have not attempted to create a combined comprehensive textbook. Instead, this textbook emphasizes those areas of mutual interest where ongoing collaboration requires a background in both fields.

Moisés A. Arriaga, M.D.

Acknowledgments

I thank Danette Knopp for her enthusiasm, guidance, and support of this project. She is a wonderful motivator who has nursed this project through to completion. The editors are grateful for the patience of the contributors as this project has evolved over the months since its inception. I also specifically thank Shirley Simonic, my academic coordinator, for her tireless efforts at organization, patience with our multiple distractions, and firm yet tactful encouragement to reach the finish line.

Neurosurgical Issues in Otolaryngology
Principles and Practice of Collaboration

Neurosurgical Issues in Otolaryngology: Principles and Practice of Collaboration,
edited by Moisés A. Arriaga and J. Diaz Day.
Lippincott Williams & Wilkins, Philadelphia © 1999.

CHAPTER 1

Cerebrospinal Fluid: Physiology, Drainage, and Leakage

Randall A. Ow, Charles A. Syms III, and Michael Gorum

APPLIED ANATOMY

Cerebrospinal fluid (CSF) is a clear, colorless fluid that bathes the brain and spinal cord. It fills the ventricles and is contained within the subarachnoid space. A major function of CSF is to cushion the brain and spinal cord against trauma. The specific gravity of the brain is within 4% of the specific gravity of CSF, and the brain literally floats within the CSF (1). Other functions of the CSF are to nourish the neural tissues of the brain and to remove waste products of neuronal metabolism.

The Meninges

The layers of connective tissue surrounding the central nervous system (CNS) include the tough fibrous dura mater, the loose connective arachnoid membrane (or arachnoidea), and the pia mater (Fig. 1-1). These layers compartmentalize both true and potential spaces with significant clinical relevance.

The epidural space is defined as the space between the inner periosteal lining of the calvarium (and vertebral canal) and the dura mater. In some places, the dura is so closely adherent to the periosteum that epidural space is actually subperiosteal. Epidural hematomas are collections of blood in this space and are commonly a result of blunt head trauma. Epidural anesthesia is a form of spinal anesthesia where anesthetic agents are placed into the epidural space. It is frequently used in obstetrics and a variety of surgical procedures requiring analgesia below the diaphragm.

R. A. Ow: Chief, Otolaryngology—Head & Neck Surgery, 3rd Medical Group, Elmendorf AFB, Alaska 99506.

C. A. Syms III: Ear Medical Group, Texas Neuroscience Institute, San Antonio, Texas 78229.

M. Gorum: Neurological Surgery, Columbus Regional Medical Center, Columbus, Georgia 31901.

The subdural space is confined between the dura mater and the arachnoid membrane. Trauma to the head is commonly associated with hematomas in the subdural space. Unlike the acute mental status changes seen with epidural hematomas, subdural hematomas can present insidiously, with fluctuations of mental status occurring over the course of days.

The arachnoid membrane and the pia mater bound the subarachnoid space. It is continuous with the ventricles (*see below*) and contains CSF. This sterile compartment with tightly regulated pressures and rigidly controlled composition is critical in the diagnosis and management of a variety of pathologic and neoplastic processes affecting the CNS.

Processes important to neurosurgeons and otolaryngologists include infections of the CNS, elevated CSF pressures, and CSF leaks. Large blood vessels of the brain traverse this space along with a delicate network of fine connective tissue. The subarachnoid space extends along the olfactory nerves to the mucoperiosteum of the nasal cavity. It also extends along blood vessels as they enter and exit the brain. Inferiorly, the subarachnoid space envelops the cauda equina and ends at the 2nd to 3rd sacral vertebra.

The pia mater is intimately associated with the convoluted undulations of the brain surface. Special extensions of the pia mater form the dentate ligaments around the spinal cord, anchoring the spinal cord to the dura.

The Ventricles

The ventricles of the brain are four fluid-filled cavities containing CSF (Fig. 1-2). They are readily identified in computed tomograms of the brain and are sensitive indicators of intracranial mass effects, exhibiting either compression or shift from their normal positions relative to the midline. Histologically, the ventricles are lined by ependyma, a

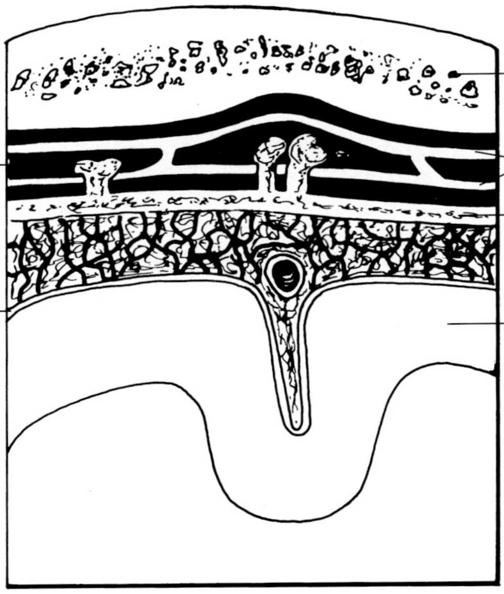

FIG. 1-1. Meningeal layers of the brain.

special simple cuboidal epithelium with limited secretory function.

The lateral ventricles are paired structures joined by the foramina of Monro to the third ventricle. Each lateral ventricle is a C-shaped cavity encased in the cerebral hemisphere. It extends from the frontal lobe, traverses the temporal lobe, and terminates in the occipital lobe. The choroid plexus of the lateral ventricle is located on the medial wall of the ventricle.

The third and fourth ventricles are unpaired, midline structures and are connected to each other by the cerebral aqueduct of Sylvius. The cerebral aqueduct is lined only by ependyma and contains no choroid. The third ventricle is a slit-like cleft lying between the two thalami of the brain. The choroid plexus of the third ventricle is located in its roof. The fourth ventricle is situated anterior to the cerebellum and posterior to the pons. It is continuous inferiorly with the central canal of the spinal cord. Importantly, the ventricles communicate with the subarachnoid space through three openings in the roof of the fourth ventricle. The foramen of Magendie is a single foramen located in the roof of the fourth ventricle; the foramina of Luschka are paired lateral openings.

At its inferior aspect, the subarachnoid space is dilated and becomes the lumbar cistern. During lumbar puncture, this cistern is accessed for diagnostic aspiration of CSF.

CSF PHYSIOLOGY

Composition

CSF is normally a clear, colorless fluid. It is composed of soluble inorganic salts similar to those found in plasma. Significant differences are summarized in Table 1-1. Notably, few cells are present in CSF. The normal lymphocyte count is 0 to 3 cells/mm^3.

CSF pressure is strictly regulated by a variety of mechanisms. Pressure is a function of CSF production, resorption, and flow dynamics. Under a wide variety of conditions, CSF pressure is maintained at 60 to 150 mm H_2O (2). It is dependent on age, position, and other factors. It is increased greatly with the Valsalva maneuver, coughing, and straining. Compressing the internal jugular veins also raises the CSF pressure. In the neonate, pressures are lower due to the pliability of the cranial cavity prior to closure of the cranial sutures.

CSF Production

The majority of CSF is produced by the choroid plexus, located in the lateral, third and fourth ventricles. Choroidal production of CSF is thought to account for approximately two-thirds of total production. Extrachoroidal formation of CSF occurs in the ventricular ependyma (3). The rate of CSF production is relatively constant throughout the day at approximately 500 cc/day or 0.30 mL/min. In adults, CSF volume averages 150 mL; therefore, CSF volume is turned over about three times a day.

The formation of CSF is a metabolically active process (4), regulated in part by the enzymes $Na\text{-}K^+$ adenosine triphosphatase (ATPase) and carbonic anhydrase. Because carbonic anhydrase is closely linked to acid-base physiology, changes in blood pH are associated with alterations in CSF production. Carbonic anhydrase inhibitors can be administered to decrease CSF production by up to 50%.

The choroid plexus is specialized tissue found in the ventricles of the brain. It is arranged as numerous villi composed of simple cuboidal epithelium surrounding a highly vascular, connective tissue core. The choroid actively modifies an ultrafiltrate of plasma and produces CSF at a steady state of 18 of 21 mL/h in both children and adults. The resulting fluid is secreted into the ventricles by the choroidal epithe-

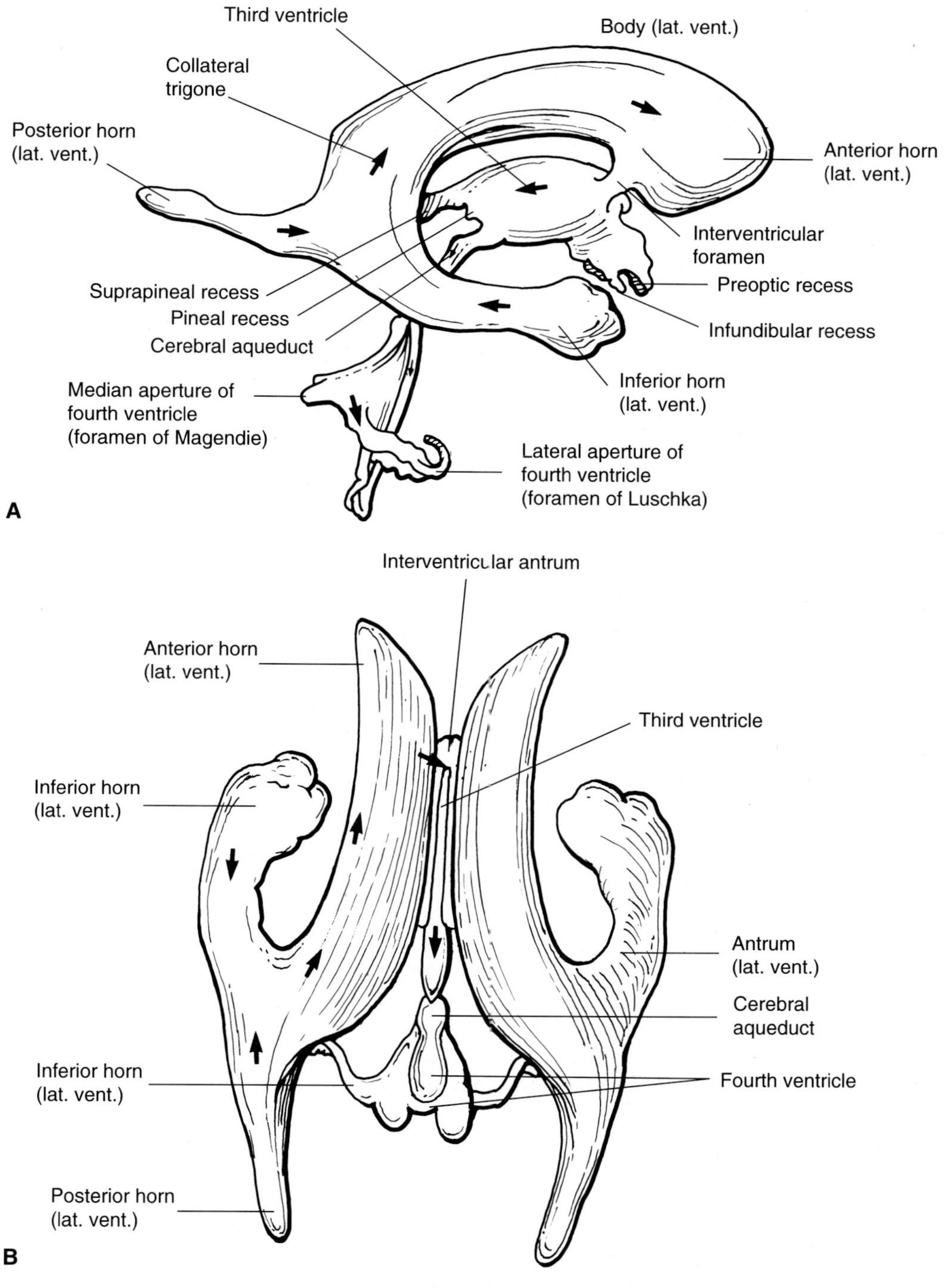

FIG. 1-2. Ventricular system of the brain.

lium. The secretion rate is not influenced by acute changes in intracranial pressure within physiologic limits, but chronic changes in intracranial pressure such as in hydrocephalus may reduce the rate of CSF formation.

CSF Resorption

The resorption of CSF classically occurs at the arachnoid villi, also known as arachnoid granulations (Fig. 1-3). These structures represent finger-like projections intimately associated with the dural venous sinuses. Resorption appears to be a passive phenomenon of CSF back into the central circulation, obeying the pressure gradient that exists between the subarachnoid space and the venous sinuses. The hydrostatic relationship is linear above a pressure threshold equal to the venous sinus pressure.

CSF Circulation

CSF flows from its site of production in the ventricles through the foramina of Magendie and Luschka, exiting the

TABLE 1–1. *Concentration of various substances in human cerebrospinal fluid (CSF) and plasma*

Substance		CSF	Plasma	Ratio CSF/plasma
Na^+	(mEq/kg H_2O)	147.0	150.0	0.96
K^+	(mEq/kg H_2O)	2.9	4.6	0.62
Mg^{2+}	(mEq/kg H_2O)	2.2	1.6	1.39
Ca^{2+}	(mEq/kg H_2O)	2.3	4.7	0.48
Cl^-	(mEq/kg H_2O)	113.0	99.0	1.14
HCD_3^-	(mEq/L)	25.1	24.8	1.01
P_{CO_2}	(mm Hg)	50.2	39.5	1.28
pH		7.33	7.40	—
Osmolality	(moem/kg H_2O)	289.0	289.0	1.00
Protein	(mg/dL)	20.0	6000.0	0.003
Glucose	(mg/dL)	64.0	100.0	0.64
Inorganic P	(mg/dL)	3.4	4.7	0.73
Urea	(mg/dL)	12.0	15.0	0.80
Creatinine	(mg/dL)	1.5	1.2	1.25
Uric acid	(mg/dL)	1.5	5.0	0.30
Lactic acid	(mg/dL)	18.0	21.0	0.86
Cholesterol	(mg/dL)	0.2	175.0	0.001

cisterna magna and the basal cisterns to enter the subarachnoid space. CSF absorption takes place at the arachnoid villi, where it is returned to the blood by way of the dural sinuses.

The driving forces behind CSF circulation remain elusive. Studies have supported various theories as to exact mechanisms. It is generally thought that arterial pulsations somehow propel CSF from the ventricles into the subarachnoid spaces overlying the cerebral convexities. Flow around the spinal cord is facilitated by vertebral column motion.

HYDROCEPHALUS

Etiology

Hydrocephalus is a condition in which the ventricular volume of CSF is enlarged in relation to brain volume. Conditions leading to white matter loss, such as stroke or head injury, may lead to *ex vacuo* hydrocephalus. In contrast to obstructive hydrocephalus, *ex vacuo* hydrocephalus is a nonobstructive form of hydrocephalus.

Obstructive hydrocephalus is classified as communicating or noncommunicating. Communicating hydrocephalus is caused by obstruction at the cisternal level, while noncommunicating hydrocephalus results from blockage of CSF flow in the ventricular system. Hydrocephalus may also result from overproduction of CSF, as well as from impaired resorption. In the practice of otolaryngology, hydrocephalus from obstruction is the most likely form to be encountered.

Noncommunicating hydrocephalus may be caused by congenital abnormalities such as aqueductal stenosis, Chiari II malformation, or vein of Galen aneurysm. In neonates, germinal matrix hemorrhage may result in obstruction at the level of the foramina of Monro, the sylvian aqueduct, or the foramina of Luschka and Magendie. Large tumors of the cerebellopontine angle, pineal region, or cerebellum may also result in noncommunicating hydrocephalus.

Communicating hydrocephalus is seen from compromised cisternal CSF circulation resulting from basal meningitis, either spontaneous or postoperative. Carcinomatous involvement of the basal cisterns in carcinomatous meningitis may also result in communicating hydrocephalus.

Signs and Symptoms

Adults may present with a variety of symptoms ranging from minor to life threatening. They include headache, nausea, vomiting, diplopia, and depressed consciousness. Signs include papilledema, gait abnormality, upgaze paresis, and sixth nerve palsy. Children may have additional symptoms related to head growth, fontanelle fullness, splayed sutures, and Macewen's sign.

Computed tomography (CT) or magnetic resonance imaging (MRI) are suggestive of hydrocephalus, and often demonstrate the etiology in cases of obstruction. Enlargement of the temporal horns, lack of visible sulci, ballooning of the third ventricle, and transependymal absorption are reliable radiographic indicators of hydrocephalus. Plain radiographs of the skull may demonstrate a beaten silver appearance of the cranium or enlargement of the sella turcica in chronic cases.

Management

The majority of cases cannot be treated with direct surgical intervention. Various CSF diversion techniques have been developed, including external drainage via lumbar or ventricular drainage, lumbar peritoneal shunting, and ventriculoatrial and ventriculoperitoneal shunting. A variety of devices are commercially available to meet these ends.

A ventriculostomy is a drainage catheter placed into the cerebral ventricular system via a burr hole. It can be used as a temporizing measure in the case of large posterior fossa lesions in hopes that normal CSF dynamics will be reestablished after successful tumor removal, or in other acute processes such as trauma or subarachnoid hemorrhage. Ventricular puncture may also be used intraoperatively to aid in exposure of circle of Willis lesions or parasellar lesions. The device may then be left in place postoperatively to function as a drain or an intracranial pressure-monitoring device. Removing the obstructing pathology will sometimes be successful in treating noncommunicating hydrocephalus.

CSF LEAKS

Pathophysiology

A CSF leak occurs when the barriers retaining CSF around the brain are violated. Normally skin, galea, periosteum, skull, dura mater, and the arachnoid membrane can all aid in the retention of CSF. In addition, the mucosal lining of the mastoid air cells and the paranasal sinuses can act as a barrier. It helps to think of these fistulas in terms of their

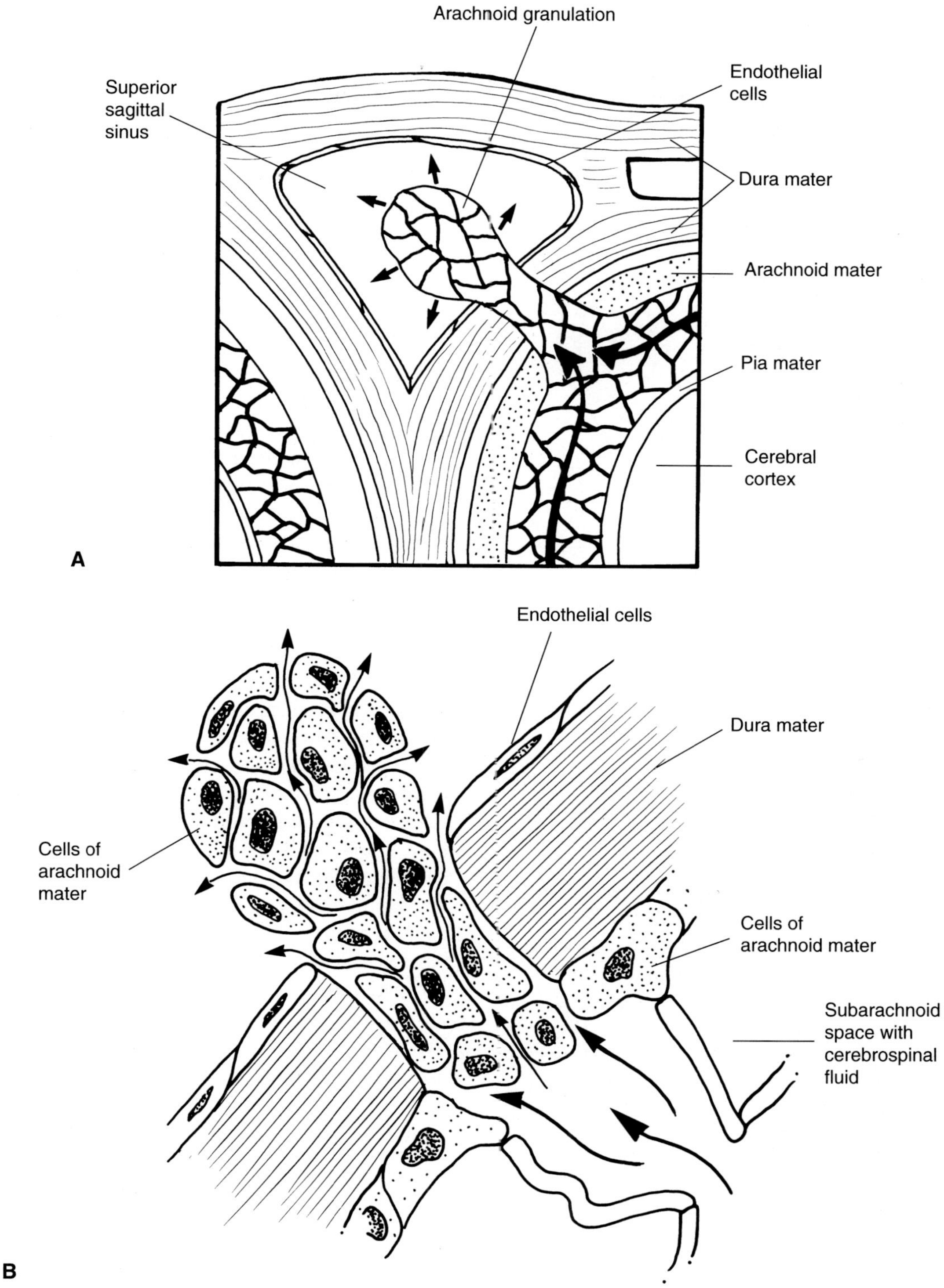

FIG. 1-3. Cerebrospinal fluid resorption in arachnoid granulation.

etiology and the localization of the site of the fistula and where the drainage comes out (Fig. 1-4). So when describing postsurgical ethmoid sinus CSF rhinorrhea or posttraumatic otorrhea the source and general location is apparent. Descriptions of a ''nontraumatic'' fistula are more difficult. Although CSF leaks can certainly occur through congenital anomalies or areas where the normal barriers are weakened or dehiscent, this is a rare situation. Most commonly a nontraumatic CSF fistula is secondary to a distant trauma that the patient may not recall except under close questioning. In these cases there was probably a small fracture that healed but remained weakened. Ommaya et al. (5) divided sponta-

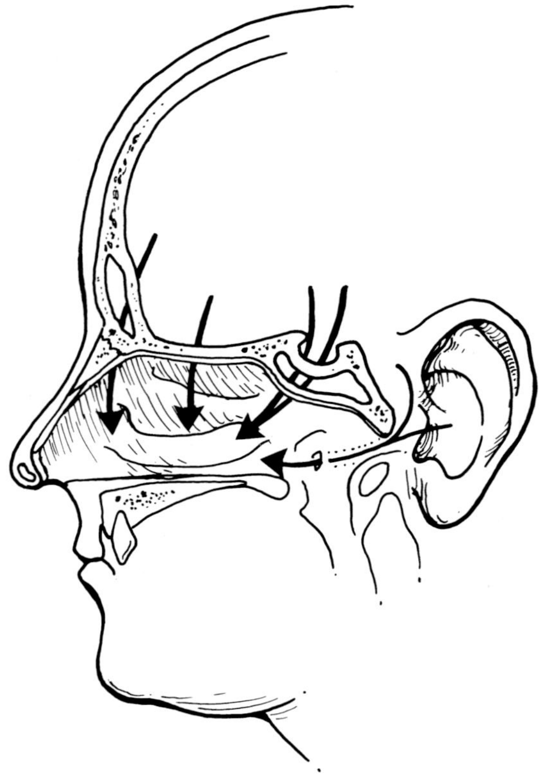

FIG. 1-4. Common sites of cerebrospinal fluid leaks.

neous CSF fistulas into high and normal pressure leaks. The high-pressure leaks are related to their concurrent hydrocephalus. Normal pressure leaks are associated with congenital dehiscence or thin bone along the skull base. Most commonly this occurs in the ethmoid sinuses adjacent to the cribriform plate or into the mastoid air cell system.

A CSF leak must be treated because of the threat of meningitis. If the CSF is escaping through a dural and skull base defect, then bacteria have a route to invade the CNS. The risk of meningitis associated with a CSF leak varies with the etiology but ranges from 4% to 50% (6,7). The leak may be obvious and follow a traumatic or surgical event, or it may present with meningitis with no obvious cause. A high index of suspicion and knowledge of the full range of diagnostic maneuvers and tests is necessary to detect fistulas that may be subtle.

Causes

A number of classification schemes have been used, but the most practical is using the cause to separate the various types of CSF leaks. The presence or absence of hydrocephalus or increased intracranial pressure must be reviewed with each individual cause of the CSF leak as either can often make the situation more difficult.

Spontaneous

Truly spontaneous fistulas are very rare. There is almost always some distant antecedent traumatic event that the patient experienced but has since forgotten. Nuss (8) has pointed out that the cause of spontaneous CSF leaks is due to the ''four Ps'': Intracranial *pressure* may be elevated. The brain continuously *pulsates* along the skull base. The degree of *pneumatization* of the paranasal sinuses and temporal bone is commonly extensive. Arachnoid *pits* or villi exist normally along the skull base, and through continued transmission of pulsations, bone is eroded away until the arachnoid communicates with a pneumatized space, with the potential to develop a fistula.

Traumatic

The most common etiology of a CSF leak is injury. Skull fractures, in addition to closed head injury, increase the incidence of CSF leaks. Lewin (9) reported CSF leaks to occur in 2% of 1,000 patients with closed head injury. In a series of 1,745 cases of skull fractures and head injuries Mincy (10) found a 3% rate of rhinorrhea. The trauma may be penetrating or blunt trauma. Most leaks develop within several days of the injury, but can be delayed by weeks, months, or even years.

Iatrogenic

Every neurosurgeon and neurotologist has experienced the difficulty of managing a postoperative CSF leak. Prevention is the key, and the incidence is greatly reduced when a dural closure is obtained. If reestablishing dural continuity is not possible, as is frequently the case in procedures involving the internal auditory canal (IAC) and skull base, then autologous fat and muscle grafts, hydroxyapatite, ionomeric bone cement, or pedicled or free tissue transfer flaps must be utilized to obtain a watertight closure. Bone wax should be used to seal all small, exposed air cell tracts. After a large extirpation and complex closure of the wound, identifying the exact site of the fistula may prove difficult. Rogers and Luxford (11) reported a 6.8% incidence of CSF leak following translabyrinthine surgery, but an incidence of up to 25% following jugular foramen surgery has been reported.

Congenital

Meningocele, meningoencephalocele, inner ear and IAC dysplasias (Mondini deformity), a patent cochlear aqueduct, Hyrtl's fissure, or petromastoid canal can all cause cerebrospinal fluid fistulas and meningitis. Spontaneous CSF leaks are a diagnosis of exclusion, and a careful search for a congenital cause must be undertaken before a leak is identified as spontaneous.

Neoplastic and Infectious

Tumors and infections both have the potential to erode all of the protective tissue surrounding CSF. Neurotologic complications of chronic otitis media do still occur and one of the authors (C.A.S.) has seen epidural and brain abscesses, meningitis, and cerebrospinal fistulas occur in patients treated with antimicrobial therapy.

Diagnosis and Evaluation

The diagnosis of a CSF leak is usually obvious in the postsurgical patient, but can present a considerable challenge in the spontaneous or congenital CSF fistula patient. Confirmation of a CSF leak usually proceeds in complexity and expense from simple bedside testing to invasive imaging.

At the bedside the simplest test is a reservoir sign (Fig. 1-5). This test is best performed upon the patient's arising in the morning. Patients place their chin to their chest and stay in this position for one minute by the clock. Although patients may complain of rhinorrhea that at times may be confusing, due to previous instrumentation of the nose, copious drainage that drips from the nose like a leaky faucet can only be due to CSF. If the leak is intermittent and a question remains, the use of topical nasal ipratropium bromide can greatly reduce nasal sources of drainage. Any drainage can be collected and tested, although we do not believe the added expense is worthwhile. The most sensitive chemical test is β_2-transferrin; tests for glucose or protein are not recommended. A ring or target sign of the drainage from a trauma patient is helpful in distinguishing simple epistaxis from a mixed rhinorrhea. The "handkerchief sign" may be helpful in patients with copious rhinorrhea due to allergic rhinitis: mucus will cause cotton or paper handkerchiefs to stiffen as they dry, but after CSF dries the handkerchief will remain soft.

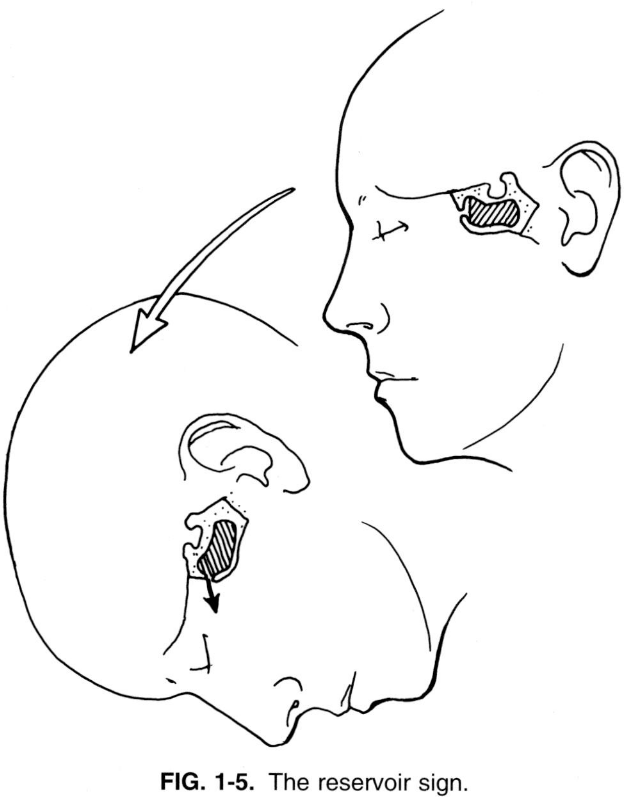

FIG. 1-5. The reservoir sign.

When the fistula is through the temporal bone, a clear effusion may be noted in the middle ear through the tympanic membrane. After placement of a pressure equalization tube, the diagnosis is usually obvious, with copious clear thin otorrhea.

The most sensitive test to detect a CSF leak is an intrathecal radionucleotide test. Unfortunately this test only localizes the leak to one side or a general area of the nose. When a leak is intermittent or consists of minute quantities, pledgets left in the different regions of the nose during the test will collect a sample that can later be measured. Although in the past this test was touted for its ability to localize the site of the leak, today there are better tests.

Localization

When attempting to determine the site of the fistula, there are three tests that we use commonly. Flow-sensitive MRI has proven useful in depicting the site of an ongoing leak (12). The leak must be active at the time of the scan to be visualized. Since this test is noninvasive, we usually attempt this first. Intrathecal administration of nonionic contrast with high-resolution CT scanning has proven to be the workhorse test for the last decade. This test is usually well tolerated and only infrequently fails to demonstrate the leak. We have not found it necessary to continuously administer the contrast, generating pressure, as described by Spetzler and Wilson (13). We frequently use intrathecal administration of low quantities of fluorescein and then view the nasal cavity or temporal bone with 490-nm light generated by optical filters (14). This has proven useful in the preoperative evaluation and especially at the time of the repair in the operating room. We use only one or two drops of 5% Fluorescite (for intravenous injection) diluted with the patient's own CSF and administered with a barbotage technique (14). This technique involves repeated partial injection and then withdrawing additional CSF to further dilute the dye. When used in this manner, we believe intrathecal fluorescein to be safe and extremely helpful in precisely identifying the site of the fistula.

Management

The management of a CSF leak depends on the cause and comorbid medical conditions. Conservative measures such as bed rest, elevating the head of the bed, stool softeners, instructions not to strain or bear down, reapplying a pressure dressing, and a short course of acetazolamide may all prove beneficial.

Continuous or daily intermittent lumbar spinal drainage has been very helpful and allowed the fistula to heal most of the time. Lumbar drainage is indicated for those failing the conservative measures mentioned above. The drains can be placed either intraoperatively or at the bedside. Sterile technique should be employed to prevent introduction of pathogens into the sterile environment of the subarachnoid space. The drain should be placed between the third and fourth lumbar vertebrae. Once free flow of CSF is established, the indwelling catheter should be advanced. Tunneling the catheter through the skin surrounding the puncture site serves several purposes. It secures the catheter in place, prevents kinking, and inhibits secondary CSF infection.

The catheter is attached to a closed drainage system and either gravity drainage or flow-regulating devices control the desired rate of evacuation. Adjusting the relative heights of the drainage bag to the patient by raising the patient's bed or lowering the reservoir bag allows control of flow without the need for mechanical devices. More precise control can be obtained by connecting the catheter tubing to intravenous pumping devices. Drainage should not exceed the rate of CSF production, which approximates 20 cc per hour. Usually, a drainage rate of 8 to 10 cc per hour is sufficient to allow most small leaks to seal.

Various problems can occur with the use of lumbar drainage. Drainage can be decreased due to migration of the catheter out of the subarachnoid space, obstruction of the catheter with blood or tissue, or kinking of the catheter itself. Leakage of CSF around the catheter site can be a misleading cause of malfunction. Too fast a rate of drainage has been associated with the development of pneumocephalus, which may be life threatening if unrecognized (15). Lastly, bacterial meningitis can be associated with the use of lumbar drains either through introduction of bacteria at the catheter site or by facilitating the ingress of bacteria at the primary leak site itself.

We do not hesitate to operate when conservative management fails. Most frequently, simply reexploring the wound and bringing fresh tissue in to seal the area is adequate. Occasionally using hydroxyapatite cement has proven beneficial in difficult cases. Obliterating the middle ear, eustachian tube, and external ear canal with oversewing of the cartilaginous canal has stopped particularly troublesome CSF leaks. In our experience, this has been necessary only in cases of severe temporal bone trauma. The technique is identical to the beginning of the infratemporal fossa approach to the jugular foramen.

Recently, CSF fistulas have been repaired from below with endoscopic techniques (Fig. 1-6). This avoids a craniotomy, but may not enjoy the same success as traditional neurosurgical approaches. We feel that this approach is best

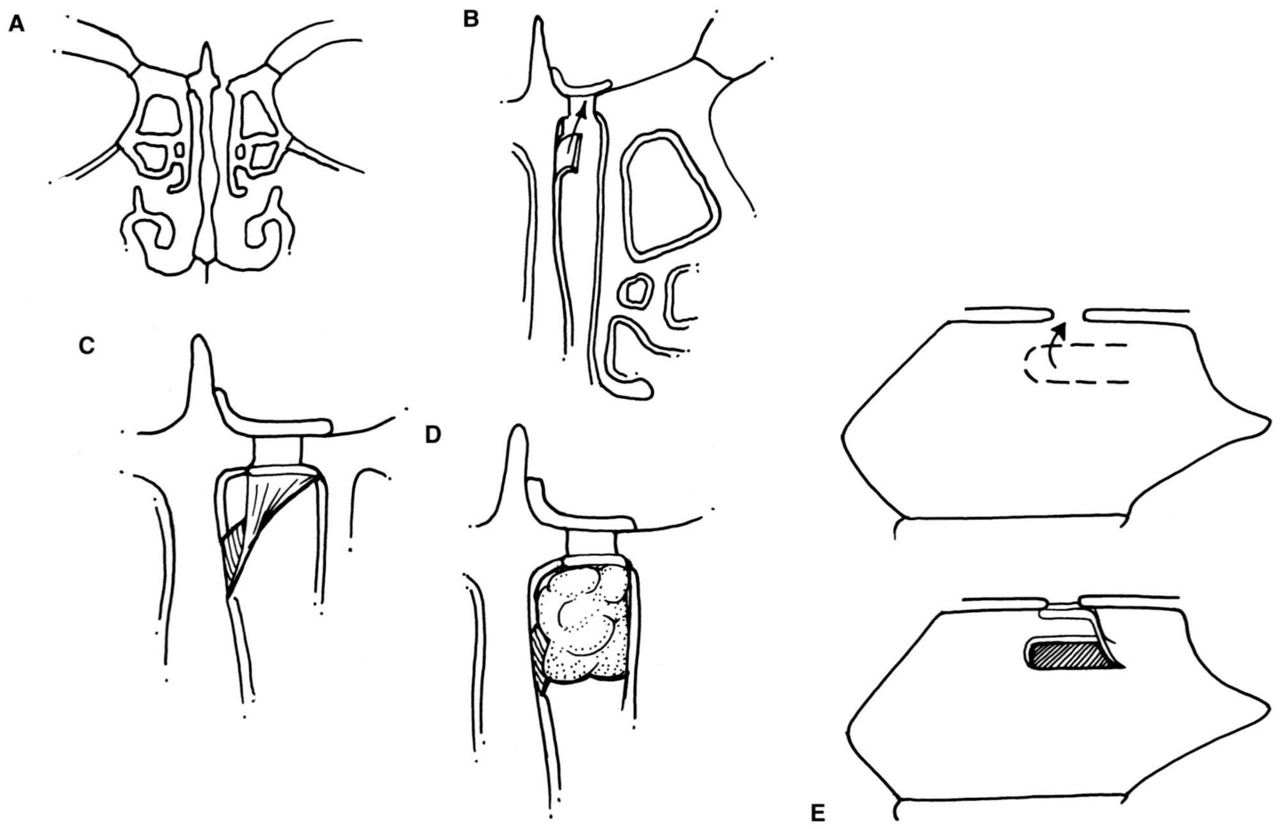

FIG. 1-6. Schematic diagram of coronal section through anterior skull base. **A:** Cerebrospinal fluid fistula at the cribriform plate. **B:** Fascia graft, larger than bony defect, placed extradurally. A flap of septal mucosa has been raised. **C:** Mucosal flap in position. **D:** Resorbable packing in place supporting the mucosal flap. **E:** Lateral view of septal mucosal flap.

reserved for an anterior cranial fossa fistula where a traditional approach will lead to anosmia in a large percentage of patients.

In trauma patients most fistulas will seal by themselves, and so they should be managed with close observation. In the past, prophylactic antibiotics were thought to do more harm than good. Brodie (16) recently did a meta-analysis of the literature on this topic and found antibiotics helpful, especially when the patient has a leak longer than 7 days or in the presence of a concurrent infection. Postsurgical patients with leaks through their nose via the eustachian tube respond to conservative management most of the time. Surgical treatment will always be required in patients with spontaneous or congenital cerebrospinal fluid fistulas.

REFERENCES

1. Kingsley RE, Gable SR, Kingsley TR, eds. *Concise text of neuroscience*. Baltimore, MD: Williams & Wilkins, 1996.
2. Guyton AC, Hall JE. *Human physiology and mechanisms of disease*, 6th ed. Philadelphia: WB Saunders, 1997.
3. Narayan RK, Wilberger JE, Povlishock JT. *Neurotrauma*. New York: McGraw-Hill, 1995.
4. Yeomans JR, ed. *Neurological surgery*, 4th ed. Philadelphia: WB Saunders, 1996.
5. Ommaya AK, Di Chiro G, Baldwin M. Non-traumatic cerebrospinal fluid rhinorrhea. *J Neurol Neurosurg Psychiatry* 1968;31:214.
6. Brisman R, Hughes JEO, Mount LA. Cerebrospinal fluid otorrhea. *Arch Neurol* 1970;22:245.
7. MacGee EE, Cauthen JC, Brackett CE. Meningitis following acute traumatic cerebrospinal fluid fistula. *J Neurosurg* 1970;33:312.
8. Nuss D. Diagnosis and management of cerebrospinal fluid fistulas. *Adv Otolaryngol Head Neck Surg* 1994;8:247.
9. Lewin W. Cerebrospinal fluid rhinorrhea in closed head injuries. *Br J Surg* 1954;42:1.
10. Mincy JE. Posttraumatic cerebrospinal fluid fistula of the frontal fossa. *J Trauma* 1966;6:618.
11. Rogers GK, Luxford WM. Factors affecting the development of postoperative CSF leak and meningitis after translabyrinthine acoustic tumor surgery. *Laryngoscope* 1993;103(9):959–968.
12. Levy LM, Gulya AJ, Davis SW, et al. Flow-sensitive magnetic resonance imaging in the evaluation of cerebrospinal fluid leaks. *Am J Otol* 1995;16(5):591–596.
13. Spetzler R, Wilson CB. Management of recurrent CSF rhinorrhea of the middle and posterior fossa. *J Neurosurg* 1978;49(3):393–397.
14. Syms CA, Syms MJ, Massey SO, Murphy TP. Cerebrospinal fluid fistulae in a canine model. *Otolaryngol Head Neck Surg* 1997;117(5): 542–546.
15. Wanamaker JR, Mehle ME, Wood BG, Lavertu P. Tension pneumocephalus following craniofacial resection. *Head Neck* 1995;17(2): 152–156.
16. Brodie H. Prophylactic antibiotics for posttraumatic cerebrospinal fluid fistulae: a meta-analysis. *Arch Otolaryngol Head Neck Surg* 1997; 123(7):749–752.

Neurosurgical Issues in Otolaryngology: Principles and Practice of Collaboration,
edited by Moisés A. Arriaga and J. Diaz Day.
Lippincott Williams & Wilkins, Philadelphia © 1999.

CHAPTER 2

Perioperative Neurophysiologic Management

Anil Nanda and Esther L. Wylen

Archaeological evidence indicates that surgical operations on the skull have been performed since antiquity. Some of these procedures may have been associated with the removal of evil spirits, rites of passage to manhood, or a cure for insanity. Simple trephination was done with a small or a large hole, and perioperative support, when provided, was minimal. Historians speculate that the earliest use of neuroanesthesia was in ancient Peru where the victim was made to chew cocoa leaves prior to trephination. From those beginnings, through the Middle Ages and the Renaissance, medications such as mandrake and opium were given, but support during intracranial procedures was insignificant. It was not until the 19th century that modern anesthesia was introduced with the use of ether and chloroform (1).

It was also during the 19th century that perioperative management techniques were first introduced. Sir William Macewen, who made remarkable contributions to neurologic surgery, was instrumental in devising the first endotracheal tubes. The father of neurologic surgery, Dr. Harvey Cushing, also introduced pulse, respiration, and temperature recordings during anesthesia, which would become the foundation for modern perioperative management. Today, neuroanesthesia and perioperative management of intracranial surgery are vital and indispensable parts of patient care. The safety of intracranial surgery has improved with understanding of the neurophysiologic basis of hyperventilation as well as with the introduction of ventilation agents that reduce intracranial pressure (ICP) and help with seizure management. This chapter discusses the physiologic management of the brain, specific techniques for brain relaxation, and the pharmacologic basis for inhalation agents, steroids, antibiotics, and seizure medications.

A. Nanda: Department of Neurosurgery, Louisiana State University Medical Center, Shreveport, Louisiana 71130-3932.

E. L. Wylen: Ochsner Medical Foundation Clinics, Department of Ophthalmology, New Orleans, Louisiana 70121.

CEREBRAL METABOLISM AND BLOOD FLOW

The central nervous system (CNS) consists of the brain and spinal cord. Its cellular components are nerve cells, which are specialized for signal transmission, and glial cells, which have structural and nutritional functions. Neurons transmit electrical and chemical messages by changing their membrane permeability to ions (Na, K, Ca) in response to stimuli. Chemical signals are carried by neurotransmitters, such as glutamate, GABA (γ-aminobutyric acid), acetylcholine, and norepinephrine, which can have an excitatory or inhibitory effect on the recipient cell (neuron), depending on the nature of the cell receptor and second messenger system. These messenger systems are the foundation for information processing, memory programming, and emotional responses. Under normal conditions, the entire energy requirement of the CNS is provided by glucose that is obtained from the degradation of glycogen from the liver and muscle. The glucose is oxidized to carbon dioxide and water in an energy-generating process. The high oxidative metabolism in the brain is reflected by its consumption of 30 to 70 mL of oxygen per minute. This elevated oxidative rate makes it highly energy dependent; oxygen or glucose deprivation for longer than 10 minutes causes irreversible damage to the cells.

The CNS consumes a high proportion of the body's energy supply. Although the brain accounts for only 2% of body weight, it receives 15% of the resting cardiac output and is responsible for 20% of the total body oxygen utilization. The energy needs of the CNS are based on the following: (a) the ion pump systems required for maintenance of transmembrane and electrochemical gradients; (b) synthesis of proteins, lipids, amines, and carbohydrates; (c) intracellular transport; and (d) glial cell function. The CNS has a unique ability to conserve energy depending on the level of cellular activity. In times of increased cerebral metabolic demands, such as mental and physical activity or seizures, the cerebral energy requirement rises because of the increased activity of ionic pump systems. In contrast, during reduced cerebral metabolic needs, as in sleep, rest, or coma, the cerebral energy requirement decreases. A concept that has been advanced is that 60% of the expenditure of energy is based on the functional activity of the CNS, which is reflected by brain and electrical activity, while the remaining 40% is devoted to basal metabolism that maintains cellular integrity (2).

VASCULAR ANATOMY

The paired internal carotid arteries, their branches, the anterior cerebral artery, and middle cerebral artery form the anterior circulation of the brain. The anterior cerebral arteries and their small perforating branches supply blood to the orbital and medial aspect of the frontal lobe and the medial aspect of the parietal lobe. The middle cerebral arteries and their perforating branches perfuse the lateral aspect of the orbital gyri and the frontal, temporal, and parietal lobes. Terminal branches of the middle cerebral arteries form anastomoses with terminal branches of the anterior and posterior cerebral arteries over the lateral surface of the brain. The choroidal arteries, anatomically variable branches of the anterior and middle cerebral arteries, supply the following important deep structures: the internal capsule, basal ganglia, thalamus, and adjacent areas. One of these vessels, the anterior choroidal artery, arises from the internal carotid artery. Other internal carotid artery branches are the ophthalmic artery (to the orbit), and the posterior communicating artery, which joins the posterior cerebral artery connecting the anterior circulation to the posterior circulation through a vascular ring at the base of the brain known as the circle of Willis. Composed of the carotid, anterior cerebral, anterior communicating, posterior communicating, and posterior cerebral arteries, the circle of Willis is the major anastomosis between the anterior and posterior circulation of the brain. The circle is complete in only 18% to 20% of the population (3). Additional extensive anastomoses exist between the major arteries of the brain; however, under conditions of low blood flow (e.g., arterial occlusion and hypotension), the collateral circulation may be insufficient to meet the metabolic requirements of the underperfused area. The paired vertebral arteries enter the cranial vault through the foramen magnum and join to form the basilar artery on the anterior surface of the brainstem at the pontomedullary junction. Branches of the vertebral and basilar arteries perfuse the brainstem, cerebellum, and part of the caudal thalamus. The basilar artery divides to form the posterior cerebral arteries, which supply portions of the brainstem, the caudal aspect of the thalamus, the occipital lobe, and the inferior posterior temporal lobe.

The brain's venous system drains into superficial venous plexuses and dural venous sinuses. The dural sinuses are valveless conduits located between two layers of the dura mater. Most of the brain's venous outflow ultimately drains into the paired internal jugular veins at the base of the skull. Venous outflow obstruction from thrombosis or structural damage can cause a venous infarct of the brain parenchyma drained by the affected vessel.

ARTERIAL GAS TENSIONS

Arterial gas tensions are primary players in the therapeutic manipulation of cerebral blood flow (CBF). Neurotransmitters have important interactions with the perivascular system; norepinephrine causes vasoconstriction and acetylcholine causes vasodilation. Yet, from a clinical standpoint, the arterial gas tensions play a pivotal role. Arterial CO_2 tension is a primary determinant of cerebrovascular resistance and CBF. Hypercapnia decreases cerebrovascular resistance by dilating cerebral blood vessels and increasing CBF. Conversely, arterial hypocapnia increases cerebrovascular resistance by constricting cerebral blood vessels and decreasing CBF. This is modulated by changes in the diameter of the cerebral blood vessels at the level of the small cortical and tissue-penetrating arteries and arterioles. The changes in CBF that occur during the changes in $Paco_2$ are associated with a nonlinear change in cerebral blood volume.

As the most potent modulator of cerebrovascular resistance, CO_2 has been used for decades in the management of head injury to decrease cerebral edema. With normotensive individuals, the change in CBF is linear to the $Paco_2$ within the range of 20 to 75 mm. However, as blood pressure decreases, this change cannot progressively compensate. The cerebral vasculature responds to systemic hypotension with autoregulatory vasodilation in an attempt to maximize CBF. Maximal vessel dilation results in loss of vascular tone, which limits the ability of the blood vessels to dilate further in response to hypercapnia (4,5). Figure 2-1 illustrates the changes in cerebral blood flow in relation to arterial carbon dioxide ($Paco_2$) and oxygen tension (Pao_2).

Studies in cats have confirmed that profound hyperventilation can decrease the CBF to below the ischemic threshold (6–8). Intraoperatively, if hyperventilation is required to decrease brain swelling, a safe $Paco_2$ range is between 25 and

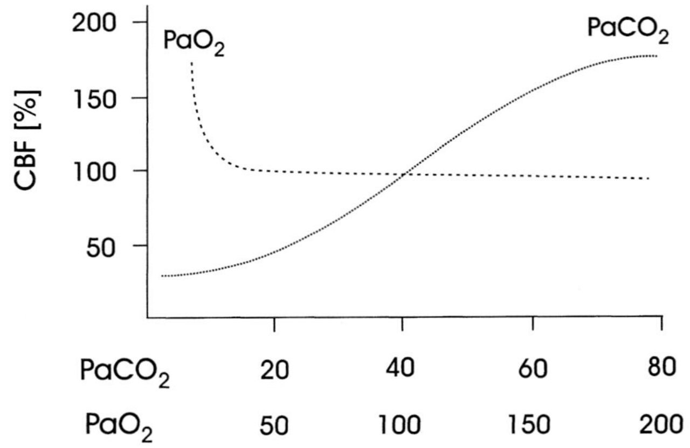

FIG. 2-1. Changes in cerebral blood flow in relation to the arterial carbon dioxide ($Paco_2$) and oxygen tension (Pao_2). (Redrawn from ref. 112.)

30 mm. Changes in oxygen tension are also associated with changes in CBF. Hypoxia tends to increase CBF, thereby increasing cerebral oxygen transportation. It is thought that this is mediated through a direct effect on the vascular smooth muscle and not through the activation of chemoreceptors, nitric oxide pathways, or α_2-adrenergic receptors (9).

AUTOREGULATION

Using autoregulation, the cerebral vasculature can tightly control CBF by altering cerebrovascular resistance (CVR) with respect to cerebral perfusion pressure (CPP). This relationship is expressed as CBF = CPP/CVR, in which CPP equals the mean arterial pressure minus the intracranial pressure (CPP = MAP − ICP). Under normal physiologic conditions, autoregulation of CBF occurs with CPPs ranging from 50 to 140 mm Hg. Autoregulation protects the brain from hypoxia under low CPPs, and from hyperemia and edema under high CPPs (10). CBF autoregulation primarily involves changes in the caliber of small arteries and arterioles, although larger cerebral arteries have been shown to contribute to this effect (11,12).

Beyond the lower limit of autoregulation, further decreases in CPP result in pressure-dependent decreases in CBF. When CPP drops too low to maintain CBF above the ischemic threshold, coma and irreversible neurologic injury can ensue (13). Conversely, increases in blood pressure or decreases in ICP produce cerebrovascular constriction to maintain constant CBF. Increases in CPP beyond the upper limit of the autoregulatory curve cause a pressure-passive vasodilation that increases the CBF. This, in turn, produces cerebral hyperemia, disruption of the blood–brain barrier (BBB), and cerebral edema resulting in a compromised mental status. The range of CPPs in which autoregulation functions (i.e., the upper and lower limits of the autoregulation curve) is affected by such factors as sympathetic activities, cerebral metabolism, $Pa\text{CO}_2$, and vasoactive substances (e.g., anesthetics). For example, in chronic severe hypertension, the autoregulation curve is shifted to the right to prevent hyperemia and brain edema in the face of chronically high CPPs. Thus, in patients with chronic hypertension, low normal blood pressure may result in CBFs in the ischemic range (14–16). Conversely, with reduced sympathetic tone, the curve is shifted to the left so that adequate CBF can be maintained despite low CPPs. If autoregulation is lost, instead of maintenance of a constant, normal CBF over a wide range of CPPs, the CBF will vary in proportion to changes in CPP (16). Autoregulation may be impaired in individuals with severe head injury or cerebral ischemia. Decreases in blood pressure or increases in ICP dilate cerebral vessels as a means of maintaining adequate CBF. Such vasodilation increases cerebral blood volume and may exacerbate pathologically elevated ICP (14,17–19). In patients with severe head injury, it has been shown that cerebral autoregulation is lost in 40% to 60% of patients while CO_2 reactivity is maintained in most of them (17).

GENERAL CONSIDERATIONS IN NEUROANESTHESIA

For all patients, the physician should perform a complete physical examination and obtain a thorough medical history including medications, allergies, and past surgical procedures and anesthetics. Routine evaluation should include plain x-ray of the chest, complete blood and platelet counts, differential blood smear, prothombin time and partial thromboplastin time, 12-lead electrocardiography (ECG), and urinalysis. Furthermore, with the possibility of using intraoperative mannitol, a screening test should include serum electrolytes, blood urine, urea nitrogen, creatinine, and glucose. Liver function tests and enzymes are valuable as baseline data as well. In all patients who are suspected to have mental dysfunction or a history of heavy smoking, pulmonary function tests including arterial blood gases before and after 100% oxygen inhalation should be performed.

Preoperative Hydration

Patients undergoing surgery for intracranial lesions frequently come to surgery with significant intravascular volume depletion. Dehydration in a neurosurgical patient has many possible causes. Patients are often intentionally fluid restricted to minimize brain edema. They may be taking diuretics (such as mannitol). They may have reduced fluid intake because of altered mental status. Reduced intravascular volume can predispose patients to perioperative hypotension, which can potentially result in brain ischemia. In patients with hypovolemia, hypotension may be precipitated by changes in position, anesthetic medication such as barbiturates, induction of anesthesia, or positive pressure ventilation. Accordingly, such maneuvers should be accompanied by careful monitoring of blood pressure. Consideration should be made on an individual basis regarding preoperative hydration.

Premedication

In general, premedication for patients with intracranial lesions should include a minimally sedating dose of a benzodiazepine such as 2 mg of midazolam or 1 mg of diazepam. Patients with a diminished mental status should not be further sedated preoperatively (20).

Monitoring

Optimal monitoring during major neurosurgical procedures (almost any craniotomy) includes monitoring of direct arterial pressure, arterial oxygen pressures, end tidal CO_2, and urinary output, as well as intermittent monitoring of arterial blood gases, electrolytes, and serum osmoles. The degree of muscle relaxation is assessed with a peripheral nerve stimulator. In select cases, precordial Doppler ultrasound imaging may be indicated to detect venous air embolism.

PERIOPERATIVE FLUID MANAGEMENT OF THE NEUROSURGICAL PATIENT

The perioperative fluid management of neurosurgical patients can involve seemingly conflicting goals. Intravascular volume and CBF must be maintained, especially in patients with aneurysmal subarachnoid hemorrhage (SAH), but cerebral edema must be minimized.

Osmolarity, expressed in osmoles per liter of solution, is a colligative property determined by the number of particles in solution. Osmolarity is key in determining fluid movement across a semipermeable membrane such as a cell membrane or blood vessel wall or an intact BBB, which is formed by the tight junctions of CNS capillaries. The osmotic gradient formed by the difference between serum osmolarity and CNS intracellular and interstitial spaces determines the movement across an intact BBB (21). Administration of hypo-osmolar fluids causes flow of water down the osmotic gradient from plasma into brain, promoting edema and elevated ICP. Because lactated Ringer's solution is hyponatremic compared with plasma, rapid large-volume infusions can promote intracranial hypertension. For this reason, normal saline (0.9%) is the intravenous fluid of choice in neurosurgical cases.

Increasing the plasma osmolarity with administration of hyperosmolar solutions such as mannitol creates an osmotic gradient from CNS tissue to plasma, thereby reducing brain water. Mannitol at 0.25 to 1.5 g/kg of a 20% solution is routinely used at the start of certain intracranial operations to relax the brain. At our institution, we administer 50 g of mannitol when the first burr hole is placed. This is standard for all intracranial procedures. It improves exposure, reduces the need to retract delicate CNS tissue, and decreases brain swelling associated with intracranial tumors or trauma. Mannitol should not be used without awareness of its side effects of hypokalemia and alkalemia (both common) and renal failure (uncommon). Accordingly, serum electrolytes, blood urea nitrogen (BUN), and creatinine should be monitored frequently in patients receiving mannitol. Because mannitol is a powerful osmotic diuretic, it can produce hypotension, especially in volume-depleted patients. Since neurosurgical patients often are managed with some degree of intravascular volume depletion to avoid inducing brain edema, blood pressure should be monitored closely while administering mannitol.

In spite of the fact that large doses of methylprednisolone have been shown to be of benefit with spinal cord injuries, routine steroid administration is not recommended with head injuries. However, in patients with vasogenic brain edema, as with gliomas or large skull base tumors, prophylactic dexamethasone helps to decrease brain swelling and may facilitate better postoperative recovery. At our institution, we routinely load patients with 10 mg of dexamethasone, then administer 6 mg every 4 hours, and taper this over the next 4 to 6 days. Although there are no data to support it, we empirically use steroids for patients with poor-grade aneurysms and severe SAH. The deleterious side effects of steroids should not be ignored. A patient's hypertension and diabetes may worsen, and insulin-dependent patients may require an insulin drip. Furthermore, gastritis or ulcers may be induced, and there is a higher incidence of infection and impaired healing with steroids. Avascular necrosis of the hip or other bones is a musculoskeletal side effect seen with steroid usage and may be associated with osteoporosis as well as muscle weakness.

The general practice has been to use caution when hydrating the neurosurgical patient who is at risk for intracranial hypertension. Head trauma, brain tumors, and other intracranial masses such as hematomas or hydrocephalus can predispose the patient to intracranial hypertension. In clinical practice, judicious use of fluids in patients with intracranial pathology is advised (22) because of the potential for ischemic brain tissue with increased permeability to ions. Colloid infusions have been used instead of crystalloid based on the presumption that the ischemic brain remains impermeable to high molecular weight (MW) molecules (23). Yet, experiments addressing the colloid versus crystalloid issue have produced conflicting results. For example, one study using middle cerebral artery occlusion in rats as an infarct model reported an increased volume of ischemic tissue when a colloid (low MW dextran) was used rather than a crystalloid (23). Most other studies addressing the question with a stroke model reported no significant differences in infarct size between animals receiving crystalloid and those given only colloid solutions (24). The advantages of colloids include a smaller infused volume and a prolonged increase in plasma volume with less peripheral edema. The disadvantages are increased cost and risk of coagulopathy, papilledema, and osmotic diuresis. Crystalloids have the advantages of lower cost, greater urinary flow, and the fact that they replace interstitial fluid. Their disadvantage is that the hemodynamic improvement is of a far shorter duration and is sometimes associated with peripheral edema as well as pulmonary edema.

Because, in theory, fluid that is isotonic (iso-osmolar) to CNS tissue should not create a significant osmotic gradient, routine use of colloid solutions in neurosurgical cases is not recommended (25). Colloid solutions in common clinical use include hetastarch (Hespan), albumin, and dextran. Both dextran and Hespan can cause allergic reactions and coagulopathy (26,27). For this reason, albumin is the volume expander of choice in neurosurgical patients (even though it is the most expensive of the three). In the postoperative management of SAH, most centers routinely administer albumin to prevent vasospasm. Caution should be exercised with any large-volume infusion of either colloid or crystalloid solutions as dilutional coagulopathy can occur.

Hypertonic saline (3% or 7.5%) is sometimes used in neurosurgical patients with intractable intracranial hypertension (usually head-injured patients). It is effective in restoring blood pressure, improving urinary output, and reducing ICP by reducing brain water contact and acting as a plasma volume expander (28). Both normal and hypertonic saline can cause hyperchloremic metabolic acidosis. Acidosis caused by the infusion of saline solutions does not normally require treatment.

Surgical stress normally causes hyperglycemia; thus only those situations associated with a risk of hypoglycemia warrant intraoperative administration of dextrose-containing fluids. This is especially important in light of evidence that hyperglycemia aggravates ischemic brain injury (29–31).

Although fluid restriction of neurosurgical patients has traditionally been emphasized, euvolemia is probably a safer goal for these patients. Hypovolemia adds risk of hypotension and hemoconcentration. Hypotension is probably the worst insult to a brain at risk for cerebral ischemia. There is indication that moderate hemodilution may improve CBF (32,33); hemoconcentration may compromise CBF with a sludging effect. In patients at risk for cerebral ischemia, the ideal hematocrit is thought to be around 35.

For most neurosurgical and skull base procedures, two to four units of blood should be reserved at the blood bank, but indications for transfusion are limited. In cases of intraoperative aneurysm rupture, it may be appropriate to start transfusion early to stay ahead of the loss. For large glomus tumors or acoustic neuromas in which some blood loss is anticipated, it may be prudent to direct the patient to donate blood 2 to 4 weeks prior to surgery. In the perioperative period, transfusion is indicated if the hemoglobin approaches 8 g/dL or if there is significant continual blood loss.

Hyponatremia is a common occurrence in neurosurgical patients. Low serum sodium states should be monitored carefully and treated, because decreases in serum sodium concentration cause increases in both intracellular and extracellular brain water. Hyponatremia may be accompanied by high, normal, or low serum osmolarity. Hyponatremia with high or normal serum osmolarity is caused by nonsodium solutes such as glucose or mannitol. In this case, the hyponatremia is due to the osmotic gradient caused by the solute that is nondiffusible across the cell membrane. Treatment entails removal of the responsible solute. Hyponatremia with hyperosmolarity can occur with high, normal, or low total body sodium (25).

Hyponatremia with high total body sodium is associated with edematous states such as cirrhosis, congestive heart failure, and renal failure. Treatment consists of improving cardiac output and renal blood flow, and restriction of sodium and water. Hyponatremia with low total body sodium occurs in hypovolemia, and can be treated by hydration with normal saline. Hyponatremia with normal total body sodium often is associated with the syndrome of inappropriate antidiuretic hormone (SIADH), which has multiple potential causes. Excessive hypothalamic secretion of antidiuretic hormone occurs with intracranial or pulmonary pathology, stress, or hypothyroidism. Certain tumors, for example bronchogenic carcinomas, can produce SIADH. The primary features of SIADH remain those described in 1967 by Bartter and Schwartz (34): (a) hyponatremia with hypo-osmolality of the serum and the extracerebellar fluid; (b) continued renal excretion of sodium, greater than 20 mg/L; (c) absence of fluid volume depletion; (d) greater osmolality of the urine than is appropriate for the osmolality of the plasma; (e) normal renal function, normal adrenal function; and (f) absence of peripheral edema. The differentiation between SIADH and hyponatremia as seen in salt depletion is clinically straightforward; none of the signs of hyponatremia (i.e., decreased blood pressure, decreased tissue turgor, and elevated BUN) are present.

In neurosurgical patients, intracranial processes are probably the primary cause of SIADH-induced hyponatremia. If laboratory findings confirm SIADH in a neurosurgical patient, the first-line treatment is fluid restriction to as little as 500 mL/day. Fluid restriction can be augmented by use of loop diuretics such as furosemide, which will cause renal loss of both water and sodium with loss of free water in excess of sodium loss. Use of a loop diuretic should be accompanied by administration of normal saline or, if the serum sodium concentration is lower than 120 mEq/L, 3% saline may be used. Demeclocycline (600 mg to 1,200 mg/day) can be used to treat SIADH, but should be used with caution and frequent monitoring of serum HCO_3, BUN, and creatinine because of the side effects of metabolic acidosis (common) and renal failure (rare).

Patients who are severely hyponatremic with serum sodium levels lower than 120 mEq/L are at risk of developing seizures or significant mental status changes. Preexisting neurologic deficits may be exacerbated or become unmasked. Patients with serum sodium levels of less than 120 mEq/L with moderate hyponatremia, or 126 mEq/L or lower that is symptomatic (e.g., seizures), should be treated emergently with infusion of hypertonic 3% saline at 1 to 2 cc/kg/h. Their plasma sodium level should not be allowed to rise more than 1 to 2 mEq/L per hour. The resulting increase in plasma sodium may be temporary, because the resulting expansion of the extracellular fluid volume increases urinary sodium excretion. Rapid increases in serum sodium also can be achieved by administration of a loop diuretic plus infusion of normal or 3% saline to replace urinary losses (25).

Correction of hyponatremia should be done with extreme caution, as an exceedingly rapid correction to normal serum sodium levels can cause central pontine myelinolysis (CPM) (35,36). CPM is an osmotic demyelination syndrome that can cause pseudobulbar palsy, quadriparesis, or death. Greater chronicity of the hyponatremia increases the risk of developing CPM, as well as the severity of its clinical effects. Sodium replacement should not proceed faster than 1 to 2 mEq/L/h, nor should it exceed a magnitude of greater than 12 mEq/L in 24 hours (37–39). Serum sodium should initially be corrected to 120 to 125 mEq/L. Once this concentration is reached, further correction can be accomplished using fluid restriction. After correction of serum sodium, fluid restriction should be continued to prevent recurrence of hyponatremia. Serum sodium need not be normalized initially. After the level has been corrected to 120 to 125 mEq/L, a serum sodium concentration of 136 mEq/L is a safe goal.

Hypernatremia (serum sodium >150 mEq/L) usually is seen in neurosurgical patients who have transient or permanent central diabetes insipidus. It also can be seen as a side effect of mannitol administration. In either case, patients typically are dehydrated. Patients with pituitary tumors or craniopharyngiomas can develop the so-called triple response, a triphasic syndrome marked by early polyuria with excessive free water loss, followed by a normalization of urine output and urine concentrating ability.

Diabetes insipidus results from inadequate amounts of antidiuretic hormone, which leads to excessive renal loss of water and electrolytes. Diabetes insipidus may result from nephrogenic causes due to resistance by the kidney to abnormally high levels of antidiuretic hormone, but it most commonly results from central neurogenic causes. Neurogenic diabetes insipidus can be seen in patients following surgery for craniopharyngiomas, pituitary tumors, and anterior communicating artery aneurysms. The diagnosis of diabetes insipidus can be made with the following criteria: (a) urine osmolality 50 to 100 mOsm/L or a specific gravity of 1.001 to 1.005, (b) urine output greater than 300 cc/hour for 2 hours, and (c) normal or above-normal serum sodium. The treatment of diabetes insipidus when patients are awake or alert includes drinking when they are thirsty; but in patients who are comatose, desmopressin [deamino-8-D-arginine vasopressin (DDAVP)] may be given 2.5 μg intranasally twice a day. DDAVP can also be given intravenously or subcutaneously at a dosage of 2 to 4 μg every 12 hours.

Hypernatremia always indicates low total body water (TBW) and is always accompanied by hypertonicity. The TBW deficit is calculated with the following equation (25): TBW deficit = [0.6][weight in kg] − {[140/actual serum (Na^+)] × [0.6][weight in kg]}. In treating hypernatremia, the hypovolemia should be corrected immediately with normal saline. The temptation to administer large quantities of dilute fluids should be avoided. Rapid correction of hypernatremia can precipitate seizures and brain edema, especially if the condition is chronic. To avoid complications, the calculated TBW deficit should be replaced every 24 to 48 hours and the serum sodium should not be corrected by more than 1 to 2 mEq/L/h. The underlying cause of the hypernatremia should be treated promptly.

Antibiotics

Most neurosurgical procedures have antibiotic prophylaxis and the general principles that apply to these are applicable to most surgical procedures (40). The antibiotics must be administered at the time of premedication and ideally should be given about 60 minutes prior to incision. Antibiotics should not be started after the surgical procedure has begun or be given more than 4 hours before the incision is initiated. In skull base or cerebrovascular procedures where the surgery may exceed 6 to 8 hours, an additional dose may be required. Typically, antibiotics should not be continued past the first postoperative day but in complex skull base procedures in which a drain is left, it may be prudent to continue antibiotics as long as the drain is present. High-risk patients, such as those with diabetes, prior radiation therapy, or infection and malnutrition, may require prolonged administration of antibiotics. In neurosurgical procedures, the risk of infection is higher in prolonged operations or in reoperations, especially in the patient with prior radiation. Although there are many antibiotic regimens, a detailed meta-analysis revealed no significant differences in specific regimens used (41).

Most neurosurgical infections are secondary to staphylococcus or the skin flora. The most widely used prophylaxis for neurosurgical procedures is cefazolin (Ancef) at a dosage of 1 g given intravenously 60 minutes before the procedure and up to every 6 hours for 24 hours postoperatively. Alternatives include vancomycin, especially when a shunting procedure is anticipated, and nafcillin.

CSF shunting procedures carry a higher rate of infection, and either cefazolin or nafcillin is the preferred prophylactic antibiotic. At times, intrathecal gentamycin (4 mg) or vancomycin can be injected into the shunt itself. In summary, for all complex and routine intracranial procedures cefazolin is the preferred prophylactic, and if reoperation or shunt placement is anticipated, vancomycin is the preferred prophylactic antibiotic.

Hypertension

Hypertension in intracranial procedures is a serious problem both intraoperatively and perioperatively. After extubation in the postoperative period, high blood pressure may cause a postoperative hematoma. Among the commonly used agents in the control of hypertension during and after craniotomy are nitroprusside, hydralazine, nitroglycerine, labetalol, enalapril maleate (Vasotec), esmolol, and propranolol (Inderal).

Historically, nitroprusside has been very popular and is still used for its quick action. However, it may dilate peripheral vessels prior to cerebral vessels thus producing a cerebral steal phenomenon. Nitroprusside acts in seconds and lasts for about 3 to 5 minutes. The main concern with nitroprusside is that it does raise intracranial pressure in patients with intracranial mass lesions due to direct vasodilation. Furthermore, it may cause thiocyanate and cyanate toxicity with prolonged usage. The dosage in intravenous drip form is 0.5 to 8 μg/kg/min.

Labetalol is replacing nitroprusside as the drug of choice; it blocks both alpha-1 selective and beta nonselective and it reduces or has no change on intracranial pressure. It can now be used in patients with congestive heart failure but is contraindicated in patients with asthma or renal failure. Intravenously, it acts in 5 minutes and peaks at about 10 minutes with a duration of about 3 to 6 hours. The initiating dose is slowly given intravenously piggybacked over 2 minutes every 10 minutes, and the dosage is increased to 20, 40, and then 80 mg; once control is accomplished that same dosage is given intravenously every 8 hours. The other option is to use an intravenous drip that is run at 2 mg/min until the blood pressure is controlled or when 300 mg have been given. Other drugs that are used are enalaprilat, enalapril maleate, and esmolol, as well as propranolol. Hydralazine and nitroglycerin are also alternatives but they may raise intracranial pressure and as such are not used as a primary drug.

Papaverine is a smooth muscle relaxant and may work by blocking calcium channels. Historically, it was used topically on arteries to reverse vasoconstriction but now is also used intraarterially to reverse vasospasm. In cerebrovascular or skull base cases where there is considerable manipulation around the major blood vessels and there is spasm that is fairly obvious, it is prudent to apply propaverine (30 mg and 9 cc), which can be applied on a cotton pledget and placed on the vessel and left in contact for about 2 minutes to reverse the spasm.

SEIZURES IN THE NEUROSURGICAL PATIENT: ANESTHETIC CONSIDERATIONS

Estimated to affect up to 10% of the population (42), seizures can manifest as the easily recognized tonic-clonic convulsions, as a subtler staring episode, or as an absence (petit mal) seizure. Seizure activity can be associated with an epilepsy disorder or a nonepileptic condition, such as hypoglycemia or alcohol withdrawal. A concise seizure classification formulated in 1981 (43) distinguishes between generalized seizures, partial seizures, and unclassified seizures. For general clinical use, a practical seizure classification considers separately epileptic and nonepileptic seizures (Table 2-1).

TABLE 2–1. *Classification of seizures*

- I. Partial seizures
  - A. Simple
  - B. Complex
  - C. Partial onset with generalization
- II. Generalized seizures
  - A. Inhibitory
    - 1. Absence
    - 2. Atomic
  - B. Excitatory
    - 1. Myoclinic
    - 2. Clonic
    - 3. Tonic
- III. Pseudoseizures
- IV. Nonepileptic seizures

From ref. 112.

Partial seizures commence within a focal site of onset. They may remain focal or become generalized. Simple partial seizures have a very limited electroencephalographic distribution in the brain. They cause altered levels of consciousness and manifest as automatisms, repetitive behaviors such as chewing or picking at clothing. Partial seizures that involve both hemispheres with seizure activity can produce generalized tonic-clonic convulsions.

Generalized seizures involve both cerebral hemispheres in epileptiform activity. The seizures can be inhibitory, resulting in absence seizures or atonic seizures in which sudden loss of muscle tone causes the patient to collapse. Excitatory generalized seizures manifest as generalized tonic-clonic or myoclonic motor activity. During a generalized tonic-clonic seizure, patients lose awareness of their surroundings due to the global disturbance of the electrical activity in both cerebral hemispheres.

Pseudoseizures can resemble any type of seizure activity. It is often difficult to distinguish between pseudoseizures and genuine seizure activity. This distinction is made even more problematic by the common existence of pseudoseizures in epilepsy patients.

Electroencephalography (EEG) measures electric potentials with electrodes placed over the scalp or over the exposed brain during epilepsy surgery. The sensitivity of EEG for detecting abnormal electric activity in an epileptic patient is greater than 90% (44). Actual seizure activity usually is not recorded on the EEG, but certain abnormal electroencephalographic patterns consistent with an underlying seizure disorder will be detected. The sensitivity of the EEG is maximized by continuous monitoring (24 hours or longer) under sleep-deprived conditions.

Seizures that are not associated with epilepsy syndromes usually stem from toxic, metabolic, structural, or traumatic causes that are to an extent age specific. Common structural abnormalities include developmental abnormalities and neuronal migration in neonates, and brain tumors and strokes in adults. Head trauma, a more common occurrence in adolescent boys and young men, causes seizure disorders in 10% of its victims (45,46). Drugs, alcohol withdrawal, and metabolic disturbances such as uremia, hypoglycemia, or hyponatremia are also important and potentially treatable causes of seizures.

Treatment of epilepsy syndromes with antiepileptic drugs proceeds according to specific guidelines. Seizures caused by structural brain lesions (stroke, tumor, mesial temporal sclerosis, and trauma) can be controlled using phenytoin (18 to 20 mg/kg loading dose, 4 to 7 mg/kg/day in children, 300 to 400 mg/day in adults). Alternative medications for control of seizures associated with structural brain lesions include carbamazepine (20 to 30 mg/kg/day in children, 600 to 1,200 mg/day in adults) or phenobarbital (3 to 5 mg/kg in children, 8 mg/kg in infants, and 60 to 200 mg/day in adults after a load of 20 mg/kg). Seizures caused by toxic insults and metabolic derangement are treated by correcting the underlying cause. For alcoholic withdrawal seizures, antiepileptic drugs (AEDs) such as phenytoin are not effective. Benzodiazepines such as lorazepam (Ativan) are the treatment of choice.

Status epilepticus occurs when seizure activity is so frequent or prolonged that the patient is continuously experiencing epileptiform activity. This condition is a neurologic emergency. The incidence of status epilepticus in the United States is approximately 100,000 to 150,000 per year; roughly 55,000 deaths per year are associated with status epilepticus (47,48). Interestingly, 12% to 30% of adult patients diagnosed with epilepsy first presented with status epilepticus. Status epilepticus can occur unexpectedly in patients with intracranial pathology or other risk factors for seizures. Definitions of status epilepticus normally include continued seizures of greater than 20 to 30 minutes' duration, but treatment should begin as soon as epileptiform activity is recognized because the mortality associated with this problem approaches almost 20%. To reduce complications such as hypoxemia and minimize the risk of hypoxic brain injury, seizure activity should be abolished as soon as possible (49,50). Clinically, status epilepticus is normally seen after head trauma, hypoxia, and massive SAH. This neurologic emergency is best managed by maintaining a proper airway and normal blood gases. Patients may have profound metabolic acidosis with a pH lower than 7. Initially, patients are given 100% oxygen, and if intubation is difficult, then neuromuscular blockage is used to facilitate intubation. Hyperthermia is a concomitant problem in the manifestation of the seizures and should be treated with massive cooling. Figure 2-2 summarizes the treatment of status epilepticus. Lorazepam is the drug of choice for the initial suppression of seizures. If that is not effective, phenytoin or fosphenytoin (Cerebyx) should be given in incremental doses. Fosphenytoin is a new water-soluble prodrug of phenytoin and is converted to phenytoin by phosphatase. Since it is not formulated in propylene glycol, up to 150 mg/min of fosphenytoin can be given, which is three times the maximum allowable rate of phenytoin. Furthermore, therapeutic concentrations of phenytoin are attained within 10 minutes when fosphenytoin is administered. If the seizures persist, phenobarbital should be given, and if they persist longer than an hour, anesthesia with midazolam or propofol should be added.

Seizure activity has been reported in association with most anesthetic agents (51). On the whole, nitrous oxide is considered to have minimal proconvulsant properties (52). However, it has been a concomitant agent in cases of anesthetic-associated seizures, so its ability to exacerbate the proconvulsant potential of other inhalational agents cannot be excluded. Both halothane and isoflurane have antiepileptic effects and can be successful in abolishing intractable status

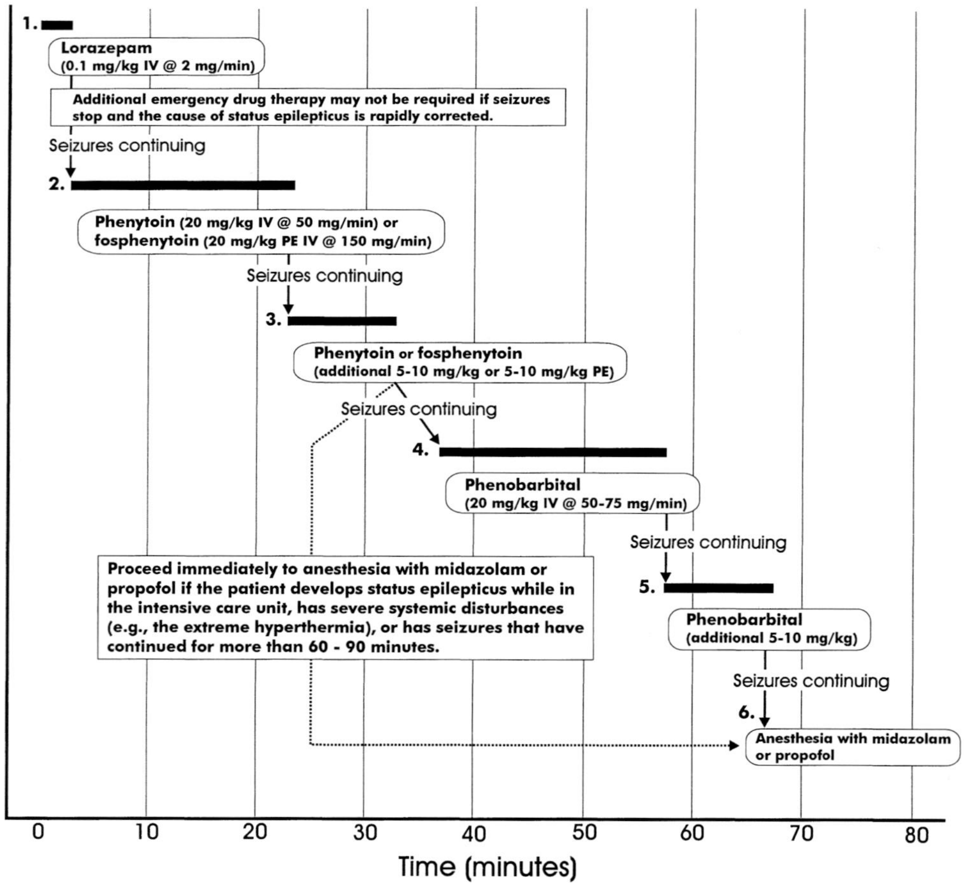

FIG. 2-2. Flow chart of antiepileptic drugs used to treat status epilepticus. (Redrawn from ref. 47.)

(53–56). Despite isolated reports of seizure activity in patients under anesthetic regimens using these agents (57–59), there is no solid evidence suggesting a consistent proepileptic effect for either halothane or isoflurane (51).

Enflurane is characterized by reproducible epileptiform EEG activity, which usually occurs at inspired concentrations of 2 to 2.5 vol%. The neuroexcitatory effect of enflurane is heightened by hyperventilation (56). Seizure activity has also been reported in postoperative patients who received enflurane. Typically, seizure activity occurred 1 to 2 hours and occasionally hours or days after emergence from anesthesia (60–62). The seizure activity caused by enflurane usually consists of tonic-clonic convulsions, although up to 25% of patients exhibit dystonic or myoclonic reactions. The mechanism of epileptogenesis for enflurane is unknown. Actual reports of enflurane-associated seizures are rare, although they are more common than similar reports for halothane and isoflurane. Paradoxically, enflurane has antiepileptic properties and has been used to treat status epilepticus (63). Enflurane use is not contraindicated in patients at risk for seizures, because in clinical practice it is used in low concentrations. Nevertheless, the use of halothane or isoflurane is preferred in this group of patients.

Desflurane and sevoflurane are newer inhalational agents, and their properties with respect to seizure termination or enhancement have not been fully characterized. Preliminary data indicate that desflurane may have an antiepileptic potential similar to isoflurane. No epileptiform activity, either clinical or by EEG, has been reported with either desflurane or isoflurane.

Several lines of evidence support both a proconvulsant and an anticonvulsant role for opioids (64,65); however, the mechanisms are complex and elusive. The practical ramifications of these phenomena are unknown. From a clinical perspective, overt seizure activity has been reported in nonepileptic patients given fentanyl (100 to 2,500 μg), sufentanil (60 to 75 μg), and alfentanil (1,500 μg) during general anesthesia (66–68). Use of anticonvulsant anesthetics such as isoflurane, thiopental, or benzodiazepines has been recommended for cases requiring high doses of opioids (69).

Morphine and meperidine both produce seizure activity in animal seizure models when administered intravenously at very high doses, which exceed clinically used doses (51). In practice, morphine appears to have no clinically relevant epileptogenic properties when administered at standard doses (70). Meperidine also lacks proconvulsant activity when administered acutely at clinically appropriate doses. With chronic meperidine administration, the neurotoxic metabolite normeperidine accumulates, possibly accounting for the myoclonus, tremor, and seizures associated with long-term meperidine use (51).

Local anesthetics have anticonvulsant effects at clinically appropriate doses (71), and proconvulsant activity at toxic doses (72). Lidocaine has been used effectively in cases of refractory status epilepticus (73) but currently is not recommended for that indication because the drug can cause seizures at high doses. Lidocaine is not approved by the Food and Drug Administration for the treatment of seizures.

Neuroepileptic medications such as haloperidol (a phenothiazine) and droperidol (a butyrophenone) lower the seizure threshold (74). For this reason, neuroepileptic drugs should be administered with caution in patients at risk for seizures. Droperidol is commonly used during epilepsy surgery in awake patients. There have been no reports of seizure activity attributable to droperidol in that setting.

Flumazenil (Romazicon) inhibits the action of benzodiazepines at the GABA receptor, reversing the sedative effects (75). Unfortunately, flumazenil also abolishes the anticonvulsant properties of benzodiazepines (76,77). Small doses of flumazenil have reportedly caused seizures in nonepileptic patients. The manufacturer of this drug discommends its use in patients at risk for seizures.

Seizures occurring during anesthesia usually are easily controlled and inconsequential (51). When seizure activity occurs during anesthesia, primary consideration should be given to stabilizing the patient's airway, breathing, and circulation. Generalized tonic-clonic seizures usually will respond to conventional AEDs such as thiopental and benzodiazepines (51). But less typical neuroexcitatory movements, such as myoclonus, and dystonic reactions, such as opisthotonus, are relatively resistant to the following standard AEDs: benzodiazepines, diphenhydramine, phenytoin, and divalproex sodium (78).

Barbiturates possess both anticonvulsant and proconvulsant properties. Thiopental, a common barbiturate, has mostly antiepileptic characteristics. It has been used in halting status epilepticus and has not been associated with seizure activity during general anesthesia (79). Methohexital appears to be specifically epileptogenic in patients with temporal lobe epilepsy, but not in patients with other seizure disorders or nonepileptic patients (78). The bulk of evidence supports a proconvulsant potential for etomidate (80–82). Etomidate should be used with caution or avoided altogether in patients at risk of seizures (83). Benzodiazepines, particularly lorazepam and diazepam, are widely used antiepileptic agents. These two agents are standard in the treatment of status epilepticus. They have not been associated with seizures in patients undergoing general anesthesia.

Ketamine, a dissociative anesthetic, is associated with seizure-like activity in nonepileptic patients, but no EEG correlates have been documented (84). Ketamine has been shown to activate seizure foci in patients with epilepsy (85). Paradoxically, ketamine also possesses antiepileptic properties. Its anticonvulsant and proconvulsant properties appear to be dose dependent, with the anticonvulsant activity occurring at subanesthetic doses, and proconvulsant activity occurring at higher anesthetic doses.

Numerous reports (86–88) document the neuroexcitatory phenomena of propofol (Diprivan) including muscular twitching, tremors, myoclonus, generalized tonic seizures, and various dystonic movements. Seizure activity has been reported in both epileptic and nonepileptic patients. Most of the episodes occur during or soon after emergence from anesthesia, and cease within 5 hours. Nevertheless, propofol has also been reported to suppress epileptiform activity in epileptic patients. Further evidence of the antiepileptic activity of propofol comes from reports of increases in seizure threshold in rat models, as well as successful termination of status in humans and animal models (89,90).

In summary, seizure activity associated with anesthesia usually occurs during induction, emergence, or in the early postoperative period. Etomidate, enflurane, ketamine, and propofol have clearly demonstrated epileptogenic potential, while halothane, benzodiazepines, isoflurane, and thiopental seem to lack neuroexcitatory properties. The mechanisms involved in seizure generation associated with general anesthetic agents remain poorly defined and uncharacterized. For the most part, when neuroexcitatory phenomena occur in association with anesthesia, they are benign and self-limited.

CONSIDERATIONS IN ANEURYSM SURGERY

Intracranial aneurysms occur as dilations at bifurcation points of major intracranial cerebral vessels. Although originally considered congenital, they are now thought to be acquired lesions often associated with hypertension. SAH is caused by a rupture of an intracranial aneurysm and has considerable morbidity and mortality. Historically, Dandy first clipped an intracranial aneurysm in 1926, and the incidence of SAH is between 10 and 28 per 100,000 patients a year. Approximately one-third of patients with SAH die prior to seeking medical attention, and only one-third of patients with SAH are functional survivors. In the International Cooperative Study on the Timing of Aneurysm Surgery, of more than 3,000 patients reviewed, only 58% returned to their premorbid neurologic condition (91,92).

The grading system most commonly used to initially evaluate patients with SAH is the Hunt and Hess classification, which indicates whether the patient is awake, alert, or in a coma (Table 2-2). Generally, patients with grade 1 to 3 are considered in fairly good neurologic condition, whereas patients with grades 4 and 5 are considered to be in a poor neurologic state. A classic presenting symptom for SAH is the "worst headache of my life" and is secondary to meningeal irritation that leads to meningismus, photophobia, and confusion. Patients may also present with focal neurologic signs such as hemiparesis secondary to a sylvian fissure hematoma or a depressed level of consciousness due to hydrocephalus. They can also have cranial nerve palsies, seizures and other metabolic effects of SAH including ECG changes, hypertension, hyponatremia, and clotting abnormalities. Computed tomography remains the best method of diagnosing SAH and arteriography can confirm location and size of the intracranial aneurysm. It may be added that 15% to 20% of patients with SAH have no identifiable aneurysm and they generally do better than those with aneurysmal SAH.

TABLE 2–2. *Clinical grading after subarachnoid hemorrhage: Hunt and Hess modification*

Grade 0	Unruptured aneurysm
Grade 1	Asymptomatic or minimal headache and slight nuchal rigidity
Grade 2	Moderate to severe headache, nuchal rigidity, no neurologic deficit other than cranial nerve palsy
Grade 3	Drowsiness, confusion, or mild focal deficit
Grade 4	Stupor, moderate to severe hemiparesis, possible early decerebrate rigidity, vegetative disturbances
Grade 5	Deep coma, decerebrate rigidity, moribund appearance

Note: Serious systemic diseases (hypertension, atherosclerotic heart disease, diabetes, chronic pulmonary disease, severe vasospasm seen on angiography) cause placement of the patient into the next less favorable category.

From ref. 113.

The urgency to treat aneurysmal SAH lies in the danger of rebleeding. The rate of rebleeding approaches almost 48% during the first 4 weeks. Consequently, most cerebrovascular centers now routinely operate on aneurysms early. Use of the Guglielmi detachable coil through interventional neuroradiology has also recently become a viable option for poor grade aneurysms.

Vasospasm is a major cause of morbidity and mortality with SAH. Angiographic vasospasm occurs in about 60% of patients and manifests in only half of them. The clinical features include focal neurologic deficits and depressed level of consciousness. The timing varies from day 3 to day 7. Bedside transcranial Doppler ultrasound imaging is a useful adjunct in the diagnosis of vasospasm. The mainstays in the management of vasospasm are Nimodipine (60 mg by mouth every 4 hours) and hypervolemic hypertensive hemodilution (HHH) therapy. Nimodipine is a calcium channel antagonist that reduces delayed ischemic deficits from vasospasm and improves the clinical outcome following SAH (93). Nimodipine does not angiographically relieve vasospasm but may act on a cellular level improving blood flow to ischemic areas and consequently improves clinical outcome. The most effective treatment besides Nimodipine is HHH therapy. The goal of this treatment is to increase cardiac output and thus increase CPP. This requires placement of a Swan-Ganz monitor and pressors to increase stroke volume and cardiac output. In older patients, this can cause problems; predominately cardiovascular and pulmonary edema and myocardial infarction may occur in a small percentage of patients.

The end point of HHH therapy is reached when neurologic deficits resolve or when they are complications ensuing from the therapy alone. As previously mentioned, the CVP guide is reasonable for volume expansion, but pulmonary artery catheterization is much more useful. The fluid used for volume expansion should be isomolar and contain adequate amounts of sodium. Although hormones such as vasopressin and fludrocortisone have been used to counteract excess volume losses, this is not part of the standard regimen. Dopamine, dobutamine, phenylephrine, isoproterenol, norepinephrine, and metaraminol have been used to artificially raise blood pressure when neurologic deficits do not respond to volume therapy. At our institution, we typically use only dopamine, dobutamine, and phenylephrine. No standard levels of blood pressure have been established, but at our institution we allow about 20 mg above the premorbid level systolic pressure or approximately 185 mm Hg. The primary goal is reversal of neurologic deficit, and if that is accomplished with volume expansion or minimal elevation of blood pressure, we are not overly zealous in continuing with blood pressure elevation.

The monitoring of the patient during aneurysm clipping includes all the routines that have been mentioned earlier in this chapter. However, in poor-grade aneurysms, the addition of a pulmonary artery catheter is helpful, if not mandatory. Intraoperative monitoring may be helpful in patients undergoing aneurysm surgery. Somatosensory-evoked potentials are a useful adjunct because they can detect ischemia during temporary vessel occlusion. However, there are high false positives and false negatives with this method, and it is not standard for all aneurysm surgery. The intraoperative EEG may also be useful to detect ischemia, and ICP monitoring is sometimes useful as well. Most patients with a poor-grade aneurysm or hydrocephalus will have a ventriculostomy with ICP monitoring, and this can be used for both CSF drainage as well as recording. At our institution, we routinely use intraoperative angiography so the patient will have a femoral sheath placed in the radiology suite before proceeding to the operating room. Placement of a lumbar drain is at the discretion of the neurosurgeon but is fairly standard in most centers. The lumbar drain is placed in the lateral position and is kept closed until the dura is open. If there is a large blood clot, lumbar drainage is contraindicated; with hydrocephalus, if the ventriculostomy has already been placed, then there is no need for a lumbar drain.

The induction of aneurysm patients is extremely important and sensitive. Rupture of an aneurysm during an induction carries high mortality. The main goal is to prevent an abrupt increase in the transmural pressure. The sympathetic response to intubation is attenuated, and anesthesia is usually induced with thiopental (3 to 5 mg/kg), although propofol (1.2 to 2.5 mg/kg) and etomidate (0.1 to 0.2 mg/kg) are reasonable alternatives. Narcotics are added to blunt the hemodynamic response to intubation; phentanyl (5 to 10 μg/kg) and sufentanil (0.5 to 1 μg) are given 5 minutes prior to laryngoscopy. To further protect the transmural pressure, concomitant hyperventilation can be used with isoflurane or addition of intravenous lidocaine, esmolol, or labetalol. Additional local anesthesia or sympathetic blockers can protect against painful stimulation that can occur during pin insertion with the Mayfield head holder. As opposed to routine craniotomies where the patient is kept dry, hypovolemia is avoided. At most institutions, prophylactic hypervolemia therapy is introduced during aneurysm clipping to maximize CBF and decrease the incidence of postoperative vasospasm.

Reduction of cerebral blood volume to facilitate dura opening can be accomplished with hyperventilation. This should be done gradually since a rapid reduction could cause changes in the transmural pressure and cause a rupture. Once the dura is open, moderate hypocarbia with P_{CO_2} of 25 to 30 should be maintained. At our institution, we routinely give mannitol prior to opening the dura, but concerns have been raised that this may cause a decrease in ICP and affect transmural pressure. Some anesthesiologists advocate using furosemide, which does not increase or decrease ICP or intravascular volume. The lumbar drain should be opened only after the dura is opened, and CSF should not be drained until the dura is opened since excessive drainage prior to opening may cause changes in the transmural pressure.

Historically, hypotension was used while dissection was done around the aneurysm dome; however, temporary clipping has moved surgeons away from that trend. At present, cerebral profusion pressures are maintained while the aneurysm is being clipped, and once it is clipped, the systolic pressure is elevated to between 140 and 160 mm Hg.

At our institution, we use controlled hypotension for large basilar artery aneurysms where proximal control is difficult. The most commonly used drugs for this are isoflurane and sodium nitroprusside. Other drugs that have been used successfully are adenosine, labetalol, esmolol. The lowest safe blood pressure should ensure a cerebral profusion pressure of at least 50 mm Hg. However, if one tends to go lower, it may be appropriate to have somatosensory-evoked potentials that may provide a warning for ischemia.

Temporary vessel clips are popular for anterior circulation aneurysms and have obviated the need for controlled hypotension. The obvious advantages of temporary clips are reduced intraoperative rupture, decrease in the transmural pressure, and easier technical clipping. They also help avoid systemic damage both to the brain and the body with controlled hypotension. It has been advocated that 15 to 20 minutes of temporary occlusion is the critical threshold for avoiding cerebral infarction (94). However, lab studies have shown that even 10 minutes of occlusion can lead to irreversible damage (95). With routine anterior circulation aneurysms such as middle cerebral or anterior communicating artery aneurysms, 15 to 20 minutes of occlusion time does not cause significant clinical problems. However, there are several risk factors associated with temporary occlusion including age over 61 years, a poor grade before surgery, and the inclusion of the nuclei of the brainstem in the vascular territory.

The goals of anesthetic management with intraoperative clipping of aneurysms include controlling the aneurysm's transmural pressure while maintaining CPP and avoiding swings in ICP. Patients with poor-grade SAH have increased ICP secondary to hydrocephalus or hematoma, and any reduction in ICP should be gradual until the dura is open.

At our institution, we induce pentobarbital coma in cases in which the temporary clip time is longer than 15 minutes or the brain looks somewhat swollen after a large arteriovenous malformation (AVM) resection. Our standard loading dosage is 3 to 5 mg/kg for an hour and then 1 to 3 mg/kg. EEG can be used to demonstrate burst suppression, but we have used it sporadically. We normally use this for up to 72 hours after surgery and then stop it. The disadvantages with pentobarbital coma are that signs of sepsis can be masked, and in patients who are obese it may take several days to reverse the effect of the coma. However, it is a useful adjunct in certain cases. Propofol is becoming the drug of choice for severe head injuries, and it may also be used in lieu of pentobarbital as a cerebroprotector. The schematic profile is similar to that of both barbiturates and etomidate and it can cause burst suppression. The dose for a drip is 5 to 10 μg/kg/min.

Aneurysm rupture during the operation or induction is a serious problem. It carries a high mortality during induction, but it can be a little more controlled during surgery. Various reports show almost a 20% rupture rate intraoperatively, but, especially with anterior circulation aneurysms, proximal control is accomplished using temporary clips. The goal of intraoperative management during rupture is to ensure adequate systemic profusion and prompt replacement of blood. Another alternative is to rapidly induce hypotension to a mean arterial pressure of 40 to 50 mm Hg, which may enable easy clipping of the aneurysm. At times, ipsilateral compression of the carotid artery for anterior circulation aneurysms may help as well.

While the patient is emerging from anesthesia, the goal is to avoid hypercarbia, straining, coughing, or wide fluctuations in blood pressure. It is important to give intravenous lidocaine to reduce coughing. With good-grade patients, it is best to proceed with extubation, but in grade 4 and 5 patients continued ventilator support is required for the next few days, depending on the outcome. Patients with posterior fossa lesions may experience difficulty with swallowing and laryngo-protective reflexes; consequently, extubation should be performed carefully.

BRAIN PROTECTION

Protection of CNS tissue from ischemic injury is a key concept in anesthetic management during neurosurgical procedures. Mechanisms to protect the brain include maintaining CPP and pharmacologic intervention for cellular protection. Ischemia results in increased concentration of extracellular glutamate, which can activate the *N*-methyl-D-aspartate (NMDA) receptors. The opening of these receptors allows an influx of sodium and can lead to lysis of the cell membrane and cell death. Thus, antagonism of the NMDA receptors, which inhibits the action of glutamate and other excitatory amino-acid neurotransmitters, confers a cerebral protective effect. Brain protection during anesthesia for neurosurgery is a common practice, the two most common modalities being hypothermia and barbiturates (96). There are, however, no convincing prospective data to support the use of brain protection measures in neurosurgical procedures (97).

In neurovascular procedures where temporary blood vessel occlusion may occur, there is an increased risk of ischemic change. Tissue stores of oxygen and glucose are virtually nonexistent in the brain, so it requires a constant and adequate delivery of energy resources. Ischemia occurs when the metabolic demands of oxygen and glucose exceed the supply. Normal CBF is 50 mL/100 g/min. Cerebral electrical activity ceases at CBFs below 16 to 18 mL/100 g/min, and cellular ion homeostasis is lost when CBF falls below 10 to 12 mL/100 g/min. Figure 2-3 represents the physiologic thresholds of CBF. The existence of two separate cellular

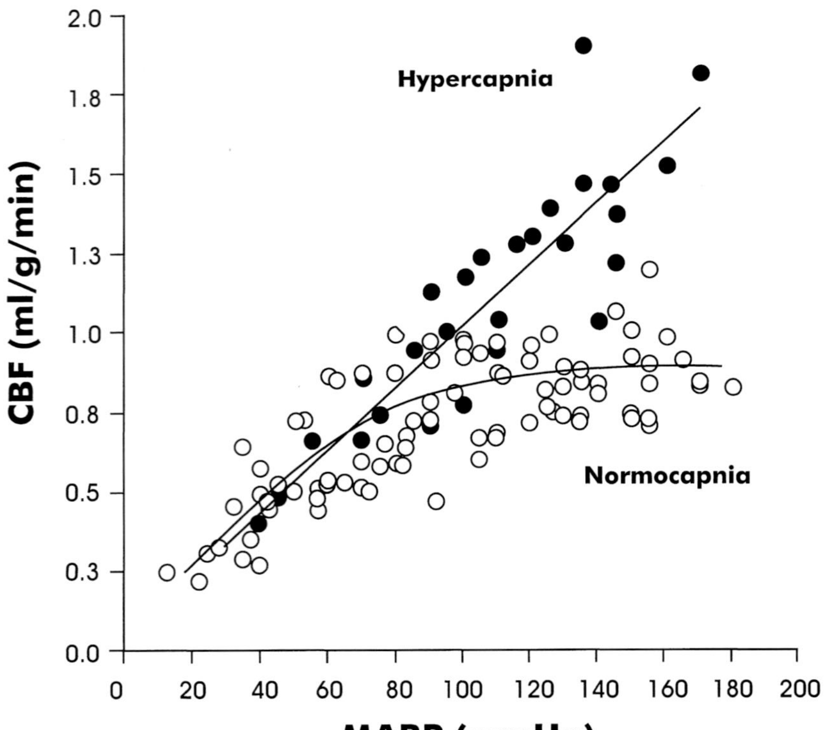

FIG. 2-3. Changes in cerebral blood flow autoregulation in relation to arterial carbon dioxide tension (Pa_{CO_2}). (Redrawn from ref. 112.)

tolerance thresholds to reduced CBF means that at certain degrees of ischemia there may be neuronal populations that have lost electrical activity and function temporarily, yet retain the potential for complete recovery of cellular function (98). This so-called ischemic penumbra (99) consists conceptually of portions of ischemic brain that are potentially salvageable utilizing brain protection techniques. Experiments confirm that both the duration and the severity of the ischemic episode affect the likelihood of subsequent infarction (95). Brain metabolism has an active component consisting of the neuron's active functions such as neurotransmission and a basal component consisting of the basic functions required for cell survival. The cerebral metabolic rate of oxygen ($CMRO_2$) consists of both components. Any technique that decreases the $CMRO_2$ will increase the tolerance of the affected neuronal population to an ischemic episode. Therapies currently in use are barbiturates and similar medications that reduce the active component of the $CMRO_2$, and hypothermia, which reduces both active and basal components.

Barbiturates reduce CBF, ICP, and cerebral metabolic rates (100). Barbiturates can cause significant cardiovascular depression. Etomidate offers a similar quality of cerebral protection without a significant risk of hypotension of cardiac depression (101). Both barbiturates and etomidate can be used to produce EEG burst suppression (102). However, there is no evidence that use of either barbiturates or etomidate reduces morbidity or mortality during neurovascular procedures (103). Propofol also can cause burst suppression, but its effect on the outcome from aneurysm surgery has not been established. Controlled hypothermia of various degrees has been used for cerebral protection during aneurysm sur-

TABLE 2–3. *Protocol for circulatory arrest*

1. Placement of arterial line and large-bore intravenous catheters prior to induction. The usual precautions with induction of patients with cerebral aneurysm apply.
2. Once anesthesia is induced and the trachea intubated, place the following: either a central venous line or pulmonary artery catheter, a second arterial line to allow phlebotomy, lumbar subarachnoid drain, and electrophysiologic monitors (EEG and/or SSEP/BAEP) nasopharyngeal/esophageal and tympanic temperature probes should be used to estimate brain temperature, whereas rectal bladder temperature probe should be placed to monitor core temperature. Anticipate periods of stimulation as during intubation, head pinning, and periosteal retraction, which can cause a hypertensive response.
3. Begin surface cooling by lowering room temperature and using a cooling blanket. Cold (refrigerated) intravenous fluids will facilitate cooling. The rate of decrease should proceed at approximately 0.2°C/min.
4. If barbiturates are to be used, administer 3 to 5 mg/kg bolus of thiopental to induce a burst suppression pattern of 1 : 5 ratio on EEG or isoelectric EEG. This can be followed with a continuous infusion of thiopental at 0.1 to 0.5 mg kg per min. Once cooling begins, the infusion is continued at this rate for the entire period on cardiopulmonary bypass.
5. Hemodilute to a hematocrit of 28% to 30% by collecting blood into an anticoagulant solution kept at room temperature. Maintain intravascular volume with up to 4 L of cold intravenous saline containing 4 to 6 mEq/L of KCl.
6. After the aneurysm is dissected and hemostasis obtained, extracorporeal circulation via femoral artery-femoral vein bypass is begun when the patient's temperature reaches 32° to 34°C. Occasionally two venous cannulas are required for adequate venous return. Just prior to initiating bypass, ensure surgical hemostasis, then heparinize with 300 to 400 IU/kg to maintain ACT of 450 to 500 s. Hetastarch should not be used to replenish intravascular volume.
7. The patient is cooled to 15° to 18°C nasopharyngeal temperature. Rectal or bladder temperature will lag behind by 5° to 7°C. Be aware of ECG changes; at 28°C, the myocardium is extremely irritable and may fibrillate continuously. Fibrillation should be stopped with 40 to 80 mEq of KCl, and, if persistent, defibrillate with 100 to 250 watts/s and administer additional doses of KCl, if necessary.
8. Circulatory arrest occurs at 15° to 18°C and should be limited to the period of clip application. EEG should be isoelectric before arrest. If barbiturates were not used earlier, they may be added at this point to achieve a silent EEG. Elevate the patient's head slightly to facilitate venous drainage, keeping in mind that too much exsanguination carries the potential risk of air embolism and a no-reflow phenomenon in small vessels.
9. The circulatory arrest time should be limited to less than 60 min for optimal results. During arrest it is critically important to keep the ambient temperature low to prevent the brain from warming up. Some surgeons advocate surgical dissection under low perfusion pressure on bypass to minimize the circulatory arrest time.
10. Once the aneurysm is clipped, bypass is reestablished and patient rewarmed at a rate of 0.2° to 0.5°C/min. Too rapid rewarming can cause tissue acidosis and hypoxia. Sodium nitroprusside may be used to allow a more homogeneous rewarming. Check ACT frequently during rewarming. Additional heparin may be necessary.
11. With rewarming, the heart will fibrillate. Cardioversion with 200 to 400 joules through external defibrillating pads and antiarrythmic agents may be required to restore a normal sinus rhythm. In addition, the patient may require inotropic support.
12. Extracorporeal circulation is discontinued when the patient's temperature is 35° to 36°C and the heart can maintain a normal cardia output and sinus rhythm. Allow an extra 20 min of rewarming before discontinuation of bypass to minimize the after-drop in temperature from heat redistribution. Supplement with warmed intravenous solutions and surface forced-air rewarming.
13. The ACT is corrected with protamine sulfate to 100 to 150 s. The autologous blood containing platelet-rich plasma is transfused as well as other blood products necessary to restore hemostasis. Full coagulation profile is determined. Two to four units of fresh frozen plasma and 6 to 12 units of platelet concentrate usually are needed.

ACT, activated coagulation time; BAEP, brainstem auditory evoked potential; SSEP, somatosensory evoked potential.
From ref. 112.

gery. Hypothermia decreases all cellular functions, resulting in a reduction in cerebral metabolism (103).

There is evidence that the neuroprotective effects of mild hypothermia rely on the inhibition of the release of excitatory amino acids, glutamate, aspartate, and glycine (104). Mild hypothermia (33–35°C) exhibited a neuroprotective effect in animals subjected to both global and focal ischemia (104–107). However, controlled studies evaluating the use of mild or moderate hypothermia in humans undergoing neurovascular surgery are lacking. Some neurovascular surgeons employ passive heat loss (i.e., avoidance of heating blankets and in-line warms) to achieve intraoperative temperatures of 33° to 35°C, but no active cooling measures are used.

Hypothermic Circulatory Arrest

The use of hypothermic circulatory arrest during repair of complex giant aneurysms has been reported to produce favorable results. Giant aneurysms are those greater than 2.5 cm in diameter. They present great technical difficulty, and surgery to repair them is associated with high morbidity and mortality. Several series have reported an operative mortality of 0% to 25% (108–110). Circulatory arrest can permit safe decompression of the aneurysm sac, better visualization of the anatomy, a bloodless field, and easier placement of the aneurysm clip. Circulatory arrest lasting up to 72 minutes has been utilized in these successful cases (111). The highly experienced team consists of a neurosurgeon, a neuroanesthesiologist, and a cardiovascular surgeon. The attendant risks of coagulopathy, cardiac arrhythmias, and postoperative intracranial hemorrhage make hypothermic circulatory arrest an option to be considered only when absolutely necessary for complex giant aneurysms.

The main advantages of hypothermic circulatory arrest for giant aneurysms include (a) ability to decompress the aneurysm sack with a Cavitron ultrasonic surgical aspirator (CUSA) or bipolar dissection without the fear of bleeding, (b) a totally bloodless field, (c) better visualization of the anatomy, and (d) easier mechanical manipulation for placement of the clip. Circulatory arrest can be performed using the closed chest femoral vein femoral artery bypass or with an open chest with a median sternotomy and ventricular stenting. The former method has a much lower morbidity and is generally preferred. Table 2-3 shows the protocol for circulatory arrest and requires the services of a cardiac surgeon and a team that is familiar with cardiopulmonary bypass. The main complication to be concerned about is postoperative bleeding. In the period of tolerated circulatory arrest, most surgeons do not feel comfortable with a circulatory arrest exceeding 60 minutes.

SUMMARY

Perioperative management in the neurosurgical patient requires attention to detail. A thorough preoperative evaluation with standard baseline laboratory values and monitoring should be performed for all cases. Seizure prophylaxis, preoperative antibiotics, steroids, and well-controlled blood pressure are part of the armamentarium. Mannitol, lumbar drainage, and hypocapnia help reduce swelling during the operative procedure, and cerebral protectants such as phenobarbital, etomidate, and propofol are useful adjuncts. The therapeutic choices currently available make the operative management of these difficult cases safer and reduce the incidence of intraoperative and postoperative complications.

REFERENCES

1. Frost EAM. History of neuroanesthesia. In: Albin MS, ed. *Textbook of neuroanesthesia with neurosurgical and neuroscience perspectives*. New York: McGraw-Hill, 1997:1–20.
2. Cucchiara RF, Michenfelder JD. *Clinical neuroanesthesia*. New York: Churchill-Livingstone, 1990.
3. Alpers BJ, Berry RG, Paddison RM. Anatomical studies of the circle of Willis in normal brains. *Arch Neurol Psychiatry* 1959;81:409.
4. Harper AM, Glass HI. Effect of alterations in the arterial carbon dioxide tension on the blood flow through the cerebral cortex at normal and low arterial pressures. *J Neurol Neurosurg Psychiatry* 1965;28:449.
5. Harper AM. Autoregulation of cerebral blood flow: influence of the arterial blood pressure on the blood flow through the cerebral cortex. *J Neurol Neurosurg Psychiatry* 1966;29:398–403.
6. Granholm L, Siesjo BK. The effects of hypercapnia and hypocapnia upon the cerebrospinal fluid lactate and pyruvate concentrations and upon the lactate, pyruvate, ATP, ADP, phosphocreatine, and creatine concentrations of cat brain tissue. *Acta Physiol Scand* 1969;75:257–266.
7. Sutton LN, McLaughlin AC, Dante S, et al. Cerebral venous oxygen content as a measure of brain energy metabolism with increased intracranial pressure and hyperventilation. *J Neurosurg* 1990;73:927–932.
8. Ruta TS, Drummond JC, Cole DJ. The effect of acute hypocapnia on local cerebral blood flow during middle cerebral artery occlusion in isoflurane anesthetized rats. *Anesthesiology* 1993;78:134–140.
9. Traystman RJ, Fitzgerald RS, Loscutoff SC. Cerebral circulatory responses to arterial hypoxia in normal and chemodenervated dogs. *Circ Res* 1978;42:649–657.
10. Paulson OB, Strandgaard S, Edvinsson L. Cerebral autoregulation. *Cerebrovasc Brain Metab Rev* 1990;2:161–192.
11. Heistad DD, Marcus ML, Abboud FM. Role of large arteries in regulation of cerebral blood flow in dogs. *J Clin Invest* 1978;62:761–768.
12. MacKenzie ET, Farrar JK, Fitch W, et al. Effects of hemorrhagic hypotension on the cerebral circulation. I. Cerebral blood flow and pial arteriolar caliber. *Stroke* 1979;10:711–718.
13. Kovach AG, Sandor P. Cerebral blood flow and brain function during hypotension and shock. *Annu Rev Physiol* 1976;38:571–596.
14. Risberg J, Ancri D, Ingvar DH. Correlation between cerebral blood volume and cerebral blood flow in the cat. *Exp Brain Res* 1969;8:321–326.
15. Barry DI, Strandgaard S, Graham DI, et al. Cerebral blood flow in rats with renal and spontaneous hypertension: resetting of the lower limit of autoregulation. *J Cereb Blood Flow Metab* 1982;2:347–353.
16. Edvinsson L, MacKenzie ET, McCulloch J. *Cerebral blood flow and metabolism*. New York: Raven Press, 1993.
17. Bouma GJ, Muizelaar JP, Bandoh K, Marmarou A. Blood pressure and intracranial pressure-volume dynamics in severe head injury: relationship with cerebral blood flow. *J Neurosurg* 1992;77:15–19.
18. Ferrari M, Wilson DA, Hanley DF, Traystman RJ. Effects of graded hypotension on cerebral blood flow, blood volume, and mean transit time in dogs. *Am J Physiology* 1992;262:H1908–H1914.
19. Gray WJ, Rosner MJ. Pressure-volume index as a function of cerebral perfusion pressure. Part 1: The effects of cerebral perfusion pressure changes and anesthesia. *J Neurosurg* 1987;67:369–376.
20. Newfield P, Hamid RKA, Lam AM. Intracranial aneurysms and A-V malformations: anesthetic management. In: Albin MS, ed. *Textbook*

of neuroanesthesia with neurosurgical and neuroscience perspectives. New York: McGraw-Hill, 1997:859–900.
21. Zornow MH, Todd MM, Moore SS. The acute cerebral effects of changes in plasma osmolality and oncotic pressure. *Anesthesiology* 1987;67:936–941.
22. Shenkin HA, Bezier HS, Bouzarth WF. Restricted fluid intake: rational management of the neurosurgical patient. *J Neurosurg* 1976; 45:432–436.
23. Korosue K, Heros RC, Ogilvy CS, et al. Comparison of crystalloids and colloids for hemodilution in a model of focal cerebral ischemia. *J Neurosurg* 1990;73:576–584.
24. Little JR, Slugg RM, Latchaw JP Jr, Lesser RP. Treatment of acute focal cerebral ischemia with concentrated albumin. *Neurosurgery* 1981;9:552–558.
25. Zornow MH, McQuitty C, Prough DS. Perioperative fluid management of the neurosurgical patient. In: Albin MS, ed. *Textbook of neuroanesthesia with neurosurgical and neuroscience perspectives.* New York: McGraw-Hill, 1997:117–148.
26. Trumble ER, Muizelaar JP, Myseros JS, Choi SC, Warren BB. Coagulopathy with the use of hetastarch in the treatment of vasospasm. *J Neurosurg* 1995;82:44–47.
27. Stump DC, Strauss RG, Henriksen RA, Petersen RE, Saunders R. Effects of hydroxyethyl starch on blood coagulation, particularly factor VIII. *Transfusion* 1985;25:349–354.
28. Worthley LI, Cooper DJ, Jones N. Treatment of resistant intracranial hypertension with hypertonic saline: report of two cases. *J Neurosurg* 1988;68:478–481.
29. Longstreth WT Jr, Diehr P, Cobb LA, Hanson RW, Blair AD. Neurologic outcome and blood glucose levels during out-of-hospital cardiopulmonary resuscitation. *Neurology* 1986;36:1186–1191.
30. Lam AM, Winn HR, Cullen BF, Sundling N. Hyperglycemia and neurological outcome in patients with head injury. *J Neurosurg* 1991; 75:545–551.
31. Lanier WL, Stangland KJ, Scheithauer BW, Milde JH, Michenfelder JD. The effects of dextrose infusion and head position on neurologic outcome after complete cerebral ischemia in primates: examination of a model. *Anesthesiology* 1987;66:39–48.
32. Wood JH, Polyzoidis KS, Epstein CM, Gibby GL, Tindall GT. Quantitative EEG alterations after isovolemic-hemodilutional augmentation of cerebral perfusion in stroke patients. *Neurology* 1984;34:764–768.
33. Wood JH, Simeone FA, Kron RE, Snyder LL. Experimental hypervolemic hemodilution: physiological correlations of cortical blood flow, cardiac output, and intracranial pressure with fresh blood viscosity and plasma volume. *Neurosurgery* 1984;14:709–723.
34. Bartter FC, Schwartz WB. The syndrome of inappropriate secretion of antidiuretic hormone. *Am J Med* 1967;42:790–806.
35. Sterns RH, Riggs JE, Schochet SS Jr. Osmotic demyelination syndrome following correction of hyponatremia. *N Engl J Med* 1986; 314:1535–1542.
36. Laureno R. Central pontine myelinolysis following rapid correction of hyponatremia. *Ann Neurol* 1983;13:232–242.
37. Berl T. Treating hyponatremia: what is all the controversy about? *Ann Intern Med* 1990;113:417–419.
38. Narins RG. Therapy of hyponatremia: does haste make waste? [Editorial]. *N Engl J Med* 1986;314:1573–1575.
39. Sterns RH. Neurological deterioration following treatment for hyponatremia. *Am J Kidney Dis* 1989;13:434–437.
40. Kaiser AB. Antimicrobial prophylaxis in surgery. *N Engl J Med* 1986; 315:1129–1138.
41. Barker FG Jr. Efficacy of prophylactic antibiotics for craniotomy: a meta-analysis. *Neurosurgery* 1994;35:484–490; discussion 491–492.
42. Hauser WA, Annegers JF, Kurland LT. Incidence of epilepsy and unprovoked seizures in Rochester, Minnesota: 1935–1984. *Epilepsia* 1993;34:453–468.
43. Anonymous. Proposal for revised clinical and electroencephalographic classification of epileptic seizures. From the Commission on Classification and Terminology of the International League Against Epilepsy. *Epilepsia* 1981;22:489–501.
44. Meglio M, Cioni B, Visocchi M, et al. Spinal cord stimulation and cerebral haemodynamics. *Acta Neurochir* 1991;111:43–48.
45. Annegers JF, Grabow JD, Groover RV, et al. Seizures after head trauma: a population study. *Neurology* 1980;30:683–689.
46. Wilberger JE. Emergency care and initial evaluation. In: Cooper PR, ed. *Head injury.* Baltimore, MD: Williams & Wilkins, 1993:27–41.
47. Lowenstein DH. Status epilepticus. *West J Med* 1998;168:263.
48. DeLorenzo RJ, Pellock JM, Towne AR, Boggs JG. Epidemiology of status epilepticus. *J Clin Neurophysiol* 1995;12:316–325.
49. Delgado-Escueta AV, Wasterlain C, Treiman DM, Porter RJ. Current concepts in neurology: management of status epilepticus. *N Engl J Med* 1982;306:1337–1340.
50. Corsellis JA, Bruton CJ. Neuropathology of status epilepticus in humans. *Adv Neurol* 1983;34:129–139.
51. Herrick IA. Seizures activity and anesthetic agents and adjuvants. In: Albin MS, ed. *Textbook of neuroanesthesia with neurosurgical and neuroscience perspectives.* New York: McGraw-Hill, 1997:613–623.
52. Modica PA, Tempelhoff R, White PF. Pro- and anticonvulsant effects of anesthetics (part I). *Anesth Analg* 1990;70:303–315.
53. Ropper AH, Kofke WA, Bromfield EB, Kennedy SK. Comparison of isoflurane, halothane, and nitrous oxide in status epilepticus [Letter]. *Ann Neurol* 1986;19:98–99.
54. Kofke WA, Snider MT, Young RS, Ramer JC. Prolonged low flow isoflurane anesthesia for status epilepticus. *Anesthesiology* 1985;62: 653–656.
55. Fiol ME, Boening JA, Cruz-Rodriguez R, Maxwell R. Effect of isoflurane (Forane) on intraoperative electrocorticogram. *Epilepsia* 1993;34:897–900.
56. Ito BM, Sato S, Kufta CV, Tran D. Effect of isoflurane and enflurane on the electrocorticogram of epileptic patients. *Neurology* 1988;38: 924–928.
57. Harrison JL. Postoperative seizures after isoflurane anesthesia. *Anesth Analg* 1986;65:1235–1236.
58. Poulton TJ, Ellingson RJ. Seizure associated with induction of anesthesia with isoflurane. *Anesthesiology* 1984;61:471–476.
59. Hymes JA. Seizure activity during isoflurane anesthesia. *Anesth Analg* 1985;64:367–368.
60. Kruczek M, Albin MS, Wolf S, Bertoni JM. Postoperative seizure activity following enflurane anesthesia. *Anesthesiology* 1980;53: 175–176.
61. Jenkins J, Milne AC. Convulsive reaction following enflurane anaesthesia. *Anaesthesia* 1984;39:44–45.
62. Yazji NS, Seed RF. Convulsive reaction following enflurane anaesthesia [Letter]. *Anaesthesia* 1984;39:1249.
63. Opitz A, Oberwetter WD. Enflurane or halothane anaesthesia for patients with cerebral convulsive disorders? *Acta Anaesthesiol Scand Suppl* 1979;71:43–47.
64. Chugani HT, Ackermann RF, Chugani DC, Engel J Jr. Opioid-induced epileptogenic phenomena: anatomical, behavioral, and electroencephalographic features. *Ann Neurol* 1984;15:361–368.
65. Kofke WA, Garman RH, Tom WC, Rose ME, Hawkins RA. Alfentanil-induced hypermetabolism, seizure, and histopathology in rat brain. *Anesth Analg* 1992;75:953–964.
66. Engel J Jr, Kuhl DE, Phelps ME, Rausch R, Nuwer M. Local cerebral metabolism during partial seizures. *Neurology* 1983;33:400–413.
67. Morris GL III, Mueller WM, Yetkin FZ, et al. Functional magnetic resonance imaging in partial epilepsy. *Epilepsia* 1994;35:1194–1198.
68. Connelly A, Jackson GD, Frackowiak RS, et al. Functional mapping of activated human primary cortex with a clinical MR imaging system. *Radiology* 1993;188:125–130.
69. Kofke WA, Tempelhoff R, Dasheiff RM. Anesthesia for epileptic patients and for epilepsy surgery. In: Cottrell JE, Smith DS, eds. *Anesthesia and neurosurgery.* St. Louis: Mosby, 1994:495–524.
70. Smith NT, Dec-Silver H, Sanford TJ Jr, et al. EEGs during high-dose fentanyl-, sufentanil-, or morphine-oxygen anesthesia. *Anesth Analg* 1984;63:386–393.
71. Modica PA, Tempelhoff R, White PF. Pro- and anticonvulsant effects of anesthetics (part II). *Anesth Analg* 1990;70:433–444.
72. Covino BG. Clinical pharmacology of local anesthetic agents. In: Cousins MJ, Bridenbaugh PO, eds. *Neural blockade.* Philadelphia: JB Lippincott, 1988:121–123.
73. Browne TR, Penry JK. Benzodiazepines in the treatment of epilepsy: a review. *Epilepsia* 1973;14:277–310.
74. Baldessarini RJ. Drugs and the treatment of psychiatric disorders. In: Gilman AG, ed. *The pharmacological basis of therapeutics.* New York: Macmillan, 1985:396.
75. Wyllie E, Awad I. Intracranial EEG and localization studies. In: Wyllie E, ed. *The treatment of epilepsy: principles and practices.* Philadelphia: Lea & Febiger, 1993:1023–1038.

76. Spivey WH. Flumazenil and seizures: analysis of 43 cases. *Clin Ther* 1992;14:292–305.
77. Hoffman EJ, Warren EW. Flumazenil: a benzodiazepine antagonist. *Clin Pharm* 1993;12:641–656.
78. Ries CR, Scoates PJ, Puil E. Opisthotonos following propofol: a nonepileptic perspective and treatment strategy [see comments]. *Can J Anaesth* 1994;41:414–419.
79. Kofke WA, Towfighi J, Garman RH, et al. Effect of anesthetics on neuropathologic sequelae of status epilepticus in rats. *Anesth Analg* 1993;77:330–337.
80. Krieger W, Copperman J, Laxer KD. Seizures with etomidate anesthesia [Letter]. *Anesth Analg* 1985;64:1226–1227.
81. Grant IS, Hutchison G. Epileptiform seizures during prolonged etomidate sedation [Letter]. *Lancet* 1983;2:511–512.
82. Laughlin TP, Newberg LA. Prolonged myoclonus after etomidate anesthesia. *Anesth Analg* 1985;64:80–82.
83. Hartzman RJ. Summary of the first international workshop on human primed LD typing. *Tissue Antigens* 1979;13:203–211.
84. Thompson GE. Ketamine-induced convulsions. *Anesthesiology* 1972; 37:662–663.
85. Ferrer-Allado T, Brechner VL, Dymond A, Cozen H, Crandall P. Ketamine-induced electroconvulsive phenomena in the human limbic and thalamic regions. *Anesthesiology* 1973;38:333–344.
86. Orser B. Propofol-induced neuroexcitation and receptor desensitization [Editorial]. *Can J Anaesth* 1994;41:366–371.
87. Bevan JC. Propofol-related convulsions [Editorial]. *Can J Anaesth* 1993;40:805–809.
88. Paech MJ, Storey JM. Propofol and seizures [Letter]. *Anaesth Intensive Care* 1990;18:585.
89. De Riu PL, Petruzzi V, Testa C, et al. Propofol anticonvulsant activity in experimental epileptic status. *Br J Anaesth* 1992;69:177–181.
90. Yanny HF, Christmas D. Propofol infusions for status epilepticus [Letter]. *Anaesthesia* 1988;43:514.
91. Kassell NF, Torner JC, Jane JA, Haley EC Jr, Adams HP. The International Cooperative Study on the Timing of Aneurysm Surgery. Part 2: surgical results. *J Neurosurg* 1990;73:37–47.
92. Kassell NF, Torner JC, Haley EC Jr, et al. The International Cooperative Study on the Timing of Aneurysm Surgery. Part 1: overall management results. *J Neurosurg* 1990;73:18–36.
93. Pickard JD, Murray GD, Illingworth R, et al. Effect of oral nimodipine on cerebral infarction and outcome after subarachnoid haemorrhage: British aneurysm nimodipine trial. *Br Med J* 1989;298:636–642.
94. Samson D, Batjer HH, Bowman G, et al. A clinical study of the parameters and effects of temporary arterial occlusion in the management of intracranial aneurysms. *Neurosurgery* 1994;34:22–28; discussion 28–29.
95. Jones TH, Morawetz RB, Crowell RM, et al. Thresholds of focal cerebral ischemia in awake monkeys. *J Neurosurgery* 1981;54: 773–782.
96. Craen RA, Gelb AW, Eliaszw M, Lok P. Current anesthetic practices and use of brain protective therapies for cerebral aneurysm surgery at 41 North American centers. *J Neurosurg Anesthesiol* 1994;6:303.
97. Gelb AW, Watts A. Anesthesia for neurovascular surgery. *Anesth Analg* 1996;82(Suppl):46S–51S.
98. Levy WJ. Neurophysiological brain monitoring: Evoked potentials. In: Cottrell JE, Smith DS, eds. *Anesthesia and neurosurgery*. St. Louis: Mosby, 1994:228–494.
99. Branston NM, Strong AJ, Symon L. Kinetics of resolution of transient increases in extracellular potassium activity: relationships to regional blood flow in primate cerebral cortex. *Neurol Res* 1982;4:1–19.
100. Spetzler RF, Hadley MN. Protection against cerebral ischemia: the role of barbiturates. *Cerebrovasc Brain Metab Rev* 1989;1:212–229.
101. Batjer HH, Frankfurt AI, Purdy PD, Smith SS, Samson DS. Use of etomidate, temporary arterial occlusion, and intraoperative angiography in surgical treatment of large and giant cerebral aneurysms. *J Neurosurg* 1988;68:234–240.
102. Frizzell RT, Meyer YJ, Borchers DJ, et al. The effects of etomidate on cerebral metabolism and blood flow in a canine model for hypoperfusion. *J Neurosurg* 1991;74:263–269.
103. Guy J, McGrath BJ, Borel CO, Friedman AH, Warner DS. Perioperative management of aneurysmal subarachnoid hemorrhage: part 1. Operative management. *Anesth Analg* 1995;81:1060–1072.
104. Busto R, Globus MY, Dietrich WD, Martinez E, Valdes I, Ginsberg MD. Effect of mild hypothermia on ischemia-induced release of neurotransmitters and free fatty acids in rat brain. *Stroke* 1989;20: 904–910.
105. Minamisawa H, Nordstrom CH, Smith ML, Siesjo BK. The influence of mild body and brain hypothermia on ischemic brain damage. *J Cereb Blood Flow Metab* 1990;10:365–374.
106. Chopp M, Chen H, Dereski MO, Garcia JH. Mild hypothermic intervention after graded ischemic stress in rats. *Stroke* 1991;22:37–43.
107. Kader A, Brisman MH, Maraire N, Huh JT, Solomon RA. The effect of mild hypothermia on permanent focal ischemia in the rat. *Neurosurgery* 1992;31:1056–1060; discussion 1060–1061.
108. Spetzler RF, Hadley MN, Rigamonti D, et al. Aneurysms of the basilar artery treated with circulatory arrest, hypothermia, and barbiturate cerebral protection. *J Neurosurg* 1988;68:868–879.
109. Solomon RA, Smith CR, Raps EC, Young WL, Stone JG, Fink ME. Deep hypothermic circulatory arrest for the management of complex anterior and posterior circulation aneurysms. *Neurosurgery* 1991;29: 732–737.
110. Ausman JI, Malik GM, Tomecek FJ, et al. Hypothermic circulatory arrest and the management of giant and large cerebral aneurysms. *Surg Neurol* 1993;40:289–298.
111. Symon L, Vajda J. Surgical experiences with giant intracranial aneurysms. *J Neurosurg* 1984;61:1009–1028.
112. Albin MS. *Textbook of neuroanesthesia with neurosurgical and neuroscience perspectives*. New York: McGraw-Hill, 1997.
113. Hunt WE, Hess RM. Surgical risk as related to time of intervention in the repair of intracranial aneurysms. *J Neurosurg* 1968;28:14–20.

Neurosurgical Issues in Otolaryngology: Principles and Practice of Collaboration,
edited by Moisés A. Arriaga and J. Diaz Day.
Lippincott Williams & Wilkins, Philadelphia © 1999.

CHAPTER 3

Neurosurgical Operative Positioning

Lokesh S. Tantuwaya and Takanori Fukushima

In neurosurgery, in particular skull-base surgery, proper operative positioning is the first step toward a successful operation. Proper positioning requires a thorough three-dimensional understanding of the relevant surgical anatomy and adherence to the basic principles of operative positioning. This chapter reviews these principles and their application in specific neurosurgical procedures that allow access to lesions at the anterior skull base, the sellar and suprasellar region, the cerebellopontine angle, and the lateral skull base.

BASIC PRINCIPLES

The basic tenets of surgical positioning include using appropriate head fixation, assuring patient safety, avoiding vascular or neural compression, providing the most direct surgical route to the lesion, allowing access to the airway and intravenous/intraarterial lines, and paying attention to surgical ergonomics. While these concepts seem relatively obvious and simple, they are frequently overlooked during the usual haste to start an operation.

In neurosurgery, head fixation is most often accomplished with either a three-point fixation system such as the Mayfield head-holder system (Ohio Medical Instruments Co., Cincinnati, OH), or a four-point fixation system such as the Sugita head-holder system (Mizuho Instrument Co., Japan). We preferentially utilize the Mayfield system for ease of use and for its compatibility with the Fukushima retractor system. Occasionally, when pin fixation is not necessary or when it may be necessary to move the head during surgery, a "horseshoe" headrest is utilized. Head fixation is addressed in more detail later in this chapter.

Attention to patient safety and comfort helps prevent easily avoidable and potentially morbid complications. The operating table is an important adjunct to a successful operation. It should be well padded and capable of allowing for Trendelenburg and reverse Trendelenburg positions, flexion and extension of the back and legs, and rotation along the longitudinal axis of the table (Fig. 3-1). Proper positioning in all cases involves assuring that all pressure points are well padded, that the position of the head does not impede venous outflow and thus potentially raise intracranial pressure, and preventing undue pressure or tension on nervous structures such as the ulnar nerve, the radial nerve, the sciatic nerve, or the brachial plexus. Additionally, the position of the patient must not place the patient at risk for air emboli nor make mechanical ventilation difficult. For this reason the sitting or "lounge chair" position is rarely used in neurosurgery. Not only have air emboli occurred during operations in this position, but also an air embolism from pin fixation has occurred in this position (1).

The concept of surgical ergonomics is an important one, and one that is often overlooked by surgeons. This concept takes into account the surgeon's comfort, his ability to view the operating field at various angles, and his ability to stabilize his hands while operating. Often complex and prolonged surgery can cause fatigue; thus, careful consideration to the comfort of the surgeon enhances the ability of the surgeon to complete the operation safely and successfully. The surgeon should arrange the operating theater in such a manner as to facilitate the unimpeded passage of instruments from the scrub nurse to himself, to allow easy access to operating microscopes, and to allow an assisting surgeon to adequately visualize the operating field (Fig. 3-2). Placement of "pockets" for frequently used surgical instruments such as suction cannulas, bipolar coagulators, and monopolar coagulators should be easily within the reach of the primary surgeon. Foot pedals for microscopes, drills, or bipolar coagulators should be easily within reach and should not require any extraneous movements to operate. In essence, the surgeon and the surgical team should arrange the surgical field and operating theater in such a way as to obviate unnecessary movement and allow for an economy of movement.

L. S. Tantuwaya: Allegheny General Hospital, Pittsburgh, Pennsylvania 15212.

T. Fukushima: Carolina Skull Base Surgery Center, Carolina Neuroscience and Ear Research Institute, Raleigh/Durham, North Carolina 27609.

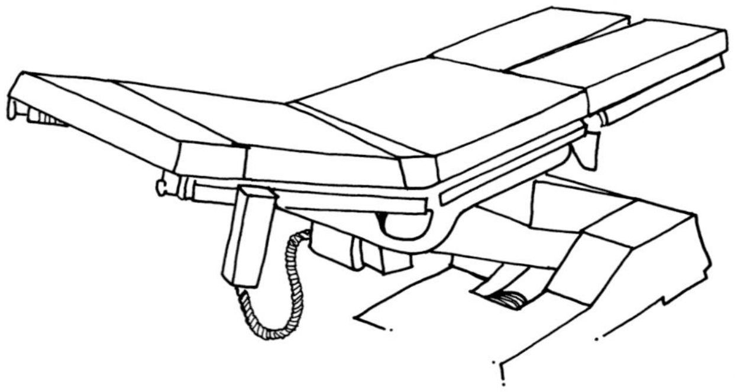

FIG. 3-1. The operating table should be well padded and mobile in multiple planes.

HEAD FIXATION

In neurosurgery, head fixation has multiple purposes. First, it stabilizes the head, preventing any unwanted movement of the operating field during surgery. Second, this stabilization allows the operating table to be moved in various directions to improve multidirectional visualization. Third, in modern neurosurgical procedures that utilize a computer-assisted frameless stereotaxic system, the head is held in a fixed three-dimensional space that is registered to a computer for the purposes of navigation within this space. There are a variety of fixation devices available, and the surgeon should choose one that is easy to use and maintain, and one that is easily adaptable to a variety of self-retaining retractor systems.

As stated earlier we preferentially use the Mayfield skull fixation device, which is a three-point fixation system. With this apparatus the head is secured using a fixator with three pins that penetrate the outer table of the skull, which is then connected through a series of movable arms to the operating table. These connectors can be individually adjusted and locked when positioning of the head is completed. One end of the fixator has two pins, and the other end has one pin with a knob that can be tightened to apply pressure (Figs. 3-3 and 3-4). We prefer to place the end with two pins posteriorly on the skull, and the end with one pin anteriorly. The posterior pins are positioned such that one pin is inserted at the external occipital protuberance, or inion, while the other is positioned in the body of the mastoid process. Of course, when the operation involves the cerebellopontine angle or the lateral skull base, the pin should be positioned in the opposite mastoid process. The anterior pin should be positioned in the frontal bone, preferably behind the hairline for cosmetic reasons. The pin should insert into the scalp in an orientation that is as orthogonal to the contour of the skull as possible; thus, only the tip of the pin will enter or touch the scalp. This prevents undue pressure on the skin from the fixation device itself—a situation that can lead to local tissue necrosis and prolonged healing. When compressing the fixator into the skull of an adult, one must apply 40 to 60 foot-pounds of pressure. In a child 20 to 40 foot-pounds of pressure is recommended. This is done by first pressing the two ends of the fixator together, then turning the knob on the single pin end of the fixator. At the tip of the knob is a

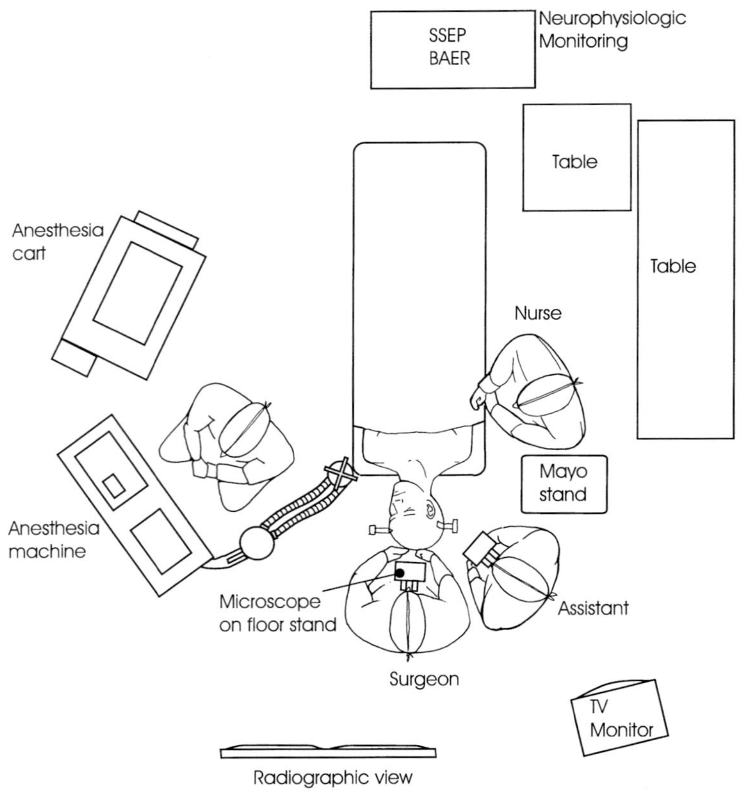

FIG. 3-2. Standard operating room arrangement for supine position surgery.

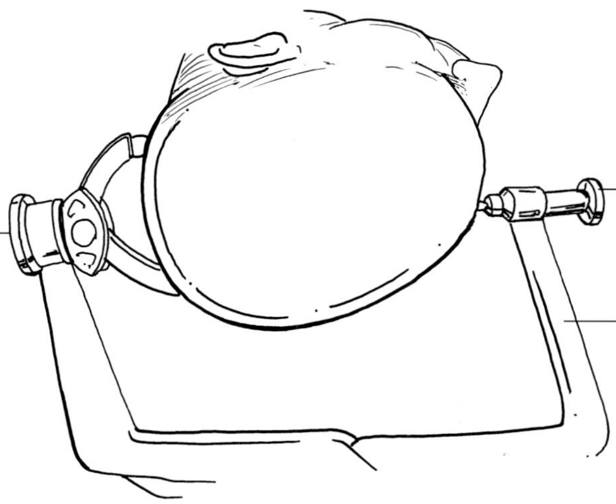

FIG. 3-3. Patient positioning for right subtemporal approach with head secured in Mayfield head holder.

pressure gauge. As the knob is tightened, lines on the pressure gauge become visible. Each line marks 20 additional foot-pounds of pressure. If more than 60 foot-pounds is applied, there is a danger of the pins penetrating the inner table of the skull and causing an intracranial hemorrhage.

Once the head pin fixator is applied, it should be secured to the table through the series of connecting arms (Fig. 3-4). Each arm should have its own tightening knob. Each knob must be tightened individually starting with the arm connecting to the three-point head fixator and proceeding to the arm connecting to the operating table. After tightening each knob, it must be checked individually. Once this is completed, the head should be held by the surgeon and checked by applying gentle pressure to be certain that it is completely immobilized.

LATERAL POSITION

One of the more commonly used positions in procedures that require the combined skills of neurosurgeons and otologists is the lateral position. This position allows access to the middle fossa, and access to the lateral skull base including the cerebellopontine angle, the jugular foramen, the lower and mid-clivus, and the anterior foramen magnum. This position can also be used for transtemporal and transcondylar approaches.

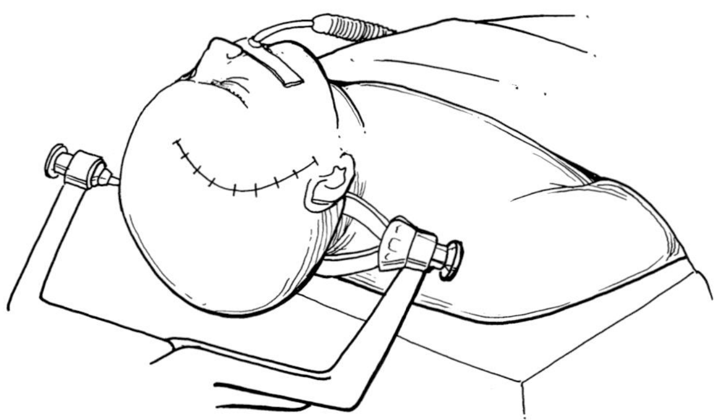

FIG. 3-4. Patient positioning for right pterional approach with head secured in Mayfield head holder. By placement of posterior pins in the mastoid body and the inion, the Mayfield is in a more horizontal positioning facilitating retraction.

Following intubation the tube is secured and the patient is placed in the lateral decubitus position. The operating table is flexed to raise the back of the table approximately 20 degrees from the floor. The patient's back is brought close to the edge of the table with the shoulders positioned to the cephalad end of the table. The body is positioned to lie obliquely across the table. This allows the back to roll slightly downward in order to expose the abdomen if it is necessary to harvest an abdominal fat graft. The lower leg, or dependent leg, is flexed 90 degrees at the knee, while the upper leg is kept only slightly flexed. After padding the heel and ankle of the lower leg, two pillows are placed transversely between the legs and one pillow placed longitudinally between the legs. A gel pad is placed underneath the hip to pad the trochanter. Improper positioning of this pad can lead to pressure sores and decubitus ulcers following prolonged operations. Next, a padded rest is positioned over the gluteal muscle to prevent the patient from rolling backward. Care must be taken to avoid compression of the sciatic nerve. An axillary roll is placed in the axilla to avoid compression of the brachial plexus. Both arms are outstretched on arm boards with care to pad the ulnar nerve at the medial epicondyle and the radial nerve at the radial groove of the humerus. The dependent arm is positioned 90 degrees to the longitudinal axis of the body while the other arm is positioned 45 degrees to the body. In positioning the nondependent arm, the shoulder must be rolled anteriorly and pulled gently in the caudal direction. Once in this position the shoulder is secured by tape to the arm board. This maneuver pulls the shoulder away from the surgeon and allows him to look up in a caudal to cranial direction if

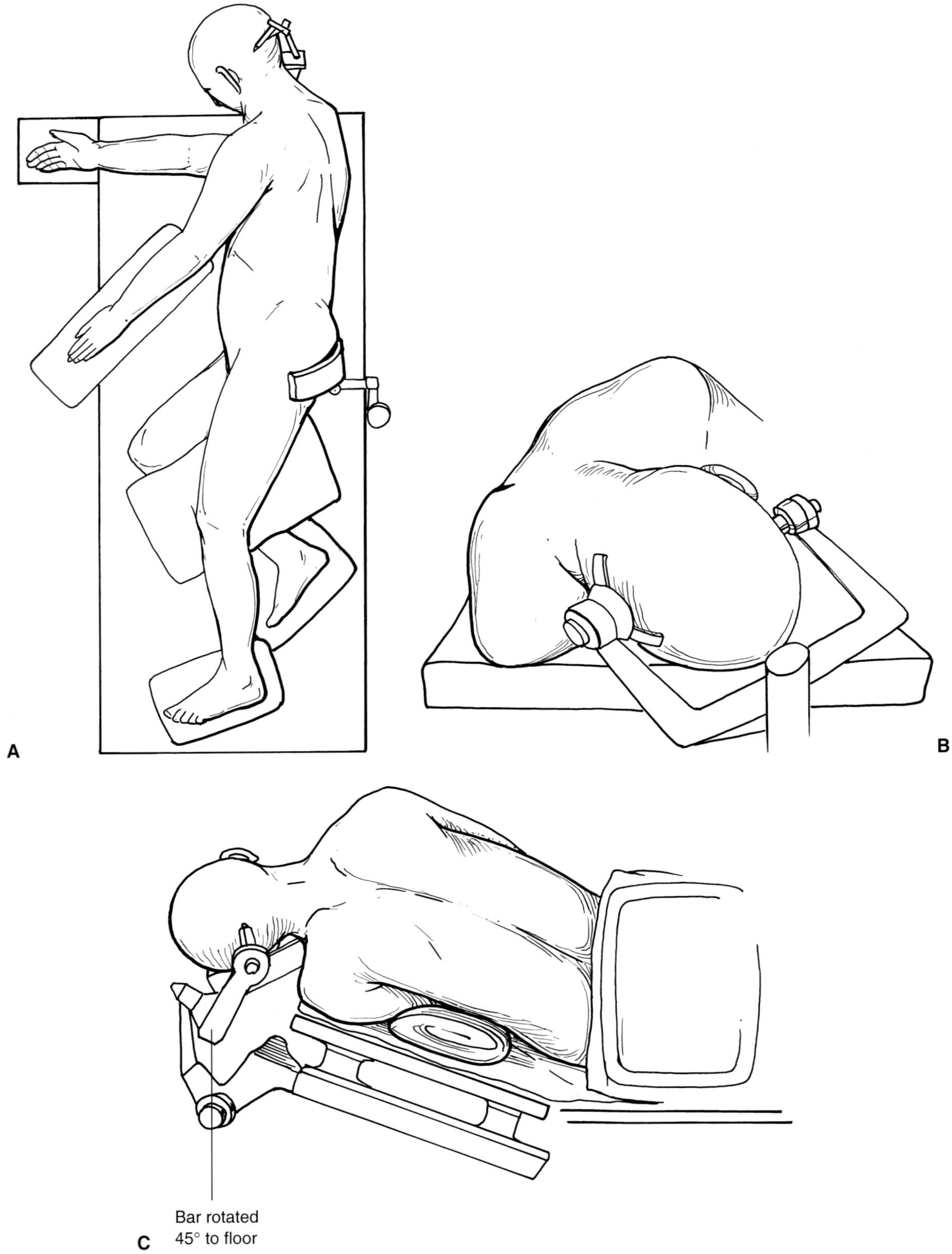

FIG. 3-5. A: The patient is positioned in the lateral position. The left arm is 45 degrees to the longitudinal axis of the body, with the shoulder pulled caudally. The body is positioned such that the abdomen is rotated posteriorly and the shoulders are rotated anteriorly with the back at the edge of the table. The abdominal region is included in the surgical field for abdominal fat harvesting. **B:** The neck is flexed and the vertex is tilted slightly downward toward the floor. The line formed from the nose to the inion is kept parallel to the floor. The back is positioned at the edge of the table. **C:** The back of the table is flexed upward 20 degrees. An axillary roll is placed in the dependent axilla and a padded rest is positioned over the gluteal region. Note the orientation of the Mayfield headrest approximately 45 degrees to the floor. This aids in placement of the self-retaining retractors.

necessary. Additionally, in positioning the arm at a 45-degree angle from the body the abdominal area is exposed if an abdominal fat graft is necessary (Fig. 3-5A).

The head is then placed in three-point fixation and positioned in such a manner as to keep the nose parallel with the floor and the cranial vertex tilted slightly down toward the floor (Fig. 3-5B,C). This position of the head allows access to the middle fossa, the cerebellopontine angle, the mastoid process, the petrous temporal bone, and the far lateral skull base extending down to the foramen magnum and upper cervical spine. For lesions of the posterior fossa or anterior foramen magnum, the head is flexed as maximally as possible to allow access to the suboccipital region. The maximum amount of flexion should allow the surgeon to pass his outstretched hand between the patient's chin and manubrium.

After the patient has been positioned, the surgeon should assure that the patient is secured with straps and adhesive cloth tape to the bed. During the course of surgery, the table may be rotated to varying degrees. This can only be done safely if the patient is fully immobilized. When placing the straps and tape, the surgeon should avoid compressing any nervous structures.

SUPINE POSITION

The supine position is the most commonly used and a versatile position in brain surgery. It is most frequently used for the "pterional" approach; however, it can be used for subtemporal or middle fossa approaches, or bifrontal and transbasal approaches. The subtemporal and middle fossa approaches can be utilized for lesions of the middle cranial fossa, the internal auditory canal (IAC), or the petrous apex and upper clival region. The bifrontal and transbasal approaches are best used for lesions of the anterior cranial fossa that also involve the cribriform plate or ethmoid sinus. Additionally, lesions involving the frontal sinus can be approached in this position.

The patient is placed on the operating table in a supine position. The patient's head is placed in a Mayfield skull fixation device with the pins inserted into the inion, the body of the mastoid process, and the frontal bone, preferably behind the hair line. In cases of a receded hair line the anterior pin can be placed in the forehead. A shoulder roll is placed underneath the shoulder along the longitudinal axis of the patient. This facilitates the placement of the head into the horizontal position with the sagittal suture parallel to the floor and the vertex tilted toward the floor so that the zygomatic process is the highest point in the field. The back of the bed should be flexed approximately 20 degrees to keep the head level with the heart (Fig. 3-6). This position requires a significant amount of rotation of the head, which in some patients can compromise the venous outflow from the contralateral jugular vein. Additionally, in elderly patients with degenerative cervical spines, this amount of rotation may be difficult to achieve. This can be overcome by placing a larger shoulder roll under the patient, rotating the operating table to position the head horizontally, or putting the patient in the lateral position as explained above.

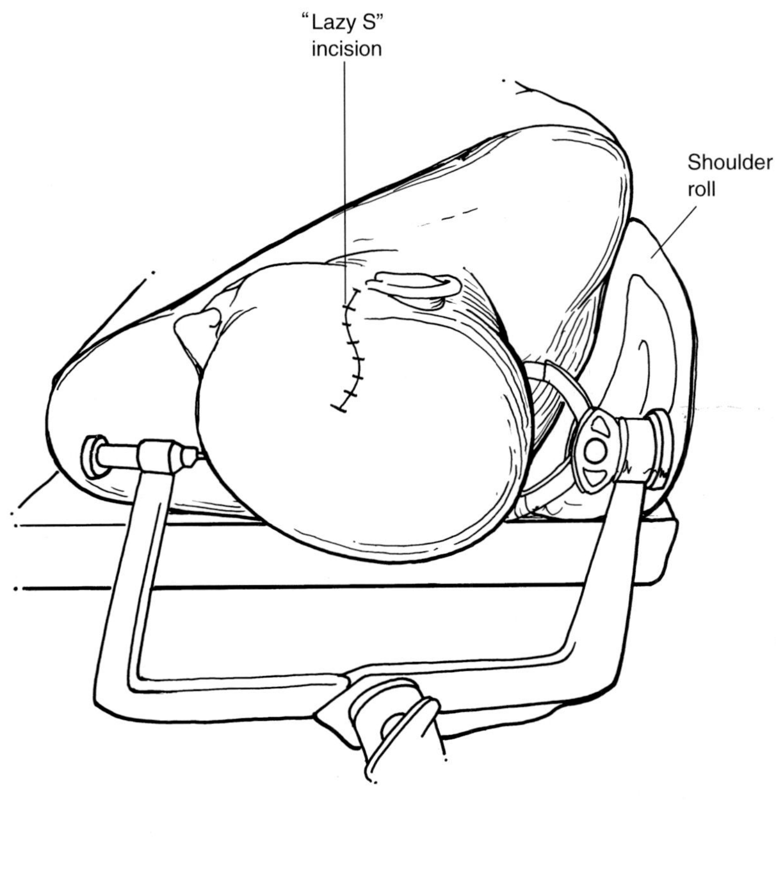

FIG. 3-6. Patient in right subtemporal position. A "lazy S" incision is made 1 cm anterior to the tragus.

For lesions or approaches involving the anterior cranial fossa, the patient is placed on the operating table in the supine position. The head is placed either in pin fixation or a horseshoe headrest. The pins cannot be inserted into the landmarks described above; instead, they are placed in the temporal and parietal bones. The pins should not be placed in the squamosal portion of the temporal bone as the bone is thin here and penetration of the inner table is more likely. The back of the table is flexed 10 to 15 degrees, and the patient's neck is flexed such that the cranial vertex is tilted up, and the nose is kept in the midline position.

TRANSSPHENOIDAL POSITION

The transsphenoidal approach to the sellar and suprasellar region is a frequently used and elegant procedure. To facilitate the exposure, the positioning of the patient is critical due to the confined corridor that is used during this approach. Additionally, to allow for a maximum viewing angle, the head must be free to rotate and tilted for adequate visualization of the deep and narrow exposure. A modified Mayfield headrest with a Hardy attachment is used. This headrest, commonly referred to as the horseshoe headrest because of its shape, does not require skull fixation with pins.

The patient is placed on the operating table in the supine position. The patient is orally intubated with an armored tube that is secured toward the left corner of the mouth. The patient is in a semirecumbent position, the back of the table is flexed approximately 20 to 30 degrees, and the knees are bent to avoid stretch of the sciatic nerve. The arms are securely tucked at the side of the patient. To provide the surgeon easy nasal access, the top of the patient's head is tilted 20 degrees toward his or her left shoulder, and the chin is rotated 20 degrees toward the surgeon, who is standing on the patient's right side. The neck should not be flexed or extended, but instead be in a neutral position parallel to the floor. The patient's abdominal region is prepped and draped into the surgical field for an abdominal fat graft that is necessary at the conclusion of the procedure (Fig. 3-7).

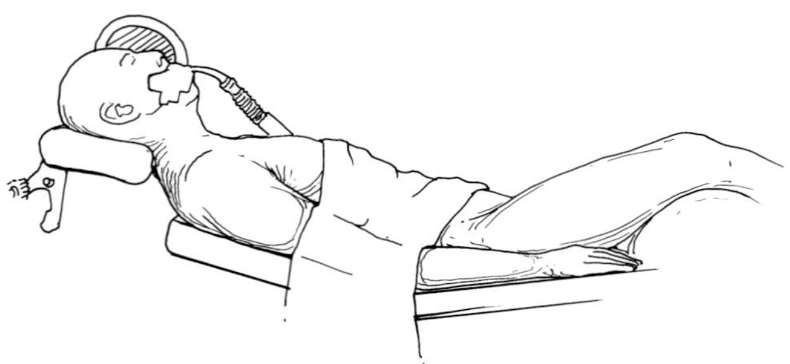

FIG. 3-7. Patient positioning for transsphenoidal surgery with the head in a Hardy horseshoe headrest. The patient is placed in a semirecumbent supine position with the head of the bed elevated 20 degrees. The endotracheal tube is secured to the left corner of the mouth. The right abdomen is prepared for possible harvest of abdominal fat. The head is turned to the right and elevated.

The arrangement of the operating room must be given careful consideration during these operations. We position the surgeon along the patient's right side and the anesthesiologist at the patient's left side. We believe that for patient safety the anesthesiologist should have easy access to the airway as well as to the intraarterial or intravenous lines. The operating microscope is brought in from a position cephalad to the patient's head. The base of the microscope stand must be positioned to allow a surgical assistant to stand above the patient's head. Additionally, the base of the stand should be positioned to allow a C-arm fluoroscope to be brought into the surgical field. In most cases, fluoroscopy is needed only during the approach to the sella, and can be removed after the approach is completed (Fig. 3-8).

RETRACTION SYSTEMS

An often overlooked and neglected aspect of surgery is the type of retraction utilized by the surgeon for both extracranial use as well as intracranial use. Kurze (2) stated, "The entire matter of retraction has been neglected in most essays about microsurgical technique . . . . Mastery of this particular element is the single most important and most difficult step in microsurgery." Greenberg (3) evaluated the idea of ergonomic variables of neurosurgery and concluded "that the combination of ergonomic analysis of surgical technique with the availability and use of specialized self retaining retractors has the enormous benefits of stimulating safer, more efficient surgery." The ideal self-retaining retractor system is one that can be placed in the surgical field from a variety of angles, is easily adjustable, and does not obstruct the view of the surgeon. Additionally, the retractor system should not prevent the surgeon from resting his hands on the patient during microsurgical maneuvers.

Chen and co-workers (4) categorized self-retaining retractors into skull/soft tissue mounted systems and flexible bar devices or "snake" retractor arms that are mounted to either the skull, operating table, or headrest. A well-known example of skull/soft tissue mounted self-retaining retractor is the House/Urban middle fossa retractor. This retractor was specifically designed for the middle fossa procedure. It employs a single blade retractor that is mechanically geared and attaches by bolts to an Adson cerebellar self-retaining retractor by means of a platform. Modifications to this retractor were made by Fisch and Garcia-Ibanez, but it remains similar to the House/Urban retractor. Another popular skull/soft tissue mounted retractor is the Janetta retractor.

The underlying limitation of self-retaining skull/soft tissue retractors is that the retractor is either very close or within the operative field. Despite the use of articulating arms, rods, and blades, these retractor systems lack versatility of placement and must be placed in a specific location. This impairs visualization of the surgical field and limits hand and instrument placement.

To surmount many of these limitations, flexible arm or snake retractors that can be made rigid through articulated

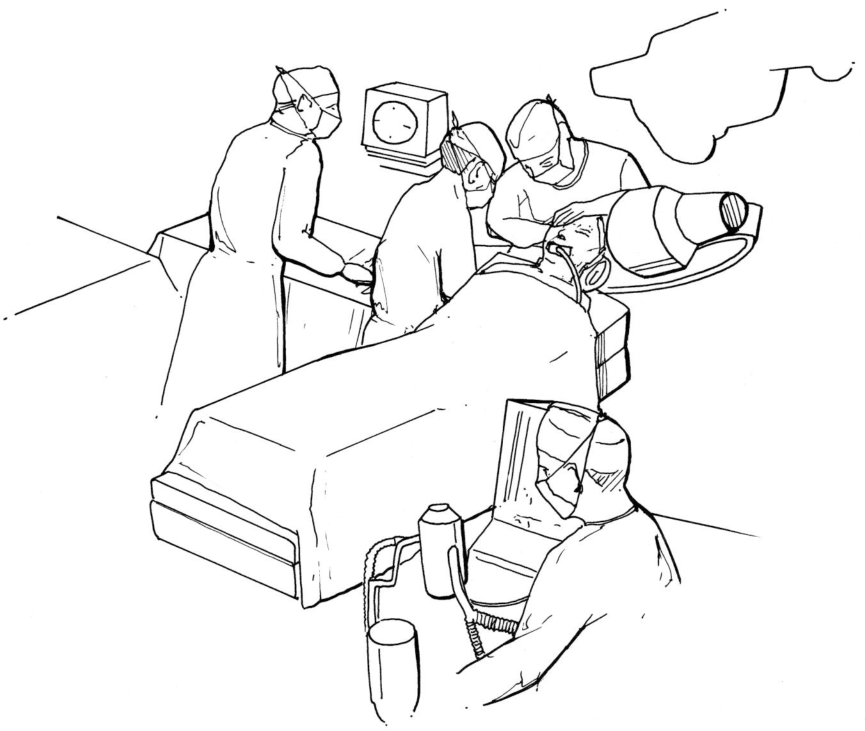

FIG. 3-8. The operating room arrangement and the position of the surgeon, anesthesiologists, and nurses are illustrated. The assistant stands at the head of the table. The fluoroscopy unit and the microscope are brought in from the head.

ball and cable mechanisms have been designed. These arms can be mounted on the skull, table, or headrest. A variety of systems have been described including, among the more popular designs, the Leyla retractor (Aesculap) introduced by Yasargil (5), the Greenberg retractor, the Sugita retractor system, and the Fukushima retractor system. The Leyla retractor mounts to the table rather than to the patient's head or a head holder. This raises the concern of independent movement of the retractor in relation to the operative site or the brain. The Greenberg retractor system utilizes lockable flexible arms and is mounted to a variety of head holders (6). The Sugita system requires a special head holder to which a multipurpose frame is attached (7). Leyla flexible arms are used with the Sugita system.

For intracranial retraction we preferentially utilize a Fukushima retractor system because of its versatility and its compatibility with the Mayfield head fixation device. Described by Fukushima and Sano (8) in 1980, this system uses two C-clamps (Elekta Instruments, Atlanta, GA) that attach to the Mayfield head holder and two adjustable and lockable retractor arms or snakes (Elekta Instruments). Each C-clamp has three positions to which a flexible retractor arm can attach, further increasing the mobility of the retractor arms. Fukushima spatula retractor blades (Elekta Instruments) are then attached to the retractor arms (Fig. 3-9). These Fukushima retractors are low profile, flexible, and tapered to varying degrees. Additionally, a set of spatula retractors has been designed for extradural retraction that is stiffer and more durable. When it is necessary to have a more mobile system of retractor arms a Fukushima J-bar (Fujita Instruments, Tokyo, Japan) can be attached (Fig. 3-10). This system allows almost 360 degrees of mobility for the retractor arms.

For extracranial retraction of scalp and muscle we utilize a Leyla bar (Aesculap), introduced by Yasargil, and Fukushima atraumatic scalp hooks, which are available in various sizes. The scalp hooks are suspended by rubber bands to the Leyla bar, to the C-clamps, or to the J-bar, thus providing 360 degrees of mobility for skin and muscle retraction that contours to the skull. By utilizing this system, we avoid

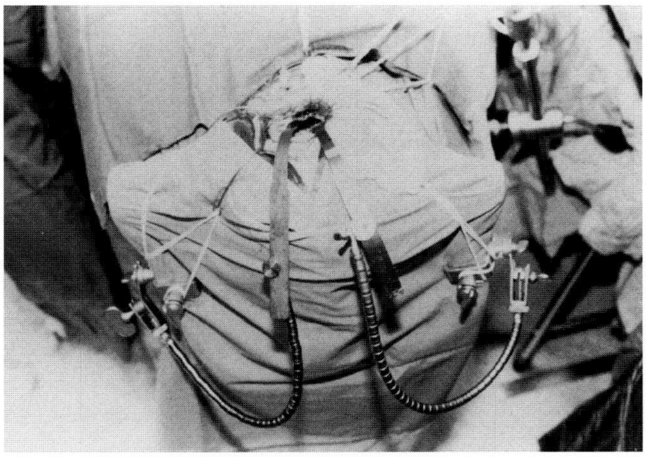

FIG. 3-9. The Fukushima retractor system with C-clamps attached to the Mayfield head holder (under the drapes) and the malleable spatulas attached to the retractor arms are illustrated. Also note the atraumatic skin hooks retracting the soft tissue. The entire system is low profile and is not obstructive.

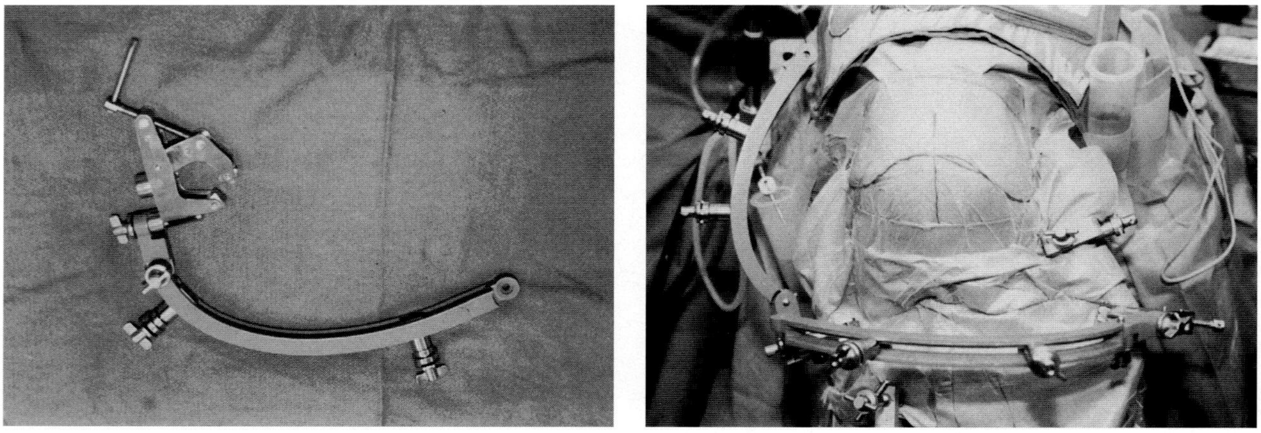

A B

FIG. 3-10. A,B: The Fukushima J-bar allows greater mobility of the retractor arms.

cumbersome self-retaining retractors that protrude from the surgical field, thereby improving surgical ergonomics (Fig. 3-9).

Neurosurgery, like otolaryngology, is a discipline that requires precise technical skills and meticulous operative planning. The operations can be prolonged and treacherous, and therefore mandate that the surgeon is comfortable and does not experience excessive fatigue, which can affect the surgeon's patience, judgment, and dexterity. Careful planning of the operating room arrangement and patient positioning, along with consideration of surgical ergonomics and retraction, will thus serve to enhance the safety, efficiency, and efficacy of the operation.

REFERENCES

1. Cabequdo JM, Carrielo R, Vognero S, et al. Air embolism from pin type head holder as a complication of sitting position: case report. *J Neurosurg* 1981;55:147.
2. Kurze T. Comment. *Neurosurgery* 1981;9:572.
3. Greenberg IM. Self retaining retractors and handrests. In: Wilkins RH, Rengachary SS, eds. *Neurosurgery*, 2nd ed. New York: McGraw-Hill, 1996.
4. Chen DA, Arriaga MA, Fukushima T. Technical refinements in retraction for middle fossa surgery. *Am J Otol* 1998;19(2):208–212.
5. Yasargil MG. *Microsurgery applied to neurosurgery*. New York: Academic Press, 1969.
6. Greenberg IM. Self retaining retractor and handrest system for neurosurgery. *Neurosurgery* 1981;8:205–208.
7. Sugita K, Hifota T, Mizutani T, et al. *J Neurosurg* 1978;48:656–657.
8. Fukushima T, Sano K. Simple retractor holder for the Mayfield skull clamp. *Surg Neurol* 1980;13:320.

Neurosurgical Issues in Otolaryngology: Principles and Practice of Collaboration,
edited by Moisés A. Arriaga and J. Diaz Day.
Lippincott Williams & Wilkins, Philadelphia © 1999.

CHAPTER 4

Neurosurgical Instrumentation

J. Diaz Day

The differences in surgical instrumentation used by the various subspecialties can be striking. Especially in comparing focused fields such as otology and intracranial neurosurgery, it is surprising the contrast between the tools individual surgeons use to meet similar ends. It is useful for members of different specialties to have some understanding of the tools that others deem necessary to performing their respective functions during the operation in combined endeavors.

Neurosurgery, possibly more than any other discipline, has realized a tremendous transformation in terms of instrumentation with recent technologic developments. Computer technology, robotics, and advanced optics are all currently changing the ways in which neurosurgeons perform surgery. Some technologic adjuncts are already proving superior to existing methods, while others are viewed as mere gimmicks with little to add to traditional methods of practice. The goal of this continual evolution of equipment is the reduction of the effects of open surgical manipulation on the surrounding brain. The development of the ultrasonic aspirator and the laser has given us the means to reduce tumor volume in an efficient manner with reduced disturbance to the surrounding structures. Developments in computer technology are contributing to a rapid evolution of stereotactic methods that are less cumbersome and are increasingly user friendly. This chapter highlights the current state of neurosurgical instrumentation for those outside of neurosurgery.

HEAD FRAMES

The demand for rigid fixation of the operative subject seems to be peculiar to neurosurgery. Neurosurgeons seem to run headlong into a debate with their colleagues in otolaryngology and plastic surgery over the necessity or desirability of rigid fixation of the patient's head. Only outside of neurosurgical circles does ''putting the patient in pins'' give rise to fears of potential morbidity. Any potential morbidity is overstated only outside of neurosurgery for this type of rigid fixation. The necessity for rigid fixation mainly stems from the demands of intracranial microsurgery. Movement of the patient during microsurgery has its disadvantages. Maneuvers performed under magnification in restricted apertures possess little room for error. Movement other than what the surgeon is responsible for could cause potential harm. Further, rigid fixation is necessary to the utilization of self-retaining retractor arms to hold brain away from the operative field. A table-mounted system is not acceptable without the patient's head in rigid fixation owing to the potential of the patient's moving against the retractor, resulting in damage to neural tissue. The retractor arms must be able to move with the patient's head, thus securing their constant position.

There exist several systems for rigid head fixation, each with various advantages and disadvantages. The most widely used system is the Mayfield fixation system [Ohio Medical Instruments Co. (OMI), Cincinnati, OH]. This system is simple and easy to apply. The frame uses three pins to fix the head with a spring-loaded mechanism. This mechanism is responsible for its ease of application. Another example is the Sugita head frame (Mizuho, Lynn, MA), which uses individual pins organized around a semicircular frame that must be individually tightened to fix the patient's head. This frame is also relatively easy to apply. The head frame is designed with an entire system of retractor arms and instrument holding pockets that makes it convenient for microneurosurgery. Most systems are also available in radiolucent models, constructed from carbon fiber materials. Such frames are more convenient for use in cases where intraoperative angiography or computed tomography scanning is used.

RETRACTOR SYSTEMS

Though the goal of contemporary skull base surgery is to limit or eliminate the necessity of brain retraction, some

J. Diaz Day: Department of Neurological Surgery, House Ear Clinic, Los Angeles, California 90057.

element of retraction remains a reality in the majority of procedures. Brain tissue often must be held away from the field to provide an adequate working space. This is accomplished utilizing self-retaining retractor arms holding the retractor blades. In microneurosurgery, an assistant holding the retractor blade is not acceptable owing to limitations in stamina, stability, and the ability to adequately view the operative field. These limitations led to the invention of such retractor arms that can be positioned securely.

Several basic systems exist that have all been modeled in one way or another after the Greenberg system (Codman & Shurtleff, Randolph, MA). The Greenberg retractor system is mounted to the head frame by clamps. Metal bars are then attached and constructed around the operative field, serving as a base for the attachment of the self-retaining retractor arms. If constructed properly, the system is not intrusive to the surgeon. A similar system is the Budde Halo (OMI, Cincinnati, OH). This is another system that attaches to the head frame by way of clamps. A ring-shaped base is mounted around the operative field. The retractor arms then attach to this "halo." When positioned properly, the system is also not intrusive. Further, the halo provides a frame for the surgeon to rest the wrists for stability.

A newer system that attempts to be the least intrusive to the surgeon is that developed by Fukushima (Fujita, Tokyo, Japan). This system (described in detail in Chapter 3) uses two C-clamps that attach to the head frame. The C-clamps contain an attachment apparatus for several retractor arms. The retractor arms may then be positioned such that they conform to the curvature of the head, staying out of the surgeon's way. This concept is also evident in the Leyla retractor system developed by Yarsargil. Retractor arms are attached to a table-mounted bar. They may also be positioned to conform to the curvature of the head. All of the above systems provide stable, secure retraction of brain tissue. When used properly, the systems are unobtrusive to the surgeon and morbidity is minimal.

DRILLS

High-speed drills have become a mainstay of instrumentation for contemporary cranial base surgery. Several drill systems have been developed for utilization in these procedures. The historical development of such systems falls outside the scope of this chapter and may be found elsewhere (1). No particular drill systems are singled out in this discussion. Those appropriate for neurosurgery generally have a craniotome attachment for cutting bone flaps. Some systems also come with a separate attachment to make burr holes utilizing a cranial perforator. Selection of a drill is based on personal preference. The individual drill's "feel" and its ease of use are important factors in selecting a system.

The most widely used systems all possess certain key attributes that make them appropriate for these procedures. One such critical attribute is their utility while working under the microscope. The drill must be designed for this use, keeping the handpiece and cord out of the surgeon's view. How comfortable the drill feels under the microscope is paramount. Drills must have proper balance and light weight, both of which decrease fatigue and enhance safety. For most situations, high speed and torque are desirable. Too little power can translate into surgeon fatigue. It also may result in the surgeon exerting too much pressure on the drill, leading to instability of the drill and loss of control. Therefore, adequate drill power is necessary to result in the surgeon's ability to exert light pressure, effecting rapid and safe bone removal. Most current systems run in the 60,000 to 80,000 rpm range, which proves adequate for neurosurgical applications.

ULTRASONIC ASPIRATORS

The most common complex instrument used in reducing tumor volume is the ultrasonic aspirator. First developed in 1947 as the CUSA (Cavitron Ultrasonic Surgical Aspirator) by Cooper instruments for removing dental plaques, its application to neurosurgical procedures began in 1976 (2–4). The technology has been produced by several different companies in various forms.

The basic unit consists of an acoustic vibrator, an irrigation system, and a suction system within a self-contained device. The acoustic vibrator converts electrical current into mechanical vibration utilizing an electric coil and a magnetostrictive transducer.

As originally produced, alternating current at 23 kHz produces a 100-μm longitudinal vibration that acts to fragment tissue within 1 mm of the tip. The irrigation fluid, emanating from near the tip, suspends the tumor fragments to be removed as an emulsion via the suction apparatus. The Selector unit manufactured by Leksell (Elekta Corp., Atlanta, GA) uses a 35-kHz acoustic vibrator. The increase in frequency translates to the delivery of greater power at lower amplitudes. This formula results in decreased tissue disruption to the surrounding area by more efficient removal of the tumor.

Studies in the laboratory have been carried out investigating the effects of the instrument on the electrical conduction properties of neural tissue. As an important initial finding, electric current is not passed from the instrument to the tissue. Also, normal electrical conduction has been demonstrated to be preserved within a 1-mm radius of the tip (5). This work has shown that the instrument may be safely used to dissect tumor adjacent to vital structures in the brain without the possibility of disrupting normal function. However, this does not apply to cranial nerves. Nerves may be damaged directly by the instrument.

The effects on surrounding tissues have also been studied pathologically. The ideal tissue for fragmentation with the ultrasonic aspirator has a high intracellular fluid content. Brain and fat are examples of two such tissues. The greater collagenous and elastic character of blood vessels make them more resistant to fragmentation by the instrument, though direct contact can still result in puncture. Cranial nerves may be damaged if coming into direct contact, being spared when only in proximity to the working instrument. Electron microscopy of adjacent tissue will show edema in both myelinated and unmyelinated axons. Large vacuoles may be present in both neurons and glial cells. Perivascular spaces will harbor an increased number of phagocytes, though the integrity of the small vessels appears preserved (6).

Wide application in neurosurgery has evolved owing to several advantages of the instrument in tumor resection. First, the ultrasonic aspirator requires little manipulation of surrounding tissues to resect tumor. There is little heat generated by the device, thus thermal damage to surrounding tissue is minimized. The device simultaneously aspirates as it irrigates and breaks up tumor; therefore, spread of tumor cells is minimized. Lastly, it is relatively easy to preserve tissue planes while using the instrument. Despite these points, the instrument does have some disadvantages. The ultrasonic aspirator is not effective in fragmenting very hard tumors. Normal structures such as vessels and nerves are not spared the destructive effects of the instrument when coming into direct contact with the vibrating tip. Hemostasis is at times problematic, as the ultrasonic aspirator can only suction blood from the field, providing no inherent hemostatic action.

From a technical standpoint, several points need to be made. The ultrasonic aspirator is in general a simple instrument to use. The instrument works quickly, and because of this rapid action it is easy to lose a controlled resection of tumor. Overly rapid and aggressive use may result in extending the fragmentation effects to surrounding tissue, not intended to be resected. Also, although vessels are resistant to the effects of the instrument, direct contact with major vascular structures may result in perforation and a potential disaster. A higher frequency vibrator helps in this regard in using lower amplitude. Third, very hard tumors are resistant to the effects of the instrument and will require an alternate strategy. The final point concerns selection of instrument design. Most instruments currently available are somewhat bulky and cumbersome, especially when working under the operating microscope. It is preferable to use one of the small numbers of designs available that incorporates a smaller, angled handpiece. Also advantageous is incorporation of suction attenuation via a slotted mechanism that the surgeon can differentially control (7).

LASERS

History and Basic Principles

Historical Aspects

The laser (light amplification by stimulated emission of radiation) has developed into a tool that has revolutionized scientific endeavors since the late 1950s. The principles upon which this device were established are derived from quantum mechanical theories originated by Bohr and Einstein. Theodore Maiman takes the credit for actually first producing laser light in the laboratory using a ruby crystal as a stimulated medium (8,9). Initial studies of the effects of this high-energy light source on biologic tissues piqued the interest of medical researchers with regard to possible "miracle cures" that could result from such application. In the 1960s, the effects of laser energy on central nervous system tissues were first investigated. The consequences of high-power laser lesions were devastating to the experimental animals treated through the intact skull. Such treatment resulted in gross hemorrhage and necrosis with signs of rapid swelling and herniation. Direct application of laser energy to the cerebral cortex through craniotomy was found to produce local necrosis and hemorrhage (10–12). These findings led to the clinical application of the medium as a means of vaporizing tumor.

Rosomoff and Carroll (13) reported the first application to the surgery of gliomas in 1966. These investigators used a low-powered ruby laser to directly deliver pulsed sequences of energy to three patients with glioblastomas. Two patients demonstrated necrosis of tumor treated by the laser at postmortem examination. This particular type of laser showed effects of deep penetration of the tissue and apparently did not instantly vaporize the tissue at surgery. The effects of this type of laser were further characterized by several groups of investigators on neural tissues in this time frame. As a result of the findings of such investigations, irreversible damage more to neurons and unmyelinated tissues than to supporting cells, this medium was largely abandoned in favor of the less penetrating CO_2 laser (9).

In 1969, Stellar (14) applied the CO_2 laser to surgical resection in three patients with malignant gliomas, taking advantage of its vaporizing effects on tissue. He reported that large blood vessels could not be coagulated using this laser. However, small vessels, 1 mm or less in diameter, were easily controlled. The result was a reduction in surgical blood loss using this tool. This was in accordance with other investigators in varying surgical specialties who found that the CO_2 laser was an efficient tool for incising and vaporizing tissues, but not coagulation (9). Despite the early reports of efficacy, widespread use was not seen until the mid-1970s. Designs took time to develop, aimed at reducing the cumbersome nature of the equipment, and adapting the laser to the operating microscope. The design flaws were largely worked out in Europe and Japan (9). Also, in this time frame, the neodymium: yttrium-aluminum-garnet (Nd:YAG) laser system was developed and applied neurosurgically in Germany by Beck (9). Since then, lasers have been variously used by many neurosurgeons as an adjunct to tumor resection operations. Because studies have not clearly demonstrated a difference in outcome, however, this is not a universally employed strategy for tumor resection.

Functional Principles

There are three main properties of laser light that make it unique. The first is monochromaticity. This means simply that the light is of the same wavelength. Ambient light, on the other hand, contains light of wavelengths throughout the visible, ultraviolet, and infrared spectra. The second feature is coherence. Coherence of light means that the waves travel in phase, both spatially and temporally. The great intensity of a laser beam is dependent on this property. The third unique property is collimation. Laser light does not diverge as it travels through space. The light can travel long distances in a strictly parallel beam.

The apparatus that produces such a beam has several key elements. The first is a medium that can be stimulated by electrical current to produce photons. The medium can exist in any of the three phases of matter: gas, liquid, or solid. The medium is housed in what is called an "optical resonator," where electrical current is passed through the medium. The energy transfer of the electrical current results in the production of electrons in an excited state. The natural laws governing matter demand that a decay process occur to restore these electrons to their lowest energy state. This process of decay results in the emission of the energy as photons. The photons may then be reflected within the chamber, striking other atoms to elevate other electrons to higher energy states, resulting in amplification of the process. The optical resonator has two mirrors, one at each end of the chamber. One mirror is only partially reflective, allowing the laser beam to be emitted. Only photons in phase and of the same wavelength are allowed to exit the chamber. This forms the highly intense laser light beam.

Tissue Interactions

The interaction of the laser beam with nervous tissue is dependent on the distribution and quantity of power within the laser beam. The area upon which the beam strikes the tissue is referred to as the laser spot. The size of the laser spot determines what effect the laser will have on the tissue, be it incision, vaporization, or coagulation. A smaller laser spot, which is finely focused, will result in vaporization or incision of the tissue in that confined area. Increasing the laser spot size will generally result in coagulation or vaporization over a wider, but more superficial, volume of tissue. The spot size is controlled via a lens system. Tissue that is positioned at the focal point of the lens will be subject to the full power of the laser beam via a finely focused, small laser spot. A larger spot is produced by "defocusing" the system. Placing tissue beyond the focal length results in coagulation or vaporization. As the beam passes through the tissue in these two modes, the energy is dissipated gradually as the beam becomes increasingly defocused. The same large spot result is obtained by placing the tissue within the focal distance of the lens. However, as the beam passes through the tissue, the power density actually increases, since the focal length lies somewhere beneath the tissue surface. This can be dangerous to underlying normal tissue (9).

Laser light may react with the tissue in four ways. The light may be transmitted, scattered, absorbed, or reflected. Application of laser light demonstrates its effect on a tissue as a combination of these four reactions. The extinction length of the particular laser is an important variable that determines this interaction. This describes the depth at which 90% of the laser light is absorbed. This length will vary for the various lasers in relation to different biologic tissues. The second important variable is the absorption coefficient of the tissue, which describes the ability of the tissue to absorb a particular wavelength of light. In a similar fashion, this varies by type of tissue and the particular laser used. This coefficient is affected by cell type, water content, temperature, and pigmentation. The extinction length values are not established for the various available lasers in neural tissues (9,15), and nor are the absorption coefficients of neural tissue. Exact determinations are not possible, as it is impossible to control for all of the factors affecting such measurements. We presently rely on some widely held general observations regarding the interactions of specific laser types to help make choices regarding the appropriate laser to employ, the spot size needed, and how to adjust the focus of the beam.

Laser Types Used in Neurosurgery

Carbon Dioxide Laser

The carbon dioxide (CO_2) laser uses a wavelength of 10.6 μm, which is invisible to the human eye. This wavelength resides in the far infrared portion of the light spectrum. Because of its invisibility, this laser must be used with a coaxial pilot beam to guide application. This laser has a short extinction length, which results in the absorption of its energy by tissue mostly at the surface. The vaporization effect on tissues is caused by the rapid heating of intracellular water, vaporizing the cell instantaneously. Because little energy is transmitted deep into tissues, this laser is ideal for tissue surface ablation. The absence of significant transmission in water or blood, however, is responsible for its poor coagulating properties. Thus, the action of this laser is dominated by its absorption by tissues (9,15).

The CO_2 laser is used either via a handheld apparatus or via attachment to the operating microscope. The microscope-mounted system is preferable and in widest use. The laser is directed via an aiming system that is attached to the body of the microscope. This system has different lenses that can be changed by the surgeon to vary the spot size of the laser beam. Precise control over the aim of the laser is through a joystick, either controlled by hand or with a mouthpiece.

This laser finds greatest utility in the debulking of large tumor masses that are in difficult areas of access. In general, this instrument is most applicable in tumors located in the ventricles, brainstem, and spinal cord. The manipulation of adjacent tissues can be decreased in these circumstances by using the laser, thus its value in these sensitive areas. The drawback of this type of laser is its inability to coagulate vessels larger than 1.0 mm. This reduces its efficacy in the case of a more vascular tumor. Reflection from shiny surfaces is an avoidable problem with this laser. Only nonreflective retractor blades and instruments should be introduced into the field when utilizing the CO_2 laser.

Kelly et al. (16,17) have developed a computer-assisted stereotaxic technique utilizing the CO_2 laser for volumetric resection of deep-seated lesions. This system helps the surgeon maintain a three-dimensional orientation during resection of such deep lesions. Kelly's technique has been reported helpful in debulking deep-seated gliomas due to the inexact nature of their boundaries.

Neodymium:Yttrium-Aluminum-Garnet Laser (Nd:YAG)

This laser possesses a wavelength in the near infrared region of the spectrum at 1.06 μm. This region is also invisible to the human eye, requiring the use of a coaxial pilot beam for this laser. The tissue interaction of this laser is dominated by its scattering through the tissue (9,15). The surgical application is enhanced by the laser's ability to be transmitted through a fiberoptic cable. It also has the ability to penetrate tissue and water deeper than the CO_2 laser, resulting in its coagulating properties. This property has made it useful in the treatment of vascular tumors. The beam is applied to the vascular tumor, coagulating and softening the tumor, so that it can be removed by mechanical suction. Little accumulated experience in the use of this type of laser in glioma surgery has been reported at this time.

Fasano (18–20) has developed a combined Nd:YAG and CO_2 laser unit that is attached to an operating microscope. This combination is used to first coagulate and devascularize the tumor with the Nd:YAG laser, then vaporize the tissue with the CO_2 laser. Fasano has reported the successful use of this combination in resecting spinal cord tumors.

Argon Laser

The argon laser falls into the visible spectrum of light at 0.488 to 0.514 μm, thus, not requiring a coaxial pilot beam for aiming. This laser also may be transmitted through a fiberoptic light cable or aimed via attachment to the microscope. This is a low-energy beam that is most useful for coagulating tissue, because the laser's action is dominated by its interaction with pigmented (red) tissue, being preferentially absorbed by hemoglobin-containing cells. Vaporization takes substantially more time with this laser as compared to the CO_2 laser. The argon laser has been reported to be used in the treatment of vascular malformations (21), acoustic neuromas (22), hemangioblastomas (21), and to make dorsal root entry zone lesions (21). This tool has not been reported to be of particular usefulness in the surgery of gliomas.

Potassium Titanyl Phosphate (KTP) Laser

The KTP laser has a wavelength of 0.532 μm. The laser beam is delivered through a fiberoptic cable that may be handheld or attached to the operating microscope. The laser may also be used through the neuroendoscope. The KTP laser has been found to be effective in coagulating and vaporizing tumor tissues (15). The extinction length in blood is 0.05 mm, which is near that of the argon laser (0.2 mm) but substantially less than the Nd:YAG laser (7.6 mm) (15). The wavelength of the KTP laser is near that of the argon laser, so the tissue effects would be predicted to be similar. The KTP laser acts on both pigmented and nonpigmented tissues.

Preliminary experience with gliomas has been reported by Gamache and Patterson (15) in the treatment of seven patients. They found this system to be more effective than the CO_2 laser at debulking masses via vaporization because of its greater ability to control blood loss through coagulation of the larger blood vessels. As this laser is more widely tested, more data should become available for the treatment of gliomas. The KTP laser is currently being most often used in endoscopic applications.

SURGICAL LOCALIZERS

The utility of intraoperative localization lies in surgical planning, sparing critical functional cortex and deep structures, and maximizing resection of tumor. The ideal system provides real-time information regarding a target volume of tissue. The systems differ from preoperative localization devices and techniques in their ability to provide dynamic output as the procedure progresses. The systems are rapidly evolving, and their utilization by an ever-increasing number of neurosurgeons is leading to an explosion in technologic improvements.

Frame-Based and Frameless Stereotaxy

Stereotactic methods are crucial for resecting or debulking gliomas that are in deep-seated areas of the brain. Applications are being expanded to increase surgical economy by limiting the size of openings and disruption of adjacent tissues. These methods allow tumor exposure with superb accuracy. The majority of stereotactic methods that are currently available, however, do not provide information in real time. Most techniques rely on preoperative imaging studies as a basis for determining specific coordinates in three-dimensional space, being largely unable to allow adjustment during the operation. Thus, the changes in spatial positioning of structures and lesions that naturally occur as a consequence of shifting fluid and brain matter during craniotomy are not compensated for by most techniques. This fact must be kept in mind when using these methods, allowing for some inaccuracies of localization during the procedure. Currently, magnetic resonance scanners have been developed that exist within the operating room environment and do provide real-time imaging information. Portable computed tomography (CT) scanners are also being used to rapidly update information during stereotactic procedures.

Frame-based stereotactic methods are currently in widespread utilization for the surgery of deep-seated brain lesions. There are a number of systems, the descriptions of which fall outside the scope of this chapter. All methods rely on preoperative imaging, either CT or magnetic resonance imaging (MRI), to generate a set of specific spatial coordinates that describe the intracranial volume. CT and MRI have been demonstrated by Kondziolka (23) to be of equal value in preoperative targeting accuracy. Novel methods of adding functional information to the targeting sequence of the procedure are under development, and include positron emission tomography (PET), magnetoencephalography, and functional MRI (24–32). These methods are adequate for localization of the tumor mass and operative planning. With respect to guiding the resection, however, the absence of real-time information is a relative limiting factor.

Kelly (33,34) is credited with the development of a system designed to define a predetermined volume of tissue in stereotactic space and resect this volume through a limited cranial opening. He has used this system to resect various types of tumors, both intracerebral and intraventricular. The main disadvantage is the lack of real-time information. Especially if used within the ventricular space, this method may offer no advantage over more traditional approaches once cerebrospinal fluid (CSF) is drained from the ventricle or a retractor blade moves adjacent tissues. The system has been used with reportedly good results in the partial resection of deep-seated gliomas.

Frameless stereotactic methods have been recently introduced that are aimed at alleviating the steps involved with image acquisition using an attached head frame as an immediate part of the operative procedure. Roberts et al. (35) were the first to use such a system, which is based on the sonic stereometric principle. This system uses spark-gap generators to produce an ultrasonic frequency signal that is received by a receiver panel mounted above the microscope. These signals are converted into spatial information regarding the relationship of the microscope to the patient's head. The three-dimensional information from the preoperative CT or MRI scans is then spatially registered with the operating microscope. Outlines of tumor margin are directed via a beam splitter back through the microscope to be superimposed on the operative field. This provides the surgeon with a comparison between the actual tissue appearance and the boundaries of enhancement, or other imaging characteristic, as seen on preoperative studies. This arrangement, although demonstrated to be reasonably accurate, does not compensate for gross intraoperative shifts of the intracranial contents.

The focus of other frameless stereotactic systems has been on an articulated arm design that acts as a pointer, called a "neuronavigator." Similar systems have been under simultaneous development since the mid 1980s (36–39). Watanabe et al. (38,39) first described the use of a six-joint sensing arm that is attached to the Mayfield pin headrest. This system is capable of displaying the location of the tip of the articulated arm in relation to the preoperative CT scan. Fiducial markers are placed at three points on the patient's head that serve to synchronize the CT image and the neuronavigator. The pointer can be used to help locate the optimal area for craniotomy, as well as its value once inside the cerebrum to locate structures. The system is also capable of interacting with other imaging modalities, making it useful in locating blood vessels using angiograms and MRI scans. Watanabe et al. have reported this instrument's use in the treatment of 35 patients with gliomas. The performance of the neuronavigator itself has been the focus of communication; therefore, the efficacy with regard to patient outcome has not been analyzed.

The question of real-time information has been addressed by this system in the form of combination with ultrasound imaging and with transcranial Doppler flowmetry (TCD). An ultrasound probe may be attached to the tip of the pointer, allowing comparison of the echographic and CT images. This has helped in terms of compensation for shifting of intracranial structures due to craniotomy. The addition of TCD helps to locate intracranial vessels that are not well demonstrated on the preoperative CT images. Localization of a vessel segment in this way has demonstrated an accuracy of within 2 mm (39). Similar methods are currently under development utilizing intraoperative CT scanning to update information, compensating for shifts in the brain. A more elaborate way to provide real-time information is the utilization of one of the currently available interventional MRI units. This is a solution that is effective at providing precise information, but at great expense.

The ISG Viewing Wand System (ISG Technologies, Mississauga, Ontario, Canada) is a Food and Drug Administration (FDA)-approved device that also makes use of an articulated arm system (36). This arrangement includes the articulated arm, acting as a three-dimensional digitizer, and a sophisticated computer graphics workstation. The images in three-dimension may by represented in several different ways to give a comprehensive display of the involved anatomy. This system also relies on preoperative imaging; however, external fiducial markers are not necessary. Rather, the computer takes reproducible anatomic points such as the eyes and nose to process targeting information. The average error of the system in testing has fallen between 1.5 to 2.5 mm (36). A component of real-time imaging is again provided by combining an ultrasound probe with the tip of the viewing wand. Various instruments can be introduced, such as an endoscope, through modified tips of the articulated arm.

Koivukangas et al. (37) have introduced a similar articulated arm system. However, this system makes use of ultrasound in a routine arrangement to make real-time confirmations and comparisons between the open intracranial and the preoperatively digitized intracranial environments. This system provides an improved sense of real-time information. The articulated arm can also be fitted with various types of adapters at the end of the probe to attach various instruments.

There are a number of stereotactic pointers that are cur-

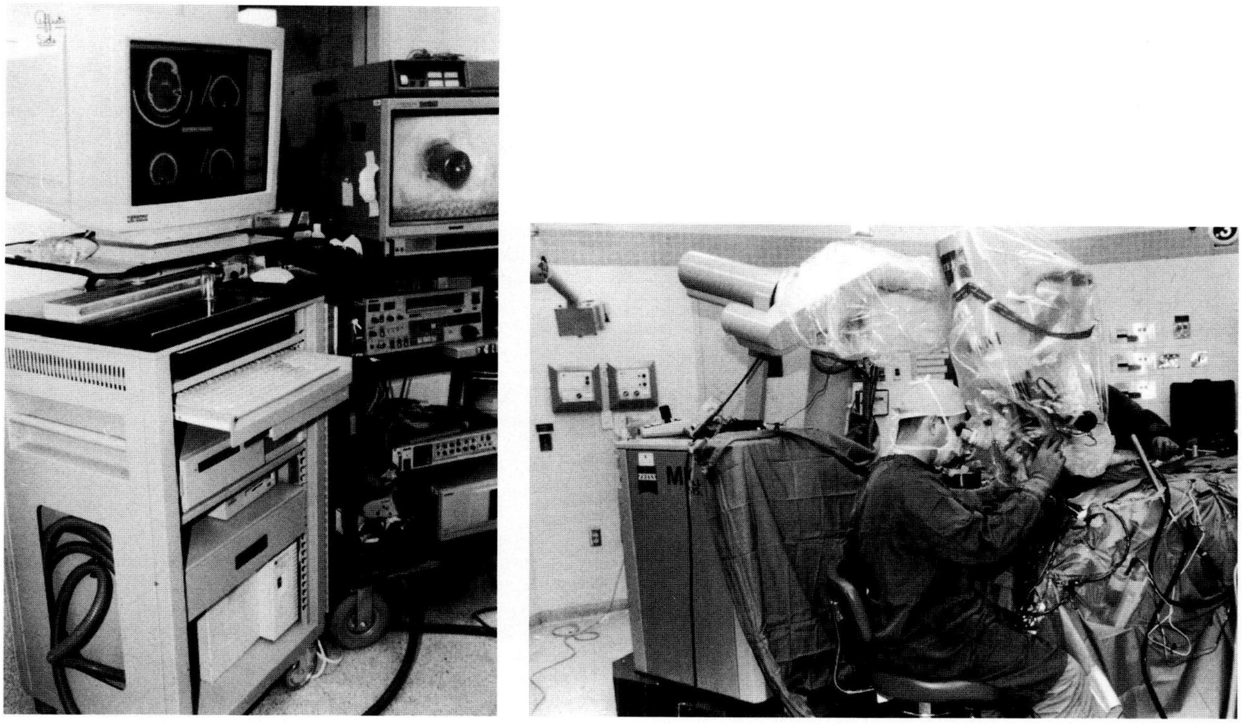

A B

FIG. 4-1. A: Computer workstation for frameless stereotactic navigation system. **B:** Zeiss MKM microscope.

rently in various stages of development and commercially available. The movement in development has been away from the instruments requiring any type of attachment. Systems now exist that are completely free of cables or other attachment to the system. Light-emitting diodes or reflective spheres arranged in patterns are used for recognition by receiving systems linked to the computer. This new direction provides greater freedom of movement and instrument selection.

Zeiss has produced the MKM model microscope, which has stereotactic capability, taking away the need for such a robotic or peripheral, passive, pointing device (Fig. 4-1). The principle of operation is much the same as the neuronavigators, with the necessary preoperative acquisition of imaging data using fiducial markers placed on the patient's head. The computer in communication with the microscope sends a signal that translates into a correction in the trajectory of the microscope to stay fixed upon any preselected target within the intracranial volume. Thus the microscope acts as its own navigator, always keeping the surgeon directed toward the target volume along a selected trajectory, no matter how the surgeon adjusts the microscope. This concept essentially renders the surgical microscope as a mechanical arm with a pointer. The pointer itself is a virtual probe. Other microscope companies have produced similar systems that take advantage of this technology. All use a "heads-up" display by which the surgeon is delivered information. This may be an outline of the target at the depth of focus, imaging studies, monitor tracings, and the like. With current optical technology, virtually any image can be superimposed or transmitted through the eyepieces along with the image of the operative field.

SUMMARY

Peculiarities of intracranial microsurgery in contrast to other disciplines have led to the development of several specialized categories of neurosurgical instrumentation. Microneurosurgery requires that the head be held perfectly still in position, thus the advent of head frames for this purpose. Brain retraction for adequate exposure and working space is also necessary in the majority of neurosurgical procedures. Special self-retaining retractor systems have been developed that are designed to be unobtrusive to the surgeon and safe when used properly. These two major systems are peculiar to neurosurgery and must be accounted for in combined endeavors with other specialists.

A principle of intracranial tumor surgery is removal of the mass with minimal manipulation of surrounding structures. To meet this end, various tumor removal devices have been developed, including the ultrasonic aspirator and laser. Surgical localizing devices are an important class of devices that serve to meet this goal. At the present time these devices consist mainly of frameless stereotactic systems. These systems help to accurately localize cranial structures from the surface to the deeper regions, helping to avoid unnecessary adjacent tissue manipulation. Rapid advancements are ongoing in this field, as is evaluation of the efficacy and benefits of such systems.

REFERENCES

1. Wirth FP. High speed drills. In: Wilkins RH, Rengachary SS, eds. *Neurosurgery update I: diagnosis, operative technique, and neurooncology*. New York: McGraw-Hill, 1990:197–200.
2. Epstein F. The cavitron ultrasonic aspirator in tumor surgery. *Clin Neurosurg* 1984;31:497.
3. Epstein F. Ultrasonic dissection. In: Wilkins RH, Rengachery SS, eds. *Neurosurgery*. New York: McGraw-Hill, 1985:476.
4. Fasano VA: Ultrasonic aspiration in neurosurgery. In: Fasano VA, ed. *Advanced intraoperative technologies in neurosurgery*. Vienna: Springer-Verlag, 1986:257.
5. Flamm ES, Ransohoff J, Wuchinich D, et al. Preliminary experience with ultrasonic aspiration in neurosurgery. *Neurosurgery* 1978;2:240.
6. Brock M, Ingwersen I, Roggendorf W. Ultrasonic aspiration in neurosurgery. *Neurosurg Rev* 1984;7:173.
7. Day JD, Fukushima T. Suction control of ultrasonic aspirators [Letter]. *J Neurosurg* 1993;78:688.
8. Hecht J, Teresi D. *Laser: super tool of the 1980s*. New York: Ticknor & Fields, 1982.
9. Tew JM, Tobler WD. The laser: history, biophysics, and neurosurgical applications. *Clin Neurosurg* 1984;31:506–549.
10. Fine S, Klein E, Novak W, et al. Interaction of laser irradiation with biological systems. *Fed Proc* 1965 (suppl 14)24:S35–S47.
11. Fox JL, Hayes JR, Stein MN, et al. Experimental cranial and vascular studies of the effects of pulsed and continuous wave laser radiation. *J Neurosurg* 1967;27:126–137.
12. Liss L, Roppel R. Histopathology of laser produced lesions in cat brains. *Neurology* 1966;16:783–790.
13. Rosomoff JL, Carroll F. Reaction of neoplasms and brain to laser. *Arch Neurol* 1966;14:143–148.
14. Stellar S. The carbon dioxide surgical laser in neurological surgery, decubitus ulcers, and burns. *Lasers Surg Med* 1980;1:15–33.
15. Gamache FW, Patterson RH. The use of the potassium titanyl phosphate (KTP) laser in neurosurgery. *Neurosurgery* 1990;26:1010–1014.
16. Kelly PJ, Goerss SJ, Kall BA. Evolution of contemporary instrumentation for computer-assisted stereotactic surgery. *Surg Neurol* 1988;30:204.
17. Kelly PJ. The stereotactic CO_2 laser: instrumentation, methodology, and clinical results. In: Fasano VA, ed. *Advanced intraoperative technologies in neurosurgery*. Vienna: Springer-Verlag, 1986:162.
18. Fasano VA. Laser neurosurgical techniques. In: Fasano VA, ed. *Advanced intraoperative technologies in neurosurgery*. Vienna: Springer-Verlag, 1986:107.
19. Fasano VA. Laser physics. In: Fasano VA, ed. *Advanced intraoperative technologies in neurosurgery*. Vienna: Springer-Verlag, 1986:53.
20. Fasano VA. Principles of laser surgery. In: Fasano VA, ed. *Advanced intraoperative technologies in neurosurgery*. Vienna: Springer-Verlag, 1986:97.
21. Edwards MSB, Boggan JE, Fuller TA. The laser in neurological surgery. *J Neurosurg* 1983;59:555–566.
22. Glasscock ME, Jackson CG, Whitaker SR. The argon laser in acoustic tumor surgery. *Laryngoscope* 1981;71:1405–1416.
23. Kondziolka D, Dempsey PK, Lunsford LD, et al. A comparison between magnetic resonance imaging and computed tomography for stereotactic coordinate determination. *Neurosurgery* 1992;30:402.
24. Barnett GH, Kormos DW, Steiner CP, Weisenberger J. Use of a frameless, armless stereotactic wand for brain tumor localization with two-dimensional and three-dimensional neuroimaging. *Neurosurgery* 1993;33:674–678.
25. Gallen CC, Sobel DF, Waltz T, et al. Noninvasive presurgical neuromagnetic mapping of somatosensory cortex. *Neurosurgery* 1993;33:260.
26. Hu X, Tan KK, Levin DN. Three dimensional magnetic resonance images of the brain: application to neurosurgical planning. *J Neurosurg* 1990;72:433.
27. Kamada K, Takeuchi F, Kurichi S, et al. Functional neurosurgical simulation with brain surface magnetic images and magnetoencephalography. *Neurosurgery* 1993;33:269.
28. Kwong KK, Belliveau JW, Chesler DA, et al. Dynamic magnetic resonance imaging of juman brain activity during primary sensory stimulation. *Proc Natl Acad Sci USA* 1992;89:5675.
29. Levivier M, Goldman S, Bidaut LM, et al. Positron emission tomography-guided stereotactic brain biopsy. *Neurosurgery* 1992;31:792.
30. Pellizzari CA, Chen GTY, Spelbring DR, et al. Accurate three-dimensional registration of CT, PET, and/or MR images of the brain. *J Comput Assist Tomogr* 1989;13:20.
31. Tan KK, Grzeszczuk R, Levin DN, et al. A frameless stereotactic approach to neurosurgical planning based on retrospective patient-image registration: technical note. *J Neurosurg* 1993;79:296.
32. Kim SG, Ashe J, Hendrich, et al. Functional magnetic resonance imaging of motor cortex: hemispheric asymmetry and handedness. *Science* 1993;261:615.
33. Kelly PJ, Kall BA, Goerss S, et al. Computer-assisted stereotaxic laser resection of intra-axial brain neoplasms. *J Neurosurg* 1986;64:427–439.
34. Kelly PJ. Stereotactic imaging, surgical planning and computer-assisted resection of intracranial lesions: methods and results. In: Symon L, ed. *Advances and technical standards in neurosurgery*, vol 18. 1991:77.
35. Roberts DW, Strohbehn JW, Hatch J, Murray W, Kettenberger H. A frameless stereotaxic integration of computerized tomographic imaging and the operating microscope. *J Neurosurg* 1986;65:545–549.
36. Drake JM, Rutka JT, Hoffman HJ. ISG viewing wand system. *Neurosurgery* 1994;34:1094–1097.
37. Koivukangas J, Louhisalmi Y, Alakuijala J, et al. Ultrasound-controlled neuronavigator-guided brain surgery. *J Neurosurg* 1993;79:36.
38. Watanabe E, Mayamagi Y, Ksougi Y, Manaka S, Takakura K. Open surgery assisted by neuronavigator, a stereotactic, articulated, sensitive arm. *Neurosurgery* 1991;28:792–800.
39. Watanabe ET, Watanabe S, Manaka S, Mayanago Y, Takakura K. Three-dimensional digitizer (Neuronavigator): new equipment for CT-guided stereotaxic surgery. *Surg Neurol* 1987;27:543–547.

Neurosurgical Issues in Otolaryngology: Principles and Practice of Collaboration,
edited by Moisés A. Arriaga and J. Diaz Day.
Lippincott Williams & Wilkins, Philadelphia © 1999.

CHAPTER 5

Monitoring: Facial Nerve and Hearing

Fred F. Telischi, Philip A. Bird, Annelle V. Hodges, and Ozcan Ozdamar

The current era of successful skull base surgery owes no small debt to the implementation of intraoperative cranial nerve monitoring. The ability to assess functional changes in structures at risk during these procedures provides an inestimable advantage for improved outcomes. This chapter focuses on intraoperative monitoring of facial and auditory function. Facial nerve monitoring has reached a level of consistency that makes it a state-of-the-art adjunct to lateral and posterior skull base approaches. Techniques for monitoring auditory function continue to evolve.

FACIAL NERVE MONITORING

Damage to the facial nerve may have devastating effects on a patient from a cosmetic, functional, and psychological perspective. In surgery for cerebellopontine angle (CPA) tumors, the introduction of microscopic techniques has dramatically improved facial nerve preservation rates. Subsequent introduction of facial nerve monitoring has further improved functional outcomes, especially in medium and large tumors.

One of the most impressive displays of the utility of facial nerve monitoring came in the report by Leonetti et al. (1). They had previously described a relatively atraumatic technique of facial nerve transposition in the approach to the jugular bulb region, which resulted in normal or near-normal immediate facial nerve function in 70% of patients (2). Following the introduction of facial nerve monitoring, 93% of patients had immediate normal or near-normal facial function postoperatively. The success of facial nerve monitoring in skull base surgery has led to the use of the same techniques to monitor other cranial nerves during a variety of head and neck procedures.

History

The first description of facial nerve monitoring was given by Krause (3) in 1912. He described unipolar faradic stimulation of the facial nerve during cochlear nerve section for tinnitus. Twitching of the ipsilateral facial muscles during stimulation helped the surgeon preserve the facial nerve, and the patient had transient facial weakness postoperatively.

Much of the other early literature describing facial nerve monitoring pertained to the preservation of anatomic neural integrity during acoustic neuroma surgery. Some authors described tumor removal under local anesthesia with a designated observer watching the patient's face for movement (4). Givre and Olivecrona (5) in 1949 used faradic stimulation both in identification of the nerve and to confirm its integrity at the end of the procedure.

In the 1960s, dedicated facial nerve monitoring systems were developed. The Hilger stimulator was used principally in the assessment of facial paralysis but was also used during surgery (6). The response to electrical stimulation still involved observation of the face. Jako (7) described a photoelectric sensing device that responded to changes in light transmission through the cheek during facial twitching. The device included production of an audible signal with facial movement. Parsons used electromyography (EMG) monitoring with recording of the EMG response on an oscilloscope (8).

Further developments in facial nerve monitoring occurred during the 1970s and 1980s. The use of EMG monitoring in CPA surgery was described by Delgado et al. (9). The response to nerve stimulation was photographed with a Polaroid camera to compare responses before, during, and after tumor dissection. Sugita and Kobayashi (10) used accelerometers attached to the orbicularis oris and orbicularis oculi

F. F. Telischi: University of Miami School of Medicine, Miami, Florida 33101.

P. A. Bird: Visiting Consultant Otolaryngologist, Christchurch Hospital, Merivale, Christchurch, New Zealand.

A. V. Hodges: Department of Otolaryngology, University of Miami School of Medicine, Miami, Florida 33101.

O. Ozdamar: Department of Biomedical Engineering, University of Miami, Coral Gables, Florida 33124.

muscles. Facial movements were converted to sound via the accelerometers, an amplifier and a speaker. Møller and Jannetta (11) combined the specificity of EMG recording with the advantage of acoustic feedback to the surgeon. The response to stimulation was displayed on an oscilloscope, amplified and made audible using a loudspeaker. Prass and Lüders (12) refined the interpretation of EMG patterns and correlated these with surgical conditions. The motion-detector device described by Jako was modified by Silverstein et al. (13), who advocated its use in a number of otologic and neuro-otologic procedures (14).

Physiology of Electromyographic Facial Nerve Monitoring

Stimulation of a motor nerve by electrical, mechanical, or thermal means results in depolarization of the nerve. If the stimulus is sufficient to reach threshold, voltage-sensitive sodium channels open, causing an action potential. The action potential then travels along the axon to the neuromuscular junction, resulting in the release of acetylcholine and subsequent depolarization of the target muscle. A wave of depolarization then spreads over the muscle fibers causing a brief muscle contraction. Facial nerve monitoring using EMG measures the electrical activity in the target muscle following nerve stimulation, as opposed to motion sensor devices that detect movement of the muscle.

A compound muscle action potential (CMAP) is the composite electrical activity within the target muscle resulting from synchronous activation of a group of motor neurons within a nerve bundle. EMG monitoring essentially measures this electrical activity in the portion of the muscle near the recording electrodes and converts the electrical activity to sound via a loudspeaker with or without visual oscilloscope display. Measuring evoked EMG activity from the muscle, rather than the nerve itself, takes advantage of the considerable magnification that takes place at the neuromuscular junction (15).

Recorded CMAPs vary in size with the density and number of contributing motor units (15). In addition, the oscilloscopic waveform morphology may vary with the degree of synchrony among contributing motor units. Synchronous activity initiated by electrical stimulation produces a biphasic and well-defined waveform. Asynchronous activity, as is generally produced by mechanical stimulation, produces a polyphasic pattern. When these response patterns are converted to sound, electrical stimulation results in well-defined pulsed sounds, whereas mechanical stimulation yields a rough, almost scratchy, burst of acoustic energy (12). The practical applications of these observations are discussed below.

Equipment and Setup for Facial Nerve Monitoring

Electrodes for EMG Monitoring

Needle electrodes are most commonly used for facial nerve monitoring. They have the advantages of ease of use, low impedance, and stability (less likely to be displaced than surface disks or cups). Electroencephalogram (EEG)-type electrodes are available in both reusable and disposable forms. Hook-wire electrodes may also be used in facial nerve monitoring, but are especially useful to record activity from sites where the mobility of the tissues causes problems for conventional needle electrodes, such as the tongue during hypoglossal nerve monitoring.

Electrode Placement

Most protocols currently use two channels for monitoring activity in two distinct muscle groups. The orbicularis oris and orbicularis oculi muscles are popular choices. Monitoring more than one muscle provides additional sensitivity and redundancy should one electrode fail (16). Since the various muscle groups exhibit different spontaneous activity, usually at least one group will be quiet enough to allow reliable monitoring. Typically, the orbicularis oris muscle is more active than orbicularis oculi when the facial nerve is irritable (16). It is also important to monitor muscle activity from both upper and lower divisions since isolated peripheral nerve branches may be injured during some skull base approaches.

For two-channel bipolar recording, a typical sensing montage includes a pair of electrodes in the orbicularis oculi approximately 1 cm apart (channel 1) and another pair in the orbicularis oris (channel 2) (Fig. 5-1). The ground electrode is placed in the forehead (ground) and the anode for

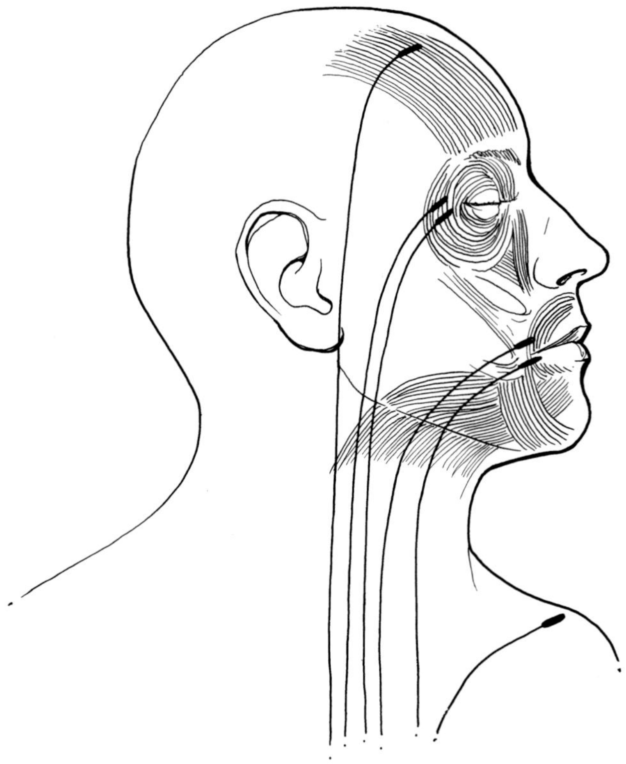

FIG. 5-1. Typical configuration for two channel bipolar facial nerve monitoring. Recording electrodes are placed in two distinct facial muscle groups for sensitivity and redundancy. Ground and reference electrodes are included.

the monopolar nerve stimulator is inserted at the ipsilateral shoulder. The electrodes are secured to the skin with tape and the wires of each of the pairs of electrodes are twisted together to reduce electrical artifact (16). Covering the ipsilateral hemiface with a clear adhesive drape further secures the electrodes and enables observation of the face for movement during electrocautery interference. The connections are checked by tapping the electrodes and observing an audible and oscilloscopic response. This mechanical CMAP results in a characteristic sound from the monitor. A second check, when available, involves testing the impedance of the inserted electrodes. Individual impedance values should be less than 5 kilo-ohm (KΩ) to avoid electromagnetic interference from other devices in the operating room. Furthermore, current instrumentation utilizes differential amplification techniques that improve signal-to-noise ratio optimally when impedance imbalance is less than 1 KΩ between the electrode pairs. Ideally, the imbalance to impedance ratio should be less than 10%.

Facial Nerve Monitoring Systems

A number of facial nerve monitoring systems are available commercially. These include the Nerve Integrity Monitor (Xomed Inc., Jacksonville, FL), Neurosign 100 (Smith and Nephew Richards Inc., Memphis, TN), Brackmann II (WR Medical Electronics Co., Stillwater, MN), and the NLI (Grass Instrument Co., Quincy, MA). All of these devices utilize EMG. The Silverstein Facial Nerve Monitor (WR Medical Electronics Co., Stillwater, MN) is an example of a motion detector device. Larger systems can monitor activity from multiple sources, including EMG and evoked potentials. Some monitoring teams have developed custom systems utilizing existing neurophysiologic electromyographic instruments.

Nerve Stimulation

Most facial nerve monitors utilize a constant current source for monopolar stimulation whereby changes in impedance are compensated for by changes in voltage so that electrical flow remains essentially constant. A typical setting for monopolar stimulation is 100-μsec pulses at a rate of four per second with a constant current of between 0.05 and 0.5 mA (see Safety Issues, below). When stimulating in the CPA, cerebrospinal fluid (CSF) can cause current shunting and consequently false-negative responses. To solve this problem, Møller and Jannetta (11) described a constant voltage system. Shunting may also be overcome by the use of a flush-tip probe (17).

Bipolar stimulators are used to limit the area of application of the stimulating current. They reduce false-positive responses caused by current spread from adjacent nerves to the facial nerve and improve the ability to distinguish a thinned facial nerve from surrounding soft tissues. Lower currents are generally needed when using bipolar stimulation.

In addition to stimulation probes, dissection instruments have been designed to allow monopolar monitoring dissection of tumor simultaneously (18). Because of the need for an adequate cutting edge, a variable part of these instruments is left uninsulated. This increases the risk of current shunting and of false-negative stimulation error (19). Insulated self-retaining retractors also have been designed to avoid static discharge interference that may be caused when two metal instruments come into contact (18).

Safety Issues

Stimulating the Nerve

Considerable experience with facial nerve monitoring suggests that the parameters of safe nerve stimulation are 100- to 250-μsec pulses with a range of 0.05 to 0.5 mA (16). Most normal facial nerves should stimulate with direct contact of the probe using a 100-μsec pulse of 0.05 mA. Settings of 0.05 to 0.1 mA are recommended when working close to the nerve. Further from the nerve, currents of 0.2 to 0.3 mA may be used. Somewhat higher settings may be required when the nerve is covered by bone, connective tissue, or granulation tissue.

Adequate Isolation and Patient Grounding

It is crucial that patients be adequately grounded to the monopolar electrocautery unit to permit safe current return. If this is not achieved, the electrocautery current may find a route through the nerve monitoring electrodes, causing severe burns. All patient connections must be optically and/or electrically isolated to prevent patient injury (15). This isolation separates the patient from power line voltages and currents. Many monitoring devices achieve this using battery power.

Pulses, Bursts, and Trains: Interpreting Responses

Evoked EMG activity measured by facial nerve monitoring may be divided into two types: repetitive (trains) and nonrepetitive (bursts) (16). Nonrepetitive responses occur in close temporal association with the stimulus and allow real-time feedback regarding the location and integrity of the nerve. As previously discussed, the nature of the nonrepetitive response and the relationship to the initiator of that response are critical. Electrical stimulation typically produces a biphasic oscilloscopic pattern and a series of precisely timed pulsed sounds via the loudspeaker when delivered via the stimulator probe (12). Mechanical stimulation produces a single polyphasic response and a burst sound (Fig. 5-2A). The initial burst response may occur as an isolated event or may be followed by a variable amount of repetitive activity depending on the stimulus.

Burst activity should be interpreted in the context of operative events. During the course of surgery, many burst poten-

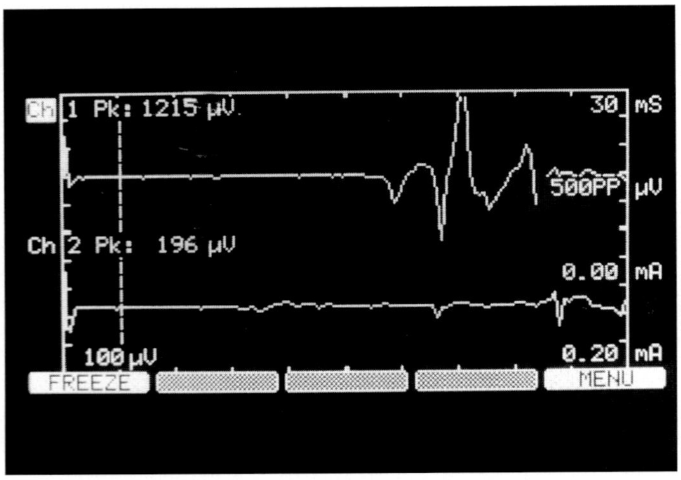

A

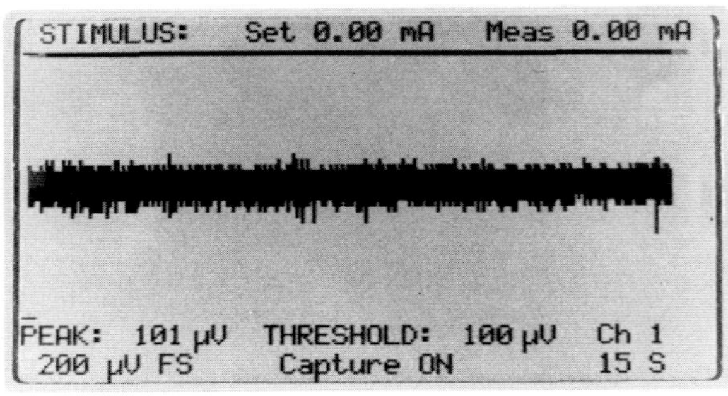

B

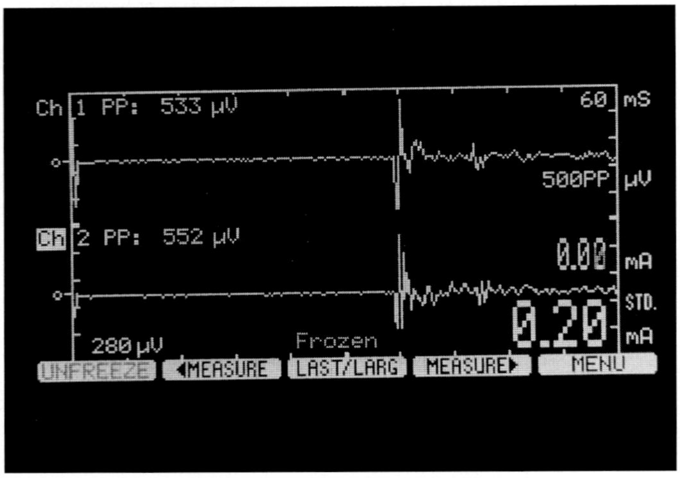

C

FIG. 5-2. Oscilloscopic representation of evoked EMG recordings. **A:** Burst response. **B:** Train response. **C:** Burst response with ongoing activity suggesting nerve irritation. (Courtesy of Xomed Inc., Jacksonville, FL.)

tials may be observed and are usually not associated with significant trauma to the nerve. Burst activity occurring with gentle manipulation suggests a healthy nerve. Very similar responses may be obtained, however, when drilling close to or after complete transection of the nerve. Lack of burst activity during dissection may be associated with minor manipulation of a healthy nerve, significant manipulation of an already injured nerve, or a problem with the monitoring connections and instruments (Fig. 5-2B). Electrically stimulating the nerve at this point will verify the integrity of the nerve.

Episodes of repetitive electromyographic activity, known as trains, may occur several seconds to minutes after the stimulus, making it difficult to identify the initiating factor or to modify dissection technique (12). Trains are caused by prolonged depolarization of the nerve beyond its threshold for developing an action potential. Subsequent repetitive firing continues until the nerve repolarizes or can no longer sustain the repetitive activation (16). The most common initiating factor is traction on the nerve. Trains may indicate significant trauma has occurred, though this is not always the case. Changes in temperature around the nerve may also precipitate train activity. When caused by cool irrigating fluid, the spontaneous activity will usually subside with warming. When a train pattern develops after laser application or cautery, however, thermal damage should be suspected. Elevated stimulation thresholds after repetitive nerve activity suggest significant injury.

Anesthetic Issues

When facial nerve monitoring is employed, neuromuscular blocking agents should not be employed following induction of anesthesia. There is some evidence to suggest that facial musculature is more resistant than other muscles to neuromuscular blockade with paralyzing agents (20,21). Blair et al. (21), using a rabbit model, found that facial EMG was measurable even with a 75% receptor blockade. Despite this evidence, there remain concerns that the monitoring system will lose the ability to detect subtle responses to mechanical stimulation with these agents (19). On occasion, paralysis may be necessary because of hemodynamic instability. When this is the case, close communication between the anesthesiologist and the surgeon is important. Constant infusion of paralytic medication is preferred over bolus injections to reduce fluctuation in neuromuscular function (16).

Antidromic facial nerve monitoring (see below) has the advantage that it may be undertaken with full paralysis.

Spontaneous repetitive responses may be observed when the level of anesthesia becomes inadequate and the facial muscles contract. This activity is commonly both the first indication that the patient is awakening and the prelude to larger movements such as coughing (''bucking'' against the endotrachial tube).

Indications for Facial Nerve Monitoring

Facial nerve monitoring should never replace anatomic knowledge, technical skill, and sound clinical judgment. It does appear to be beneficial during procedures that carry a higher risk for facial nerve injury, such as those involving the internal auditory canal (IAC)/CPA and lateral skull base. Otologic procedures where the nerve is at risk include cochlear implantation, revision tympanomastoidectomy, and repair of external auditory canal bony stenosis.

Advocates for routine monitoring of all otologic and neuro-otologic surgery emphasize that abnormalities in facial nerve anatomy and unusually severe temporal bone pathology may not be identifiable preoperatively (13). Routine use of the monitor also enables the surgical team to develop expertise with the techniques and response patterns. Routine monitoring may also be of benefit in training centers where some portions of operations are performed by less experienced surgeons (22).

Practical Application in Surgery

Although the following description pertains to the use of facial nerve monitoring during acoustic neuroma surgery, the principles are the same for other procedures. Monitoring has three primary uses: locating the nerve, avoiding trauma, and assessing nerve integrity (18).

Locating the Facial Nerve

Electrical stimulation is an adjunct to anatomic landmarks in locating the facial nerve. Monopolar stimulation is especially useful for mapping the nerve throughout its course (11). A stronger stimulus is used to confirm that the nerve is not in close proximity to an area of tumor to be removed. When the nerve is injured or transected proximal to the site of stimulation, however, a misleading negative response will be obtained when attempting to localize a more distal segment.

Care should be taken when interpreting stimulation results. As previously discussed, both false-positive and false-negative responses may occur. False-positive responses may be obtained from stimulation of the superior vestibular and cochlear nerves due to electrical current dispersion, especially within the IAC where the nerves lie in close proximity to one another. This is most effectively overcome by using bipolar stimulation or a flush-tip monopolar stimulator on the lowest possible setting. False-negative responses are usually related to technical errors such as failure to connect the stimulus probe. A useful method to check the monitoring system is to stimulate the nerve where it is known to be available and intact. If no response can be obtained at that location, then the entire setup should be inspected from the electrode placements in the facial muscles to the recording instrument. Once a reliable response is elicited from the nerve, then stimulation may be resumed with confidence. To provide a redundant system check, some newer-generation monitors emit a characteristic sound when the stimulating probe is in good contact with the patient's tissues but no facial nerve activity is present. With attention to detail, most false responses can be avoided, improving the sensitivity and specificity of stimulation.

Avoiding Trauma

Continuous EMG monitoring provides real-time feedback, enabling the surgeon to immediately alter technique when a burst response occurs. The inciting factors for repetitive activity should be sought and corrected. Temporary cessation of dissection and irrigation, or loosening of the retractors, may lessen the ongoing trauma to the nerve. When performing lateral skull base surgery, it is important to maintain monitoring during wound obliteration and closure to avoid trauma to the nerve.

Assessing Nerve Function: Postoperative Prognosis

Although the primary aim of facial nerve monitoring is to prevent iatrogenic nerve injury, it may also be of value in the prognostic assessment of acute injury. The threshold for stimulation has been shown to correlate with postoperative facial nerve function. Using constant current stimulation with a 50-μsec pulse, Selesnick et al. (23) found that when the threshold for facial nerve stimulation at the brainstem was 0.1 mA or lower, 90% of patients exhibited House-Brackmann (HB) grade I (normal) or II (near normal) function at 1 year following CPA surgery. Thresholds of 0.1 to 0.2 mA were associated with grade I or II function in 78% of cases. The amount of energy delivered to the nerve using a 50-μsec pulse of 0.1 mA is equal in magnitude to a 100-μsec pulse of 0.05 mA as delivered by many commercial facial nerve monitors. Silverstein et al. (24), using a 200-μsec pulse, found that at 1 year 95% of patients had HB grade I facial function if the stimulation threshold was 0.1 mA or lower.

Another technique for prognosticating postoperative facial nerve function is to measure the amplitude of the evoked CMAP. Because the size of the CMAP is proportional to the number of muscle fibers stimulated, the position of the needle electrodes must be consistent among patients in order to compare. This may be difficult to achieve (23).

When testing the nerve at the root entry zone of the brainstem to determine threshold at the conclusion of the procedure, it is important to contact the nerve long enough to confirm the precisely timed pulses of electrical stimulation. A single noise could be a mechanically evoked burst, which may give the surgeon a falsely optimistic estimate of nerve function. When damage to the nerve is severe, it may lose the ability to conduct an action potential past the site of the injury. Thus, neuropraxia, axonotmesis, and neuronotmesis may be indistinguishable by monitoring alone (16). Decisions regarding nerve repair or grafting should only be made by direct visual inspection. Monitoring can still be of value in locating the distal segment of an acutely transected nerve. In cases of established injury, following wallerian degeneration, facial nerve monitoring is not helpful unless there are a proportion of axons with neuropraxia rather than more severe injury. For example, facial nerve monitoring has been used to identify the area of maximal constriction of facial nerve fibers during decompression for Bell's palsy (25).

Artifactual Responses

Artifacts (i.e., monitor activity not due to facial nerve stimulation) are relatively common and may cause confusion. Electrocautery obliterates facial nerve responses by saturating the monitor with electrical noise. Some instruments incorporate a muting circuit so that monitoring is discontinued during cautery. Ultrasonic aspirators also cause a large electrical artifact and may trigger a muting circuit. When accurate monitoring cannot be performed, many surgeons engage a member of the team to visually observe or palpate the patient's face. Monopolar cautery may charge the nerve stimulator so that positive responses are obtained when the probe discharges by contacting any soft tissue. Observation of the oscilloscopic display reveals a direct current (DC) shift of the EMG baseline in this situation.

Static discharge may be caused by contact between two metal instruments. This results in a single polyphasic response that can be distinguished on oscilloscopic display from a true burst by its very abrupt onset and short duration. As previously mentioned, the monitor may demonstrate activity reminiscent of a train if there is inadequate anesthesia and facial muscle fasciculations begin. Although true facial EMG activity, these responses are not due to surgical stimulation of the facial nerve.

Antidromic Facial Nerve Monitoring

When a nerve is stimulated, in addition to conduction distally (orthodromic), an action potential is conducted proximally (antidromically). The antidromic electrical activity can be measured and used to assess neural function. A major advantage of this technique, first described by Richmond and Mahla (26), is that it may be performed under neuromuscular blockade. Colletti et al. (27) have been involved with ongoing research into this technique, with some promising results. Their protocol involves bipolar stimulation of the marginal mandibular branch and recording the antidromic potentials via an electrode placed close to the root entry zone of the facial nerve at the brainstem. Antidromic potentials have also been utilized by Møller and Jannetta (28) during microvascular decompression operations for hemifacial spasm. They found that a compressed facial nerve exhibited abnormal antidromic responses whereby stimulation of an upper face muscle gave rise to a burst of EMG activity in the mentalis muscle. Decompression of the facial nerve abolished this ''lateral spread'' phenomenon.

Another use for antidromic potentials was described by Arriaga et al. (29). During middle fossa craniotomy with conventional facial nerve monitoring, antidromic potentials were used to locate the geniculate ganglion. Stimulation of the greater superficial petrosal neurectomy (GSPN) caused facial EMG activity, presumably via antidromic conduction along the parasympathetic fibers with electrical stimulation of adjacent motor nerve fibers in the region of the geniculate ganglion.

Conclusion

Facial nerve monitoring is a well-established and effective means of preventing facial nerve injury during skull base and otologic surgery. Although a number of different techniques and devices may be employed, of prime importance is that the surgical monitoring team fully understand its particular system. Consistent technique and an understanding of the limitations will result in a successful program of facial nerve monitoring.

MONITORING HEARING

Many surgical approaches risk damaging the anatomic structures related to hearing. Modern microsurgical techniques have advanced expectations from ensuring life and major neurologic function to preserving sensory functions such as auditory perception. Dissection within the IAC and CPA places cranial nerve VIII and the internal auditory artery (IAA) at risk. Even painstakingly careful dissection can result in loss of function since damage may not be readily visible even under high magnification. Techniques for providing the surgeon feedback regarding the physiologic status of the auditory system may improve hearing outcome. Monitoring also may result in improved surgical technique by helping identify particular maneuvers that tend to injure auditory structures. Ultimately, the goal of intraoperative monitoring of auditory function is to preserve hearing, not just anatomy.

Hearing depends on the integrity of the peripheral and central auditory structures and their vascular supplies. Conductive hearing losses occur lateral to and at the level of the stapes footplate. Sensory hearing losses involve the cochlea, while neural losses arise from dysfunction of the cochlear nerve, nucleus, and central auditory pathways. Some of the surgical approaches described in other chapters in this book involve removal or reconfiguration of various parts of the temporal bone, including the ossicular chain and cochlea.

Generally, the skull base surgeon knows what effect these procedures will have on a patient's hearing. It is more difficult to predict the effect on hearing of manipulations within the IAC, CPA, and brainstem. A variety of techniques have been applied to the challenge of monitoring the integrity of the auditory system during posterior fossa surgery. The measures reviewed here include standard and rapid auditory brainstem response (ABR), electrocochleography (ECochG), direct eighth nerve compound action potentials, otoacoustic emissions (OAEs), and laser-Doppler cochlear blood flow (CBF).

Indications

Selecting appropriate cases for monitoring involves analysis of preoperative hearing, disease prognosis, and surgical approach. Operations in which monitoring of auditory function has been reported include microvascular decompression to treat hemifacial spasm, trigeminal neuralgia, glossopharyngeal neuralgia (30,31) and disabling positional vertigo (32), vestibular nerve section (33), and removal of acoustic neuromas (ANs) (34–38) and other CPA masses (39). When at risk, hearing should be tested preoperatively at least with pure-tone and speech audiometry. In appropriate candidates, preoperative values are also obtained for the measures to be monitored. Consideration should be given to the impact of hearing loss on the overall postoperative outcome, with particular reference to the disease and quality of life. The probabilities for preserving hearing in both the literature and the surgeon's experience are also important factors.

The likelihood of success for hearing conservation AN removal improves with smaller tumors (40–43). More extensive tumor involvement of the IAC, including erosion of the bony walls and impacting into the fundus of the canal, seems to make hearing preservation less likely (44,45). The prognostic value of preoperative audiometric and vestibular tests remains in doubt. Some authors have reported higher rates of hearing preservation with better preoperative hearing (46,47). In other series, no such relationship could be identified (40,42,45,48). Markedly abnormal ABR with or without intact behavioral thresholds portends low probability of retaining hearing postoperatively (48,49). One report, however, did not find preoperative ABR to be predictive of hearing outcome (50). A reduced vestibular response by preoperative caloric testing with electronystagmography (ENG) suggests involvement of the superior vestibular nerve by tumor since the ENG measures horizontal (lateral) semicircular canal function. A normal caloric test may imply that the tumor arises from the inferior vestibular nerve adjacent to cochlear nerve in the inferior compartment of the IAC. Some studies have found that hearing preservation rates are lower for tumors arising from the inferior vestibular nerve and that this condition can be identified preoperatively with ENG testing (40). In other centers, ENG has not been predictive (49).

The issue of how much residual hearing is worth preserving, however, should be individualized for each patient. It is important to consider the hearing in the opposite ear. The generally accepted limits of serviceable hearing have been 50-dB pure-tone average (PTA) threshold and 50% speech discrimination score (SDS). Patients with auditory sensitivity at or below these levels usually consider the ear to be useless, but a few individuals will want to maintain even that amount of perception. Tumors in only-hearing ears and bilateral tumors warrant special consideration. Worse hearing may indicate a more severe insult of auditory structures by disease and poor prognosis for hearing conservation. Exceptions exist, however, for hearing improvement when, for example, tumor removal alleviates eighth nerve conduction block.

In some cases, preoperative audiometric tests suggest a site of the lesion for the hearing loss. Inappropriately large reduction in SDS with relatively good PTA suggests tumor effect on the eighth nerve or brainstem rather than on the cochlea. Intact OAEs with poor ABR suggests the same. The prognostic value of these interpretations remains unknown.

Another indication for intraoperative monitoring of auditory function is to provide prognostic information about postoperative hearing. Loss of responses during the operation may allow the surgeon greater freedom to more completely resect tumor without further concern of preserving auditory structures. Also, when no hearing is expected postoperatively, preparations can be made sooner to compensate for the situation.

To summarize, hearing preservation rates for surgical extirpation vary inversely with tumor size. There appears to be little reason to monitor hearing during planned total removal of a 4 cm or larger tumor. Conversely, auditory monitoring is ideal when removing smaller tumors or sectioning the vestibular nerve in the face of serviceable hearing. A number of other factors may suggest a better prognosis for hearing preservation, including lack of both tumor extension into the lateral IAC and erosion of bony walls, low behavioral thresholds (i.e., good hearing), normal ABR, and reduced caloric response on ENG. Some methods of monitoring have alternative benefits. For example, measuring the ABR during CPA surgery may also alert the surgical team to potentially catastrophic manipulations of the brainstem. Monitoring auditory function makes sense during attempts at hearing preservation surgery, but becomes irrelevant during destructive procedures such as the translabyrinthine approach to tumor removal.

Pathophysiology of Sensorineural Hearing Loss During Skull Base Surgery

Operating in the IAC/CPA poses two potential mechanisms for hearing loss: interruption of blood flow to the cochlea and cochlear nerve, and injury to neural structures of the auditory pathway (51). The IAA arises from a loop of the anterior inferior cerebellar artery (AICA) to supply the cochlea via the cochlear artery. Though there may be more than one parallel vessel, the usual configuration is that of a single artery coursing in the anterior or anteroinferior aspect of the IAC. There are no collateral or other primary arteries that supply the cochlea. Permanent interruption of the IAA leads to complete and irreversible sensory deafness. Experimental occlusion by pressure or vasospasm lasting more than 4 to 5 minutes causes a variable amount of permanent hearing loss (52). Topical application of a vasodilator has been shown to reverse a sudden deterioration of measured auditory responses (46). Alternatively, mechanical trauma to the cochlear nerve or brainstem may also result in hearing loss. Even using meticulous technique, dissection on or near these structures may cause injury. Retraction of the cerebellum during the early stages of the operation may stretch and damage the eighth nerve, which is particularly vulnerable in the CPA (53). In short, surgeons need an objective measure of hearing preservation since visual confirmation of intact anatomic structures alone is inadequate to ensure postoperative auditory function.

Preoperative Testing

Preoperative evaluation of hearing begins with the history and physical examination. It is important to document not only the presence but also the degree of disability caused by the hearing loss. Retaining binaural hearing is more crucial for some than for others. The risk of further hearing loss from either disease progression or treatment may be the deciding factor in some cases for choosing a treatment modality. Preliminary assessment of hearing acuity may be obtained during the initial visit using tuning fork tests such as the Weber and Rinne. Patients are often referred to the specialist with some type of audiometric evaluation since hearing loss is a common presenting symptom of IAC/CPA pathology.

Objective measurement of hearing begins with behavioral audiometry and speech testing. A standard audiogram displays auditory thresholds at frequencies important to language (500–8,000 Hz). A variety of word-list tests may be administered to corroborate pure-tone threshold averages and quantify speech discrimination ability. Acoustic reflex tests examine the integrity of the seventh and eighth cranial nerve reflex arc. Further testing varies according to behavioral measurements and institutional practices and the type of intraoperative auditory monitoring planned. Patients with profound hearing loss or anacusis discovered on behavioral audiogram need nothing further. Cochlear potentials, ABRs, and OAEs are useful both to further evaluate the integrity of the auditory pathways and to establish a baseline for intraoperative monitoring. It is important to know preoperatively whether the physiologic measures to be monitored are abnormal.

METHODS OF INTRAOPERATIVE AUDITORY MONITORING

General Considerations

Many lateral skull base approaches involve temporal bone dissection. Fluid and bone dust may accumulate in the middle ear and external auditory canal, resulting in a conductive hearing loss (CHL). ABR, ECochG, and direct eighth nerve potentials are delayed in the presence of CHL. Interpeak latencies and waveform configurations, however, remain unchanged (54). OAEs generally cannot be measured in the presence of significant CHL. Whenever possible, the middle ear and external canal should be isolated from manipulation when monitoring auditory function.

The field of intraoperative monitoring of auditory function continues to evolve. One or more of the techniques described below are commonly employed in hearing preservation procedures. Obtaining these neurophysiologic responses in the controlled conditions of the office requires training and experience. Attempting to interpret these signals in the electrically and acoustically hostile environment of the operating room demands professionals highly familiar with the equipment, techniques, and potential problems. Personnel from a range of backgrounds, including physicians from a variety of specialties, audiologists, nurses, and medical technicians, may be enlisted to man the monitoring station, depending on their knowledge and interest. To prevent failure or inaccurate monitoring, only those with experience and proper education should engage in this activity.

Anesthetic Effects

None of the methods for measuring auditory function during surgery should be affected by the use of routine anesthetics, including neuromuscular blockade (55). Even OAEs, which are especially sensitive to changes within the middle ear, appear to be unaffected by the use of inhalation agents that may accumulate and alter middle ear pressure (56). Patient factors such as core temperature, muscle activity, blood pressure, and oxygenation may alter electrophysiologic responses. For example, relatively small decreases in core body temperature to 34.5°C result in delays of ABR waves (57). Similarly, increased muscle activity (e.g., fasciculations in a nonparalyzed patient) or hypotension and hypoxia may interfere with accurate measurements. Therefore, the person monitoring the case should be observant of the patient's vital signs and ever alert to significant changes that may affect auditory responses.

Auditory-Evoked Brainstem Response

The use of the ABR as a method for ongoing assessment of auditory system integrity during posterior fossa surgical procedures has been described in numerous reports since the mid-1980s (58–62). For a number of years, it was the standard by which other methods were compared. In spite of its history, there appears to be no consensus regarding the usefulness of ABR monitoring during hearing preservation operations. Reports such as that of Kveton (63) support the position that ABR monitoring is of little benefit, while other reports such as those by Slavit et al. (64) and Harper et al. (65) present a more positive view. What is often not clear in such studies is whether the actual goal of monitoring is prediction of outcome or modification of surgical technique during the procedure based on the monitoring information. Additionally, these series are often difficult to compare due to differences among researchers on what constitutes a significant change in the ongoing response and in the criteria defining a successful outcome. Such criteria range from an SDS of greater than 40% to a more conservative criterion of 15%, while others regard changes in pure tone averages as the determining factor. Nevertheless, ABR monitoring remains the most commonly used technique for monitoring the peripheral and central auditory pathways during surgical procedures.

Basis of the Response

Ongoing random bioelectric activity from the brain is represented by the EEG, a relatively large and irregular pattern of responses that varies with the patient's state of arousal. Development of signal averaging techniques has enabled the much smaller synchronous electrical activity associated with a sensory stimulation to be extracted from the EEG. All such stimulus-related changes within the EEG are termed evoked-potentials as they are seen only in response to an external stimulus. Much too small to be seen within the ongoing EEG, responses to repeated stimuli presented at regular intervals can be summed, while the random background noise tends to cancel during averaging, thus producing a regular pattern discernible from the EEG. When the stimulus used is auditory, the response is referred to as an auditory-evoked potential.

Auditory-evoked potentials are classified as early, middle, or late, depending on the time poststimulation in which the response occurs. Since effective use of monitoring information requires the fastest indication of change, the most useful responses for monitoring surgical procedures are the earliest of the potentials that occur within the first 10 to 15 msec poststimulation. The ABR includes the earliest of the auditory-evoked potentials. Components prior to and including wave I of the ABR are measured through ECochG, which is discussed below. The ABR is considered a far-field response since it represents activity measured between scalp electrodes that are placed at relatively large distances from the eighth nerve and brainstem generator sites. Far-field recordings have the disadvantage of relatively larger amplitude background electrical activity with which to contend and require more careful recording techniques including signal averaging. The advantages of far-field measurements are accessibility of recording sites and acquisition of responses from a larger number of structures associated with auditory function that may be at risk during surgery.

The ABR response consists of seven peaks, of which the first five are considered more useful diagnostically. Wave I is believed to correspond to the proximal cochlear nerve. Wave II is generated at the cochlear nerve near the brainstem. Waves III to V probably represent contributions of activity from multiple sites in the brainstem including the cochlear nucleus. In normal ears, amplitudes and morphology of component waves vary considerably. Latencies, both absolute and the more important interpeak, are of the greatest diagnostic significance. In pathologic ears, morphology is likely to deteriorate and become even more variable. Amplitude is likely to decrease, especially in the presence of peripheral hearing loss, and latencies may increase based on the location and size of the lesion. Consequently, during monitoring of a previously impaired ear, changes from a well-established baseline are generally of more use than comparison to a norm. Since wave I is less likely to be present in an impaired ear, monitoring decisions may often depend on wave V. Enhancement of the wave I response can be achieved through ECochG recordings. Techniques for recording the ABR and ECochG simultaneously have been described by Hall (66).

The Intraoperative ABR

Selection of testing parameters must be made with the goal of optimizing the recording of the desired response while minimizing the interference inherent in the electrically hostile operating room environment. This must be accomplished rapidly if the information is to be of use to the surgeon. It is difficult to suggest a single protocol since both the surgical suite and the patient present a dynamic situation in which the test environment changes from moment to moment. The most important factor in establishing a monitoring protocol is a competent examiner who is able constantly to assess the testing situation and immediately modify procedures as indicated. Møller (67) listed factors that should be considered by the monitoring team for minimizing time delays in updating data during ABR monitoring. Click stimuli should be present at sufficiently high rates and intensities. Wherever possible, background noise must be eliminated at the source. Finally, state-of-the-art signal processing techniques should be employed to enhance the signal-to-noise ratio and minimize the number of responses averaged to obtain an adequate waveform.

Notwithstanding the above discussion, there are certain recording and stimulus parameters that represent the most effective starting points for intraoperative recordings. Commercial evoked-response recording instruments for the office continue to improve and may be adapted to the operating room. An excellent discussion of these parameters and the rationale behind their selection was delineated by Hall (66). Summarized briefly, the suggested initial stimulus parameters are high-level rarefaction clicks presented at 21.1/sec with the use of ER-3A transducers with TIPtrodes (Etymotic Research Corporation, Elk Grove Village, IL) for signal presentation. As stressed above, these parameters are subject to such changes as differing click polarity and decreased rate whenever necessary to improve the response. Other recommended recording parameters include a 15-msec time window, filter settings of 30 to 3,000 Hz, and acquisition of at least 1,500 samples.

Surface or subdermal needle-recording electrodes transmit responses from the patient to the amplifier. The needle variety seem to be more stable and provide a uniform impedance. Hall (66) suggested initially recording between electrodes placed at the ear (e.g., external auditory canal, lobule, or tragus) and in the midline between the vertex (Cz) and forehead (Fpz). Ground can be located near the recording electrodes at a convenient spot (e.g., ipsilateral shoulder or contralateral forehead).

It is important to keep in mind that none of these parameters is absolute, and that manipulation of one or more may be necessary to maintain an adequate response throughout the procedure. To maximize the amplitude of the response, stimuli may be varied between intensities of 100–120 dB sound pressure level (SPL) and rates of 20 to 50 clicks per second. Repetitive clicks or tone bursts are presented in the test and contralateral ears. Broad-band clicks probably make the better stimulus since they activate more of the cochlea and result in more robust responses. Data from the contralateral ear distinguishes changes in auditory function in the operated ear from patient factors such as decrease in brain temperature.

Interpretation of Results

During posterior fossa surgery, damage is most likely to occur at the cochlea, eighth nerve proper, or its root entry zone at the brainstem (68). Disruption of the cochlear blood supply produces a relatively sudden and complete loss of the ABR. Rapid response by the surgeon to restore the blood supply, if possible, is vital to prevent permanent damage. Other types of insults such as stretching, compression, manipulation, or heat from the drill can affect the eighth nerve and its root entry zone. The ABR responses to these insults are neither as quick nor as easily interpretable as those produced by the loss of blood flow. Further compounding the difficulty is that currently there are no uniform criteria for interpreting the information gained from ABR monitoring during surgery.

Much is dependent on obtaining an optimal preoperative baseline response before entering the operating room and again after induction of anesthesia prior to initiation of the procedure. Criteria for judging that a change has occurred varies from increases in absolute latency of wave V from 0.5 msec (69) to 2.0 msec (70). The strongest change, of course, is the loss of a repeatable wave V after all potential sources of interference have been ruled out. This should be the only basis for recording a change according to Friedman et al. (71). If a clear wave I is present, Hall (66) suggested that either I to III or I to V delays, based on the anatomic area of interest, are both more stable as indicators of actual injury and less affected by external influences. Harper et al. (65) and Slavit et al. (64) used criteria of greater than a 0.1-msec increase in latency or greater than a 50% decrease in amplitude to identify a change in the response. Figure 5-3 demonstrates progressive changes in the ABR during IAC tumor dissection.

Future Directions in ABR Monitoring

Significant progress has been made in response acquisition time and evaluation to speed up the process of obtaining reproducible ABR data. Rapid acquisition of ABRs for intraoperative monitoring can be achieved using two approaches: high stimulus rates and digital signal-enhancing methods. Increasing stimulus repetition rates generally changes the physiologic characteristic of the system, reducing the usefulness of the responses. Typically, at high stimulus rates, neural adaptation takes place and responses are reduced and prolonged. This effect, however, can be reduced or eliminated by taking advantage of the special characteristics of the sensory organ. For the auditory system, intensity and frequency of tonal stimuli can be ordered such that adaptation is kept at a minimum (72,73).

A second approach involves the use of a variety of innovative acquisition processes other than traditional averaging. Limitations of the traditional ensemble averaging method in evoked-potential acquisition have long been recognized, and numerous attempts have been made to overcome them. Most problems arise from poor signal-to-noise ratio (SNR), the nonstationary nature of the noise, and the small amplitude of the single response. Many alternatives, such as Wiener filtering, adaptive filtering, and weighted averaging, have been proposed but none has yet been shown to offer a distinct advantage over traditional averaging. Advantages offered by these proposed methods are generally lost due to variations of the signal or lack of a true reference signal that does not contain part of the evoked response.

A variety of new methods for recording and evaluating ABR waveforms are currently under investigation (74–76). In general, these techniques utilize creative signal processing strategies in an attempt to reduce or eliminate time delay between adverse surgical manipulation and changes in measured response.

Electrocochleography

Basis of the Response

ECochG is a method of measuring the most peripheral of the auditory-evoked responses. The ECochG response consists of three primary components: cochlear microphonic (CM), summating potential (SP), and action potential (AP). The CM is generated within the organ of Corti by outer hair cells and follows the stimulus sound wave as an alternating current. The SP is a direct current potential that produces a baseline shift following the envelope of the stimulus. The AP is another alternating current potential that is associated with the synchronous discharge of numerous neural fibers located in the basal region of the cochlea. The AP represents the same activity as wave I of the ABR. It is the AP component that is most useful for intraoperative monitoring.

The ECochG has the advantage of being a near-field recording and as such requires fewer averages and less time to obtain a response. In addition, the response obtained is

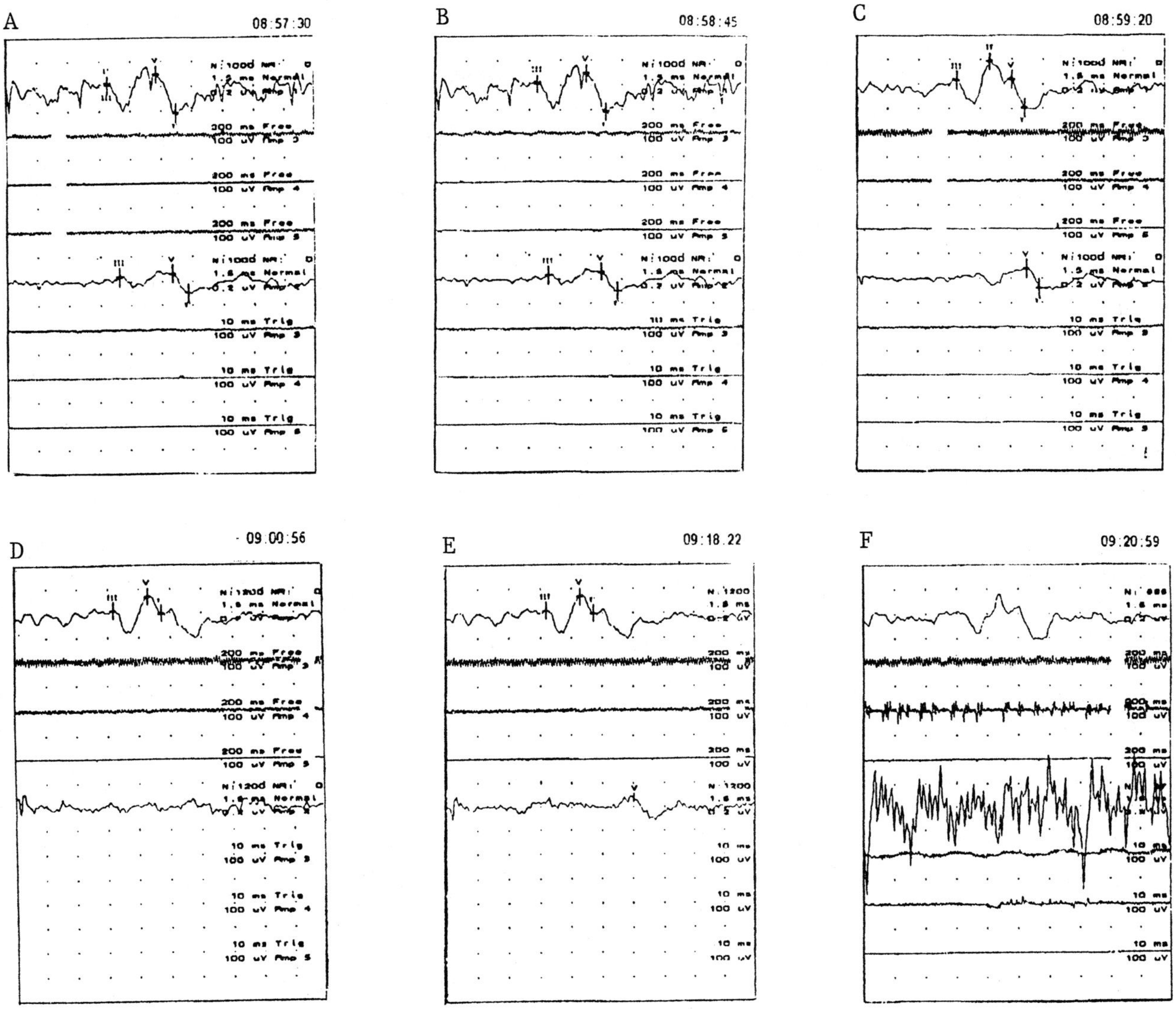

FIG. 5-3. Auditory brainstem response (ABR) monitoring recordings obtained during acoustic neuroma (AN) tumor dissection. The upper tracing in each panel shows the normal response of the unoperated ear. Each panel depicts a response obtained at approximate 1-minute intervals. The bottom tracing of panel **A** shows a normal, though slightly decreased in amplitude, response from the affected ear. The response in the lower tracing is seen to gradually disappear within a 3-minute period during tumor dissection **(B–D)**. Some recovery of the response is demonstrated in panel **E**. Panel **F** illustrates the effect of irrigation, which obscures the ABR response.

larger and easier to interpret. The ECochG can be recorded using a noninvasive technique in which either an ear canal or tympanic membrane electrode are used as the positive recording site. The response can also be recorded using an invasive technique in which the positive recording site is on the promontory of the cochlea within the middle ear reached by means of a transtympanic needle electrode. Ruth (68) compared the time and number of sweeps required to obtain a response using both techniques. Noninvasive extratympanic recordings require 250 to 1,200 samples over a 12- to 60-second time course, while transtympanic needle electrodes require only 40 to 100 sweeps over a 2- to 5-second time period. The improved SNR of the transtympanic placement resulted in more efficient recording.

The Intraoperative ECochG

The instrumentation used to record the ECochG is similar to that used to obtain the ABR. Recording parameters vary depending on the purpose of the test. Enhancement of the SP/AP is needed in evaluation of endolymphatic hydrops (e.g., Meniere's disease), while the AP is the more important factor for intraoperative monitoring. Detailed descriptions of stimulus and recording parameters can be found in Hall (66). Briefly, the stimulus should be a broad-band rarefaction click of high intensity [85 to 95 dB normalized hearing level (nHL)] with a rate of 21.1/sec. Recording parameters differ from those of the ABR primarily in that the positive recording site is the ipsilateral promontory as opposed to a distant surface placement. Negative and ground electrodes remain the same. Another difference is that the number of samples may be reduced to fewer than 100 compared to the 1,500 suggested for the ABR. According to Ruth (68), an impedance of as high as 100 KΩ may be acceptable in a transtympanic montage as compared to the need for extremely low impedance of less than 5 KΩ required for surface electrodes.

Interpretation of Results

As with the ABR, an adequate preoperative baseline response must be obtained against which to judge changes observed during the procedure. Zappia et al. (77) suggest that latency changes of greater than 1 msec and an amplitude decrease of greater than 50% should be considered significant changes in the response, although any measurable deviation should be reported immediately to the surgeon. Significant changes in the AP indicate, and can be used to differentiate between, cochlear and neural injury. Twenty seconds or more must elapse before changes in the ECochG response can be detected (78). This delay presumably occurs as a result of metabolic reserves that sustain cochlear function until their depletion from prolonged ischemia causes failure of electrophysiologic activity (79).

It has been suggested that simultaneous recording of the ABR and ECochG would result in the most effective monitoring system (66). The ECochG provides an interpretable wave I in cases where it cannot be identified in the ABR. Using the responses in combination, it would be possible to monitor changes in interpeak latencies, which could not be done using either alone. On the other hand, ECochG alone is not reflective of activity in the proximal region of the eighth nerve or the brainstem. It is possible to record a normally appearing ECochG in the presence of significant eighth nerve dysfunction. Monitoring of the ABR wave V provides information related to these more central areas of auditory processing.

Direct Eighth Nerve Recording

In an effort to gather information regarding the cochlear nerve and brainstem auditory structures more rapidly than could be obtained by ABR, surgical teams in the 1980s began recording from electrodes placed directly on the proximal eighth cranial nerve during posterior fossa surgery (32,36,80,81). It was found that potentials measured directly from the cochlear nerve required significantly fewer averages than those of an ABR (0 to 100 vs. hundreds to thousands) to display a recognizable wave pattern. This suggested that responses could be updated every few seconds under ideal circumstances. The rapidity of these near-field recordings also allowed progressive changes in responses to be better appreciated than with ABR, in which the averaging paradigm assumed a constant response (32). In addition, cochlear nerve action potentials (CNAPs) were found to be present when ABR and ECochG recordings had been eroded by tumor or other pathology (36). The disadvantage of this type of recording in acoustic neuroma surgery became evident during procedures to treat larger tumors that extended to or into the brainstem. There must be some portion of uninvolved cochlear nerve on which to place the electrode. Practically, many larger tumors are unsuitable for hearing conservation surgery anyway. If auditory function is to be monitored in a larger tumor, an electrode can be placed into the lateral recess adjacent to the cochlear nucleus (35,82), or one of the other techniques for auditory monitoring may be employed.

For direct eighth nerve monitoring, recording electrodes are most commonly placed on or around the intracranial segment of the cochleovestibular nerve. Recording should take place at a location on the nerve promixal to surgical manipulations. This fragile portion of the nerve lacking a fibrous sheath must be protected and handled gently in order to avoid injury during electrode positioning. A cotton or fibrous wick sutured to the tip of a Teflon-insulated wire secures the electrode to the nerve atraumatically. Møller et al. (35) suggested suturing the cotton to the electrode with 5-0 silk. The wire should be secured to the wound edge or suitable place to avoid inadvertent traction. During middle fossa exposure to remove intracanalicular acoustic neuromas, the electrode may be placed extradurally adjacent to the cochlear nerve, between bone and dura (83). The locations of the reference and ground electrodes are similar to those described for recording ABR. Recording instrumentation may be customized or that for ABR can be employed. The same wide-band click stimulus as that for ABR is presented by external auditory canal insert earphones.

The response waveforms obtained from direct recordings of the cochlear nerve typically exhibit triphasic patterns (Fig. 5-4) (84). The initial positive deflection (defined as downward) represents nerve activity approaching the recording site. The generally larger negative (upward) deflection occurs as the impulse passes under the electrode. As the depolarization moves away (more central) from the recording electrode, another positive wave results, thus completing the triphasic complex. Electrode position strongly influences the appearance of waveforms. Hearing loss and patient variabil-

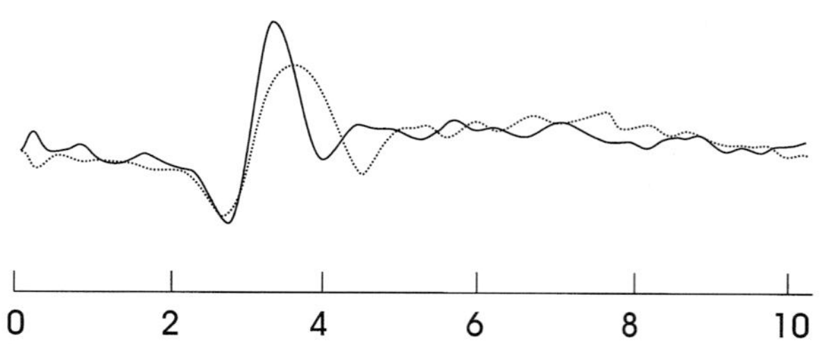

FIG. 5-4. Characteristic compound action potential recorded from the cochlear nerve. The waveforms will differ in amplitude and latency depending on the stimulus and recording parameters. Therefore, comparisons should be made using baseline responses obtained after exposure of the nerve but before tumor dissection.

ity also affect response patterns. As with other monitoring techniques, changes should only be reported using comparisons to baseline measurements. In the case of eighth nerve monitoring, baseline recordings are obtained after craniotomy but prior to tumor dissection.

Surgical manipulations can distort CNAPs in several ways. Stretching the cochlear nerve causes increased latency and broadening of the response waveforms. Partial block of conduction, as may occur with direct pressure by a surgical instrument on the nerve, results in lower amplitude of the prominent negative peak. Only the initial positive (downward) deflection is seen after complete conduction block or transection of the nerve. Møller (84) provided an excellent review of the physiology behind these waveforms and the responses to operative maneuvers.

Otoacoustic Emissions

Otoacoustic emissions (OAE) are low-level sounds measured from the ear canals of humans and animals with intact cochlear function (85). Evidence suggests that they arise from motion of the outer hair cells within the organ of Corti (86). OAEs have found utility in the detection of a variety of sensory hearing losses, such as noise exposure, aging, ototoxicity, endolymphatic hydrops (Meniere's disease), genetic hearing disorders, and others (87). Of the various types, transient or click-evoked (TEOAE) and distortion-product (DPOAE) emissions appear to be the most useful clinically. Both TEOAEs and DPOAEs may be useful in differentiating sensory (cochlear) from neural (retrocochlear) hearing losses (88). Poor behavioral hearing thresholds and good emissions suggest a retrocochlear site of lesion. Reduced OAEs indicates at least cochlear dysfunction. These stimulus-evoked OAEs have been measured preoperatively in patients with acoustic neuromas (89,90). Otoacoustic emissions were absent in more than half of the ears, suggesting a negative effect on cochlear function by these tumors.

Distortion-product OAEs have been shown to be very sensitive to hypoxia (91) and interruption of inner ear blood flow (92). Being sound waves, OAEs are described by amplitude, frequency, and phase measures. The frequency of the responses varies with that of the stimulus. Amplitude and phase are affected by manipulations that alter cochlear (and presumably outer cell) function. Studies of interruption to CBF in rabbits demonstrated the onset of reduction of DPOAE amplitudes to occur reliably 15 to 25 seconds after the onset of cochlear ischemia (92). Subtle early changes in amplitude were measurable in some subjects within the first 10 seconds after IAA occlusion (93). More recently, phase changes have been noted within 2 to 3 seconds of IAA compression, suggesting that phase measures may be the most sensitive OAE parameter for monitoring cochlear function during surgery (94).

OAEs have been measured in the operating room during surgery (Fig. 5-5) (56,95). Emissions were stable during a variety of procedures over many hours. Inhalation and intravenous (narcotic) anesthetics did not appear to affect the recording of emissions. Acoustic noise has the potential to undermine the recording of OAEs. This effect was particularly prominent when measuring emissions at frequencies below 2 KHz (56). Based on numerous recordings from various operating rooms, the majority of background acoustic noise energy appeared consistently concentrated below 2 KHz (Fig. 5-5C). Therefore, the SNR became too low to judge the presence of or changes in OAE amplitude. Based on these results, the authors recommended choosing patients for surgical OAE monitoring with preoperatively intact hearing and emissions above 2 KHz.

To date, low-frequency (below 2 KHz) background noise remains an obstacle to monitoring auditory function with OAEs in ears with hearing predominantly in that range. The patient's vital functions and life support systems used during general anesthesia contribute a significant amount of this acoustic energy. Some of the noise can be eliminated from the ear canal by sealing the probe and the meatus. A surgical scrub sponge has been used with some success (56). Silicone, wax, and other substances have also been employed in an attempt to solve this problem. Current electronic signal processing techniques are better at rejecting higher frequency noise. DPOAEs have been monitored during loud suctioning of CSF (relatively high frequency) from the operative field (Telischi et al., unpublished data). Emissions could not be monitored during drilling (large amplitude noise of both low and high frequency) (Fig. 5-5B). Studies in animals have not shown any temporary threshold effects on DPOAEs after temporal bone drilling that would affect monitoring (Telischi et al., unpublished data). Mechanical interference with the conductive hearing mechanism would affect measurement of OAEs. Fluid or debris such as bone dust in the external auditory canal or middle ear would interfere with emissions. For this reason, OAE monitoring is not suitable for many transmastoid surgical approaches.

Emissions can be elicited using the previously mentioned stimuli: clicks (TEOAEs), single frequency tones (stimulus frequency), and two tones (DPOAEs). TEOAEs result in an amplitude-weighted frequency spectrum that may be repeated throughout the critical portion of the operation (95). The number of averaged sweeps, and hence the time it takes to update data, depends on the background noise. Generally, reliable TEOAEs can be obtained in 30 to 40 seconds in ideal conditions and longer intervals in noisy situations. Devices under development promise to be able to capture responses more quickly. Pure-tone stimuli also require multiple averages depending on the resonance characteristics of the test ear and sound environment. Measuring stimulus-frequency emissions usually requires half a minute or more. An unexplored advantage of using single-frequency stimuli lies in the ability to focus recordings at a particular frequency and perhaps allow monitoring below 2 KHz.

Using a customized software PC-based system, DPOAEs

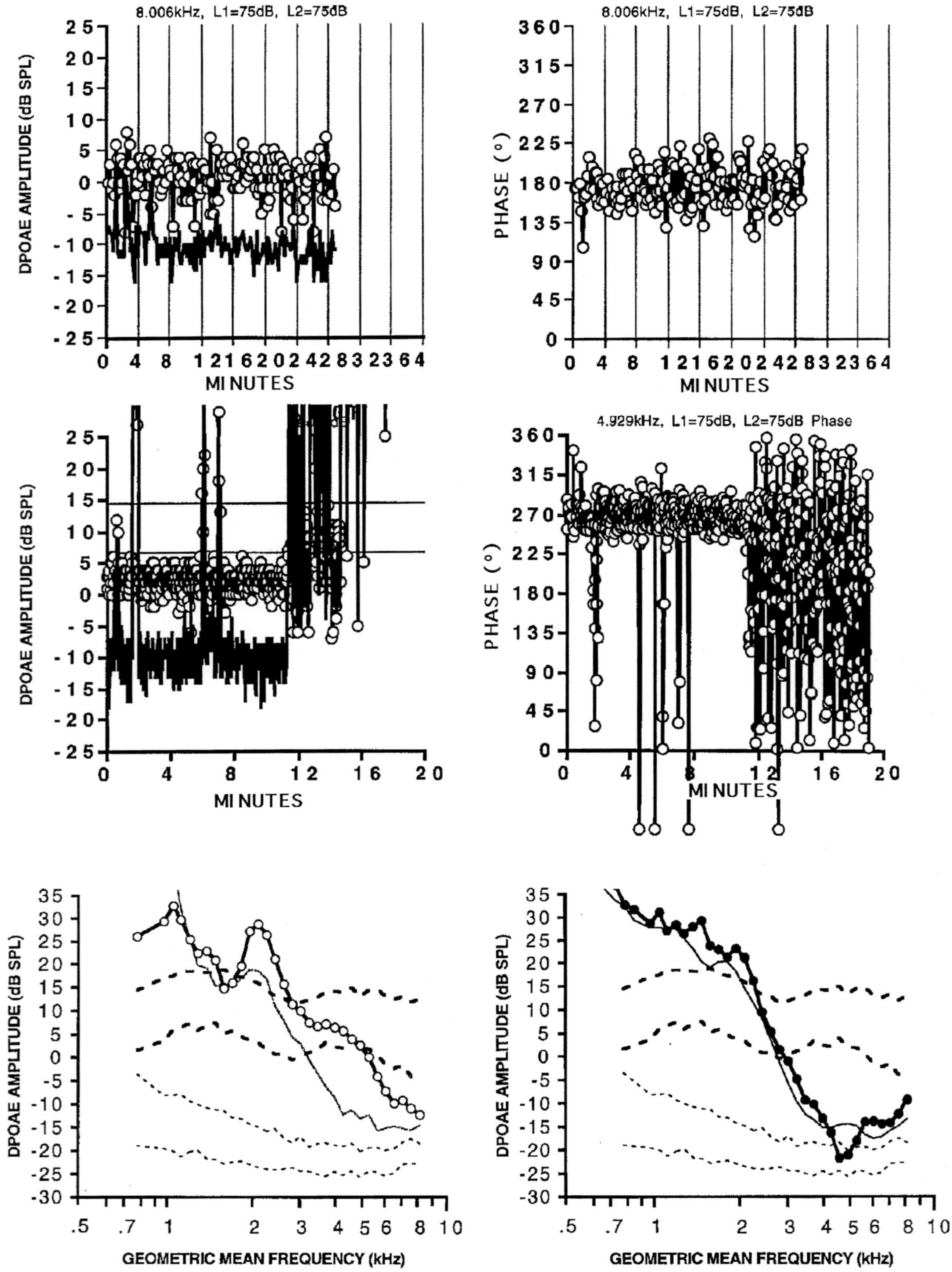

A B C

FIG. 5-5. Otoacoustic emissions (OAEs) monitored during surgery to remove AN. **A:** Distortion-product OAE (DPOAE) amplitude and phase measures at 8 KHz. Data were obtained every 2 to 5 seconds. **B:** DPOAE amplitude and phase measures demonstrating the effects of drilling noise. **C:** DPOAE frequency graphics obtained intraoperatively post-AN removal. The *left* graph shows emissions present at 3 to 7 KHz. The patient retained some hearing in that range. The *right* graph demonstrates no emissions in a patient with no hearing postoperatively. Note the elevated background noise floor (*solid line*) below 2 to 3 KHz.

have been monitored during surgery as rapidly as every 2 seconds (56). During experimental operations, DPOAEs were obtained several times per second (94). As mentioned above, DPOAEs appear to be more robust than other types of emissions and are expected to be present in ears with mild to moderate sensory hearing loss (pure-tone thresholds up to 45 dB). Also, monitoring programs can be designed to monitor a single or any number of frequency locations of the cochlea. This flexibility allows monitoring those frequencies that demonstrate the greatest amplitude on the day of surgery. The best frequency for monitoring may change during the case, and the program can be modified to reflect this. Because of these properties, DPOAEs at this time appear to be best suited for intraoperative OAE monitoring.

Since OAEs reflect only cochlear function, a complete monitoring regimen should also include information regarding the auditory nerve and brainstem structures if they will be at risk during the operation. ABR or direct eighth nerve techniques would be appropriate to combine with emissions monitoring. DPOAEs and ABR have been measured during acoustic neuroma surgery using the same acoustic probe (ER 10-B, Etymotic Research Corp., Elk Grove Village, IL), which contained two speakers and a microphone (56). Rapid switching between the two recording instruments allowed comparisons of the responses. Studies are under way to test a prototype system that monitors rapid ABR and TEOAEs simultaneously. In the meantime, a number of commercial OAE instruments may be employed for the operating room. A high-quality speaker/microphone probe like the one mentioned above will enhance the recordings. The probe should be secured in the ear canal at the level of the meatus. The pinna, probe, and tubing may be prepped out of the field by folding and securing (with tape or suture) the pinna anteriorly. The tubing should be secured to the patient or operating table in a location to prevent pulling or other disturbance. Baseline measurements obtained after probe insertion and after sterile draping of the operative field help ensure successful monitoring. For DPOAEs, the best frequencies to monitor are selected from these baseline measurements. A complete DPOAE response graphic helps to identify any changes in other frequencies. As the operation proceeds, the frequency to be monitored may be changed based on these graphics. As with the other methods of intraoperative monitoring of auditory function, experience and improvements in technology will guide the evolution of OAE techniques.

Laser-Doppler Cochlear Blood Flow

Interruption of CBF probably causes a significant number of cases of postoperative hearing losses after IAC/CPA surgery. A direct method of monitoring CBF has been described using laser-Doppler (LD) measurements (96). The technique involves positioning the end of a needle probe, housing both emitter and collector optical fibers, against the cochlear promontory in the middle ear. The angle of the probe is adjusted to obtain maximal flow readings. Moving blood within the cochlear circulation causes a Doppler shift in the light returning to the collector. Signal processing of the light reflected by the static tissues (nonshifted) and moving blood (Doppler shifted) gives a relative velocity of flow. Laser-Doppler measurements are useful only to detect changes in flow. Because of extreme variability in responses with minor changes in probe position, absolute flow rates cannot be compared among subjects to obtain normal values. Levine et al. (96) were able to obtain good correlation between ECochG and LD measurements during animal surgery that occluded CBF. Though the potential application of this technology is exciting, transferring LD flow measurement techniques developed in the animal model to human surgery has proved a difficult task and awaits further study before it can be practically applied during tumor removal operations.

Results of Surgery Performed Using Intraoperative Auditory Monitoring

The main goal of monitoring auditory function during posterior fossa surgery is to prevent hearing loss. To achieve this goal, the monitoring paradigm must provide the surgeon with timely and accurate information both to prevent, or repair, reversible injuries to auditory structures and to identify those maneuvers that cause hearing loss so that they may be avoided or modified in the future. In general, the loss of a physiologic response correlates with poor postoperative hearing. Irrespective of the monitoring technique used, the presence of an unchanged or reduced response is not predictive of hearing, which limits the prognostic accuracy of current monitoring techniques. There appears to be a consensus to use auditory monitoring during nerve section and microvascular decompression procedures where hearing preservation rates are quite high (32,97). A review of the current literature suggests that techniques in use today have only begun to meet the stated objectives in operations to remove acoustic neuromas (34,77,98,99). Studies generally compare rates of hearing preservation using current auditory monitoring techniques with historical control groups with the potential confounding variables of improved surgical skills and instrumentation. Some studies frankly do not find any advantage to monitoring at this time (43,63,100).

As previously discussed, technologic advancements in each type of monitoring have increased the timeliness of information fed back to the surgeon. The ideal monitoring system would provide real-time feedback of the functional status of both the cochlea and the central auditory structures including the cochlear nerve. It is important to separate and distinguish changes in sensory and neural auditory responses to understand how a particular surgical manipulation will affect hearing. In the future, probably a combination of two or more of the methods described in this chapter will be the standard. Although each has theoretical advantages, use of no one technique to date has resulted in statistically improved hearing outcomes compared to the others (77).

Approximately one-third of all patients retain hearing

after planned hearing preservation AN operations (77,101,102). Hearing preservation rates improve considerably for intracanalicular tumors, with rates of up to 50% to 60% (103). Jackler's (104) review of the subject emphasizes the disparity of results among published reports. It is clear that hearing outcomes depend on many factors, including surgeon's experience, tumor size and location, tumor invasiveness, surgical approach, and preoperative hearing levels. Jackler concluded that only about 5% of all patients maintain useful hearing after AN removal. Certainly this leaves considerable room for improvement. Refining techniques of intraoperative auditory monitoring may ensure better hearing outcomes in the future.

The recording and interpretation of auditory-evoked potentials in an operating room setting is technically difficult. In the hands of knowledgeable and competent clinicians, the response can provide useful information in the detection of surgically induced dysfunction. It is important that each team establish goals and expectations for monitoring, and evaluate the measurement and interpretive techniques suggested in the literature to select those that best meet their needs.

REFERENCES

1. Leonetti JP, Brackmann DE, Prass RL. Improved preservation of facial nerve function in the infratemporal approach to the skull base. *Otolaryngol Head Neck Surg* 1989;101:74–78.
2. Brackmann DE. The facial nerve in the infratemporal approach. *Otolaryngol Head Neck Surg* 1987;97:15–17.
3. Krause F. *Surgery of the brain and spinal cord.* New York: Rebman, 1912.
4. Hullay J, Tomits GH. Experiences with total removal of tumors of the acoustic nerve. *J Neurosurg* 1965;22:127–135.
5. Givre A, Olivecrona H. Surgical experiences with acoustic neuroma. *J Neurosurg* 1949;396–407.
6. Hilger JA. Facial nerve stimulator. *Trans Am Acad Ophthalmol Otolaryngol* 1964;68:74–76.
7. Jako GJ. Facial nerve monitor. *Trans Am Acad Ophthalmol Otolaryngol* 1965;69:340–342.
8. Parson RC. Electrical stimulation of the facial nerve. *Laryngoscope* 1966;76:391–406.
9. Delgado TE, Buchheit WA, Rosenholtz HR, Chrissian S. Intraoperative monitoring of facial muscle evoked responses obtained by intracranial stimulation of the facial nerve: a more accurate technique for facial nerve dissection. *Neurosurgery* 1979;4:418–421.
10. Sugita K, Kobayashi S. Technical and instrumental improvements in the surgical treatment of acoustic neurinomas. *J Neurosurg* 1982;57: 747–752.
11. Møller AR, Jannetta PJ. Preservation of facial function during removal of acoustic neuromas: use of monopolar constant-voltage stimulation and EMG. *J Neurosurg* 1984;61:757–760.
12. Prass RL, Lüders H. Acoustic (loudspeaker) facial electromyographic monitoring: part 1. Evoked electromyographic activity during acoustic neuroma resection. *Neurosurgery* 1986;19:392–400.
13. Silverstein H, Smouha E, Jones R. Routine intraoperative facial nerve monitoring during otologic surgery. *Am J Otol* 1988;9:269–275.
14. Silverstein H, Rosenberg SI, Flanzer J, Seidman MD. Intraoperative facial nerve monitoring in acoustic neuroma surgery. Am J Otol 1993; 14(6):524–532.
15. Prass RL. Intraoperative electromyographic recording. In: Kartush JM, Bouchard KR, eds. *Neuromonitoring in otology and head and neck surgery.* New York: Raven Press, 1992:81–97.
16. Prass RL. Iatrogenic facial nerve injury: the role of facial nerve monitoring. *Otolaryngol Clin North Am* 1996;29:265–275.
17. Prass RL, Lüders H. Constant-current versus constant-voltage stimulation. *J Neurosurg* 1985;62:622–623.
18. Kartush JM. Electroneurography and intraoperative facial monitoring in contemporary neurotology. *Otolaryngol Head Neck Surg* 1989;101: 496–503.
19. Kartush JM, Bouchard KR. Intraoperative facial nerve monitoring: otology, neurotology, and skull base surgery. In: Kartush JM, Bouchard KR, eds. *Neuromonitoring in otology and head and neck surgery.* New York: Raven Press, 1992:99–120.
20. Lennon RL, Hosking MP, Daube JR, Welna JO. Effect of partial neuromuscular blockade on intraoperative electromyography in patients undergoing resection of acoustic neuromas. *Anesth Analg* 1992; 75:729–733.
21. Blair EA, Teeple E, Sutherland RM, Shih T, Chen D. Effect of neuromuscular blockade on facial nerve monitoring. *Am J Otol* 1994;15: 161–167.
22. Pensak ML, Willging JP, Keith RW. Intraoperative facial nerve monitoring in chronic ear surgery: a resident training experience. *Am J Otol* 1994;15:108–110.
23. Selesnick SH, Carew JF, Victor JD, Heise CW, Levine J. Predictive value of facial nerve electrophysiologic stimulation thresholds in cerebellopontine-angle surgery. *Laryngoscope* 1996;106:633–638.
24. Silverstein H, Willcox TO, Rosenberg SI, Seidman MD. Prediction of facial nerve function following acoustic neuroma resection using intraoperative facial nerve stimulation. *Laryngoscope* 1994;104: 539–544.
25. Fisch U. Surgery for Bell's palsy. *Arch Otolaryngol* 1981;107:1–11.
26. Richmond IL, Mahla M. Use of antidromic recording to monitor facial nerve function intraoperatively. *Neurosurgery* 1985;16:458–462.
27. Colletti V, Fiorino FG, Policante Z, Bruni L. New perspectives in intraoperative facial nerve monitoring with antidromic potentials. *Am J Otol* 1996;17:755–762.
28. Møller AR, Janetta PJ. Monitoring facial EMG responses during microvascular decompression operations for hemifacial spasm. *J Neurosurg* 1987;66:681–685.
29. Arriaga M, Haid R, Masel D. Antidromic stimulation of the greater superficial petrosal nerve in middle fossa surgery. *Laryngoscope* 1995;105:102–105.
30. Møller AR, Jannetta PJ, Moller MB. Neural generators of brainstem evoked potentials: results from human intracranial recordings. *Ann Otol Rhinol Laryngol* 1981;104:841–859.
31. Møller AR. *Evoked potentials in intraoperative monitoring.* Baltimore, MD: Williams & Wilkins, 1988.
32. Møller AR, Jannetta PJ. Monitoring auditory functions during cranial nerve microvascular decompressions operation by direct recording from the eighth nerve. *J Neurosurg* 1983;59:493–499.
33. Winzenburg SM, Margolis RH, Levine SC, Haines SJ, Fournier EM. Tympanic and transtympanic electrocochleography in acoustic neuroma and vestibular nerve section surgery. *Am J Otol* 1993;14(1): 63–69.
34. Nedzelski JM, Chiong CM, Cashman MZ, Stanton SG, Rowed DW. Hearing preservation in acoustic neuroma surgery: value of monitoring cochlear nerve action potentials. *Otolaryngol Head Neck Surg* 1994;111:703–709.
35. Møller AR, Jho HD, Jannetta PJ. Preservation of hearing in operations on acoustic tumors: an alternative to recording brain stem auditory evoked potentials. *Neurosurgery* 1994;34:688–693.
36. Silverstein H, Norrell H, Hyman S. Simultaneous use of CO_2 laser with continuous monitoring of eighth cranial nerve action potential during acoustic neuroma surgery. *Otolaryngol Head Neck Surg* 1984; 92:80–84.
37. Slavit DH Harner SG, Harper CM, Beatty CW. Auditory monitoring during acoustic neuroma removal. *Arch Otolaryngol Head Neck Surg* 1991;117:1153–1157.
38. Yingling CD, Gardi JN. Intraoperative monitoring of facial and cochlear nerves during acoustic neuroma surgery. *Otolaryngol Clin North Am* 1992;25(2):413–448.
39. Stanton SG, Cashman MZ, Harrison RV, Nedzelski JM, Rowed DW. Cochlear nerve action potential during cerebellopontine angle surgery: relationship of latency, amplitude, and threshold measurements to hearing. *Ear Hear* 1989;10:23–28.
40. Shelton C, Brackmann DE, House WF, Hitselberger WE. Acoustic tumor surgery: prognostic factors in hearing conservation. *Arch Otolaryngol Head Neck Surg* 1989;115:1213–1216.
41. Shelton C. Hearing preservation in acoustic tumor surgery. *Otolaryngol Clin North Am* 1992;25:609–621.

42. Cohen NL, Lewis WS, Ransoff J. Hearing preservation in cerebellopontine angle tumor surgery: the NYU experience 1974–1991. *Am J Otol* 1993;14:423–433.
43. Rowed DW, Nedzelski JM. Hearing preservation in the removal of intracanalicular acoustic neuromas via the retrosigmoid approach. *J Neurosurg* 1997;86:456–461.
44. Jackler RK, Pitts LH. Selection of surgical approach to acoustic neuroma. *Otolaryngol Clin North Am* 1992;25:361–387.
45. MacDonald CB, Hirsch BE, Kamerer DB, Sekhar L. Acoustic neuroma surgery: predictive criteria for hearing preservation. *Otolaryngol Head Neck Surg* 1991;104:128.
46. Nadol JB, Levine R, Ojemann RG, et al. Preservation of hearing in surgical removal of acoustic neuromas of the internal auditory canal and cerebellar pontine angle. *Laryngoscope* 1987;97:1287–1294.
47. Josey AF, Glasscock ME, Jackson CG. Preservation of hearing in acoustic tumor surgery: audiological indicators. *Ann Otol Rhinol Laryngol* 1988;97:626.
48. Glasscock ME, McKennan KX, Levine SC. Acoustic neuroma surgery: the results of hearing conservation surgery. *Laryngoscope* 1987; 97:785.
49. Kanzaki J, Ogawa K, Shiobara R, et al. Hearing preservation in acoustic neuroma surgery and postoperative audiological findings. *Acta Otolaryngol (Stockh)* 1989;107:474.
50. Kemink JL, LaRouere MJ, Kileny PR, et al. Hearing preservation following suboccipital removal of acoustic neuromas. *Laryngoscope* 1990;100:597.
51. Levine RA, Ojemann RG, Montgomery WW, McGaffigan PM. Monitoring auditory evoked potentials during acoustic neuroma surgery: insights into the mechanism of the hearing loss. *Ann Otol Rhinol Laryngol* 1984;93:116–123.
52. Mom T, Avan P, Ropmand R, Gilain L. Monitoring of functional changes after transient ischemia in gerbil cochlea. *Brain Res* 1997; 751:20–30.
53. Sekiya T, Møller AR, Jannetta PJ. Pathophysiological mechanisms of intraoperative and postoperative nearing deficits in cerebellopontine angle surgery: an experimental study. *Acta Neurochir* 1986;81: 142–151.
54. Moore EJ. *Bases of auditory brain-stem evoked responses*. New York: Grune & Stratton, 1983.
55. Stockard JJ, Rossiter VS, Jones TA, Sharbrough FW. Effects of centrally acting drugs on brainstem auditory responses. *Electroencephalogr Clin Neurophysiol* 1977;43:550–551(Abst).
56. Telischi FF, Widick MP, Lonsbury-Martin BL, McCoy MJ. Monitoring cochlear function intraoperatively using distortion product otoacoustic emissions. *Am J Otol* 1995;16(5):597–607.
57. Stockard JJ, Sharbrough FW, Tinker JA. Effect of hypothermia on the human brain stem auditory response. *Ann Neurol* 1978;3:368–370.
58. Levine RA, Montgomery WW, Ojemann RJ. Evoked potential detection of hearing loss during acoustic neuroma surgery. *Neurology* 1978; 28:339.
59. Grundy BL, Jannetta PJ, Lina A, et al. Intraoperative monitoring of brainstem auditory evoked potentials. *J Neurosurg* 1982;57:674–681.
60. Hardy RW, Kinney SE, Luders H, et al. Preservation of cochlear nerve function with the aid of brain stem auditory evoked potentials. *Neurosurgery* 1982;11:16–19.
61. Abramson M, Stein BM, Pedley TA, Emerson RG, Wazen JJ. Intraoperative BAER monitoring and hearing preservation in the treatment of acoustic neuromas. *Laryngoscope* 1995;95:1318–1321.
62. Cohen NL, Hammerschlag P, Berg H, Ransohoff J. Acoustic neuroma surgery: an eclectic approach with emphasis on preservation of hearing: the New York University-Bellevue experience. *Ann Otol Rhinol Laryngol* 1986;95:21–27.
63. Kveton JF. The efficacy of brainstem auditory evoked potentials in acoustic tumor surgery. *Laryngoscope* 1990;100:1171–1173.
64. Slavit DH, Harner SG, Harper CM, Beatty CW. Auditory monitoring during acoustic neuroma removal. *Arch Otolaryngol Head Neck Surg* 1991;117:1153–1157.
65. Harper CM, Harner SG, Slavit DH, et al. Effect of BAEP monitoring on hearing preservation during acoustic neuroma resection. *Neurology* 1992;42:1551–1553.
66. Hall JW. *Handbook of auditory evoked responses*. Boston: Allyn and Bacon, 1992.
67. Møller AR. Monitoring auditory function during operations to remove acoustic tumors. *Am J Otol* 1996;17:452–460.
68. Ruth RA. Electrocochleography. In: Katz J, ed. *Handbook of clinical audiology*. Baltimore, MD: Williams & Wilkins, 1994.
69. Little JR, Lesser RP, Lueders H, Furlan AJ. Brainstem auditory evoked potentials in posterior circulation surgery. *Neurosurgery* 1983; 12:496–502.
70. Schwartz DM, Bloom MJ, Dennis JM. Perioperative monitoring of auditory brainstem responses. *Hear J* 1985;38:9–13.
71. Friedman WA, Kaplan BJ, Gravenstein D, Rhoton AL. Intraoperative brainstem auditory evoked potentials during posterior fossa microvascular decompression. *J Neurosurg* 1985;62:552–557.
72. Hoke M, Pantev C, Ansa L, Lutkenhoner B, Herrmann E. A timesaving BEAR technique for frequency-specific assessment of the auditory threshold through tone-pulse series stimulation (TOPSTIM) with simultaneous gliding high-pass noise masking (GHINOMA). *Acta Otolaryngol Suppl (Stockh)* 1991;482:45–56.
73. Hamill TA, Hussung RA, Sammeth CA. Rapid threshold estimation using the ''chained-stimuli'' technique for auditory brain stem response measurement. *Ear Hear* 1991;12:229–234.
74. Ozdamar O, Delgado RE, Eilers RE, Widen JE. Computer methods for automated hearing determination with auditory brainstem responses. *Ear Hear* 1990;11:417–429.
75. Ozdamar O, Delgado RE, Eilers RE, Urbano R. Automated electrophysiologic hearing testing using a threshold-seeking algorithm. *J Am Acad Audiol* 1994;5:77–88.
76. Don M, Eberling C. Use of quantitative measures of auditory brainstem response peak amplitude and residual background noise in the decision to stop averaging. *J Acoust Soc Am* 1996;99:491–499.
77. Zappia JJ, Wiet RJ, O'Connor CA. Intraoperative monitoring in acoustic neuroma surgery. *Otolaryngol Head Neck Surg* 1996;115: 99–106.
78. Levine RA. Surgical monitoring applications of the brainstem auditory evoked response and electrocochleography. In: Owen J, Donohoe C, eds. *Clinical atlas of auditory evoked potentials*. New York: Grune & Stratton, 1988:103–116.
79. Perlman HB, Kimura R, Fernandez C. Experiments on temporary obstruction of the internal auditory artery. *Laryngoscope* 1959;69: 591–613.
80. Jannetta PJ, Møller AR, Moller MB. Technique of hearing preservation of small acoustic neuromas. *Ann Surg* 1984;200:513–523.
81. Silverstein H, McDaniel A, Norrel H, Haberkamp T. Hearing preservation after acoustic neuroma surgery with intraoperative direct eighth cranial nerve monitoring: part II. A classification of results. *Otolaryngol Head Neck Surg* 1986;95:285–289.
82. Kuroki A, Møller AR. Microsurgical anatomy around the foramen of Luschka with reference to intraoperative recording of auditory evoked potentials from the cochlear nuclei. *J Neurosurg* 1995;82:933–939.
83. Roberson J, Senne A, Brackmann D, Hitselberger W, Saunders J. Direct cochlear nerve action potentials as an aid to hearing preservation in middle fossa acoustic neuroma resection. *Am J Otol* 1996;17: 653–657.
84. Møller AR. Physiology of the auditory system and recording of auditory evoked potentials. In: Kartush JM, Bouchard KR: *Neuromonitoring in otology and head and neck surgery*. New York: Raven Press, 1992:163–198.
85. Lonsbury-Martin BL, Harris FP, Hawkins MD, Stagner BB, Martin GK. Distortion product emissions in humans: I. Basic properties in normally hearing subjects. *Ann Otol Rhinol Laryngol* 1990; 99(suppl)147:3–13.
86. Brownell WE. Outer hair cell electromotility and otoacoustic emissions. *Ear Hear* 1990;11:82–92.
87. Lonsbury-Martin BL, Martin GK. The clinical utility of distortion-product otoacoustic emissions. *Ear Hear* 1990;11:90–99.
88. Olms LA, Lonsbury-Martin BL, Martin GK. Acoustic-distortion products: separation of sensory from neural dysfunction in sensorineural hearing loss in humans and rabbits. *Otolaryngol Head Neck Surg* 1991;104:159–174.
89. Robinette MS, Bauch CD, Olsen WO, Harner SG, Beatty CW. Use of TEOAE, ABR, and acoustic reflex measures to assess auditory function patients with acoustic neuromas. *Am J Audiol* 1992(Nov)ə–74.
90. Telischi FF, Roth J, Stagner BB, Lonsbury-Martin BL, Balkany TJ. Patterns of evoked otoacoustic emissions associated with acoustic neuromas. *Laryngoscope* 1995;105(7):675–682.
91. Rebillard G, Lavigne O, Rebillard M. Effect of reversible hypoxia

on the compared time courses of endocochlear potential and 2f1-f2 distortion products. *Hear Res* 1992;62:142–148.

92. Telischi FF, Widick MP, Stagner BB, Martin GK, Lonsbury-Martin BL. Effects of vascular compromise on rabbit DPOAEs: implications for cerebellopontine angle surgery. *Abstr Assoc Res Otolaryngol* 1994; 17:46.
93. Widick MP, Telischi FF, Lonsbury-Martin BL, Stagner BB. Early effects of cerebellopontine angle compression on rabbit DPOAEs: a model for monitoring cochlear function during acoustic neuroma surgery. *Otolaryngol Head Neck Surg* 1994;111:407–416.
94. Telischi FF, Stagner BB, Widick MP, Balkany TJ, Lonsbury-Martin BL. Distortion-product otoacoustic emission monitoring of cochlear blood flow. *Laryngoscope* 1998;108:837–842.
95. Cane MA, O'Donoghue GM, Lutman ME. The feasibility of using oto-acoustic emissions to monitor cochlear function during acoustic neuroma surgery. *Scand Audiol* 1992;21:173–176.
96. Levine RA, Bu-Saba N, Brown MC. Laser-Doppler measurements and electrocochleography during ischemia of the guinea pig cochlea: implications for hearing preservation in acoustic neuroma surgery. *Ann Otol Rhinol Laryngol* 1993;102:127–136.
97. Rowed DW, Nedzelski JM, Cashman MZ, et al. Cochlear nerve monitoring during cerebellopontine angle operations. *Can J Neurol Sci* 1988;15:68–72.
98. Matthies C, Samii M. Management of vestibular schwannomas (acoustic neuromas): the value of neurophysiology for intraoperative monitoring of auditory function in 200 cases. *Neurosurgery* 1997; 40(3):459–468.
99. Nadol JB, Chiong CM, Ojemann RG, et al. Preservation of hearing and facial nerve function in resection of acoustic neuroma. *Laryngoscope* 1992;102:1153–1158.
100. Torrens M, Maw R, Coakham H, Butler S. Facial and acoustic nerve preservation during excision of extracanalicular acoustic neuromas using the suboccipital approach. *Br J Neurosurg* 1994;8: 655–665.
101. Gardner G, Robertson JH. Hearing preservation in unilateral acoustic neuroma surgery. *Ann Otol Rhinol Laryngol* 1988;97:55–66.
102. Glasscock ME III, Hays JW, Minor LB, Haynes DS, Carrasco VN. Preservation of hearing for acoustic neuromas. *J Neurosurg* 1993;78: 864–870.
103. Brackmann DE, House JR III, Hitselberger WE. Technical modifications to the middle fossa craniotomy approach in removal of acoustic neuromas. *Am J Otol* 1994;15:614–619.
104. Jackler RA. Acoustic Neuroma (vestibular schwannoma). In: Jackler RA, Brackmann DE, eds. *Neurotology*. St. Louis: Mosby-Year Book, 1994:729–785.

Neurosurgical Issues in Otolaryngology: Principles and Practice of Collaboration, edited by Moisés A. Arriaga and J. Diaz Day. Lippincott Williams & Wilkins, Philadelphia © 1999.

CHAPTER 6

Monitoring: Somatosensory Evoked Potentials, Cranial Nerve, and Micro Doppler Sonography

Gary W. Schurman and Paul A. Lobaugh

The rapid advancement of neurosurgical and combined neurosurgical and neurologic techniques over the past several decades has led the surgeon into regions of the central nervous system (CNS) previously deemed inaccessible. These surgical advances have been accompanied by the ever-present possibility of inadvertent damage to neural and/or vascular structures, which may compromise the postoperative outcome. Historically, surgeons relied on direct visualization, preoperative x-ray, and experience to guide them past the structures at risk whose compromise might lead to unfavorable neurologic sequelae. Unfortunately, anatomic integrity doesn't always predict functional integrity. The need for intraoperative functional assessment and monitoring of neural pathways became increasingly acute.

As surgeons turned toward neurophysiology seeking techniques for neuromonitoring, they found two existing clinical strategies—electroencephalography (EEG) and electroneuromyography (ENMG). There were many drawbacks to each approach, the primary one being inability to assess conduction through the spinal cord. Rapid advances in both quality and quantity of spinal cord surgical procedures necessitated the development of a reliable and accurate neurophysiologic measure of cord functional status in the anesthetized patient. The pioneering investigators of the 1960s began to evaluate the emerging technology of sensory evoked potentials, which were obtained using computer averaging of EEG epochs following stimulation of a distal neural receptor (1).

EVOKED POTENTIALS

The development of knowledge regarding evoked potentials is analogous to the course of development of the computer, the prerequisite tool for acquisition of the responses.

G. W. Schurman and P. A. Lobaugh: Neuromonitoring Services, Allegheny General Hospital, Pittsburgh, Pennsylvania 15212.

The first published evoked potential tracings appeared shortly after the Second World War. Dawson (2) applied electrical stimulation to the median nerve and recorded EEG from electrodes over the contralateral parietal scalp. Observation of EEG tracings led him to suspect the presence of an extremely small amplitude response that appeared to be related to the stimulus but was mainly obscured by the much larger amplitude EEG.

Dawson theorized that a small-voltage response that occupied a fixed position in time following a brief stimulus existed beneath the large-voltage, random electrical brain activity seen on the electroencephalogram. Utilizing a primitive vacuum-tube computer, he triggered the computer to sweep $\frac{1}{10}$ second of EEG data coincidental to the onset of the shock at the wrist. A series of several dozen such samples were then overlaid so that the random EEG were essentially canceled out, while the synchronous, recurrent wave (occurring about 20 msec after delivery of the shock to the wrist) grew larger in size up to a maximal amplitude of approximately 5 mV. Thus, the first recorded somatosensory evoked potential (later identified as generated from primary sensory cortex hand area of the post central gyrus) was reported.

Research activities into basic properties of evoked potentials (EPs) multiplied in the 1950s as investigators observed the EP recorded over the occipital scalp. The visual evoked potential to pattern-reversal stimulation was first described by Van Der Tweel and Spekreijse (3). Davis (4) published EP tracings recorded from the scalp in response to an auditory tone burst. Somesthetic responses to more natural stimuli such as cutaneus taps, painful pinch, and near-threshold electrical shock were revealed. Somatotopic mapping of sensorimotor cortex was conducted using electrodes in direct contact with cortical tissue by neurosurgeons. The period of basic discovery of EPs culminated in the study by Jewett

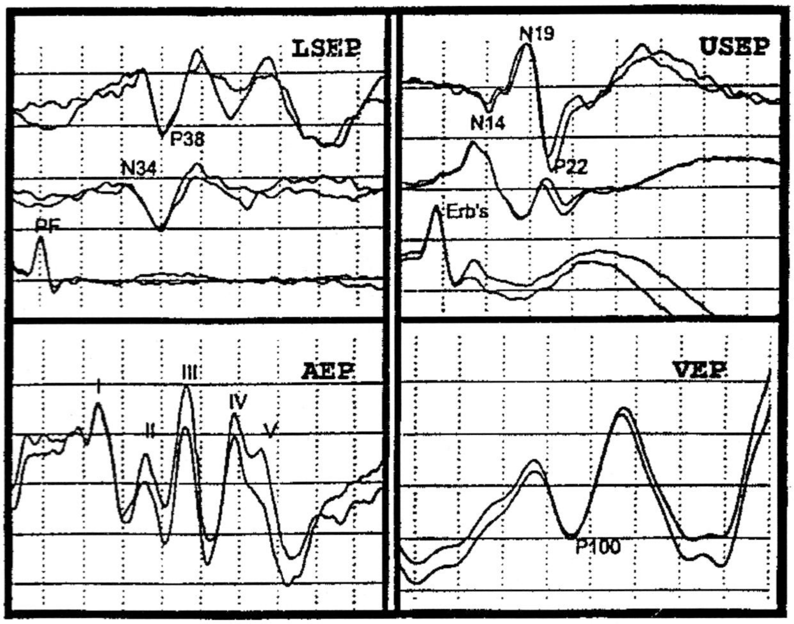

FIG. 6-1. Examples of normal visual evoked potential (VEP), somatosensory evoked potential (SSEP), and auditory evoked potential (AEP).

(5,6) describing the short latency auditory EP generated from cochlea, eighth nerve, and brainstem structures. Figure 6-1 provides an illustration of the visual, upper and lower extremity somatosensory, and auditory brainstem evoked potentials as they are typically displayed in current clinical practice.

This chapter presents a broad picture of intraoperative somatosensory evoked potential and cranial nerve monitoring, and emphasizes the role of the surgeon as the end-user of data supplied by the neurophysiologic monitor. In addition, intraoperative Doppler, a technique only recently introduced into the intraoperative arena of neurologic surgery, is explained. A loop system analogy is often helpful as an illustrative aid for describing the acquisition, interpretation, and application of neurophysiologic monitoring data in the operating room. To this end the focus here is on the importance of proper technique to acquire quality data, the interpretation of normal versus abnormal responses, the interaction of anesthetic agents with central and peripheral nervous system responses, and the applicability of monitoring to various neurosurgical cases.

ACQUISITION OF EVOKED POTENTIALS

Sensory evoked potentials recorded from the scalp have amplitudes of less than 100 nanovolts. For comparison, the EEG is measured in microvolts while the electrocardiogram is measured in millivolts (7). Consider that the operating room is filled with multiple sources of extraneous electrical "noise" emanating from electrocautery, anesthesia monitoring, fiberoptic light sources, etc. The challenge of acquiring such minute bioelectric signals in this busy electrical environment may be intimidating. Fortunately, instrumentation technology has grown in quality over the past decade, allowing the EP monitor to satisfactorily collect these signals using commercially available equipment at a reasonable cost. A caveat of successful monitoring and data collection is strict attention to detail such as preparation and application of stimulating and recording electrodes, proper amplifier gain and band pass, stimulus delivery rate, and rejection of artifact. Preoperative and intraoperative communication with the anesthesiologist is also critical. This section describes these interactive variables in greater detail.

The system required for collecting and analyzing EPs is based on a microprocessor. The various stimulation modalities (electrical shock, auditory click, visual flash) are controlled from the computer. The EP workstation is typically located 20 to 30 feet from the patient in the operating room, so appropriate extension cables are required for stimulus delivery (Fig. 6-2). The stimulus/patient interface requires bipolar, disposable 2 × 2 cm pregelled electrodes that are applied over the surface of the skin above a mixed nerve at either the wrist or the ankle with the cathode proximal and a 3-cm separation between the two electrodes for somatosensory evoked potential (SSEP).

Patient responses are collected using sterile needle electrodes that are inserted subdermally (NeuroSupplies, Inc., Waterford, CT) at sites that are appropriate for the far-field generators of the EP under study. These are typically referenced to cephalic electrode recording locations from the International 10-20 Nomenclature System. Bipolar electrode derivations are used with multiple recording sites for each component EP. An EP system must be capable of acquiring a minimum of four channels of activity, therefore the electrode leads (48-inch length) are led from the patient to an electrode "headbox." This interface connects patient electrodes to the analog-to-digital (A/D) converter of the computer. Some commercial systems currently integrate the A/D converter

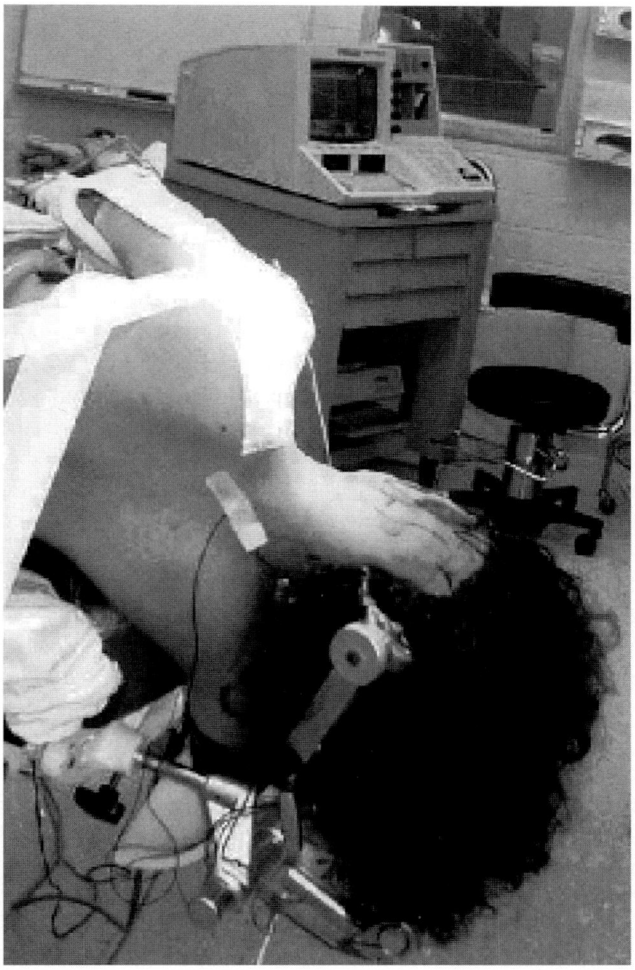

FIG. 6-2. Typical arrangement of intraoperative EP monitoring instrumentation.

within the electrode interface box. A single common ground (4 × 4 cm) plate electrode is attached in a proximal position on an extremity and connected to the interface box. As a cautionary note, only a single ground is placed on the patient, as multiple grounds create the possibility of a "ground loop," which is a patient safety hazard and must be avoided. A heavy, shielded cable feeds the signal back to the microprocessor for A/D conversion and band pass filtering following preamplification. The digitized signals are averaged and displayed on the screen for visual inspection. Information on EP status can be updated to the surgeon or anesthesiologist throughout the surgical case. Thus, the EP loop is completed.

A brief explanation of signal averaging is necessary, as it is directly relevant to the means and timing of information made available to the surgeon. Signal averaging is a common method of separating the desired signal from background noise. The number of epochs of data needed to be averaged is directly related to the original size of a single response and the size of the background noise. This may be expressed as:

$$\frac{S}{N} = \frac{1}{\sqrt{n}}$$

where S = signal (EP), and N = noise (EEG, electrical, EMG, etc.), and n = number of sweeps.

Thus, if the original signal is large amplitude and the background noise small, only a few (10 to 20) sweeps are required, allowing the monitor to update the response every 5 seconds. However, if the original signal is small and extraneous noise large, then 100, 500, or even 1,000 responses may have to be averaged, requiring several minutes instead of seconds to acquire an interpretable response.

The implication for the surgeon, then, is that careful and appropriate monitoring techniques will yield electrophysiologic information in a nearly real-time fashion, as opposed to poor quality data with excessive noise contamination. The difference between seconds and minutes in the notification of significant EP changes makes careful and consistent technique imperative.

ANESTHETIC EFFECTS ON NEUROELECTRIC ACTIVITY

General anesthetic agents alter cortical EPs by producing latency increase and amplitude decrease. The effects of most agents are additive, and the dose-related effects of inhaled anesthetics have been well documented (8–13). For example, nitrous oxide alone slightly depresses amplitude but has little effect on latency (12). Since changes in the EP relative to preoperative baseline may appear similar whether the cause is surgical or anesthetic, one needs to be able to differentiate between sources of alteration. Better still, the monitoring individual and anesthesiologist should plan in concert for an optimal anesthetic protocol that will produce the least EP alteration during the surgical case.

Cortically generated waves of SSEP are affected by the volatile inhalation anesthetics. Grundy (14) provides an excellent review of studies of the EP changes due to various minimal alveolar concentration (MAC) of halothane, enflurane, and isoflurane. Although there is considerable individual patient variation (due to age, general health, neuropathology, etc.) to end-tidal MACs, general patterns and subsequent guidelines are apparent. More than half of patients demonstrate SSEP cortical waveform decrement at 1.0% MAC of isoflurane with 60% nitrous oxide (NO_2), while all patients demonstrate severe alteration to complete abolition of cortical EPs at 2.0% MAC with 60% $N0_2$. These waveform alterations are most pronounced for tibial nerve SSEP and less for median nerve SSEP. Although effects of NO_2 are minimal, they are additive when combined, e.g., with isoflurane (15–17).

Inhalation anesthetics have little, if any, effect on brainstem components of SSEP (11,18,19). This interesting phenomenon regarding the brainstem response behaviors may presumably be related to that fact that fewer synapses are traversed than with cortical generators, and general anesthetics affect synaptic transmission to a larger extent than single nerve fiber transmission (14,20). Despite knowledge of the mechanisms of action of anesthetic agents on these synaptic transmissions, these observations indicate that brainstem EPs can be effectively monitored in conjunction with high-dose inhalation anesthesia.

Intravenous anesthetics affect cortical SSEP significantly less than do inhalation anesthetics. Narcotics such as fentanyl or sufentanil alter cortical SSEPs only in high doses, but responses can still be visualized (17,21,22). To our knowledge, there are no effects of narcotics on brainstem SSEP in human SSEP effects (10). Interestingly, bolus-administered fentanyl has a much greater effect on cortical EPs than does a steady-state infusion (23). We have recorded a number of cases in which a narcotic bolus suddenly reduced amplitude and shifted latency in a manner that mimicked a traumatic surgical event. Thus, we routinely request that the anesthesiologist notify the EP monitor of any bolus narcotic administration in excess of 5 cc. Barbiturates such as either thiopental or pentobarbital have little effect on cortical and no effect on subcortical SSEP (24). Reports indicate that SSEP can be adequately monitored in barbiturate-induced coma (25,26). Propofol, a relatively new intravenous anesthetic agent, has recently been studied for effects on SSEP and motor evoked potentials (15,27). Initial reports suggest that propofol with nitrous oxide has minimal latency shift/amplitude reduction effects on the SSEP and offers promise as an effective adjunct to neuroanesthesia.

Optimal anesthetic protocol in conjunction with EP monitoring then is the balanced technique of narcotic with nitrous oxide. Taniguchi et al. (27) proposed a total intravenous anesthesia to provide large amplitude median nerve cortical SSEP, which is extremely helpful in cerebrovascular surgeries. At the least, shared communication between the individual performing the monitoring and the anesthetist with a coordinated plan stressing safe and effective anesthesia with adequate EP signals will lead to the optimal protocol. While no single technique will perfectly satisfy each member of the neurosurgical team, compromise through common goals will usually provide for an effective neuromonitoring environment.

GENERATORS OF EVOKED POTENTIALS

A great deal of basic and clinical research has been applied to the task of localization of the anatomic generator sources of the far-field scalp-recorded EPs during the past 20 years. Various approaches have been employed to isolate neural structures believed responsible for specific EP components. These include electrode mapping, intra- and extracellular microelectrode recordings, ablation studies, surgical-electrophysiologic correlation with known pathology intraoperatively, and postmortem studies. Understanding the neural generator of a specific EP provides the neurosurgeon a neuroanatomic basis for preoperative planning and intraoperative decision making for the utilization of various EP monitoring techniques. There are three components of the SSEP: peripheral, subcortical, and cortical. The sources of surface-recorded SSEP are well documented for peripheral components, namely, the brachial plexus volley and the tibial nerve propagated volley. The N10 component from median or ulnar nerve stimulation occurs between sensory depolarization at the axilla and arrival of the volley at the brachial plexus (1). This large amplitude wave represents the final response from the peripheral nervous system and is often referred to as the Erb's point potential, owing to the electrode recording site at the supraclavicular fossa used to optimally visualize this brachial plexus component. The propagated volley recorded at the popliteal fossa following stimulation of the posterior tibial nerve at the ankle is generated in the same manner as other sensory nerve conduction velocity measurements. Both of these EP components are examples of propagated action potential waveforms. Peripheral and spinal volleys differ significantly from waveforms arising from stationary intracranial generators. The salient difference is that latency of response for a propagated volley will vary depending on the proximity of recording electrodes to stimulus onset, while latency of a generator potential is invariable with respect to proximity and stimulus onset.

The subcortical component of the SSEP recorded from the posterior neck referenced to forehead is visualized at 13 to 14 msec for median and 29 to 34 msec for posterior tibial stimulation. This stationary potential is most likely generated in the medial lemniscus (1,28,29) or just caudal to this structure (30). There is high probability that the brainstem wave seen in bipolar scalp recordings is a composite of multiple generator sources between the foramen magnum and the ventrobasal thalamus (31).

The cortical components of median and tibial SSEP are of maximal amplitude at locations C4′, CZ′, and C3′ referenced to Fz. All electrode locations follow the international 10–20 system of nomenclature. These responses at 20 msec (median) and 40 msec (posterior tibial) operate in a manner consistent with functional dipoles situated in the postrolandic gyrus at Brodmann's area 3 (28) and the leg and foot area on the mesial aspect of the postcentral gyrus (31), respectively. These are the primary cortex-generated components of SSEP and are robust despite general anesthesia, as previously mentioned. These generator sites lie within perfusion fields supplied from middle cerebral artery (median SSEP) and anterior circulation to midline (tibial SSEP). Cerebrovascular/SSEP correlates have been investigated most notably by Symon et al. (32,33) and others and have useful implications for SSEP monitoring in aneurysm and arteriovenous malformation (AVM) surgery (see below).

A summary of the generator sites for primary peak components of SSEP is presented in Table 6-1. We do not assume that these anatomic locations represent the sole and complete source of generation; however, the tabular summary is as complete and accurate as our present review can be. The reader should refer to Table 6-1 as a guide when considering intraoperative monitoring anatomic pathways relevant to specific neurosurgical applications.

TABLE 6–1. *Generator sights for primary peak components of somatosensory evoked potentials (SSEPs)*

Lower SSEP	Upper SSEP
N9—tibial nerve	N10—brachial plexus
N13—lateral lemniscus	N14—lateral lemniscus
P38—cortex	N19—cortex
N45—cortex	P22—cortex

SSEP MONITORING IN CEREBROVASCULAR

A wealth of data has been published and the authors have extensive experience monitoring cerebrovascular procedures that may help explain the dynamics of monitoring changes in skull base surgery. Branston et al. (34) first noted a causal relationship between cortical SSEP and local cerebral blood flow during middle cerebral artery occlusion in the baboon. Subsequent studies related the application of SSEP and auditory evoked potential (AEP) monitoring to patients undergoing temporary and/or permanent arterial occlusion (32,35–39).

The SSEP is sensitive to changes in neural pathways resulting from hypoperfusion. Median SSEP has been most effective with middle cerebral artery distributions, while tibial SSEP has been more specific to anterior cerebral artery territories. Little et al. (7) reported false negatives (failure to identify ischemic events) in 4 of 16 patients undergoing basilar aneurysm clipping using AEP and SSEP. Schramm et al. (38) noted more sensitivity of SSEP to changes and eventual neurologic outcome in basilar tip aneurysm. They noted that in aneurysms involving the posterior circulation, the surgeon should be very concerned if SSEPs disappear, but not feel confident if SSEPs persist. Symon et al. (33) reported that median SSEPs were helpful during temporary occlusion prior to ablation of feeding vessels to AVMs.

Various criteria for observed SSEP changes consequent to cerebral hypoperfusion during surgery have been described. Wang et al. (40) described central conduction time (CCT) as being the time required for the SSEP signal to travel from the lateral lemniscus to the primary sensory cortex and expressed as the difference, in milliseconds, between the cortex (N20 peak) and brainstem (N14 peak). The authors proposed use of this conduction time to measure cortical SSEP changes in aneurysmal subarachnoid hemorrhage (SAH) (40). Symon et al. (32) first proposed this measure based on studies of SAH where CCT delays correlated with clinical outcome. Further intraoperative studies of CCT confirmed the usefulness of this SSEP technique (39). Friedman et al. (35) applied CCT monitoring to a series of patients who underwent cerebrovascular surgery requiring temporary and/or permanent vascular occlusion. They concluded that amplitude decreases as well as subtle morphologic changes to the cortical N20 waveform, in conjunction with CCT calculations, provided an even more sensitive method of recognizing neuroelectric alteration following clipping. Taniguchii et al. (27) further report that anesthetic protocols that allow for identification of the second cortical SSEP peak (N27) provide even greater sensitivity to the effects of cerebrovascular ischemia on neuroelectric response.

In summary, EPs may be used as a monitor of cerebral perfusion by recording the neuroelectric response. Care must be taken to apply the appropriate EP for anatomic correlation with the region of possible disruption of cerebral blood flow. The following case description with SSEP waveforms (Fig. 6-3) is illustrative of the results of posterior tibial nerve response change during clipping of a basilar artery bifurcation aneurysm and the time course of recovery of SSEP to normal. The surgeon was able to successfully reposition the aneurysm clip to occlude the aneurysm without SSEP change. The patient had no permanent postoperative deficit. The surgeon would not have altered his clip position had EPs not been monitored.

In our experience, the value of SSEP monitoring in skull base surgery falls into three distinct areas. The first is during the positioning stage of surgery. We have found changes in the evoked potentials due to lateral or modified lateral positioning of patients prior to incision. The change is unilateral and can involve the arm in either the lateral up or lateral down position. A shift of 1.5 to 3 msec of the N10 or brachial plexus response and all subsequent waves is readily apparent. This situation is easily remedied by adjusting the involved arm. Typically, the response returns to normal levels within 1 to 5 minutes. This situation must be addressed immediately, otherwise a potential brachial plexopathy will develop given the extended length of these surgeries.

The second area where we see changes in the SSEP is in the brainstem or N14 response. This signal complements the auditory evoked potential with information from a different pathway through the brainstem. Changes in the somatosensory brainstem response can either be diminished amplitude or prolonged latency. Changes in the brainstem response cannot occur without concurrent changes in the later cortical waves. Desynchronization at the brainstem level can cause severe amplitude or latency changes of the cortical response or total abolition of the same. In most cases brainstem changes are due to compression caused by surgical retractors. When brainstem changes occur, the retractors should be immediately adjusted or removed. Our experience indicates that the brainstem response will return to baseline values within 3 to 6 minutes. A distinguishing factor of retraction-induced brainstem changes is the relatively gradual onset and progressive nature of the SSEP changes.

More immediate and profound brainstem changes can occur with surgical brainstem trauma and ischemic insults. The immediate and often total abolition of the brainstem and later waves gives the distinguishing feature of these types of lesions. Recovery of the brainstem and cortical response following traumatic or vascular insult has nonspecific but positive predictive value. Nonrecovery of the brainstem or cortical response suggests a potentially catastrophic outcome.

Cortical changes without alteration of the peripheral and

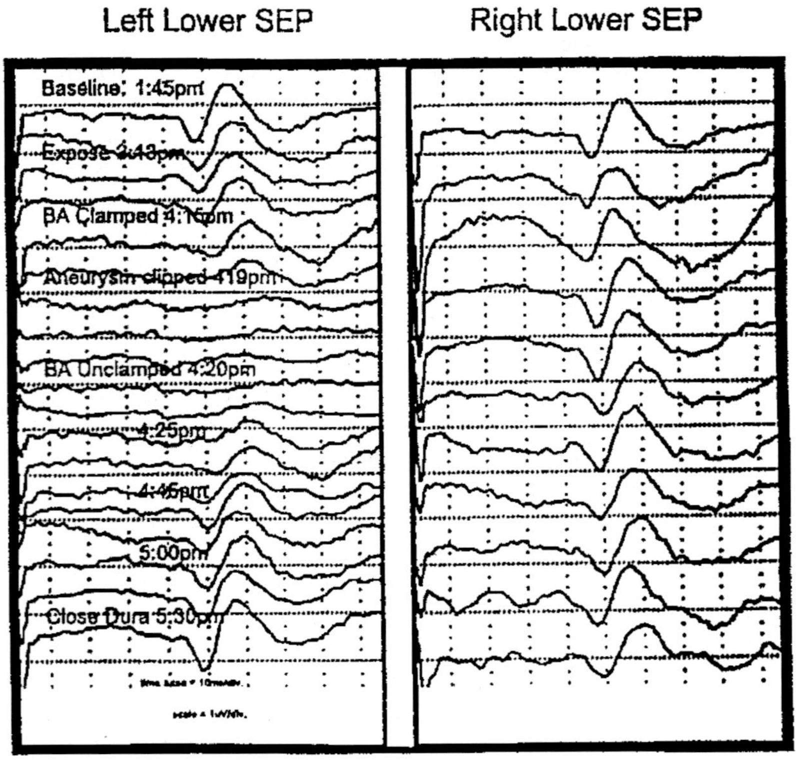

FIG. 6-3. SSEP monitoring changes following aneurysm clipping.

brainstem responses are often confounding and provide little predictive value other than those instances when the cortical responses are lost completely and do not recover. We believe that the majority of pure cortical deficits relate to ischemic changes due to surgical manipulation, such as retraction, vessel oblation, and vessel compression, or relate to infarct due to brain tissue expansion following large tumor excision. There are limited published data on outcomes following cortical changes during skull base surgery. However, our own experience and that of others during aneurysm clipping surgeries suggests a similar process. We can consistently say, however, that complete loss of the lower extremity SSEP response with or without loss of the upper extremity response will result in a poor neurologic outcome—typically hemiplegia.

INTRAOPERATIVE CRANIAL NERVE MONITORING

Surgical procedures of the cranial base often place one or more of the cranial nerves at risk particularly when in the cerebellopontine angle and the areas of the cavernous and sphenoidal sinuses, jugular foramen, and foramen magnum. Conditions in these areas that may require neurosurgical intervention include entities such as tumors, aneurysms, adenomas, and microvascular compression.

Cranial nerves can be purely afferent (olfactory, optic, and vestibulocochlear), or efferent (oculomotor, abducens, accessory, and hypoglossal). But many are mixed, providing both sensory and motor innervations (trigeminal, facial, glossopharyngeal, and vagus) (41). The auditory branch of the vestibulocochlear nerve is routinely monitored utilizing brainstem evoked potentials and is discussed elsewhere in this volume. ENMG techniques can only be used intraoperatively to preserve neural function of a cranial nerve if the nerve innervates a muscle and is accessible to the clinician. Of the 12 cranial nerves, nine can be monitored intraoperatively.

ENMG assesses lower motor neuron (LMN) tracts from the brainstem to their peripheral innervations (42). Any damage to these LMNs or their axons results in an LMN lesion that can include complete paralysis, loss of muscle tone, loss of tendon reflexes, and rapid atrophy and fasciculation of the innervated muscle. Cranial nerves carry three distinct modalities in the motor realm: somatic motor (which innervate muscles that develop from somites); branchial motor (which innervate muscles that develop from the branchial arches); and visceral motor (which innervate the viscera, including glands and all smooth muscle). Cranial nerves that innervate muscles that arise from somites and from the branchial arches are suitable for ENMG assessment and monitoring may include cranial nerves III, IV, V, VI, VII, IX, X, XI, and XII.

Cranial nerve ENMG monitoring records electrical potentials generated by the muscle that the nerve innervates by utilizing the muscle as an amplifier of the neural activity. The fundamental unit of ENMG activity is the motor unit action potential (MUAP), which is the result of electrical activity in the muscle when it is activated from a single motor neuron. The number of muscle fibers activated by a single motor neuron varies widely from one muscle group to another and can significantly affect the sensitivity and potential benefit of intraoperative monitoring. In theory, small highly coordinated muscles performing very fine movements can contain as few as three fibers per unit, whereas larger gross activity muscles may contain as many as 2,000 fibers per unit. The myogenic electricity generated from the same amount of nerve activation may increase as the ratio of muscle fibers to motor unit increases. In all instances the electrical display of the action potential is representative of the summated discharge of many fibers.

When a normal muscle is at rest, there should be electrical silence; hence, quiet ENMG recordings. However, potentials from many sources are present in the surgical theater—physiologic and artifactual. It is not uncommon to encounter spontaneous muscle activity such as muscle fibrillations, positive sharp waves, and high-frequency discharges. Electrical noise from various lighting sources and medical equipment, interference from nerve stimulators and electrocautery, and movement artifact can limit the benefit of monitoring if not recognized and properly managed. The monitor and surgeon are only interested in what have been termed *neurotonic discharges*, potentials that are the result of mechanical or metabolic irritation of the nerve (43). Therefore, they must be able to determine what information is important within the context of the particular surgical manipulation.

Neurotonic is a clinical needle electromyography (EMG) term that is somewhat of a misnomer when used to describe muscle potentials evoked during surgery, since the response observed results from the examiner's monopolar needle contacting the nerve supplying the muscle under investigation (44). The responses seen intraoperatively during cranial nerve monitoring may or may not be neurologic in origin, and it is unlikely that the type of recording electrodes used would come in contact with the nerve. Møller and Jannetta (45) classified these same responses as injury potentials even though there has been little evidence that such activity necessarily results in damage to the nerve.

Prass and Luders (46) proposed that the more descriptive generic term *evoked electromyographic activity* be adopted and subclassified as either nonrepetitive or repetitive. Nonrepetitive activity generally provides more useful information for the surgeon as to causative effects. ENMG responses to specific mechanical and electrical stimulation of the nerve can be invaluable in identifying it and determining its location and course. However, persistent repetitive responses may represent established or developing nerve damage that might affect the surgeon's technique.

A compound muscle action potential (CMAP) is the composite electrical response from a muscle to the rapid synchronous depolarization of its innervating nerve bundle (42). The integrity of motor axons can be tested directly by stimulating the nerve in the surgical field and recording the CMAP from the muscle. Activating an exposed cranial nerve requires minimal electrical stimulation (≤0.1 mA) (47–50).

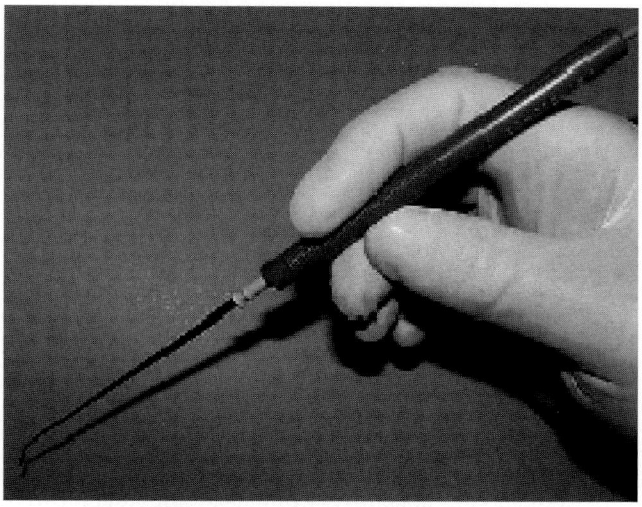

FIG. 6-4. Photograph of monopolar probe stimulator.

Using a handheld microstimulator as illustrated in Fig. 6-4, the surgeon can probe the surgical site to objectively identify the nerve(s) in question from surrounding tissue. Segmental stimulation may help to identify axonal damage. It is also possible to obtain useful prognostic information about postsurgical nerve damage when pre- and posttreatment recording can be acquired proximal and distal to the operative site.

Instrumentation

Most good-quality commercially available EMG machines that meet the electrical safety standards required in the operating room environment can be used for monitoring of the cranial nerves. Often, EMG capability is incorporated into evoked potential instrumentation already being used for recording auditory, visual, and somatosensory EPs. They generally provide the appropriate time base, band pass filter adjustments, and amplifier characteristic for recording EMG signals. Two channels of data acquisition are minimally satisfactory but multiple channels (up to eight) are desirable. The instrument should be capable of clearly displaying all of the channels simultaneously for easy identification of the muscle activated. Event capture and rapid magnetic storage and retrieval capability are useful for review and documentation purposes. Two items that will likely require modification are the audio feedback speaker and the electrical stimulation source.

The loudspeaker provides direct auditory feedback to the operating surgeon, who, with experience, is able to immediately discriminate useful information about the nerve in question. There is no time delay between the surgical event and the instrument response, and there is seldom need for interpretation by the monitoring individual. Appropriate integration of this information permits timely modification of surgical technique, often reducing the risk of permanent neural damage.

Delivering a safe, appropriate level of electrical stimulation requires a second modification to almost all available EMG instrumentation. Specifically, the stimulator should produce a constant voltage electrical signal with a variable pulse width at low voltage levels that can be precisely adjusted between 0 and 1 V, in 0.1V or smaller steps. Intact cranial nerve thresholds range from 0.05V to 0.2V, whereas the compromised nerve may require a voltage level as high as 1 V for activation. A signal pulse width of 100 μsec to 200 μsec is satisfactory in either case (47–50). When stimulating through bone or other tissue in an attempt to locate a particular nerve, stimulation levels up to 10 V may be required.

Battery-operated constant current stimulation has also been used successfully and incorporated into some dedicated cranial nerve monitoring equipment. Again, discrete low-level stimulation capability is critically important. Direct cranial nerve stimulation should not exceed 0.2 mA. A healthy nerve will respond to 0.05-mA stimulation at a rate of four pulses per second and a 100-sec pulse width (50).

Both monopolar and bipolar probes have been used to apply electrical stimulation within the surgical wound either directly to the nerve or to the surrounding tissue. Bipolar stimulators possess the advantage of minimizing current spread throughout adjacent nerves that produces responses that may be incorrectly interpreted. The disadvantage of most bipolar stimulators is current shunting caused by pooling of blood and spinal fluid. If the wound is kept reasonably dry, any appropriately sized bipolar probe yields satisfactory results. A small diameter coaxial bipolar stimulator has been designed that eliminates most problems associated with current shunting by separating, with insulation, concentric anode and cathode rings (47,51).

Various recording electrodes can be successfully employed during intraoperative ENMG monitoring. Typically, 1-cm, 26-gauge subdermal EEG paired electrodes are utilized to detect the electromyographic potentials. These needles are inserted into the belly of the studied muscle, parallel, approximately 2 cm apart, ensuring their tips do not come into contact. If placed on the skin, they can be carefully secured with tape. Small paired EEG disk electrodes applied over the muscle with electrode gel and taped can also be used to record the CMAPs, but additional artifacts may be introduced if the disks shift or as the electrolyte gel dries. Surface electrodes are also more likely to be dislodged during the monitoring. Where electrode placement is difficult, such as in the tongue, pharynx, and larynx, paired hook-wire electrodes may be considered (43). They can be fashioned out of thin-gauged Teflon-coated wire. The recording end is stripped and hooked while a standard ⅛-inch jack is attached to the opposite end for insertion into the preamplifier of the EMG machine. Placement is accomplished by threading the hooked end of the electrode into the tip of a hypodermic needle and then inserting the needle and electrode into the muscle (44).

More attention has been directed toward maintaining the integrity of the facial nerve (VII) than any other cranial nerve (47,51–55). Dating as far back as 1898, a variety of techniques have been developed to intraoperatively monitor facial nerve function (56,57). In 1979, Delgado et al. (58) were the first to use EMG recording during cerebellopontine angle surgery. Sugita et al. (59) introduced the loudspeaker to provide acoustic feedback even though they recorded facial activity with motion detectors. In 1986, Prass and Luders (46) correlated specific patterns of EMG activity to surgical manipulations and described what is probably the most universally used facial nerve monitoring technique currently. Of equal importance, their techniques can be applied either directly or indirectly to the intraoperative monitoring of every cranial motor nerve.

Intramuscular subdermal or hook-wire electrodes are inserted in bipolar pairs into the superior-lateral area of the orbicularis oculi and in the orbicularis oris at the nasolabial fold on the operative side. Two needle electrodes are placed in the forehead—one to serve as a ground, the other as a return (anode) if a monopolar stimulator is used. Additional recording sites innervated by the facial nerve can be utilized to improve sensitivity, or at a noninnervated site such as the contralateral side to service as a control measure if more recording channels are available (51,60,61).

Trigeminal nerve (V) motor function and spinal accessory nerve (XI) ENMG monitoring can be accomplished similarly to that for the facial nerve. Cranial nerve V supplies motor function to the muscles of mastication—the tensor tympani, tensor palatini, mylohyoid, and the anterior belly of the digastric. CMAP responses can be recorded from paired bipolar electrodes placed in the temporalis and masseter muscles. A ground electrode is placed in the forehead. Cranial nerve XI is branchial motor, supplying function to the sternomastoid and trapezius muscles. Both of these muscles are easily accessible, and electrode choice is based on preference. Again, a ground electrode is place in or on the forehead.

Recording from the extraocular muscles can be monitored to help identify the trochlear nerve (IV), which innervates the superior oblique muscle; the abducens (VI), the lateral rectus muscle; and the oculomotor nerve (III) and all other extraocular muscles. Satisfactory recordings from these muscles using fine platinum needles percutaneously placed near the muscle have been reported by Møller (45,62). The method of choice, however, is to place paired hook-wire electrodes directly into the muscle.

Intraoperative monitoring of the glossopharyngeal (IX), vagus (X), and hypoglossal (XII) nerves is rare and requires extreme care and skill to successfully position the thin hooked-wire electrodes. The stylopharyngeus muscle is deep in the pharynx and difficult to locate due to its size and proximity to the other pharyngeal muscles. It is nearly impossible to determine correct placement and maintenance of electrode integrity is difficult.

The vagus and hypoglossal nerves are often grouped for cranial nerve monitoring purposes. Insertion of the hooked-wire recording electrodes into the cricothyroid of the vocalis muscles (vagus nerve) is accomplished using direct laryn-

TABLE 6–2. *Suitable recording electrodes*

Cranial nerve	Choice innervated muscle(s)	Choice recording electrodes
Oculomotor (III)	Superior rectus, medial rectus, inferior rectus, and inferior oblique	Hooked wire
Trochlear (IV)	Superior oblique	Hooked wire
Trigeminal (VI)	Masseter	Hooked wire or paired subdermal
Abducens (VI)	Lateral rectus	Hooked wire
Facial (VII)	Frontalis, orbicularis oculi, and orbicularis oris	Hooked wire, paired subdermal, or surface disk
Glossopharyngeal (IX)	Stylopharyngeous	Hooked wire
Vagus (X)	Cricothyroid and vocalis	Hooked wire or endotrachial tube
Accessory (XI)	Sternomastoid and trapezius	Hooked wire or paired subdermal
Hypoglossal (XII)	Genioglossus, styloglossus, and hypoglossus	Hooked wire

goscopy through the mouth or needle puncture through the skin of the neck and the cricothyroid membrane (43,62–65). An experienced otolaryngologist should perform this task to avoid possible vocal cord paralysis. In recent years we have abandoned the use of needles for cranial nerve X monitoring. We now use a specially designed endotracheal tube equipped with bipolar exposed wire electrodes on either side for direct contact with the vocal folds (Xomed-Treace, Jacksonville, FL). This eliminates the need of an otolaryngologist for electrode placement and the risk of iatrogenic injury. There is no greater risk inserting this special tube than there is with a standard endotracheal tube. The muscles innervated by cranial nerve XII (genioglossus, styloglossus, and hypoglossus) are easily accessible through the mouth into the posterior pharyngeal wall (Table 6-2).

General anesthetic agents do not adversely affect the ENMG response during intraoperative cranial nerve monitoring. Neuromuscular blocking agents must be avoided, however, so that the CMAP is not obliterated. This requirement can cause practical problems during delicate microsurgeries when attempting to acquire SSEP simultaneously. Applying electrical stimulation to the extremities can cause significant patient movement and thus potential interference to the surgeon and risk to the patient. The surgeon must weigh the benefit of monitoring multiple modalities against the inconvenience and risk of patient movement. The surgeon must also be warned whenever SSEP stimulation is pending.

MICRO-DOPPLER SONOGRAPHY

The Doppler effect is a wave theory that describes the change in frequency of a sound wave when the transmitter, the receiver, and the reflecting object move in relation to one another. Austrian physicist Christian Doppler (66) first reported this phenomenon as it relates to moving objects at the Royal Bohemian Society of Science in Prague in 1842. We experience the Doppler effect when listening to the change in tone (frequency) of a train whistle as the train approaches, passes by us, and proceeds down the track. Changes in the frequency of the sound wave relate to movement of the sound source, the listener or sensor, and the reflecting object, one to another. This frequency change is proportional to the velocity of the movement. When we apply this theory to human blood flow through vessels, the frequency shift produced by red blood cells traveling past an ultrasound microprobe is described in the following formula:

$$F = \frac{2Fo \cdot v \cdot cosa}{C}$$

where F = the Doppler frequency, Fo = the frequency of the transmitted ultrasound, v = the blood flow velocity, $cosa$ = the angle between the transmitted sound beam and the direction of the blood flow and C = the velocity of sound in the tissue (67). The Doppler effect is the difference in frequency of transmitted sound waves and received sound waves and is proportional to the blood flow velocity (68). It is within the audible range and, with the aid of spectrum analysis, can be visualized to show waveform characteristics such as flow direction and velocity (cm/sec).

Doppler sonography has been used in medicine for many years and is now a tool for virtually all specialties including radiology, cardiology, neurology, urology, obstetrics, and surgery. Early Doppler instrumentation utilized continuous wave ultrasound signals with probes in the 4- to 9-MHz frequency range, which were effective for measuring blood flow in peripheral limb arteries. Development of pulsed wave signal presentation and lower frequency probes (1–2 MHz) allowed investigators to delve into the skull to measure intracerebral vessels, particularly those in the circle of Willis. These two enabling technical advances provided for precise depth of insonation and permitted penetration through thin segments (windows) of the developed skull.

In 1965, Miyazaki and Kato (69) were the first to investigate cerebral hemodynamics using Doppler sonography by recording blood flow velocity in extracranial arteries supplying the brain. In 1979, Nornes et al. (70,71) published two articles of their pioneering work in the *Journal of Neurosurgery* reporting Doppler sonography recording taken intraoperatively during AVM and aneurysm surgeries. Two years later, the first transcranial (TCD) recordings of intracerebral vessels were made by Rune Aaslid in his laboratory. The primary focus of his work was assessment of vasospasm following subarachnoid hemorrhage (72). The work of Aas-

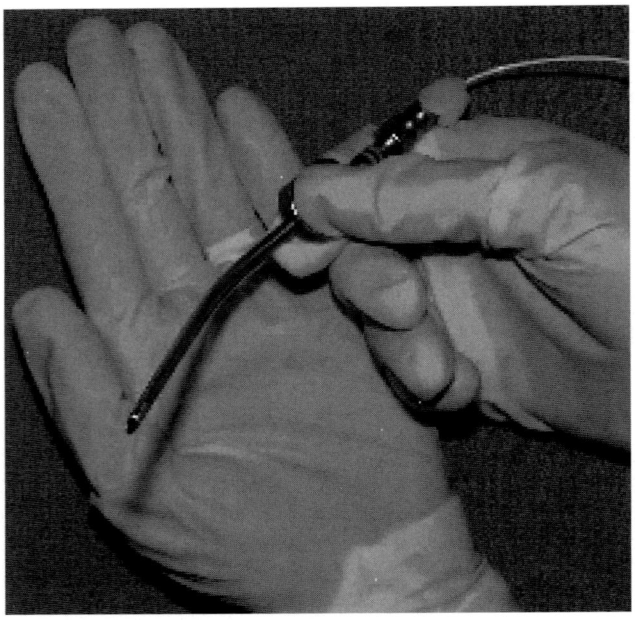

FIG. 6-5. Photographs of 1-mm, 20-MHz Doppler probe in suction tip.

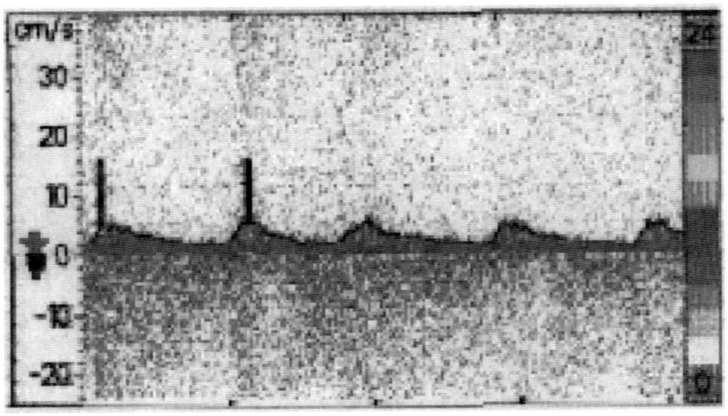

FIG. 6-7. Doppler recording of vessel of Hubner.

lid and his colleagues led to the development of the first small and simple, microprocessor-controlled clinical Doppler instrument with digital output and video display, which greatly facilitated the use of this technique for monitoring of cerebral hemodynamics (TCD-64, Medical Electronics, Uberlingen, Germany).

The most significant advancement for neurologic surgery application of Doppler sonography was put forward by German neurosurgeon Joachim Michael Gilsbach (68) in his now classic monograph published in 1983. He used a prototype pulsed Doppler ultrasound instrument with one of the first developed 20-MHz transmission frequency probes during neurosurgical procedures for microvascular anastomoses, bypass, and aneurysms. The small probe diameter (2–3 mm) was well suited for use deep inside the subarachnoid space, and the ultrahigh probe frequency was ideal for small vessel investigation.

Microvascular Doppler sonography instruments are commercially available from several manufacturers today. Most of these units are multiple probe frequency capable, usually supplied with 2-MHz, 4-MHz, 8-MHz, and 16- or 20-MHz transducers. Microvascular probes can be sterilized and reused, and are available in 1-mm, 2-mm, and 3-mm tip diameters. We have found the 1-mm probe to be best suited for intracranial applications. For the surgeon's convenience, the probe is passed through an appropriately sized suction tip and secured at the base with bone wax. For direct intracerebral vessel insonation, recording parameters are rarely altered from the following: depth = 1 mm, sample volume = 0.5 mm, and power <20% (Fig. 6-5).

At our institution, microvascular Doppler sonography has become the preferred method for evaluating pre- and postaneurysm clipping patency of parent vessel and branching arteries, including small perforators (Figs. 6-6 to 6-8).

With exception of those vessels that are inaccessible to direct or optimal probe placement (angle of insonation between 40 and 60 degrees), microvascular Doppler is reliable and effective, and can, in certain instances, replace intraoperative angiography during the surgical treatment of aneurysms (73).

Another useful application of microvascular Doppler is during extracranial-intracranial bypass for occlusions and stenoses of the cervical or cavernous internal carotid artery, and giant aneurysms of the cavernous carotid artery (67). The donor superficial temporal artery can be identified and its path mapped by transcutaneous insonation. Depth of insonation should be between 1.4 mm and 1.8 mm with a sample

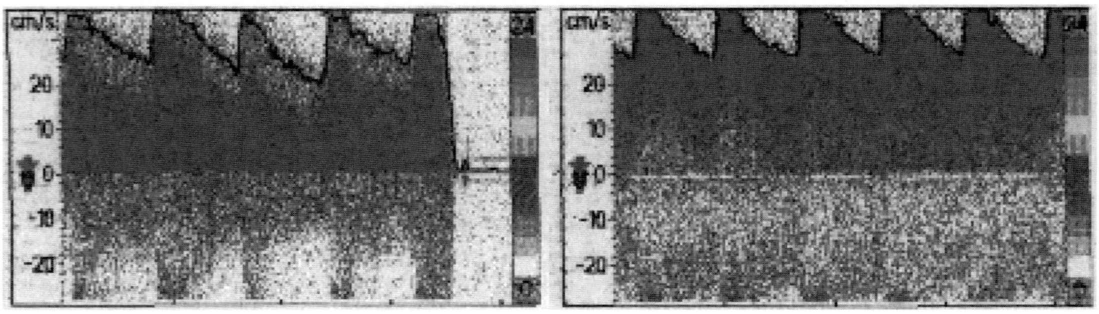

FIG. 6-6. Doppler waveform of parent vessel, pre- and postclip.

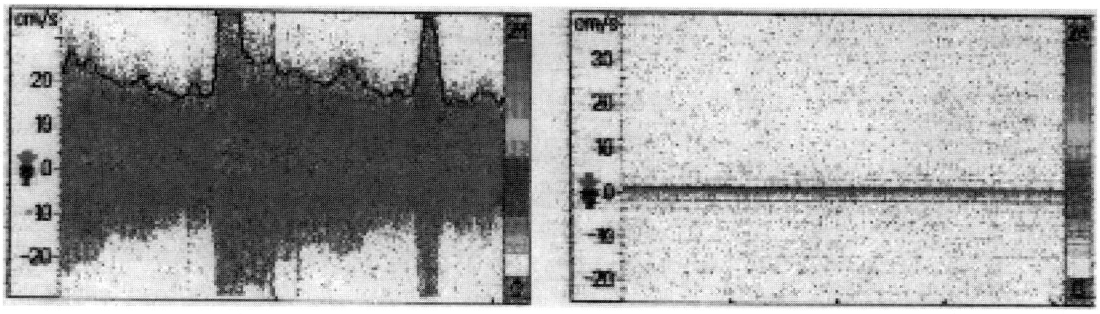

FIG. 6-8. Doppler recording of aneurysm dome, pre- and postaneurysm clipping.

volume of 0.5 mm and a power setting of 20% to 35%. Once the bypass is completed, the entire length to the donor vessel needs to be examined for consistent patency and flow using the same instrument parameter described earlier for aneurysm surgery. Careful attention should be paid to both anastomotic sites for possible occlusions and areas of stenosis (Fig. 6-9).

Microvascular Doppler is a safe, reliable, and effective tool for direct intraoperative measurement and recording of blood flow velocities of intracranial vessel. It is used primarily during aneurysm surgeries to assess blood flow before and after clipping, but can also be helpful in locating arteries and veins, determining the direction of blood flow within a vessel, and assessing vessel anastomosis and bypasses.

CONCLUSION

As evidenced in this review, current technique and knowledge allow for extensive intraoperative neurophysiologic monitoring. Nevertheless there are philosophical differences over the need for monitoring and its practical application in routine neurosurgical practice. In addition, the cost/benefit ratio of monitoring has come into question.

The primary goals of intraoperative monitoring are to facilitate the neurosurgical procedure and ultimately reduce the neurologic risks. The available literature indicates that both goals can be reliably accomplished as long as there is cooperation among the surgical, anesthesia, and monitoring teams. Utilization of electrophysiologic changes as an early warning system allows for constant reassessment of surgical technique and objectives since anatomic preservation does not necessarily ensure functional integrity.

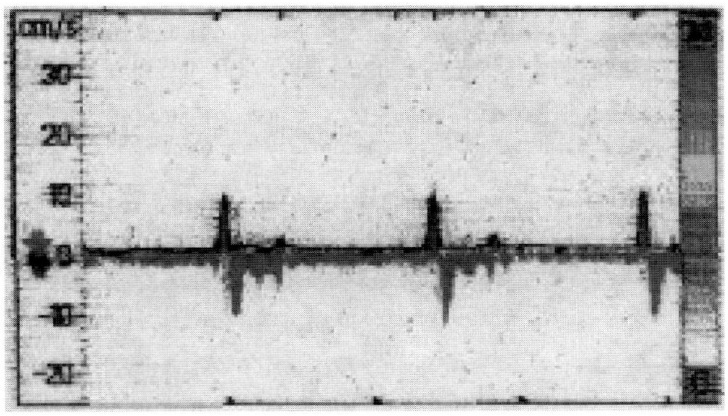

FIG. 6-9. Doppler of stenoic vessel.

The application of intraoperative neurophysiologic monitoring on a selective basis as part of an overall neurosurgical management schema will likely assume increasing importance in the future. The choice of monitoring modality, quality of ongoing data collection, collaboration with the anesthesiologist, and timely, accurate interpretation of neuroelectric and hemodynamic events are the key elements of successful monitoring. When considering surgery of the cranial base, these elements combine into a valuable adjunct to the reduction of postoperative neurologic morbidity.

REFERENCES

1. Desmet JE, Cheron G. Prevertebral (esophageal) recording of subcortical somatosensory evoked potentials in man: the spinal P13 component and the dual nature of the spinal generators. *Electroencephalogr Clin Neurophysiol* 1981;52:257–275.
2. Dawson GD. Investigation on a patient subject to myoclonic seizures after sensory stimulation. *J Neurol Neurosurg Psychiatry* 1947;10: 134–140.
3. Van Der Tweel LH, Spekreijse H. Visual evoked responses. *Iscerg Symp Ghent* 1966;83–94.
4. Davis PA. The electrical response of the human brain to auditory stimuli. *Am J Physiol* 1939;126:475–476.
5. Jewett DL. Volume-conducted potentials in response to auditory stimuli as detected by averaging in the cat. *Electroencephalogr Clin Neurophysiol* 1970;28:609–618.
6. Jewett DL, Williston JS. Auditory evoked far-fields averaged from the scalp of humans. *Brain* 1971;94:681–696.
7. Little JR, Lesser R, Luders H. Electrophysiological monitoring during basilar aneurysm operation. *Neurosurgery* 1987;421–427.
8. Pathak KS, Amaddio MD, Scoles PV, Shaffer JW, Mackay W. Effects of halothane, enflurane, and isoflurane in nitrous oxide on multilevel somatosensory evoked potentials. *Anesthesiology* 1989;70:207–212.
9. Salzman SK, Beckman AL, Marks HG, Naidu R, Bunnell WP, Macewen GD. Effects of halothane on intraoperative scalp-recorded somatosensory evoked potentials to posterior tibial nerve stimulation in man. *Electroencephalogr Clin Neurophysiol* 1986;65:36.
10. Samra SK, Krutak-Krol H, Pohorecki R, Domino EF. Scopolamine, morphine, and brain stem auditory evoked potentials in awake monkeys. *Anesthesiology* 62:437–441.
11. Samra SK, Vanderzant CW, Domer PA, Sackellares JC. Differential effects of isoflurane on human median nerve somatosensory evoked potentials in humans. *Anesthesiology* 1986;66:29–35.
12. Sebel PS, Flynn PJ, Ingram DA. Effect of nitrous oxide on visual, auditory, and somatosensory evoked potentials. *Br J Anaesth* 1984;56: 1403–1407.

13. Wolfe DE, Drummond JC. Differential effects of isoflurane/nitrous oxide on posterior tibial somatosensory evoked responses of cortical and subcortical origin. *Anesth Analgesia* 1988;67:852–859.
14. Grundy BL. Effects of anesthesia and hypothermia [lecture]. University of Florida College of Medicine, 1989.
15. Jellinek D, Jewkes D, Symon L. Noninvasive intraoperative monitoring of motor evoked potentials under propofol anesthesia: effects of spinal surgery on the amplitude and latency of motor evoked potentials. *Neurosurgery* 1991;29:551–557.
16. Kalkman CJ, Traast H, Zuurmond WA, Bovill JG. Differential effects of propofol and nitrous oxide on posterior tibial nerve somatosensory cortical evoked potentials during alfentanil anesthesia. *J Anesthesia* 1991;483–489.
17. Peterson DO, Drummond JC, Todd MM. Effects of halothane, enflurane, isoflurane, and nitrous oxide on somatosensory evoked potentials in humans. *Anesthesiology* 1986;65:35–40.
18. Manninen PH, Lam AM, Nicholas JF. The effects of isoflurane and isoflurane-nitrous oxide anesthesia on brain stem evoked potentials in humans. *Anesth Analg* 1985;64:43–47.
19. Thornton C, Heneghan PH, James PFM, Jones JG. Effects of halothane or enflurane with controlled ventilation on auditory evoked potentials. *Br J Anaesth* 1985;56:315–323.
20. Ueda I, Kamaya H. Molecular mechanisms of anesthesia. *Anesth Analg* 1984;63:929.
21. McPherson RW, Sell B, Traystman RJ. Effects of thiopental, fentanyl, and etomidate on upper extremity somatosensory evoked potentials in humans. *Anesthesiology* 1986;65:584–589.
22. Schubert A, Drummond JC, Peterson DO, Saidman LJ. The effect of high-dose fentanyl on human median nerve somatosensory-evoked responses. *Can J Anaesth* 1987;34:35–40.
23. Bird J, Donegan J, Rupp S, White P, Sessler D. Effects of sufentanil bolus and two steady state infusions on median nerve evoked potentials. *Anesthesiology* 1986;65:A341.
24. Koht A, Schutz W, Schmidt G, Schramm J, Watanabe E. Effects of etomidate, medazolam, and thiopental on median nerve somatosensory evoked potentials and the additive effects of fentanyl and nitrous oxide. *Anesth Analg* 1988;67:435–441.
25. Drummond JC, Todd M, U HS. The effect of high dose sodium thiopental on brain stem auditory and median nerve somatosensory cortical evoked responses in man. *Anesthesiology* 1985;63:249–254.
26. Drummond JC, Todd MM, Schubert A, U HS. The effect of acute administration of high dose pentobarbital on human brainstem auditory and median nerve somatosensory evoked responses. *Neurosurgery* 1987;20:830–835.
27. Taniguchi M, Nadstawek J, Pechstein U, Schramm J. Total intravenous anesthesia for improvement of intraoperative monitoring of somatosensory evoked potentials during aneurysm surgery. *Neurosurgery* 1992; 31:891–897.
28. Allison T, Hume AL. A comparative analysis of short-latency somatosensory evoked potentials in man, monkey, cat, and rat. *Exp Neurol* 1981;72:592–611.
29. Mauguiere F, Courjon J. The origins of short-latency somatosensory evoked potentials in humans. *Ann Neurol* 1981;9:607–611.
30. Emerson R, Pedley T. Generator sources of median somatosensory evoked potentials. *J Clin Neurophysiology* 1984;203–218.
31. Seyal M, Emerson R, Pedley T. Spinal and early scalp-recorded components of the somatosensory evoked potential following stimulation of the posterior tibial nerve. *Electroencephalogr Clin Neurophysiol* 1983; 55(3):320–330.
32. Symon L, Momma F, Murota T. Assessment of revisable cerebral ischaemia in man: intraoperative monitoring of the somatosensory evoked response. *Acta Neurochir Suppl (Wien)* 1988;42:3–7.
33. Symon L, Wang AD, Costa E, Silva IE, Gentili F. Perioperative use of somatosensory evoked responses in aneurysm surgery. *J Neurosurg* 1984;60:269–275.
34. Branston NM, Symon L, Crockard HA, Pasztor E. Relationship between critical evoked potential and local critical blood flow following acute middle cerebral artery occlusion in the baboon. *Exp Neurol* 1974; 45:195–208.
35. Friedman WA, Chadwick GM, Verhoeven F, Mahla M, Day AL. Monitoring of somatosensory evoked potentials during surgery for middle cerebral artery aneurysms. *Neurosurgery* 1991;29:83–88.
36. Friedman W, Kaplan B, Day A, Syper G, Curran M. Evoked potential monitoring during aneurysm operation: observations after fifty cases. *Neurosurgery* 1987:678.
37. Kidooka M, Nakasu Y, Watanabe K, Matsuda M, Handa J. Monitoring of somatosensory-evoked potentials during aneurysm surgery. *Surg Neurol* 1987;27:69–76.
38. Schramm J, Koht A, Schmidt G, Pechstein U, Taniguchi M, Fahlbusch R. Surgical and electrophysiological observations during clipping of 134 aneurysms with evoked potential monitoring. *Neurosurgery* 1990; 61–70.
39. Symon L, Hargadine J, Zawirski M, Branston N. Central conduction time as an index of ischaemia in subarachnoid hemorrhage. *J Neurol Sci* 1979;44:95.
40. Wang AD, Cone J, Symon L, Costa E, Silva IE. Somatosensory evoked potential monitoring during the management of aneurysmal SAH. *J Neurosurg* 1984;60:264.
41. Wilson-Pauwels L, Akesson EJ, Stewart PA. *Cranial nerves: anatomy and clinical comments*. Toronto: B.C. Decker, 1988.
42. Mann MD. *The nervous system and behavior*. New York: Harper & Row, 1981.
43. Daube JR. Intraoperative monitoring of cranial motor nerves. In: Schramm J, Moller AR, eds. *Intraoperative neurophysiologic monitoring in neurosurgery*. Berlin: Springer-Verlag, 1991;246–247.
44. Prass R. Intraoperative electromyographic recording. In: Kartush JM, Bouchard KR, eds. *Neuromonitoring in otology and head and neck surgery*. New York: Raven Press, 1991;81–97.
45. Møller AR, Jannetta PJ. Microvascular decompression in hemifacial spasm: intraoperative electrophysiologic observations. *Neurosurgery* 1985;16:612–618.
46. Prass RL, Luders H. Acoustic (loud speaker) facial electromyographic monitoring: part evoked electro-myographic activity during acoustic neuroma resection. *Neurosurgery* 1986;19:392–400.
47. Kartush JM. Electroneurography and intraoperative facial monitoring in contemporary neurotology. *Otolaryngol Head Neck Surg* 1989;101: 496–503.
48. Møller AR, Jannetta PJ. Preservation of facial function during removal of acoustic neuromas: use of constant-voltage stimulation. *J Neurosurg* 1984;61:757–760.
49. Parsons RC. Electrical stimulation of the facial nerve. *Laryngoscope* 1966;76:391–406.
50. Prass R, Luders H. Constant current versus constant voltage stimulation. *J Neurosurg* 1986;19:392–400.
51. Kartush JM, Bouchard KR. Intraoperative facial nerve monitoring: otology, neurotology, and skull base surgery. In: Kartush JM, Bouchard KR, eds. *Neuromonitoring in otology and head and neck surgery*. New York: Raven Press, 1991;99–120.
52. Hammerschlag PE, Cohen NL. Intraoperative monitoring of facial nerve function in cerebellopontine angle surgery. *Otolaryngol Head Neck Surg* 1990;103:681–684.
53. Hilger J. Facial nerve monitor. *Trans Am Acad Ophthalmol Otolaryngol* 1964;68:74–76.
54. Jako G. Facial nerve monitor. *Trans Am Acad Ophthalmol Otolaryngol* 1965;69:340–342.
55. Møller AR, Jannetta PJ. Monitoring of facial nerve function during removal of acoustic tumor. *Am J Otol* 1985:27–29.
56. Dickens JR, Graham SS. A comparison of facial nerve monitoring systems in cerebellopontine angel surgery. *Am J Otol* 1991;12:1–6.
57. Krauze F. *Surgery of the brain and spinal cord*, 1st English ed. London: Rebman, 1912.
58. Delgado TE, Buchheit WA, Rosenholtz HR, Chrissian S. Intraoperative monitoring of facial muscle evoked responses obtained by intracranial stimulation of the facial nerve: a more accurate technique for facial nerve dissection. *Neurosurgery* 1979;4:418–420.
59. Sugita K, Kobayashi S, Matsuga N, Suzuki Y. Microsurgery for acoustic neurinoma-lateral position and preservation of facial and cochlear nerves. *Neural Med Chir (Tokyo)* 1979;19:637–641.
60. Møller AR. *Evoked potentials in intraoperative monitoring*. Baltimore, MD: Williams & Wilkins, 1988.
61. Schwartz DM, Rosenberg SJ. Facial nerve monitoring during parotidectomy. In: Kartush JM, Bouchard KR, eds. *Neuromonitoring in otology and head and neck surgery*. New York: Raven Press, 1991;121–130.
62. Møller AR. Electrophysiologic monitoring of cranial nerves in operations of the skull base. In: Sekhar LN, Schramm VL Jr, eds. *Tumors of the cranial base: diagnosis and treatment*. Mt. Kisco, NY: Futura, 1987.

63. Gavilan J, Gavilan C. Recurrent laryngeal nerve: identification during thyroid and parathyroid surgery. *Arch Otolaryngol Head Neck Surg* 1986;112:1286–1288.
64. Lennquist S, Cahlin C, Smeds S. The superior laryngeal nerve in thyroid surgery. *Surgery* 1987;102:1000–1008.
65. Lipton RJ, McCaffrey TV, Litchy WJ. Intraoperative electrophysiologic monitoring of laryngeal muscle during thyroid surgery. *Laryngoscope* 1988;98:1292–1296.
66. Doppler C. Ueber das farbige Licht der Doppelsterne und einiger anderer Gestirne des Himmels. *Abh Kgl Boehm Ges Wissensch (Prag)* 1842; 465–482.
67. Ausman JI, Diaz FG. Correlation of noninvasive Doppler and angiographic evaluation of extra-intracranial anastomoses. In: Peerless SJ, McCormick CW, eds. *Microsurgery for cerebral ischemia.* Berlin: Springer, 1980:125–127.
68. Gilsbach JM. *Intraoperative Doppler sonography in neurosurgery.* New York: Springer-Verlag, 1983.
69. Miyazaki M, Kato K. Measurement of cerebral blood flow by ultrasonic Doppler technique. *Jpn Circ J* 1965;29:375–382.
70. Nornes H, Grip A, Wikeby P. Intraoperative evaluation of cerebral hemodynamics using directional Doppler technique: 1. arteriovenous malformations. *J Neurosurg* 1979;50:570–577.
71. Nornes H, Grip A, Wikeby P. Intraoperative evaluation of cerebral hemodynamics using directional Doppler technique: 2. saccular aneurysms. *J Neurosurg* 1979;50:570–577.
72. Aaslid R, Markwalder TM, Nornes H. Noninvasive transcranial Doppler ultrasound recording of flow velocity in basal cerebral arteries. *J Neurosurg* 1982;57:769–774.
73. Bailes JE, Fukushima T, Tantuwaya L, Schurman G, Davis DL. Intraoperative microvascular Doppler sonography in aneurysm surgery. *Neurosurgery* 1997;965–972.

Neurosurgical Issues in Otolaryngology: Principles and Practice of Collaboration, edited by Moisés A. Arriaga and J. Diaz Day. Lippincott Williams & Wilkins, Philadelphia © 1999.

CHAPTER 7

Endovascular Diagnosis and Management

In Sup Choi and Jarturon Tantivatana

Since the 1970s, endovascular intervention has been developed as the primary management, preoperative adjuvant therapy, and palliative treatment in neurosurgery and otolaryngology. New technology and equipment provide much improvement in endovascular treatment and outcome.

TECHNIQUES FOR ENDOVASCULAR DIAGNOSIS

Endovascular Access

Seldinger's technique is generally used for percutaneous endovascular access. The preferred site of puncture is the common femoral artery. An alternative site for arterial access is the axillary artery. Puncture of the superficial femoral, external iliac, or brachial or carotid arteries should be avoided since complications such as hemorrhage, dissection, and thrombosis occur significantly more often than in puncture of the common femoral artery. A puncture needle with stylet is advanced into the arterial lumen. The stylet is removed and then a guidewire is introduced through the needle until it is placed in the abdominal aorta under fluoroscopic guidance. The puncture needle is removed with the guidewire maintained in place. The catheter is advanced to the desired position and the guidewire is removed.

The femoral endovascular sheath is routinely introduced for the interventional procedure. The catheter can be removed or exchanged while maintaining vascular access. The sheath is constantly flushed with heparinized saline solution to prevent clot formation.

Catheters

Endovascular therapy requires catheters to deliver contrast material and therapeutic agents at the desired vascular target. There are many types of catheters that differ in size, shape, proximal and distal diameter, outer and inner diameter, length, and consistency. Size and length are measured in French (Fr) units and centimeters, respectively. Generally, the catheters can be divided into three categories.

Diagnostic Catheter

Diagnostic catheters are used for endovascular access for diagnostic purposes. They consist of variable stiffness, elasticity, and thickness, and have a tapered end. The tip of the catheter is preshaped into various angles and configurations depending on the vascular anatomy. The inner diameter and distal lumen of the catheter are rather narrow. Examples are the modified Head-Hunter, Cobra, Simmons, and Sidewinder.

Guide Catheter

Guide catheters are nontapered catheters with extremely thin walls and wide inner luminal diameters. The inner surface is coated with low-friction material to facilitate coaxial system. It provides support for the microcatheter. The tip of the guide catheter can be shaped under hot steam by the operator. This type of catheter was developed for endovascular treatment using the coaxial microcatheter. The guide catheter must be placed in secured position prior to coaxial introduction of the microcatheter.

Microcatheter

Microcatheters were developed for superselective catheterization of small vessels. The size of the microcatheter ranges from 1.0 to 1.8 Fr. The microcatheter must be longer than the guide catheter. Embolic material such as particle, glue, or coil can be introduced through the microcatheter. Recently, a hydrophilic-coated microcatheter was released that is easier to manipulate and propagate. The operator can

I. S. Choi: Interventional Neuroradiology, Lahey Clinic Medical Center, Burlington, Massachusetts 01805.

J. Tantivatana: Department of Radiology, Faculty of Medicine, Chulalongkorn University, Bangkok 10120, Thailand.

make a suitable curve on distal portion of the microcatheter with the shaping mandril. An exaggerated curve is formed to compensate for catheter relaxation after being shaped under hot steam. Two types of design are available.

Infusion Microcatheter

Infusion microcatheters are designed for delivery of particles, coils, chemical agents, and glue. Manual steering and manipulation with a compatible microguidewire is required. The infusion microcatheter has relatively large lumen and good stability. Examples are the Excel-Tracker (Target Therapeutics, Fremont, CA) and Prowler (Cordis, Miami, FL).

Flow-Guided Microcatheter

Flow-guided microcatheters are designed for embolization with glue or particles. The tip is bulb-shaped, and it facilitates propulsion by intravascular flow. Advancement of and navigation with the microcatheter depends on the direction and amount of flow. This catheter is useful in distally navigating through a small tortuous artery. Examples are the Regatta (Cordis) and the Spinnaker (Target Therapeutics).

Balloon Catheter

The balloon catheter was invented with an inflatable balloon at distal portion. Different models of balloon catheters vary in diameter and length of the balloons, length of the tip, size, and total length of the catheter. The standard inflation medium is a 1 : 1 mixture of contrast medium and normal saline. Any air bubble should be removed from the balloon prior to inflation. The following balloon catheters are available.

Occlusion Balloon Catheter

Typically, a balloon catheter contains a single lumen connected to the distal balloon. Inflation and opacification of the balloon is obtained by injection of contrast material through the catheter. The Cirrus temporary occlusion balloon catheter (Medtronic, Boston, MA) is a special occlusion balloon catheter designed for use in small and tortuous vessels. When the guidewire is retracted, the central lumen is open for infusion. The central lumen is closed for balloon inflation when the guidewire is advanced beyond the distal tip.

Double-Lumen Balloon Catheter

The double-lumen balloon catheter contains two lumina, one connected to the distal balloon and the other connected to the tip of the catheter. The parent vessel is occluded with inflation of the balloon by injection of the first lumen. Administration of contrast material, embolic agents, or heparinized saline can be obtained by injection of the second lumen. The double-lumen balloon catheter provides several advantages. A vascular structure distal to the occluded segment can be evaluated during contrast injection without the effect of dilutional inflow washout. Artificial flow arrest can be induced in order to gain more control of histoacryl glue injection. An example is the 5-Fr OB5-2-100 double-lumen balloon catheter (Meditech, Boston, MA).

Balloon Dilatation Catheter

The balloon dilatation catheter consists of a distal inflatable balloon and a distal lumen at the catheter tip, similar to the double-lumen balloon catheter. The balloons are designed to achieve their nominal diameters and length over a range of inflation pressure, usually within 3 to 20 atmospheres, depending on the manufacturer. The maximal practical pressure generated should not exceed the rated burst pressure stated in the instructions. The inflation pressure is determined by the size of the syringe. The smaller the barrel of the syringe, the greater the pressure generated. Usually a 10-cc syringe can generate a maximum practical pressure of 11 atmospheres; therefore, it is considered safe and optimal for balloon inflation. A 1-cc syringe can generate pressure up to 40 atmospheres, which entails the danger of balloon rupture. A typical balloon dilatation catheter consists of radiopaque makers inside the balloon to provide reference points for positioning the balloon across the stenosis prior to inflation. The balloon catheter is placed at the target site under a guidewire. Examples are the symmetry balloon dilatation catheter (Meditech) and the FasStealth dilatation catheter system (Target Therapeutics).

Guidewires

A guidewire may be needed to manipulate a diagnostic or infusion catheter. The diameter and length of the guidewire and the catheter must be compatible. Hydrophilic guidewires are available, providing better mobility and advancement. The preshaped tips of regular guidewires are either straight, angled, or C- or J-shaped. Tip of the guidewire can be shaped to the desired curve to match the vascular anatomy in each case.

Contrast Material

Contrast material provides luminal opacification of the vascular structure. Non-ionic contrast medium is more suitable for endovascular procedures than ionic contrast medium. Low incidence of adverse reaction and good patient tolerance are observed. Premedication with corticosteroid is administered to patients with a history of allergic reaction to iodine or contrast material if endovascular intervention is necessary.

Imaging

Conventional Angiography

Images of the vascular structures are recorded during contrast injection of the catheterized vessels. Rapid sequential x-ray exposure is performed with images developed directly on radiographic films. Bony and contrast opacities are shown. A subtracted image can be obtained by radiographic masking.

Digital Subtraction Angiography (DSA)

Angiographic images are recorded digitally with computer facility. Live subtracted images showing only vascular structures are displayed on the monitor. The systems also provide road-mapping fluoroscopy with maintained visualization of the vascular tree during selective catheterization. The operator can manipulate and advance the catheter by following the mapped route without the necessity of continuous contrast injection. Although the spatial resolution of the digital image is less than with conventional radiographic film, vascular opacity is displayed instantaneously without superimposed bony opacity. Other advantages are the ease of saving films and the reduced storage space needed. A disadvantage is that under minimal motion of the patient, subtraction artifacts become obvious, with degradation of image quality.

MATERIAL USED IN ENDOVASCULAR TREATMENT

Particles

Particles are used to embolize the desired vascular territory. Occlusion of the vessels depends on the size of the particles, the concentration of the particle mixture, and the rate of injection. Particles are mixed with contrast medium to provide opacity on fluoroscopy. Smaller particles can reach smaller and more distal vessels. A particle mixture with low concentration can penetrate deeply into distal and small branches. A slower injection rate can perfuse the particle mixture into more distal territory. Large particles block proximal branches, therefore allowing distal collateral flow, which is an advantage in high-risk situations of concurrent normal territory embolization.

Polyvinyl Alcohol (PVA) Particles

Polyvinyl alcohol particles are inert and nonabsorbable. Sizes of particles are available from 50 to 1,000 μm. PVA particles are mainly used for embolization of arteriovenous malformations or fistulas with numerous small feeders. PVA embolization is also very helpful in preoperative devascularization of meningiomas or hypervascular tumors of the head and neck, including the skull base. PVA can be used even in highly vascular tumors with a shunt. Blood loss and operating time are significantly reduced. Hemorrhage is possible although rare, secondary to increase resistance and pressure in the proximal arterial feeder after peripheral occlusion with particles. For skull base lesions with intracranial extension, the patient should be kept in low blood pressure after extensive embolization with PVA particles, in order to reduce the risk of hemorrhage.

Gelfoam

Gelfoam is an absorbable embolic material, supplied in forms of sheet and powder. Recanalization is observed in 7 to 21 days after embolization. Gelfoam powder is available with very small particle size of 30 to 60 μm. It penetrates deeply into the lesion at the precapillary and capillary levels. Gelfoam powder easily escapes into dangerous anastomosis. The incidence of cranial nerve deficit and scalp necrosis of Gelfoam powder embolization is higher when compared with PVA particles. Gelfoam powder is mainly used in preoperative devascularization of vascular tumors such as meningiomas and juvenile angiofibromas. Gelfoam sheets are cut into small strips and injected one by one for occlusion of the main feeder after microparticle embolization. Gelfoam strips may be used to temporarily occlude normal vessels for protection and redirection of flow. It is also a good choice of embolic material in cases of traumatic arterial hemorrhage. Late recanalization provides restoration of flow into the normal vessel previously occluded.

Organic Particles

Silk particles were used in the past but are rarely used today. Silk particles induce intense inflammatory response and are highly thrombogenic. Biologic dural particles are more biocompatible than silk, but also out of date.

Coils

Coils are made of platinum for optimal radiographic opacity and biocompatibility. Typical configurations of coils are simple straight, single-diameter helix, two-diameter helix, vortex, and complex. The size of a coil is described in length, loop, and core diameters. Coils act as permanent occlusive devices with mechanical and thrombogenic blockage. Coils may be used for primary occlusion, flow diversion, territory protection, and flow reduction prior to glue or particle embolization. Different types of coils are invented.

Fibered Coil

Fibered coil is used for occlusion of arterial or venous vascular structures. Fiber material attached to the coil promotes thrombosis. A coil pusher is required to push the fibered coil through the catheter.

Liquid Coil

Liquid coil is soft, of low friction, and injectable. It is propagated into the catheter and target vessel by flow from injection. It is useful in reduction of rapid flow prior to glue embolization and occlusion-protection of the normal vascular territory.

Guglielmi Detachable Coil (GDC)

Detachable coil was developed by Guglielmi et al. (1,2) in 1991. The GDC works by the principles of electrothrombosis and electrolysis. The GDC consists of four components: (a) a proximal guiding wire, made of stainless steel coated with Teflon for electric insulation, 175 cm in length, which functions as a delivery system; the proximal end is uninsulated for connecting to a battery; (b) an intermediate platinum marker, 5 mm in length; (c) a 3-cm intermediate stainless steel coil with an uninsulated distal 2 mm for electrolytic detachment; and (d) an extremely soft platinum coil with preformed helix, which is located distally. Detachment is achieved by applying direct current of 1 mA to the system. The anode connects to the GDC and the cathode connects to the patient. The uninsulated steel wire in the third portion undergoes electrolysis and the platinum coil is subsequently detached. At the same time, electrothrombosis occurs at the positively charged platinum coil with attracted negatively charged red blood cells, white blood cells, and platelets. The GDC is used with a two-tip marker microcatheter. The distal tip marker of the microcatheter is obscured by a pack of coils. Proper positioning of coils is assured by advancing the GDC wire until the wire marker overlaps the proximal marker of the two-tip microcatheter. The GDC is used primarily in the packing of aneurysms and the occlusion of arteriovenous fistulas and venous sinuses. A fibered GDC is also available.

GDCs are available in 0.01- and 0.015-inch diameters, for use with the Tracker or Prowler 10 and 18, respectively. The platinum coils are extremely soft and preformed in a helix of 2 to 14 mm. Once extruded from the catheter tip, the coil forms loops to prevent unnecessary stress to the aneurysm wall. When a proper-size coil is introduced into the aneurysm, it adapts to the shape of the lumen, not deforming the aneurysm. If a coil is not in proper position or not a suitable size, it can be withdrawn and then repositioned or exchanged for a different size.

Glue

Histoacryl glue, *N*-butyl cyanoacrylate (NBCA), is a stable nonabsorbable liquid polymerizing embolic agent commonly used in the treatment of arteriovenous malformations or fistulas. NBCA becomes polymerized when it comes into contact with ionic solution or blood. NBCA is mixed with Ethiodol by a 1 : 4 to 1 : 2 volume ratio. The greater the Ethiodol proportion, the slower the polymerization and liquidity. Ethiodol also provides opacification for the glue mixture. Dense opacification of the glue mixture can be obtained by adding tantalum powder.

Balloons

Detachable balloons were invented by Serbinenko (3) in Kiev, Russia. Debrun studied the technology and introduced it to the Western world in 1975. Detachable balloons come in various diameters, lengths, and configurations. The balloon can be expanded to the desired size by controlling the inflating volume injected through the delivery catheter. The limited maximum inflating volume with corresponding maximal diameter and length is described in the product manual. The balloon is mounted to the tip of the catheter. Two major types of delivery systems are used. The simple system consists of a traction-resisted variable stiffness microcatheter with a distal extended mounting tip for installation of the balloon. Examples are the Hieshima Taper Select Infusion Catheter (Meditech) and the Tracker (Target Therapeutics). The balloon is detached by friction-traction force during gentle traction of the catheter. Another system is the coaxial catheter composed of a sliding stiff outer sheath and a soft inner catheter (CC0L2S, Nycomed, Paris, France). A balloon is mounted on the inner catheter. The outer sheath gives support during introduction and manipulation, and stabilizes the balloon in position during detachment. The balloon is detached by a counteracting force applied to the neck of the balloon, generated by the stabilized outer sliding sheath and traction of the inner coaxial catheter. There are two types of balloon available.

Latex Balloon

The latex balloon is made of elastic latex. The earlier version of balloon had to be tied manually with latex thread to the tip of the delivery catheter for assembly. Latex is photosensitive; thus, it becomes degraded under light exposure and must be kept away from the light. The latex balloon accommodates to fit the shape of vascular space better than the silicone balloon. The new generation of latex balloon, the gold valve latex balloon (GVB), consists of an inner small balloon acting as a check valve when the balloon is inflated, and it prevents deflation after detachment. The GBV can be mounted simply to the tip of the delivery catheter. Elongated oval and round shapes are available.

Silicone Balloon

The silicone balloon is made of semipermeable silicone membrane. It has to be inflated with isotonic or slightly hyperosmolar medium to prevent diffusion and deflation. The miter valve is incorporated for sealing after detachment. The traction force required for detachment depends on the type of valve installed.

Eventually, both types of balloons will deflate. Deflation

of the latex balloon usually occurs in 4 to 8 weeks. The silicone balloon lasts longer, and it may remain inflated for more than 24 weeks. Taki et al. (4) introduced the use of hydroxyethlymethacrylate (HEMA) for solidifying medium inflation of the silicon balloon for the purpose of preventing balloon deflation, with later components for polymerization modified by Hieshima to gain more reliability. HEMA is a liquid monomer that can be cross-linked and catalyzed to produce polymerization, eventually becoming solid in 20 to 40 minutes. Multiple exchanges are required to increase the concentration of HEMA in the balloon.

Sclerosing Agents

Sclerosing agents are used for closing the vascular or lymphatic space in cases of venous or lymphatic malformation. The chemical agent induces inflammation of the intimal lining as well as thrombosis. The space is subsequently collapsed with adhesion of the internal wall. Two types of sclerosing chemical agents are currently used.

95% Ethyl Alcohol

Ethyl alcohol is a strong cytotoxic agent. It induces anoxic cell damage, protein precipitation, and fibrinoid necrosis of the intimal lining. Aggregation of red and white blood cells as well as platelets are noted with thrombosis. Ninety-five percent ethyl alcohol or absolute ethanol is effective in closing of vascular space. Absolute dehydrated ethanol is mixed with metrizamide powder for opacification. Mixing absolute ethanol with contrast medium solution dilutes the ethanol concentration and impairs the sclerosing property. Tissue necrosis may occur if the injected ethanol leaks outside the pocket. Ethanol injection is used to treat slow to moderate flow vascular lesions. Treatment of very high flow lesions is not effective. Ethanol can be used in transarterial injection or direct intralesional injection into venous malformations. Severe local pain was observed during ethanol injection. The procedure must be done under general anesthesia. Local induration and swelling occurs almost immediately after intralesional injection and becomes maximal in 3 to 7 days (5). The process usually resolves in 6 to 8 weeks. Complications of transarterial ethanol injection are vasospasm and mucocutaneous necrosis. Systemic complication is unusual. Ethanol is diluted and becomes nontoxic when it reaches venous outflow.

Sotradecol

Sotradecol, sodium tetradecyl sulfate, is a mild liquid sclerosing agent available in concentrations of 1% and 3%. Sotradecol is mixed with contrast medium for opacification. Sotradecol is used in sclerotherapy for lymphatic malformations or slow flow venous malformations.

BALLOON OCCLUSION TEST

The balloon occlusion test is a method of predicting tolerance to surgical ligation or endovascular occlusion of the carotid artery. Several other methods have been used in conjunction with temporary occlusion of the internal carotid artery, such as testing of neurologic function, electroencephalography (EEG), regional cerebral blood flow (CBF), venous blood gas, and carotid stump pressure. Many factors determine the tolerance, including cerebral blood flow, blood volume, oxygen extraction and saturation, regional metabolism, and cerebrovascular regulatory response. Reliability of the test is high if it is performed under a complete set of measurements, but this is impractical. Choi et al. (6) reported that 31 patients tolerated temporary occlusion, three developed transient symptoms, and two developed permanent ischemic symptoms in 30 minutes to 18 hours following acute occlusion of the internal carotid arteries with detachable balloons. Analysis of preembolization angiograms of the patients with postocclusion ischemic symptoms revealed insufficient collateral flow through the circle of Willis. Delivery of blood flow will be inadequate if the anterior or posterior communicating arteries are not of reasonable size. Keller et al. (7) used enlarged hemodynamic monitoring in balloon occlusion test with patients monitored under EEG, neurologic examinations, transcranial Doppler sonography (TCD) of the ipsilateral middle cerebral artery, and 99m-technetium (Tc)–HMPAO–single photon emission computed tomography (SPECT) imaging for cerebral perfusion. Of their 24 patients, three were excluded from permanent occlusion since one developed acute neurologic deficit and two had pathologic results in SPECT and TCD.

The temporary occlusion test should be assessed by the principles of anatomical evaluation and hemodynamic investigation (8). For anatomical evaluation, high-volume angiography of the contralateral carotid and vertebral arteries is necessary. A larger volume of contrast medium is injected to show better opacification of the collateral circulation through the circle of Willis, 10 cc in 1 second for the internal carotid artery, and 12 cc in 2 seconds for the vertebral artery, instead of the usual 8 cc in 1 second and 10 cc in 2 seconds for the internal carotid and vertebral arteries, respectively. Three sources of collateral circulation in the cerebral hemisphere are leptomeningeal, transcerebral, or through the circle of Willis. The most important collateral route is the circle of Willis in cases of internal carotid artery occlusion. If spontaneous filling of the M1 segment of the middle cerebral artery from the anterior or posterior communicating arteries is revealed on angiography, tolerance of acute carotid occlusion can be safely predicted. If no opacification of the ipsilateral anterior cerebral artery is seen, prophylactic external to internal carotid artery bypass surgery should be considered prior to occlusion of the internal carotid artery. After a successful bypass, the patient undergoes a functional investigation. The patency of the bypass is routinely studied and the degree of revascularization is evaluated by a common carotid angiogram with similar temporary balloon occlusion of the internal carotid artery. Permanent occlusion is usually performed on the 5th to 7th day after bypass, rather than in the immediate postoperative period. Although this may increase the chance of closure of the bypass, it is more important to be able to use systemic anticoagulation to prevent postocclusion thromboembolic complications, which can occur in up to 40% of cases. Although there is no general consensus, systemic heparinization is probably safe as early as 5 days after craniotomy.

Hemodynamic investigation includes physiologic tolerance tests performed in conjunction with temporary occlusion of the ipsilateral internal carotid artery. A basic neurologic test is to constantly monitor sensory, motor, and cognitive functions in an awake patient during temporary occlusion for a period of 15 to 20 minutes. EEG can be monitored to detect any ischemic focus that may precede clinical symptoms. Measurement of systolic blood pressure in the distal segment of the internal carotid artery can be recorded through a double-lumen balloon catheter or a directly inserted needle. Many authors suggest a slightly difference level of stump pressure acceptable for safety. Ehrenfeld et al. (9) use a systolic stump pressure over 70 mm Hg as an adequate limit for safe ligation, with pressure below 55 mm Hg constituting an unacceptable vulnerability to stroke. Jawad et al.'s (10) criterion for safety is a stump pressure of more than 60 mm Hg. Generally, a systolic stump pressure below 50 mm Hg is considered a high risk for postembolization stroke. Quantitative measurement of regional cerebral blood flow may yield a more accurate prediction of tolerance, but it is not widely done since it is complicated, requiring special equipment and radiopharmaceuticals. Jawad et al. concluded that the internal carotid artery could be safely sacrificed when CBF is greater than 40 mL/100 g/min. In the study by Erba et al. (11), patients with less than 30 mL/100 g/min of flow in the middle cerebral artery distribution were considered to have a moderate to high risk of stroke.

The patient is prepared in the same manner as for routine angiography. Femoral artery access is used with introduction of an 8-Fr sheath. The internal carotid artery is selectively catheterized using an 8-Fr guide catheter. The guide catheter is positioned in the cervical segment of the carotid artery; 10,000 units of heparin are administered intravenously to achieve full systemic heparinization. Then a 5-Fr double-lumen balloon catheter is coaxially introduced and the balloon is positioned approximately 1 cm distal to the end of the introducing guide catheter. The occlusion balloon is inflated with contrast material until the flow in the internal carotid artery is completely stopped. Contrast material can be injected through the second lumen to confirm occlusion, to visualize the exact geometry of the aneurysm, and to evaluate the collateral circulation by observing flow washout. The internal carotid artery proximal to the balloon is constantly flushed with heparinized saline to prevent any formation of thrombus. A neurologist evaluates neurologic functions continuously for 20 minutes. The author does not use EEG monitoring, stump pressure measurement, or CBF study. If there is any doubt, a challenge hypotensive test may be induced by decreasing blood pressure to approximately 80 mm Hg. If the patient can tolerate this occlusion and the high volume angiogram reveals sufficient collateral circulation, permanent occlusion is possible.

ENDOVASCULAR MANAGEMENT OF VARIOUS PROBLEMS IN HEAD AND NECK INCLUDING SKULL BASE

Epistaxis

Epistaxis commonly occurs in the anterior septal network of blood vessels and is easily controlled with simple local treatment. However, in cases of severe epistaxis, hemorrhagic foci are located posteriorly in the nasopharynx. Massive posterior epistaxis may require hospital admission and blood transfusion. Surgical treatment includes ligation of the internal maxillary or ethmoidal arteries, which may be neither easy nor effective since there are numerous anastomoses in the ethmoidonasal region. The role of embolization is accepted in emergency massive nasal bleeding or in recurrent or persistent epistaxis.

The etiologies of epistaxis are spontaneous, traumatic, neoplastic, hereditary hemorrhagic telangiectasia (Rendu-Osler-Weber disease), coagulopathy, pseudoaneurysms, aneurysms, arteriovenous malformations, and fistulas.

The goal of embolization is to achieve devascularization and control of the suspected bleeding site while preserving blood supply to the critical structures. The ethmoidonasal and nasopharyngeal mucosa usually tolerate ischemia, with good recovery and regeneration. Medium-sized particles, 250 to 500 μm, are used. The arterioles are reached and blocked while capillaries and sinusoids are mostly preserved. The site of bleeding is suggested by the focal area of increased vascular blush at the nasal, ethmoidal, or nasopharyngeal mucosa. Extravasation of contrast material is observed in active bleeding (Fig. 7-1A,B). The specific origin of bleeding is occasionally not shown on angiography, so the embolization is directed toward the suspected territory. Generally, branches of the distal internal maxillary artery, the sphenopalatine artery, and the descending palatine artery are embolized (Fig. 7-1C). Dangerous anastomoses are in the anterior deep temporal artery to the ophthalmic artery and the artery of foramen rotundum to the C4 branches of the internal carotid artery. The superior and middle pharyngeal branches of the anterior division of the ascending pharyngeal artery may be embolized if they are sources of bleeding. Bleeding from the superior portion of the nasal septum and the ethmoidal region is difficult to embolize since the supply is from the ethmoidal branches of the ophthalmic artery, and surgical clipping of the ethmoidal arteries is indicated. Massive hemorrhage from a ruptured cavernous or petrous carotid aneurysm or pseudoaneurysm is often fatal. Endovascular treatment of this condition includes occlusion of the parent artery with detachable balloon or coils, or GDC pack-

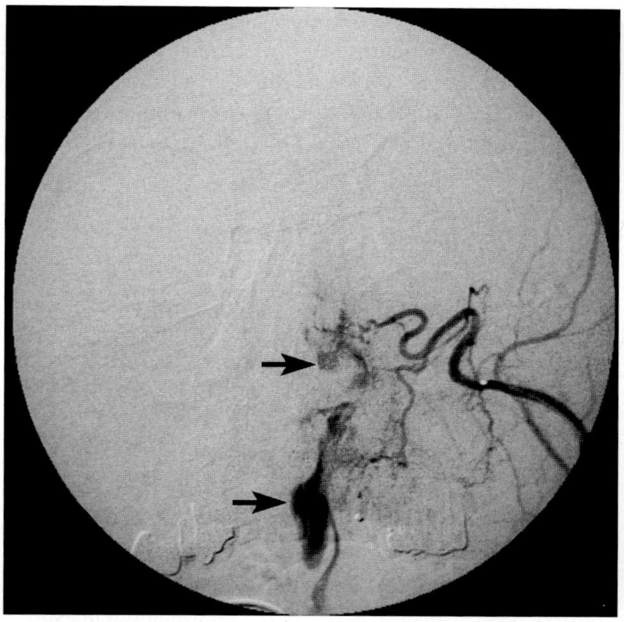
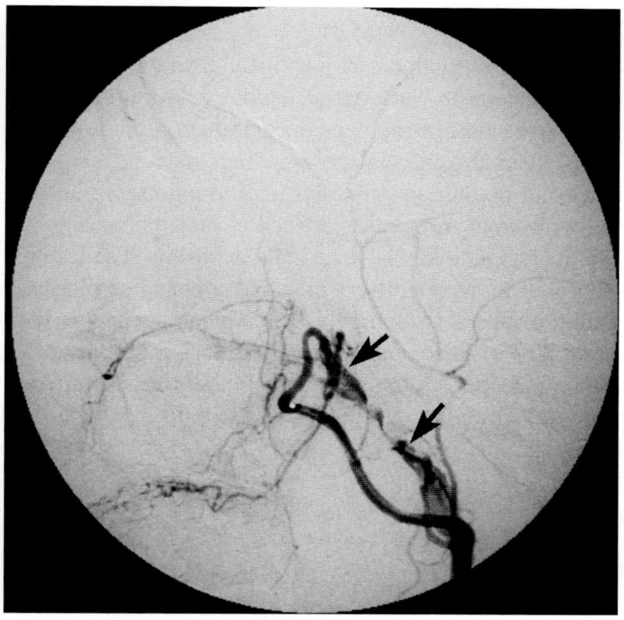
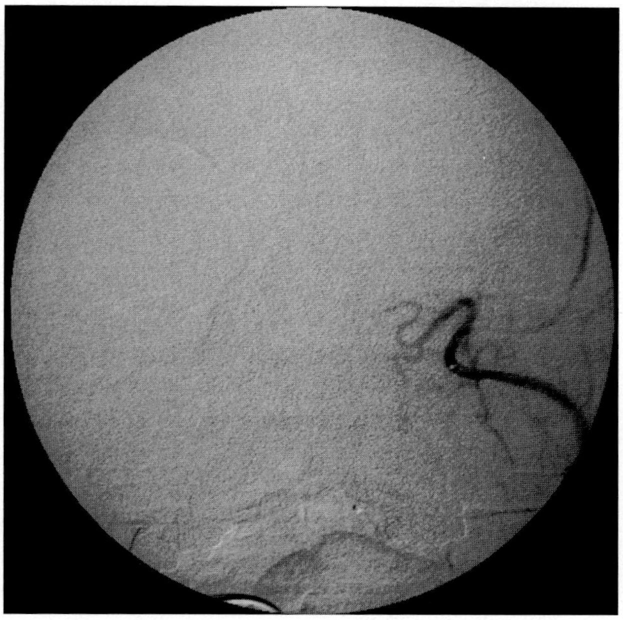

FIG. 7-1. A 74-year-old woman with persistent epistaxis despite nasal packing. **A,B:** Frontal and lateral digital subtraction angiography (DSA) of the left internal maxillary artery demonstrates extravasation of contrast material from the sphenopalatine artery into the nasopharynx, which indicates active bleeding (*arrows*). **C:** Bleeding is controlled after embolization of bilateral sphenopalatine and descending palatine arteries with polyvinyl alcohol (PVA) particles.

ing of the aneurysm, depending on the vascular anatomy of the lesion and the condition of the patient. Carotid-cavernous fistulas also produce fatal epistaxis from rupture of the engorged draining pterygoid venous plexus. Posterior nasal packing is not effective. Closure of the fistula site is the treatment of choice.

Elahi et al. (12) studied 54 patients with intractable epistaxis who underwent embolization of the distal internal maxillary arteries. Successful control of epistaxis was observed in 96% and the major neurologic complication rate was 6% without permanent deficits. Klein et al. (13) reported a series of 26 cases with persistent epistaxis even after anterior and posterior nasal packing. The technical success rate was 96% and the clinical success rate was 100%, with neither complication nor delayed hemorrhage. Chen et al. (14) reported a series of six patients having skull base internal carotid pseudoaneurysms who presented with delayed life-threatening epistaxis; they were treated successfully with detachable balloons and coils. Tseng et al. (15) reviewed 112 patients who underwent selective arterial embolization for epistaxis. The immediate success rate was 93%, with long-term success achieved in 88% of the patients. The overall complication rate was 17%, and the long-term morbidity rate less than 1%.

The patients may experience sore throat after embolization due to mucosal ischemia, which usually resolves within 1 to 2 weeks. Repeat embolization is still effective in recurrent bleeding.

Vascular Malformations

Vascular malformations are a congenital anomaly of vascular morphogenesis. The arterial, capillary, venous, or lymphatic channels may be involved in combination. The natural history of the malformation shows neither spontaneous proliferation nor involution. Vascular malformations are histologically different from vascular tumors such as hemangiomas by the fact that they have no cellular stroma. The lesion presents at birth, with a history of stable or changing phases. Alteration in size is secondary to hemodynamic change. Increase in size of the lesion is observed during outflow obstruction induced by thrombosis, infection, inflammation, or dependent positioning. Hormonal changes during puberty, menstruation, and pregnancy also influence the size of the lesion.

Arteriovenous Malformations

Arteriovenous malformations of the head and neck manifest as masses with pressure effects, cosmetic disturbance, ulceration, or hemorrhage. Profuse bleeding may follow dental extraction, caries, or minor trauma. Dural arteriovenous malformations of the posterior fossa and skull base present with pulsatile tinnitus, hearing loss, temporo-occipital pain, and headache.

Embolization is effective in control of bleeding. The size and vascularity of the lesions decrease after preoperative embolization, thus reducing blood loss and operating difficulty. Small nonresorbable particles or glue can be used, depending on the location, flow, and the presence of dangerous anastomosis. Associated arterial or venous aneurysms usually resolve after the nidus is treated but may require obliteration if they are persistent or large. In a high-flow lesion, the component of arteriovenous fistulas often exists.

Venous and Lymphatic Malformations

Developmental anomalies of venous and lymphatic malformations are closely related. Either the venous or lymphatic component may be dominant. Venous malformations show ectatic tortuous venous channels that may connect with normal venous drainage or be isolated as a venous pouch. Lymphatic malformations often communicate with systemic veins.

The goal of interventional sclerotherapy is to obliterate the ectatic venous or lymphatic channel by induction of intimal inflammation and thrombosis. The procedure is performed under general anesthesia. Percutaneous puncture of the lesion is performed using a 20- to 24-gauge needle with stylet. Proper positioning is assured by fluoroscopy. When the tip of the needle is within the space, serous fluid or venous blood comes out in cases of lymphatic or venous malformation, respectively. The location and size of the pocket is evaluated with contrast injection. The sclerosing agent is administered into the lesion. Ninety-five percent alcohol is preferred in high-flow venous malformations. Large lesions usually require multiple punctures and injections. Sotradecol is used in cases of lymphatic malformation or slow-flow venous malformation. Swelling of the treated lesion develops almost immediately after the procedure and gradually resolves in 4 to 8 weeks. Minimal pain related with severe swelling is occasionally experienced by the patient and may need symptomatic treatment. Sclerotherapy and embolization of the deep cervical or parapharyngeal lesion can cause temporary airway obstruction and may require prolonged intubation after the procedure.

Aneurysms

Obliteration

The ideal goal of aneurysm treatment is to occlude the lumen of the aneurysm while preserving the patency of the parent artery. In 1982 Romodanov and Shchegelov (16) reported the occlusion of cerebral saccular aneurysms with detachable balloons. Since then several methods based on this principle have been developed. Hilal et al. (17) developed a method that involves placing multiple short coils with or without a fiber in the aneurysm. The most recent advance in the field is the development of the detachable coil system by Guglielmi in 1991. The new system has proven safer and more effective in the treatment of intracranial and extracranial aneurysms. Indications for endovascular therapy of aneurysms include unfavorable location for surgical clipping, previously failed clipping, technical difficulties, and a poor medical status that precludes surgery. Contraindications are critical perforators and dangerous arterial branches arising from the aneurysms.

Detachable Balloons

The balloon is navigated into the aneurysm by partial inflation and deflation, facilitated by laminar flow in the lumen of the aneurysm. If the lumen is difficult to enter, two separate balloons, one detachable and one fixed, can be employed, with the fixed balloon positioned beyond the neck of the aneurysm, occluding distal flow. Then, the detachable balloon is advanced into the aneurysm. Schegelov used balloons of various shapes to fit the differing geometries of the aneurysm. Hieshima et al. (18) fill the entire lumen; therefore, giant aneurysms require more than one balloon. Moret has developed a technique to close only the entrance of the aneurysm with a single balloon.

After the balloon is properly positioned, the volume at which it properly occludes the lumen is measured and then it is filled with permanent solidifying agent HEMA by the method of volume exchange. Despite technologic advances, balloons have two fundamental disadvantages. First, since the geometry of an aneurysm does not always match the configuration of the balloons, complete obliteration of the lumen is often difficult. Second, the wall of the aneurysm is fragile and undergoes excessive stress during manipulation of the balloons, exchange of HEMA, and traction of the catheter for detachment, thus increasing the risk of rupture.

In 1989, Romodanov and Shchegelov presented the largest series of balloon occlusion of the aneurysms with a total of 671 cases. The aneurysms were successfully occluded in 91% of patients. Their mortality rate was 1.7% in 338 patients who were in fair to good condition and 22% in 71 patients in poor condition. Higashida et al. (19) reported their results in 84 patients with unclippable aneurysms due to location, shape, and size of the ill-defined neck. Complete occlusion was achieved in 65 patients (77.4%) and incomplete in 19 (22.6%). The mortality rate related to treatment was 17.9%. Nine patients had cerebral infarcts, caused by thrombi in five cases, occlusion of the parent artery in two cases, leakage of semisolid HEMA in one case, and premature balloon detachment in one case. In 1991, Moret (20) reported the results of 93 cases that included small clippable aneurysms. Treatment was successful in 73 patients, with preservation of the parent artery in 66 cases. His complication rate was 11%, including four deaths.

Detachable Coils

Guglielmi et al. developed detachable coils in 1991 based on the principles of electrothrombosis and electrolysis. The goal of treatment is to exclude the aneurysm from circulation by packing its neck and lumen. Obstructed inflow and an occluded cavity prevent pulsation, expansion, and rupture.

Proper angiographic evaluation of the aneurysm is performed with analysis of its size, the neck, involvement of parent artery, nearby perforators, and vascular territory. A two-tip microcatheter is coaxially advanced into the aneurysm through the guide catheter. A soft tip guidewire is used when entering the aneurysm not only to guide the catheter into the lumen but to prevent inadvertent rupture of the wall by a relatively stiffer catheter tip. A coil of proper diameter and length is introduced into the lumen. If the coil migrates or does not adapt to the aneurysm, it can be repositioned or changed. A proximal maker of the two-tip microcatheter must be overlapped with the marker on the wire to ensure that the detaching segment is beyond the catheter tip. The coil is detached after it is placed at a satisfactory position by connecting with a direct current generator of 0.5 to 1.0 mA. Detachment is accomplished when the potential difference or voltage peaks up to 6 V and the electric current is reduced. Tight packing up to 50% of volume may be necessary to prevent reopening of the lumen caused by recanalization of migration of coils toward the dome of the aneurysm. The patient is kept under heparinization during the procedure and throughout the following 48 hours with a retained introducing sheath in order to decrease the incidence of thromboembolism. A follow-up angiogram is performed before sheath removal and discharge for evaluation of the parent vessel, critical perforators, coil migration, or any residual lumen. Repeat follow-up angiogram is usually performed in 6 months or 1 year. Skull radiographs are considered in long-term follow-up of stable patients.

We have treated 144 patients with aneurysms using GDC. Complete occlusion (100%) was achieved in 48 cases. Near total occlusion (90%–99%) was noted in 89 cases. There were 21 patients with cavernous and cervical carotid artery aneurysms treated with GDC. These aneurysms were totally occluded in 12 cases and satisfactory near-total occlusion was achieved in nine cases. Minor stroke developed in three cases and resolved with minimal morbidity.

Malisch et al. (21) reported a prospective study in a series of 100 patients who underwent endovascular embolization of 104 intracranial aneurysms using GDCs. They concluded that the GDC procedure is a safe, effective, and reliable means of preventing aneurysm hemorrhage in patients with small and large intracranial aneurysms, but the results were less satisfactory in cases involving giant lesions. Patients with grade IV or V subarachnoid hemorrhage in this series generally had poor outcomes even if the procedure was successful in occluding the aneurysm. Halbach et al. (22) reported 35 cases of cavernous carotid aneurysms treated with GDC. All four patients who presented with epistaxis had no bleeding after treatment. Complete resolution and dramatic improvement were noted in 58% and 38% of patients with cranial nerve palsy.

Complications directly related to the procedure include rupture of the aneurysms, coil fracture, coil misplacement, thrombosis, embolism, and protrusion of the loop of the coil with compromised flow of the parent vessel and critical branches. Coil migration is observed in partially thrombosed aneurysms despite tight packing, probably secondary to intraaneurysmal clot lysis generating more space. The packed coils become loose and displaced by inflow toward the inside of the reopening lumen of the aneurysm. Increase in size of lumen of the residual aneurysm in cases of near-total packing is also noted. Further packing of coils toward the dome of the aneurysm caused by constant pulsation is believed to cause regrowth of the lumen. Choi reported six cases of recurrent aneurysms after coil packing, and four of them required second treatment.

Occlusion of Parent Vessel

Indications for occlusion of the parent vessel are unclippable aneurysms at an inaccessible location, giant cavernous or petrous carotid artery aneurysms, dissecting aneurysms of the internal carotid or vertebral arteries, and fusiform aneurysms without a well-defined neck (Fig. 7-2). The advantage of detachable balloon occlusion over surgical ligation is that balloons can trap the neck of the aneurysm, thereby ensuring complete occlusion and preventing refilling of the aneurysm by reverse blood flow. If a balloon cannot be navigated to this position because of geometric or hemodynamic difficulties, it can occlude the parent artery close to the aneurysm and its origin, hence reducing the length of the throm-

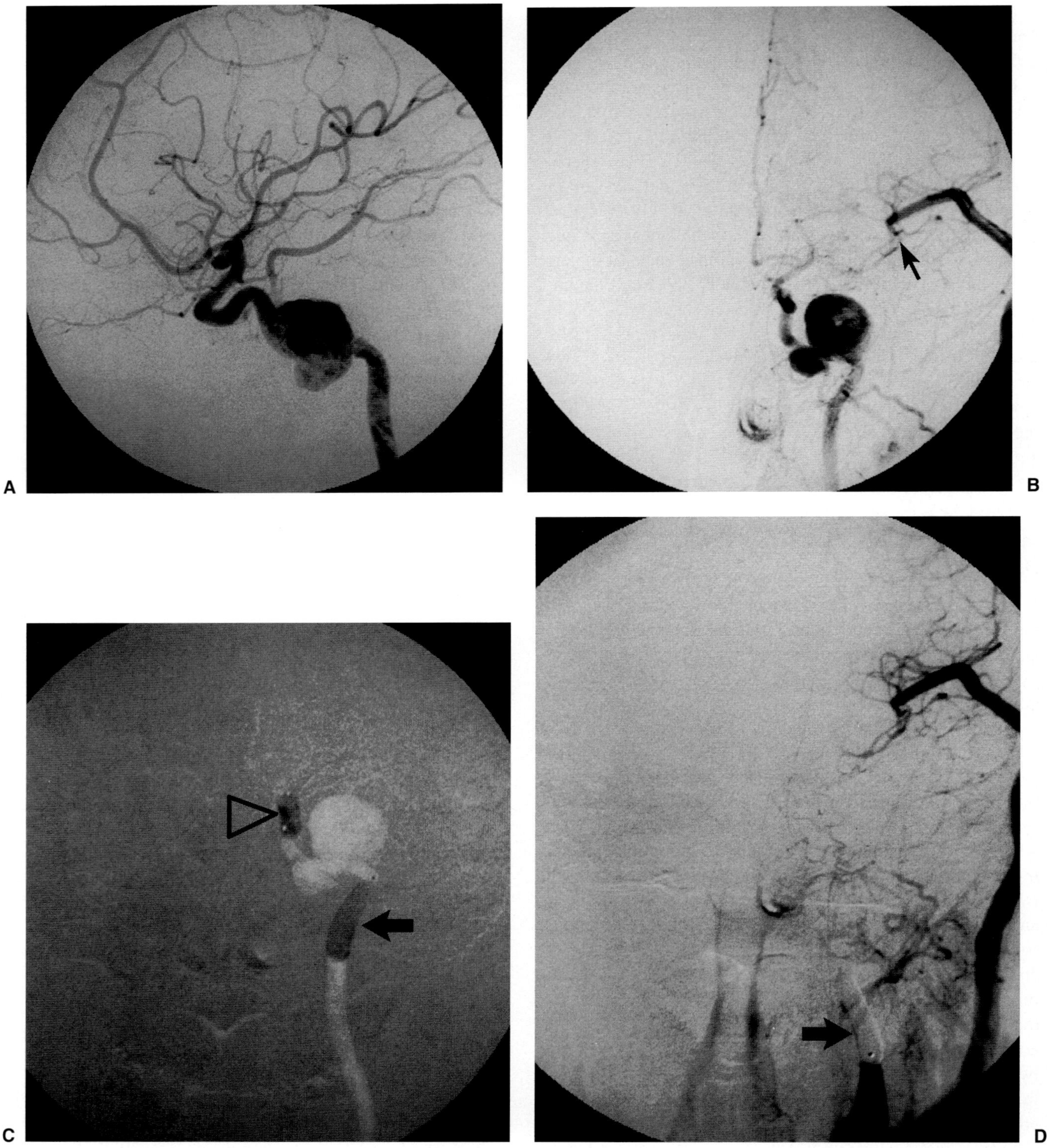

FIG. 7-2. Parent vessel occlusion after external-internal carotid bypass for treatment of the giant left carotid aneurysm in a 35-year-old man who did not pass the occlusion test. **A:** Lateral DSA of the left internal carotid artery shows giant aneurysm at petrous segment. **B:** Frontal DSA of the left common carotid artery shows external to internal carotid bypass performed prior to balloon occlusion (*arrow*). **C:** Frontal road-mapping image demonstrates occlusion of the parent artery with balloons trapping at petrous portion proximal to the aneurysm (*arrow*) and cavernous portion distal to the aneurysm (*arrowhead*). **D:** Frontal DSA of the left common carotid artery shows placement of the third balloon at the proximal left internal carotid artery with complete occlusion (*arrow*).

bus in the parent artery, which can be a source of future embolic complications.

The balloon is mounted on the tip of the catheter, either of variable stiffness or with a coaxial catheter. Elongated GBV no. 16 is preferred since it accommodates the contour of the artery and provides more surface contact between the vessel wall and balloon, therefore reducing the chance of distal migration of the detached balloon. The preparation and guiding catheter is similar to that used in the balloon occlusion test. The detachable balloon catheter system is advanced coaxially through the guiding catheter. The ideal position of the first balloon is just distal to the neck of the aneurysm without occlusion of normal arteries. The position of the detachable balloon should be proximal to the origin of the ophthalmic artery. In cases of wide-neck aneurysms, the balloon catheter may not be advanced distally and may be curled within the aneurysm under turbulent flow. In this situation, the balloon has to be positioned close to the neck of the aneurysm. When the balloon is in the desired position, it is inflated with isosmolar contrast material. Hieshima (23) used HEMA as a solidifying agent to prevent deflation of the detached balloon by exchange replacement with contrast medium. The detached balloons filled with contrast material gradually deflate without contrast opacification after 2 to 3 months. Only radiopaque metallic markers at the tip of the balloon are left visualized on radiograph. During this period, complete thrombosis of the occluded segment and reendothelialization of the stumps have occurred. The rate of recanalization is not significantly higher even when the balloon is filled only with contrast material. The second balloon is immediately introduced after detachment of the first balloon to prevent possible migration of the first one. The second balloon is usually positioned proximal to the neck for the trapping procedure or next to the first balloon for proximal occlusion of the parent artery. The first or second balloon may be inflated across the neck of the aneurysm if it is narrow enough. The last balloon should be detached as close as possible to the origin of the parent artery to minimize the length of the stump (balloon stumpectomy), since many authors believe that the residual stump may be the source of thromboemboli and subsequent late embolic complications.

Postocclusion care is required with low-level heparinization maintained for 4 to 5 postoperative days. Patient activity is strictly regulated, with complete bed rest for the first 48 hours. The patient's head is gradually elevated beginning on the 3rd day, and the patient subsequently ambulates on the 6th or 7th day. If any symptoms of cerebral ischemia develop, blood pressure is elevated and blood volume is expanded by increasing fluid intake. Activity is gradually increased to facilitate adjustment of the postocclusion cerebral hemodynamic changes; therefore, the incidence of cerebral ischemia is decreased.

Clinical improvement depends on the location and degree of obliteration of the aneurysm and initial symptoms. All patients who were treated for cavernous aneurysms had complete resolution of pain. Ocular motor dysfunction was improved in 81% of patients. Follow-up studies demonstrated reduced mass effect after the aneurysms were completely obliterated.

Aneurysms of the internal carotid artery below the ophthalmic artery or of the vertebral artery undergo complete obliteration if proximal occlusion of the parent artery is achieved. Fox et al. (24) reported complete obliteration in 37 cases of internal carotid artery aneurysm below the ophthalmic artery and in one case of vertebral aneurysm. The rate of complete obliteration drops to 50% in cases of aneurysms above or at the ophthalmic artery or basilar aneurysms, due to persistent flow in the aneurysm lumen through collateral circulation. Larson et al. (25) reviewed 58 patients who had aneurysms of the internal carotid artery treated by intravascular balloon occlusion with median follow-up of 76 months. They reported a morbidity rate of 10% caused by transient ischemia. The permanent morbidity rate is 5%, and the mortality rate is 5%.

We have seen four patients with dissecting aneurysm of the vertebral artery who presented with subarachnoid hemorrhage and have had no recurrence of hemorrhage following proximal occlusion in a period of 1 to 6 years, with complete clinical recovery. Tsukahara et al. (26) reported five cases of dissecting vertebral aneurysm with subarachnoid hemorrhage treated by endovascular proximal balloon occlusion of the extracranial vertebral artery after the potentially dangerous period of cerebral vasospasm. No patients showed postoperative hemorrhages or progression of the dissection during 19 to 48 months of follow-up, even though four of them had residual aneurysms on angiograms.

The most common complication following parent vessel occlusion is cerebral ischemia, transient or permanent. The incidence of complication is up to 16% despite preocclusion tolerance testing. Landolt and Millikan (27) suggested several mechanisms of cerebral ischemia and concluded that early ischemic insult most likely results from insufficient collateral circulation caused by preexisting structural constraints that later regress. They also concluded that late cerebral infarction that occurred from a few hours to days after the procedure can be explained by the thromboembolism theory. Procedure-related complications are uncommon and occurred in less than 1% of cases, and include occlusion of the distal artery caused by premature balloon detachment, dislodging of a thrombus from a partially thrombosed aneurysm lumen, and thromboembolism attributable to the catheter system.

Tumors

Meningioma

Meningiomas are relatively common intracranial extraaxial tumors, accounting for 13% to 18% of the primary intracranial neoplasm (28). Female to male incidence is 2:1. Most of the meningiomas are vascular lesion. The tumor blush is visualized on angiogram in the early arterial phase through the late venous phase. Meningiomas can be categorized by location as parasagittal, convexity, falcine, tentorial, peritorcular, anterior cranial fossa, olfactory groove, sphenoid ridge, clinoid, cavernous, petroclival, posterior cranial fossa, cerebellopontine angle, and foramen magnum.

Surgical removal of meningiomas is not always easy since some of the tumors are hypervascular, fragile, and subject to bleeding. Adjuvant preoperative embolization is considered advantageous by several authors as a combined therapeutic approach for meningiomas. Preoperative embolization is also effective in controlling the supply from a surgically inaccessible area, especially in cases of skull base involvement. Reduction in blood loss and operating time has been documented (29). In cases of extensive parasellar involvement or carotid encasement, in which it is inevitable to sacrifice the carotid artery, a preoperative balloon occlusion test is performed to evaluate collateral blood flow and the patient's tolerance.

Diagnostic or preoperative angiograms are required for evaluation of tumor location, arterial supply, vascular displacement or encasement, dangerous anastomosis, venous drainage, dural sinus involvement, and normal brain circulation. Meningiomas usually gain arterial contribution from dural vessels supplying the adjacent meninges. Arterial feeders enter the tumor at the meningeal or osseous attachment and supply it in radial fashion with a sunburst appearance on the angiogram. Branches of the external and internal carotid arteries can supply the tumor depending on its location. The usual arterial supplies are branches of the middle meningeal artery. Large meningiomas may acquire additional pial blood supply. Bitzer et al. (30) suggested that pial blood supply may be associated with the development of peritumoral brain edema in meningiomas.

Parasagittal and high-convexity meningiomas receive blood supplies from branches of the ipsilateral middle meningeal artery and the artery of the falx cerebri, with supplemental supplies from corresponding contralateral arteries. Frontal convexity and anterior falcine meningiomas may be supplied from meningeal branches of the anterior ethmoidal or anterior falcine branches of the ophthalmic artery. Olfactory groove meningiomas derive supply from branches of the anterior and posterior ethmoidal arteries. The recurrent meningeal branch of the ophthalmic artery and sphenoidal branches of the middle meningeal artery may supply sphenoid wing meningiomas. Parasellar meningiomas recruit complex supplies from branches of the C5 portion of the internal carotid artery, cavernous branches of the middle meningeal artery, cavernous branches of the accessory meningeal artery, the distal internal maxillary artery via artery of the foramen rotundum, and the neuromeningeal trunk of the ascending pharyngeal artery. Tentorial meningiomas receive arterial supply from the marginal tentorial artery and the inferolateral trunk. Meningiomas of the cerebellopontine angle may derive supplies from petrosal, petrosquamosal, and occipital branches of the middle meningeal artery as well as transmastoid branches of the occipital artery, subarcuate branches of the anterior inferior cerebellar artery, and jugular branches of the neuromeningeal trunk of the ascending pharyngeal artery. Occipital and foramen magnum meningiomas may be supplied by the posterior meningeal branch of the vertebral artery, the artery of the falx cerebelli, or the hypoglossal division of the neuromeningeal trunk.

The goal of embolization is to devascularize the tumor capillary bed while preserving normal arterial territory (Fig. 7-3). PVA particles are generally used for arterial embolization. Small particles, 150 to 250 μms, are preferred since

A 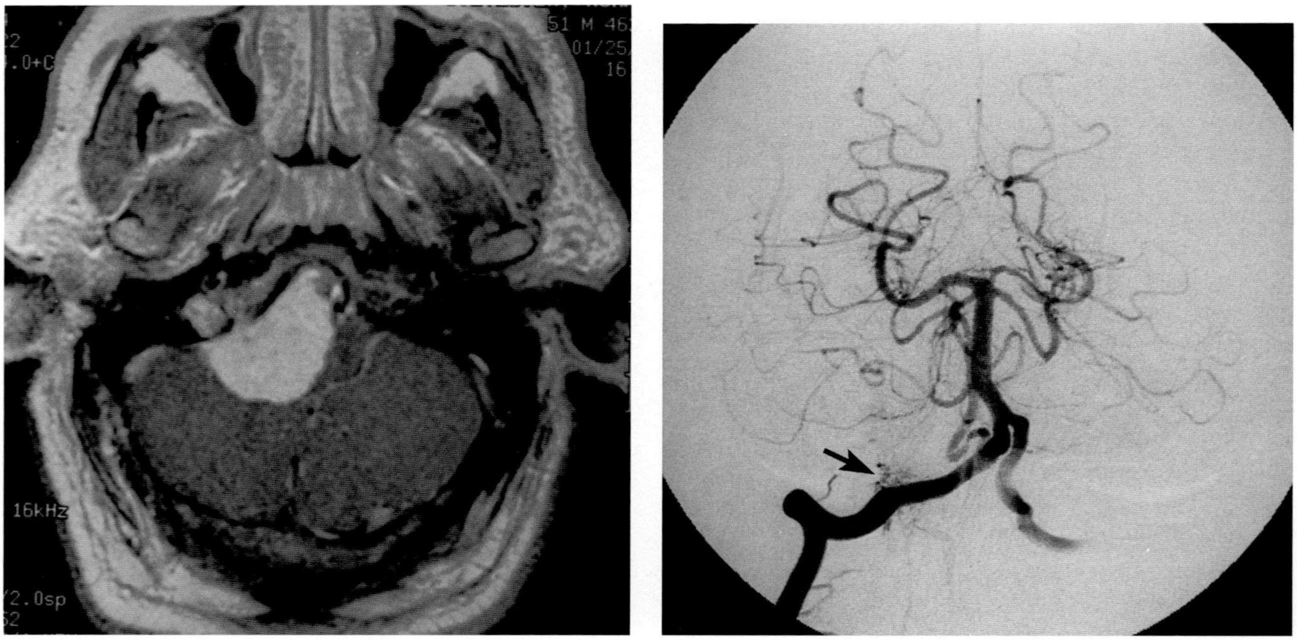 B

FIG. 7-3. Cerebellopontine angle meningioma in a 53-year-old man. **A:** Axial T1-weighted magnetic resonance imaging (MRI) with gadolinium shows enhancing right cerebellopontine angle mass with involvement of the right petrous and internal acoustic meatus. *(Continued.)*

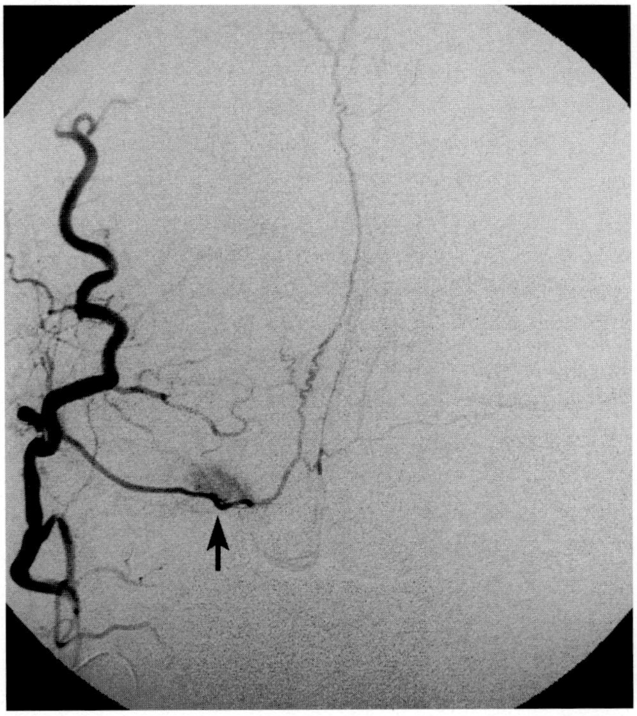

C

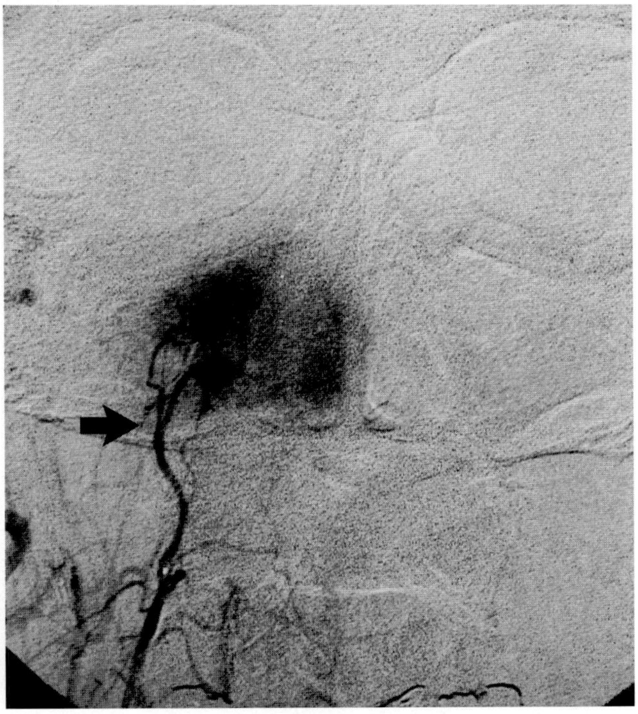

D

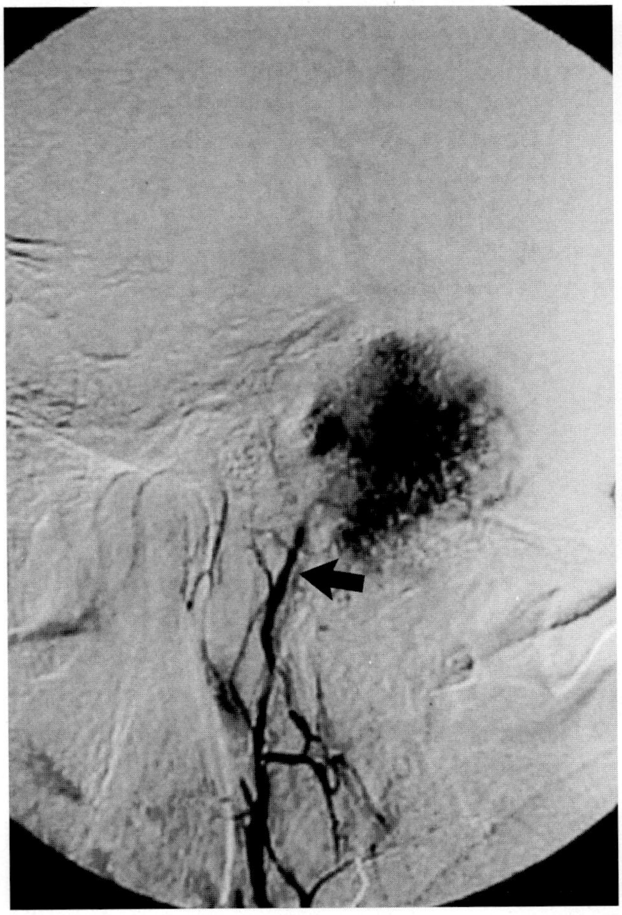

E

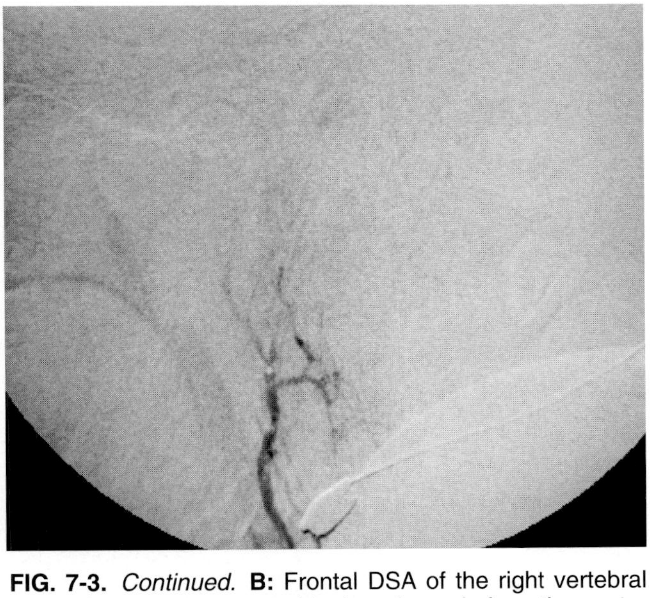

F

FIG. 7-3. *Continued.* **B:** Frontal DSA of the right vertebral artery demonstrates tumor blush and supply from the posterior meningeal artery (*arrow*). **C:** Supply from the artery of the falx cerebelli is also noted on frontal DSA of the right occipital artery (*arrow*). **D,E:** Frontal and lateral DSA of the right ascending pharyngeal artery show major blood supply from the neuromeningeal trunk with intense tumor staining (*arrow*). **F:** Lateral DSA of the right ascending pharyngeal artery after preoperative embolization with PVA particles demonstrates successful devascularization of the tumor.

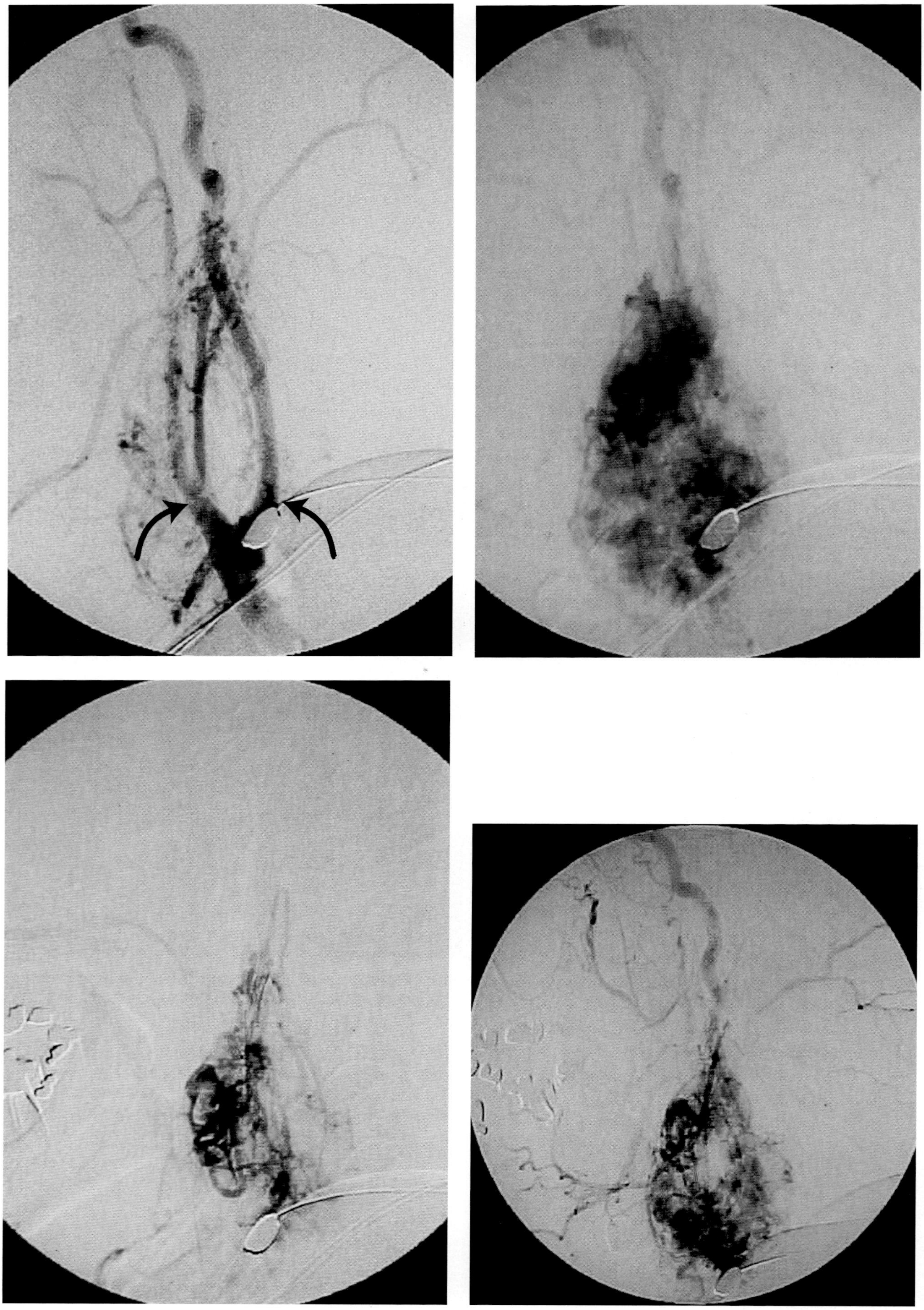
A
B
C
D

the particles penetrate deeply into the tumor and result in more complete devascularization. Preferential perfusion of the tumor is augmented by flow control. Particle size is gradually increased in the later stages of embolization. The procedure should be stopped if significant reflux or change in flow pattern is noted. Use of particle size larger than the anastomotic channel should be considered if there is visible dangerous anastomosis or when the chance of reflux into normal territory is likely. During embolization, the critical territory can be protected by temporary balloon occlusion, detachable balloon, coil, or macroparticle. The proximal middle meningeal artery may be occluded at the level of foramen spinosum with Gelfoam or coil at the end of embolization to reduce hemorrhage during subsequent skull base surgery and craniotomy.

The most common histopathologic findings of postembolized meningiomas is necrosis, in the form of confluent necrosis as well as micronecrosis (31). Other characteristic features included florid ischemic changes, intravascular PVA particles, and fibrinoid necrosis of vascular walls.

In cases of preoperative embolization, surgery is optimal on the 3rd to 5th day. Nelson et al. (32) and others suggest a period of at least 24 hours between embolization and subsequent operation. Patients with significant intracranial extension are placed on corticosteroids and anticonvulsant medication. Recanalization and collateral blood supply may develop after a postembolization period of more than 1 week. Complications of embolization in treatment of meningiomas include intratumoral hemorrhage, postembolization swelling of the tumor, and perilesional and subarachnoid hemorrhage. There were seven cases of hemorrhage associated with embolization of meningiomas reported from 1986 to 1997 (33). Large tumor size and dense vascular blush were noted in all cases. Most authors have implicated small-diameter embolic agents or cystic change within the tumor as risk factors for hemorrhage (34,35).

Paragangliomas

Paragangliomas or glomus tumors are encapsulated neuroendocrine neoplasms derived from paraganglionic cells. Branchial paragangliomas arise in the head and neck, most commonly in the temporal region. Brachial paragangliomas are practically approached as temporal (tympanic and jugular) and cervicocarotid. Patients with tympanic paragangliomas present with pulsatile tinnitus aggravated by exertion and decreased by cervical vascular compression or the Valsalva maneuver. The typical presentation of jugular paraganglioma is the jugular foramen syndrome with paralysis of the 9th, 10th, and 12th cranial nerves. Carotid paragangliomas present as expansile pulsating masses, but involvement of the cranial nerve is rare. Vagal paragangliomas present with a cervical or pharyngeal mass with cranial nerve impairment manifested by neck hypoesthesia and pharyngeal pain.

Differential diagnosis of temporal paragangliomas includes prominent jugular bulb, intratympanic course of the internal carotid artery, persistent stapedial artery, tympanic granuloma, neurogenic tumors, meningiomas, hemangiomas, and metastasis. Mass effect of carotid and cervical paragangliomas must be differentiated from aneurysms, ectatic carotid bulb, neurogenic tumors, lymphadenitis, and metastasis.

The most constant supply of brachial paragangliomas is the ascending pharyngeal artery (36). Other possible feeders of temporal paragangliomas are branches of the vertebral, posterior auricular, and occipital arteries. Typical angiographic features of paraganglioma include moderate enlargement of the feeding arteries, early intense parenchymal blush, and rapid venous filling. Intradural posterior fossa extension is indicated by the presence of supplies from the anterior and posterior inferior cerebellar arteries. Invasion of the carotid canal is suggested if the petrous internal carotid artery is narrow, or an enlarged caroticotympanic artery is noted. Venous invasion is diagnosed by the presence of an intraluminal filling defect and consistent tumor blush within the vein.

Complete removal of the resectable tumor is the treatment of choice. Preoperative embolization is helpful in diminishing the intraoperative blood requirement (37). Decrease in size of the lesion is observed and an initially large inoperable tumor may become resectable after embolization (Fig. 7-4).

The technique of embolization in paragangliomas is similar to that of meningiomas. PVA particles of 150 to 250 μm are used for superselective embolization, which is completed with proximal occlusion by Gelfoam strips or coils. Embolization is contraindicated in cases of arterial supply from the anterior or posterior inferior cerebellar arteries. Reported complications include lower cranial nerves palsies, especially in cases of embolization using liquid agents.

Juvenile Angiofibroma (JAF)

Juvenile angiofibromas, which are benign nonencapsulated fibrovascular tumors with red-purple color and rubbery consistency, typically develop in boys at puberty. The lesions usually arise in the nasopharynx and may invade the nasal cavity, nasal septum, ethmoid air cells, sphenoid sinus, orbit, middle cranial fossa, soft palate, pterygopalatine fossa,

FIG. 7-4. Carotid body paraganglioma in a 56-year-old man with preoperative embolization. **A,B:** Lateral DSA of the left common carotid artery shows hypervascular mass in the left carotid space with splaying of the internal and external carotid arteries (*arrow*). **C:** Lateral DSA of the left ascending pharyngeal artery demonstrates major blood supply from the inferior pharyngeal and muscular branches. **D:** Postembolization of the left ascending pharyngeal artery with PVA particles shows decrease tumor vascularity.

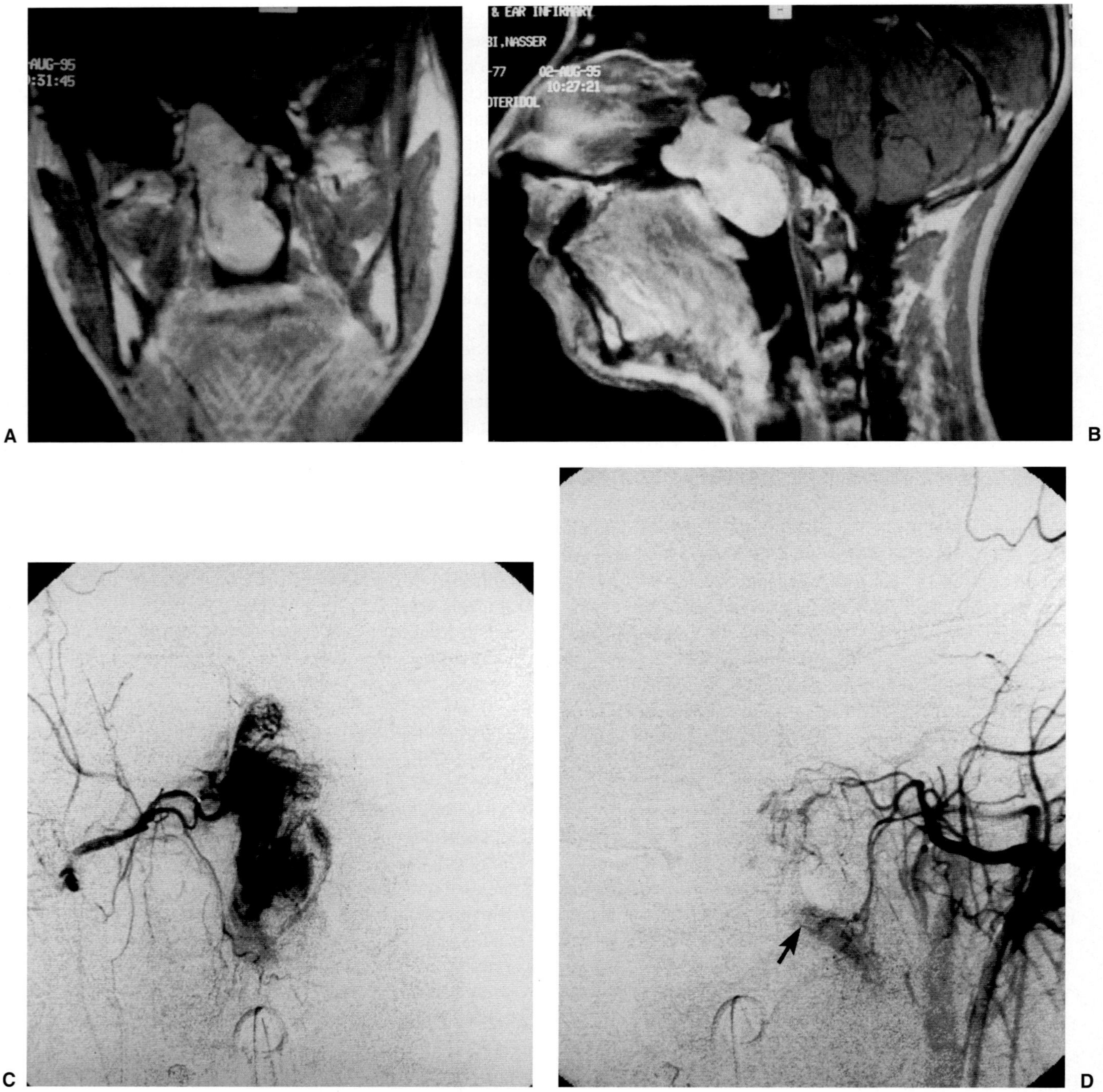

FIG. 7-5. Preoperative embolization of juvenile angiofibroma in an 18-year-old man. **A,B:** Coronal and sagittal T1-weighted MRI with gadolinium shows intensely enhancing mass involving the right nasopharynx and right sphenoid sinus. Inferior extension across midline is also noted. **C:** Frontal DSA of the distal right internal maxillary artery demonstrates hypervascular tumor with dense staining fed by the right sphenopalatine and descending palatine arteries. **D:** Anastomotic channels across the midline from the left sphenopalatine artery, and contralateral supply from the left descending palatine artery to the inferior portion of the tumor are noted on frontal DSA of the left internal maxillary artery (*arrow*). *(Continued.)*

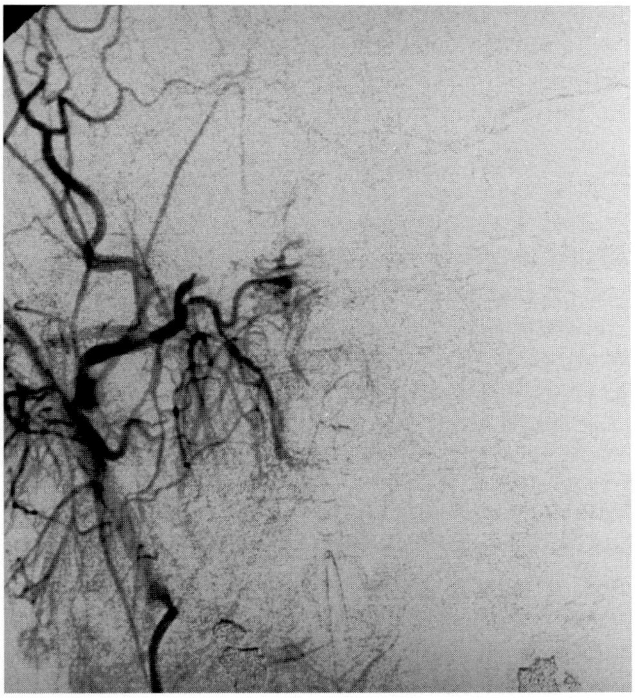

E

FIG. 7-5. *Continued.* **E:** Postembolization of bilateral sphenopalatine and descending palatine arteries with PVA particles shows markedly decreased tumor vascularity.

and parapharyngeal space. The major presentations are sinonasal obstruction and recurrent epistaxis. Hemorrhage in JAF can be fatal and uncontrollable by nasal packing. Superselective embolization is effective in the treatment of bleeding. Surgical removal is facilitated by preoperative embolization (38).

Pretherapeutic evaluation includes computed tomography (CT) or magnetic resonance imaging (MRI), and angiogram (Fig. 7-5A,B). Usual angiographic findings are hypervascular mass with intense parenchymal blush and no demonstrable arteriovenous shunt (Fig. 7-5C). The tumor derives blood supply from branches of the distal internal maxillary artery, the accessory meningeal artery, the ascending palatine artery, and the superior pharyngeal division of the ascending pharyngeal artery. Contralateral supplies are also noted in large lesions (Fig. 7-5D).

The goal of embolization is to devascularize the tumor as much as possible while preserving blood supply to the critical territory (Fig. 7-5E). Small PVA particles, 150 to 250 μm, are the agents of choice for embolization. Glue or 95% alcohol may be used in large or nonresectable tumors. Dangerous anastomosis normally exists between the external and internal carotid arteries. Orbital branches of the anterior deep temporal artery anastomose with the ophthalmic artery, the accessory meningeal artery anastomoses with cavernous branches of the internal carotid artery, the artery of the foramen rotundum anastomoses with cavernous branches of the internal carotid artery, and the ascending pharyngeal artery anastomoses with the vertebral artery as well as petrous and cavernous branches of the internal carotid artery. Larger particles may be used instead in cases of a visible dangerous anastomosis. Moulin et al. (39) reported significant reduction of blood loss in patients with high-grade tumors who underwent preoperative embolization compared with a nonembolized group.

Malignant Tumors of the Skull Base

Many malignant tumors involve the skull base, such as hemangioendothelioma, neurogenic tumor, chordoma, osteosarcoma, chondrosarcoma, and metastasis. Embolization of malignant skull base tumors can be performed as preoperative or palliative treatment (Fig. 7-5A–D). Hypervascular metastasis to the skull base from, for example, the thyroid, kidney, melanoma, and breast, responds well to embolization. The goal of embolization is to cease local growth, stop bleeding, relieve pain, and permit resection if possible. Histoarcyl glue, 95% ethanol, chemotherapeutic agents, or nonabsorbable microparticles are used. Attention should be paid during embolization since these aggressive embolic agents may cause a disaster if they reflux into the normal territory or escape into the dangerous anastomosis. Protection of the anastomosis and critical territory is accomplished by temporary balloon occlusion, detachable balloon, or coils (Fig. 7-5E). The lesions may be stabilized but not cured in most cases.

Preoperative Venous Occlusion

Surgery of the skull base often involves the regions of the jugular foramen and jugular bulb. Retrograde hemorrhage from jugular tributaries includes inferior petrosal sinus, anterior and posterior condylar veins, and posterior cervical venous anastomosis. Transvenous occlusion of these tributaries eases surgery and reduces blood loss. Angiographic study of cerebral venous system is mandatory for evaluation of drainage routes of the normal brain. Occlusion of the venous pathway used by the normal brain causes venous infarction. The anastomotic channels are catheterized and occluded with detachable coils. Carrier et al. (40) described three cases of preoperative venous embolization without significant blood loss during subsequent surgery of the jugular bulb.

COMPLICATIONS AND SIDE EFFECTS OF ENDOVASCULAR TREATMENT

Dissection

Dissection of the catheterized vessels can occur during the procedure. Dissecting the false lumen and the true lumen of the carotid or vertebral artery is usually not visualized on angiography, contrary to that frequently seen on aortic dissection. Common findings are irregularly narrow segment, flame or pencil-shaped narrowing, or complete occlusion. Three factors influence the occurrence of dissection.

First is the technique of vascular catheterization. Vigorous manipulation of the catheter and forceful selective catheterization results in intimal damage. Misplacement or improper positioning of the catheter or guidewire also induces dissection. Second is the guidewire and the catheter. A damaged tip of the catheter or a defect at the tip of the guidewire may injure the intima. Stiffness and sharpness of the guidewire and the catheter also contribute to dissection. Third is the underlying vascular disease of the patient. Patients with fibromuscular dysplasia, vasculitis, and atherosclerosis are prone to develop intimal dissection.

Vasospasm

Direct intimal injury from the catheter tip during difficult selective catheterization may cause vasospasm. Secondary vasospasm follows rupture of the aneurysm or subarachnoid hemorrhage. Usually, the vasospasm is transient. The patient should be kept under heparinization, good hydration, and high blood pressure (so-called triple-H therapy). Mathis et al. (41) reported the use of intraarterial infusion of papaverine hydrochloride for subarachnoid hemorrhage-induced vasospasm. In severe cases with poor response to conservative or medical treatment, balloon angioplasty should be considered.

Embolism

Embolic material such as particles or glue mixture may be propagated into undesired vascular territory during the procedure via improper catheter placement, reflux, or dangerous anastomosis. Air bubble or blood clot may escape into the vascular system. Any air bubble or blood clot in the endovascular device and catheter system must be removed. Careful evaluation of the position of the catheter tip and dangerous anastomosis should be taken prior to embolization. If the risk of embolism is expected or inevitable, the patient should be kept under elevated blood pressure and systemic heparinization in order to promote collateral circulation and prevent aggravating thrombosis.

Rupture and Hemorrhage

Rupture of the aneurysm during coil packing may happen, usually at the tip of the aneurysm. Coils may migrate out of the aneurysmal sac. Rupture of the parent artery may occur during balloon occlusion or dilatation. Contrast extravasation can be visualized on DSA or CT scan. Rupture of the intradural vascular lesion can produce subarachnoid hemorrhage. Localized intramuscular or compartmental hematoma may develop after extradural rupture.

Thrombosis

Thrombosis or distal thromboemboli of the femoral, popliteal, anterior, and posterior tibial arteries may develop during or after endovascular procedure. Popliteal or dorsalis pedis pulsation should be checked during the procedure, as well as during and following compression of punctured femoral artery at the end of the procedure. The affected vessel is evaluated with Doppler auscultation or Doppler sonography. Emergency thrombolysis or vascular surgery may be needed.

Tissue Necrosis

Skin necrosis may follow extensive embolization of the external carotid territory or sclerotherapy using 95% ethanol. Necrosis and ulceration usually heal with granulation, occasionally with possible scarring. Care should be taken to prevent or treat superimposed infection.

IMPACT OF ENDOVASCULAR INTERVENTION ON MANAGEMENT OF PATIENTS

Many studies indicate decreased operating time, reduced blood loss, shortened period of hospitalization, and improved outcome (37–40). Surgical resection of the large or hypervascular tumor becomes possible after preoperative embolization. Endovascular procedure can be done on an outpatient or ambulatory basis.

SUMMARY

Endovascular treatment shows promise as a multimodality treatment of various vascular diseases. It is the treatment of choice in vascular malformations, arteriovenous fistulas, aneurysms, and emergency hemorrhage. Preoperative embolization benefits tumor removal by shortening the operating time and reducing blood loss. Palliative embolization is also helpful in cases of inoperable lesion with relief of symptoms. Initially assumed unresectable tumors may become resectable after embolization.

Although innovative technology and equipment are available and helpful in endovascular treatment, basic vascular anatomic knowledge and interventional skill are still the most important necessity for safe intravascular procedures.

REFERENCES

1. Guglielmi G, Vinuela F, Septeka I, et al. Electrothrombosis of saccular aneurysms via endovascular approach. Part 1: electromechanical basis, technique, and experimental results. *J Neurosurg* 1991;74:1–7.
2. Guglielmi G, Vinuela F, Dion J, et al. Electrothrombosis of saccular aneurysms via endovascular approach. Part 2: preliminary clinical experience. *J Neurosurg* 1991;75:8–14.
3. Serbinenko FA. Balloon catheterization and occlusion of major cerebral vessels. *J Neurosurg* 1974;41:125–245.
4. Taki W, Handa H, Yamagata S, et al. Radiopaque solidifying liquids for releasable balloon technique: a technical note. *Surg Neurol* 1980; 13:140–142.
5. Lasjaunias P, Berenstein A. Technical aspects of surgical neuroangiography. In: Lasjaunias P, Berenstien A, eds. *Surgical neuroangiography*, vol 2. New York: Springer-Verlag, 1987:40–43.
6. Choi IS, Berenstein A, Eskridge J, et al. *Value of temporary balloon occlusion test of major cerebral arteries in predicting tolerance*. Presented at 1986 ASNR annual meeting, Orlando, FL.

7. Keller E, Ries F, Urbach H, et al. Endovascular balloon occlusion test of the internal carotid artery with increased hemodynamic monitoring for determination of circulatory reserve before planned carotid occlusion. *ROFO* 1996;164:324–330.
8. Choi IS. Endovascular treatment of aneurysms. In: Ojemann RG, Ogilvy CS, Crowell RM, Heros RC, eds. *Surgical management of neurovascular disease.* Baltimore, MD: Williams & Wilkins, 1995: 138–150.
9. Ehrenfeld WK, Stoney RJ, Wylie EJ. Relation of carotid stump pressure to safety of carotid artery ligation. *Surgery* 1983;93:299–305.
10. Jawad K, Miller JD, Wyper DJ, et al. Measurement of CBF and carotid artery pressure compared with cerebral angiography in assessing collateral blood supply after carotid ligation. *J Neurosurg* 1997;46:185–196.
11. Erba SM, Horton JA, Latchaw RE, et al. Balloon test occlusion of the internal carotid artery with stable xenon/CT cerebral blood flow imaging. *AJNR* 1988;9:533–538.
12. Elahi MM, Parnes LS, Fox AJ, Pelz DM, Lee DH. Therapeutic embolization in the treatment of intractable epistaxis. *Arch Otolaryngol Head Neck Surg* 1995;121:65–69.
13. Klein GE, Kole W, Karaic R, Szolar DH, Hausegger KA, Scheryer HH. Endovascular embolization treatment for intractable epistaxis. *Laryngorhinootologie* 1997;76:83–87.
14. Chen D, Concus AP, Halbach VV, Cheung SW. Epistaxis originating from traumatic pseudoaneurysm of the internal carotid artery: diagnosis and endovascular therapy. *Laryngoscope* 1998;108:326–331.
15. Tseng EY, Narducci CA, Willing SJ, Sillers MJ. Angiographic embolization for epistaxis: a review of 114 cases. *Laryngoscope* 1998;108: 615–619.
16. Romodanov AP, Shchegelov VI. Intravascular occlusion of saccular aneurysms of the cerebral arteries by means of detachable balloon catheter. In: Krayenbuhl H, ed. *Advances and technical standards on neurosurgery*, vol 9. New York: Springer-Verlag, 1982:25–48.
17. Hilal SK, Khandji, AG, Chi TL, et al. Synthetic fiber-coated platinum coils successfully used for endovascular treatment of arteriovenous malformations, aneurysms, and direct arteriovenous fistulas of CNS. *AJNR* 1988;9:1030.
18. Hieshima GB, Higashida RT, Wapenski J, et al. Balloon embolization of a large distal basilar aneurysm: case report. *J Neurosurg* 1986;65: 413–416.
19. Higashida RT, Halbach VV, Barnwell SL, et al. Treatment of intracranial aneurysms with preservation of the parent vessel: results of percutaneous balloon embolization in 84 patients. *AJNR* 1990;11:633–640.
20. Moret Y. Endovascular treatment of berry aneurysm by endovascular occlusion. *Acta Neurochir* 1991;53:48–49.
21. Malisch TW, Guglielmi G, Vinuela F, et al. Intracranial aneurysms treated with the guglielmi detachable coil: midterm clinical results in a consecutive series of 100 patients. *J Neurosurg* 1997;87:176–183.
22. Halbach VV, Higashida RT, Dowd CF, et al. Cavernous internal carotid artery aneurysms treated with electrolytically detachable coils. *J Neuro-ophthalmol* 1997;17:231–239.
23. Hieshima GB. Therapeutic embolization of vascular injuries. In: Tsai FY, ed. *Neuroradiology of head trauma*, pp. 72–85. Baltimore, MD: University Park Press, 1985.
24. Fox A, Vinuela F, Pelz D, et al. Use of detachable balloons for proximal artery occlusion in the treatment of cerebral aneurysm. *J Neurosurg* 1987;66:40–46.
25. Larson JJ, Tew Jm, Tomsick TA, Van Loveren HR. Treatment of aneurysms of the internal carotid artery by intravascular balloon occlusion: long-term follow up of 58 patients. *Neurosurgery* 1995;36:26–30.
26. Tsukahara T, Wada H, Satake K, Yaoita H, Takahashi A. Proximal balloon occlusion for dissecting vertebral aneurysms accompanied by subarachnoid hemorrhage. *Neurosurgery* 1995;36:914–919.
27. Landolt AM, Millikan CH. Pathogenesis of cerebral infarction secondary to mechanical carotid artery occlusion. *Stroke* 1970;1:52–62.
28. Capps JJ. *Meningiomas: biology, pathology, and differential diagnosis.* New York: Masson, 1982.
29. Manelfe C, Lasjaunias P, Ruscalleda J. Preoperative embolization of intracranial meningiomas. *AJNR* 1986;7:963–972.
30. Bitzer M, Wockel L, Luft AR, et al. The importance of pial blood supply to the development of peritumoral brain edema in meningiomas. *J Neurosurg* 1997;87:368–373.
31. Ng HK, Poon WS, Goh K, Chan MS. Histopathology of post-embolized meningiomas. *Am J Surg Pathol* 1996;20:1224–1230.
32. Nelson PK, Setton A, Choi IS, Ransohoff J, Berenstein A. Current status of interventional neuroradiology in the management of meningiomas. *Neurosurgery Clin North Am* 1994;5:235–259.
33. Kallmes DF, Evans AJ, Kaptain GJ, et al. Hemorrhagic complications in embolization of a meningioma: case report and review of the literature. *Neuroradiology* 1997;39:877–880.
34. Suyama T, Tamaki N, Fijiwara K, et al. Peritumoral and intratumoral hemorrhage after gelatin sponge embolization of malignant meningioma. *Neurosurgery* 1987;21:944–946.
35. Halbach VV, Hieshima GB, Higashida RT, et al. Endovascular therapy of head and neck tumors. In: Vinuela F, ed. *Interventional neuroradiology: endovascular therapy of the central nervous system.* New York: Raven Press, 1992:17–28.
36. Lasjaunias P, Berenstein A. Temporal and cervical tumors. In: Lasjaunias P, Berenstein A, eds. *Surgical neuroangiography*, vol 2. New York: Springer-Verlag, 1987:127–162.
37. Liapis C, Gougoulakis A, Karydakis V, et al. Changing trends in management of carotid body tumors. *Am Surg* 1995;61:989–993.
38. Ungkanont K, Byers RM, Weber RS, Callender DL, Wolf PF, Goepfert H. Juvenile nasopharyngeal angiofibroma: an update of therapeutic management. *Head Neck* 1996;18:60–66.
39. Moulin G, Chagnaud C, Gras R, et al. Juvenile nasopharyngeal angiofibroma: comparison of blood loss during removal in embolized group versus nonembolized group. *Cardiovasc Intervent Radiol* 1995;18: 158–161.
40. Carrier DA, Arriaga MA, Gorum MJ, Dahlen RT, Johnson SP. Preoperative embolization of anastomoses of the jugular bulb: an adjuvant in jugular foramen surgery. *ANJR* 1997;18:1252–1256.
41. Mathis JM, Jensen ME, Dion JE. Technical considerations of intraarterial papaverine hydrochloride for cerebral vasospasm. *Neuroradiology* 1997;39:90–98.

Neurosurgical Issues in Otolaryngology: Principles and Practice of Collaboration, edited by Moisés A. Arriaga and J. Diaz Day. Lippincott Williams & Wilkins, Philadelphia © 1999.

CHAPTER 8

Complications in Skull Base Surgery: Prevention, Recognition, and Management

Peter D. Costantino and Matthew E. Wolpoe

Skull base surgery has seen a rapid progression in technology and technique over the last 15 years, which has been aided by the development and implementation of several medical modalities. These advances now enable surgeons in this new surgical subspecialty to resect extensive lesions in anatomically complex areas most often with minimized morbidity and postoperative complications. Among these developments are advanced imaging techniques such as magnetic resonance imaging (MRI), high-resolution computed tomography (CT) scanning, and angiographic techniques that permit highly accurate localization and characterization of skull base tumors. Modern anesthetic techniques permit safe conduction of lengthy cranial procedures. The surgical microscope now facilitates precise surgical resection of skull base lesions while leaving uninvolved surrounding structures intact.

With the increasing numbers of skull base procedures performed each year, cranial base surgeons are gaining considerable experience in treating and resecting numerous tumor types in disparate anatomic locations. This experience also has aided these surgeons in developing methods to deal with a myriad of intraoperative and postoperative complications. Furthermore, modern reconstructive techniques, which include the use of local and regional flaps as well as the more recently developed free flap and microvascular technology, permit reconstruction of significant defects to produce good aesthetic and functional continuity. But perhaps most importantly, the interdisciplinary nature of skull base surgery, which includes neurosurgeons, neuropathologists, plastic and reconstructive surgeons, neurologists, neuroanesthesiologists, as well as numerous other specialists and support staff, has contributed greatly to the successes of this new subspecialty. In no other area of medicine today have so many different specialties cooperated in such a comprehensive manner to achieve a common goal. These factors taken as a whole have created impressive 5-year survival rates and now make feasible the extraction of neoplastic lesions that were considered unresectable even a decade ago.

Unfortunately, despite these facts, the inherent nature of skull base procedures makes the avoidance of complications a virtual impossibility. This is due to many factors, many of which are unique to the skull base. Surgery in this region requires addressing tumors in a gravity-dependent area of the brain, which predisposes to leakage of cerebral spinal fluid. In addition, tumors are often localized within an intricate system of vital neurologic structures, cranial nerves, major arteries, and venous sinuses. This often makes resection exceedingly difficult. These problems are confounded by large tumors that may directly invade any skull base structure. Furthermore, the close proximity of the skull base to contaminated aerodigestive structures such as the paranasal sinuses, palate, and pharynx puts many postoperative wounds at a high risk of infection.

The primary goal of the surgeon must be to prevent complications with technical skill, proper instrumentation, and cooperation of a competent support staff. In addition, extensive preoperative planning based on the physical exam, radiographic studies, histology of the lesion, and location and size of the tumor is essential. Such an evaluation allows the surgeon to choose the appropriate surgical approach, and, in cases of especially large tumors, to decide if two approaches will be necessary. In addition, proper screening also aids the reconstructive surgeon in formulating a plan to restore cranial continuity. Furthermore, proper preoperative evaluation enables the surgeon to inform the patient and the family of the risks and potential sequelae of any skull base procedure. This gives the patient and family an opportunity

P. D. Costantino and M. E. Wolpoe: Department of Otolaryngology, Mount Sinai Medical Center, New York, New York 10029.

TABLE 8–1. *Potential complications in cranial base surgery*

Category	Complication	Treatment options
Mass lesions	Brain edema	Mannitol, diuretics, barbiturate coma, occasionally lobectomy
Vascular	Hematomas	Evacuation
	Carotid or vertebral artery rupture	Reexploration and repair or occlusion
	Arterial thrombosis	Microvascular bypass Anticoagulation
	Arterial dissection	Anticoagulation
	Cerebral infarction	Induced hypertension
	Venous thrombosis	Volume expansion Diuretics, heparinization
	Air embolism	Left lateral decubitus position, occlusion of venous defect
Other cerebral	Seizures	Anticonvulsants
Cerebrospinal fluid	Cerebrospinal fluid leakage—wound, ear, nose nasopharynx	Reexploration and repair: spinal fluid drainage; vascularized flap
Infections	Meningitis	Antibiotics
	Wound abscess	Drainage
	Epidural, subdural or brain abscess	Antibiotics
Wound	Flap necrosis	Local or distant flap repair
Cranial nerve palsies	Cranial nerves I through XII	Nerve reconstruction; compensatory procedures (e.g., vocal cord injection) Rehabilitation
Metabolic	Diabetes insipidus (DI)	Fluid replacement, vasopressin
	Syndrome of inappropriate antidiuretic hormone secretion (SIADH)	Fluid restriction, hypertonic saline

From ref. 8, with permission.

to develop realistic expectations of the outcome of the procedure and helps avoid undue postoperative strain on the doctor–patient relationship.

However, due to the issues mentioned earlier, even with careful and thorough preoperative planning it is impossible to anticipate and avoid all complications. Therefore, the skull base surgeon should be prepared to deal with complications of any contingency. This chapter addresses many of the most common complications associated with skull base procedures and discusses ways of preventing and managing these potential pitfalls as they arise (Table 8-1).

CEREBROSPINAL FLUID (CSF) LEAK

Since the pioneering skull base procedures described by Ketchum et al. (1) in 1966, CSF leak has been acknowledged as one of the most commonly encountered postoperative complications. While boundless technical advances have been made since these early procedures (Ketchum reported CSF leak or infection in almost 70% of his cases), CSF leak remains the most commonly encountered and one of the most frustrating postoperative sequelae. In fact, CSF leak is still reported to occur in approximately 20% of cranial base procedures (2).

Prevention, or, if not possible, prompt recognition and closure of CSF leaks is extremely important, as meningitis complicates as many as one-third of these fistulas. In addition, CSF leak has also been associated with headaches, hearing loss, hydrocephalus, and intracranial hematomas. These postoperative sequelae are a great source of morbidity, can significantly extend a patient's stay in the hospital, and in some cases can be life threatening.

Although the location of many skull base lesions and the surgical manipulations required to remove them make preventing all CSF leaks impossible, by being aware of the factors that play a role in the development of this complication, the risk of developing a CSF leak can be reduced significantly. Some of the factors that increase the risk of CSF leak include large tumor size, prior irradiation and/or surgery, poor nutritional status, and the presence of dead space following ablation. In addition, certain surgical approaches, such as transphenoidal, transoral, and subfrontal with breach of the frontal sinus, as well as translabyrinthine approaches to acoustic neuromas carry an inherently higher risk of CSF leak (3). Similarly, tumors involving the sella turcica, temporal bone, nasopharynx, paranasal sinuses, or clivus, or lesions in close proximity to the basal cisterns are associated with high rates of CSF leaks.

Through knowledge of these risk factors, and a thorough preoperative patient evaluation including radiographic studies, comprehensive medical history, and a complete head and neck exam, the surgeon should be able to recognize when risk of postoperative CSF leak is high and arrive at an effective plan for prevention and management. Prophylactic lumbar drainage may lower CSF pressure and allow the dura to heal.

While preoperative planning is essential, the single most important measure a surgeon must take to prevent CSF leak is meticulous, watertight closure of the dura. Whenever possible, the surgeon should take great efforts to preserve the dura for adequate closure. However, in cases of intracranial extension, large meningiomas, or extensive dural involvement, this may be impossible. While a detailed description of reconstruction of skull base defects is beyond the scope of this chapter, some general principles that should be followed to avoid complications are worth mentioning.

We advocate reconstructing most dural defects in a layered fashion. Most dural defects in the anterior skull base can be closed primarily with a locking 5-0 suture and supported with a layer of pericranium. This can be facilitated by making the bicoronal incision sufficiently behind the hairline as to preserve an expanse of pericranium and galea adequate for use as a reconstructive flap. There is an increased risk of developing CSF leak if reconstruction is done with a pericranial flap alone since a galeal-pericranial flap has superior vascular supply. Larger dural defects that cannot be closed primarily can be repaired with fascia lata or AlloDerm (Life Cell Technologies, The Woodlands, TX). If extensive portions of the bony orbit are involved, it will be necessary to support cranial structures with a bone graft to prevent herniation, CSF fistulization, and transmission of vascular pulsations. Similarly, if the mucosa covering the frontal sinus has been disturbed, this structure should be filled with autogenous fat, fascia, or hydroxyapatite cement (Bone Source-Leiginger Corp., Rutherford, NJ).

To lessen the chance of leakage and brain herniation in the middle and posterior skull base as well as the infratemporal fossa, similar techniques can be employed. Large defects can be fixed with temporalis muscle, or alternatively by vascularized free flaps. Muscle or soft tissue should not be used as the sole method to cover dural defects, as this is often inadequate. As in the anterior skull base, pericranium, fascia lata, and AlloDerm are all viable options to repair larger dural defects.

A great deal of attention has been paid to the repair of lateral skull base defects following removal of acoustic neuromas and glomus tumors, as localization near the mastoid air cells and eustachian tube is associated with a high rate of CSF leaks (4). In these situations, fat, fascia, and often fibrin glue have been used traditionally to obliterate mastoid air cells, middle ear, and eustachian tube (5). In contrast, we advocate obliterating these structures instead with Bone Source (6). This substance has been shown to provide stable volume while exhibiting low complication rates. These reconstructive techniques should be coupled with the use of lumbar spinal drainage intraoperatively to lower CSF pressure and lessen the likelihood of postoperative leaks.

Even with meticulous closure of the dura and reconstruction of skull base defects, CSF leaks are inevitable in cranial base surgery. Therefore, knowledge of how to recognize and treat them is of paramount importance. The most salient principle in early recognition of CSF leaks is continuous postoperative monitoring of the patient, aided by support staff trained in critical care. Symptoms of CSF leak include pain or headache (especially positional), unexplained fever, and, more seriously, meningitis. In addition, rhinorrhea may present as a sweet or salty taste in the patient's mouth, or alternatively may produce hoarseness or coughing. Otorrhea, although more subtle, may be described as a fullness in the patient's ear or intermittent dizziness. Such signs and symptoms should be taken with extreme seriousness and aggressive measures should be taken to rule out a leak.

Once a CSF leak is suspected, two primary questions must be answered: Is it a high- or low-flow leak, and where is it coming from? These questions are important as they determine the type and timing of treatment. High-flow leaks can be seen actively draining from the wound ear canal or nasal cavity; if active drainage is not visible, the leak must be considered low flow.

Before any treatment is employed, efforts should be made to verify that the fluid leaking is in fact CSF, but in some situations this is difficult to do. Fluid that contains glucose is most likely CSF, since this is not present in nasal secretions. However, because nasal secretions may be mixed with a glucose containing serous exudate, this criteria is not entirely specific. Traditionally, CSF leak was diagnosed by eliciting the halo sign, which results from the mixture of blood and CSF. The halo is formed when the blood/CSF mixture spreads out on an absorbent surface. A dark ring of blood will encircle a center of more lightly stained CSF. While this sign is fairly specific, it has a relatively low sensitivity. Therefore, we recommend performing a β-transferrin electrophoretic assay. This test is both highly sensitive and specific for CSF.

In addition to recognition of CSF leaks, it may also be necessary to localize low-flow leaks. Several methods are currently available to do this accurately. One highly effective technique is gamma cisternography. In this procedure pledgets are first packed into both of the patient's nostrils. A lumbar puncture is then made, during which an infusion of radioactive albumin is infused into the subarachnoid space. Twenty-four hours later the cotton pledgets are removed and examined for radioactivity. Since albumin induces meningeal irritation, indium may be used instead.

A second technique for localization, metrizamide CT cisternography, employs similar concepts to those used in gamma cisternography. In this procedure, following lumbar puncture metrizamide is infused in the subarachnoid space. Activity is detected later with axial and coronal CT scans by a neuroradiologist. In the proper hands it has been reported that this method is highly sensitive at localizing CSF leaks (7).

A third method for CSF localization is by detection with low-concentration fluorescein dye. In this procedure, a sterile dilution of 0.3 mL of fluorescein in 10 mL of CSF is prepared and then infused intrathecally. It can be expected that the fluorescein will become visible in 20 to 30 minutes. If necessary, visualization may be enhanced with the aid of a Wood's lamp.

Once a CSF leak is identified, to prevent potential infectious sequelae immediate steps must be taken to stop the leak. High-flow leaks should be fixed in the operating room as soon as is feasible. However, there is much less consensus among surgeons on how to treat low-flow leaks. Since as many as 70% of CSF leaks close spontaneously, a short trial of conservative therapy should be attempted before more invasive measures are taken. This consists of a several-day trial of bed rest, head elevation, and warnings about sniffing, sneezing, and coughing. CSF pressure may be reduced pharmacologically with Lasix, Digitalis, or acetazolamide in selected patients. Prophylactic antibiotics may promote development of resistant organisms.

Low-flow leaks should be treated immediately by elevating the patients head 20 to 50 degrees and inserting a lumbar spine drain (some advocate use of continuous lumbar cerebrospinal drainage) for a period of 3 to 5 days. The egress of CSF through lumbar drain must be controlled strictly to avoid the development of pneumocephalus (.50 mL of CSF should be removed, .50 mL every 8 hours, to allow the leak to seal). The patient should also be given stool softeners and cough suppressant as needed to prevent staining. Furthermore, he or she should be monitored continuously for changes in mental status and evidence of air within the subarachnoid space. Sudden rapid drainage of spinal fluid may result in brainstem herniation and death.

If spinal drainage is unsuccessful in stopping the leak, surgical intervention must be employed. Although there is increasing experience repairing CSF fistulas endoscopically, currently the most reliable technique is to open the wound, identify the leak, and repair the defect. If the fistula is large or in a compromised area, vascularized tissue should be considered.

If the predisposing element for the leak is elevated spinal fluid pressure, this must be evaluated, since increased intracranial pressure may be associated with grave consequences. If this is suspected, the patient should be treated immediately with a ventriculoperitoneal shunt.

One last point that merits consideration is that due to the inherent time length of skull base procedures, the surgical team often may be tired at the end. Thus, errors might be committed during closure and reconstruction. While it is imperative to achieve clear margins following tumor removal, even if the patient is cancer free, he or she may still suffer great morbidity if meticulous closure and repair of operative defects is not employed. Therefore, concentration, while always important, is essential near the completion of cranial base procedures.

MENINGITIS

As the majority of cases of meningitis can be linked directly to a persistent CSF fistula, the methods described in the previous section to prevent and treat this complication will also lower the risk of infectious meningitis. Meningitis can complicate as many as one-third of CSF fistulas. Although many skull base procedures are performed in a clean-contaminated environment, where the wound is in close contact with the aerodigestive tract the rate of infectious complications is surpassingly low, occurring in only 5% of skull base procedures. This is due in large part to the efforts by surgeons to achieve complete postoperative separation of the palate, paranasal sinuses, and nasopharynx from the intracranial environment.

Also, in an effort to prevent postoperative infection and meningitis, it is our common practice to employ intraoperative antibiotics routinely. These should be started on the day of the operation and continued for 48 hours postoperatively. Lengthier courses of antibiotic therapy have not been shown to decrease the rates of infection. The antibiotics used should offer broad coverage to include both aerobic and anaerobic organisms. Penicillin, clindamycin, and aminoglycosides such as tobramycin, ceftriaxone, and vancomycin are commonly used for this purpose. When infection is suspected, the therapeutic regimen should be modified by postoperative cultures. If preoperatively the patient is recognized as a high-risk candidate for postoperative infection, many surgeons advocate doing a preoperative resistance analysis on cultures taken from the nose, mouth, and pharynx. It should be noted that while this is a commonly accepted practice, some authors contend that perioperative antibiotic prophylaxis increases the risk of opportunistic organisms and fungal growth (4).

To prevent gross contamination of tissues intraoperatively, it is also wise to irrigate the subarachnoid space and exposed structures with a bacitracin solution. Similarly, only well-vascularized tissues should be placed into or near the wound site, as ischemic tissues serve as a nidus for bacterial growth. Also, drains and catheters should be removed as soon as is feasible. Other risk factors for meningitis that have appeared in the literature include prior irradiation, longer operative procedures, and poor nutritional status.

It is not possible to overstate the importance of having a high index of suspicion for meningitis, as early recognition of infection is imperative to ensure patient survival. We routinely obtain cultures on the second postoperative day, prior to stopping prophylactic antibiotics. Cultures should be repeated every 48 to 72 hours until the patient is discharged. If the patient develops signs of altered mental consciousness, fever, headache, nausea and vomiting, or nuchal rigidity, meningitis should be suspected until proven otherwise. Kernig's sign (pain in the hamstring muscles on attempted extension of the leg after flexing the thigh), and Brudzinski's sign (either passive flexion of the legs with flexion of the neck or the passive flexion of one leg when the other is bent) may be elicited, and should be used as clues to confirm suspicions of meningitis.

Treatment of meningitis includes similar broad-spectrum antibiotics as used for prophylaxis but are tailored to the results of susceptibility cultures. Additionally, since CSF leaks are frequently a cause of meningitis, vigorous efforts should be made to diagnose, locate, and close them. Surgical treatment should include debridement of necrotic and ischemic tissues and replacement by fresh vascularized tissues to insulate the CNS and obliterate dead space. Free, nonvascularized bone flaps should be removed, but osteotomized facial pieces should be left in place as these resist infection.

It is worth noting that not all meningitis is infectious in origin. Aseptic meningitis, which is the result of meningeal irritation, is a commonly encountered complication of skull base surgery. Signs and symptoms are similar to infectious meningitis, but cultures are typically negative, and there is absence of significant pyrexia (8). Repeatedly negative cultures, CSF with normal sugar, and slightly increased white blood cell count and protein, in the face of signs of low-grade fever and mild nuchal rigidity, should raise suspicions of aseptic meningitis.

As a preventative measure, since bone dust and sharp edges have been shown to cause meningeal irritation, they should be removed after craniotomy has been completed. Several types of tumors, including craniopharyngiomas, epidermoid tumors, cholesteatoma, and cholesterol granulomas, are of particularly high risk of inducing aseptic meningitis since spillage of cystic fluid within these tumors into the subarachnoid space can result in acute irritation. Treatment of aseptic meningitis is conservative because the condition almost always resolves spontaneously, although death has been reported in rare cases.

CRANIAL NERVE DEFICITS

Cranial nerve deficits are potentially the most debilitating complication encountered in skull base surgery. Since preoperative functioning is usually a good indicator of postoperative outcome, a thorough preoperative head and neck exam is essential to estimate the degree of postoperative morbidity. In addition, the location of tumor and its extension confirmed by MRI, as well as the type of approach or approaches that will be attempted, should give the surgeon a good idea of the type and severity of deficits to expect postoperatively. Furthermore, the patient and family should be informed of this expected outcome as it is important for them to have realistic expectations of the limits and pitfalls of the intended procedure.

Cranial nerve and sensory function should be monitored intraoperatively with somatosensory evoked potentials (SSEPs) and electromyographic (EMG) potentials. SSEP is useful in tracking the general status of the neuraxis by electrically stimulating sensory nerves and recording responses. Changes in wave forms may suggest ischemia or improper manipulation. EMG is useful in detecting functional impairment of motor nerves and may allow detection of impairment of even smaller branches of cranial nerves.

Olfactory Nerve

The olfactory nerve is often involved in tumors of the anterior skull base (e.g., in ethesioneuroblastoma) and may be injured during removal of tumors in this region or the paranasal sinuses. Unfortunately, at present there is no treatment for anosmia. While this is true, although anosmia is usually uncomfortable initially to the patient, overall it is fairly well tolerated. Anosmia is associated with some morbidity since patients will be unable to detect rancid food or potentially dangerous problems like gas leaks, unless these substances cause irritation to trigeminal nerve fibers within the nasal mucosa and palate. The patients should be made aware of these potential complications in order to avoid any unfortunate sequelae.

Optic Nerve

The optic nerve is purely a special sensory nerve, which, like the olfactory nerve, is enveloped by central myelination. Therefore, this nerve also has very poor regenerative capacity. The optic nerve may be compressed as a result of craniopharyngiomas, pituitary adenomas, and some meningiomas. In addition, vision may be jeopardized by a transsphenoidal approach to the sella turcica, manipulation of the ethmoid system, or surgery in the maxillary antra.

If there is a potential for visual loss in any procedure, visual potentials should be monitored during surgery. Furthermore, as is true of all cranial nerves, sharp dissection around the optic nerve under direct visualization of the operating microscope will lower the risk of injury. If direct irreversible injury to the eye occurs, it should be recognized that blindness in the contralateral eye may occur due to sympathetic uveitis.

In addition to the aforementioned causes, vision loss has also been reported because of suprasellar hematoma, optic nerve migration into an empty sella turcica, and most importantly from ischemia. If visual loss occurs as a result of hematoma, it should be evacuated immediately, because return of vision after decompression is possible. In addition, since the decussating fibers of the optic chiasm are supplied uniquely by inferior arteries from the circle of Willis, these arteries should be identified and preserved to avoid ischemic nerve injury.

Cranial Nerves III, IV, V, and VI

Cranial nerves III, IV, V1, V2, and VI all course within the confines of the cavernous sinus and exit the skull via the superior orbital fissure. Therefore, surgery in or around the cavernous sinus, the petrous apex, and in the anterior skull base risks injuring any or all of these nerves. Unlike the optic and olfactory nerves, as long as these nerves are in relative continuity, there is a good chance of at least some recovery if anastomosis can be performed. Realistic expectations of postoperative function can be gauged by the preoperative degree of impairment. Patients should undergo a comprehensive ophthalmic evaluation, and a history of diplopia, eye injuries, or surgery should be documented so they will not be wrongly construed as a surgical complication.

Injury to the oculomotor nerve is relatively uncommon, but when it does occur a significant degree of morbidity may ensue. If this nerve is sectioned, a primary anastomosis should be attempted if the fibers can be sewn under minimal tension. If this cannot be done because portions of the oculomotor nerve are missing or damaged, primary anastomosis should not be contemplated. Instead, a cable graft composed of the greater auricular or sural nerve should be interposed between the severed ends. Because the oculomotor nerve innervates multiple, highly intricate extraocular muscles as well as being the parasympathetic control to the pupillary and ciliary muscles, these repairs are associated with varying levels of recovery.

Paralysis of the oculomotor nerve causes binocular diplopia strabismus, ptosis, and mydriasis. Under the supervision of an ophthalmologist, persistent postoperative diplopia can be managed with patches, occlusive lenses, special glasses, and prisms (9). Other therapies that have been described include botulinum toxin, which is used to weaken antagonistic muscles, and strabismus surgery to restore binocular vision in a functional position of gaze. Surgery has been successful in treating ptosis, and sympathomimetic eye drops are usually effective in treating mydriasis.

Unlike the oculomotor nerve, cranial nerves IV and VI are purely motor nerves; each innervates a single muscle. Because of this, diplopia induced by injury or compression of these nerves is usually well tolerated. While the trochlear nerve exits the brainstem posteriorly and therefore has a long intracranial course, it is relatively well protected within the tentorium and is injured infrequently. In contrast, the abducens nerve, which also has a long intracranial course, may be injured during temporal bone resection and in surgery of the posterior fossa, especially if Dorello's canal is disturbed.

Injuries to both the trochlear and abducens nerves cause diplopia but are often corrected by the patient's turning his or her head when gazing in the region of the paralysis. As with the oculomotor nerve, if possible primary anastomosis should be attempted, if either nerve is injured, or if anastomosis is not feasible, a cable graft should be used. Both nerves typically respond quite well to these types of reconstructions. If function of the nerve does not resume, treatment is nearly identical to that for the oculomotor nerve. This can include paralysis of antagonistic muscles with botulinum toxin as well as surgical alterations of the lengths of various extraocular muscles to achieve better visual alignment. The surgeon should be aware that various conditions such as Duane's syndrome (congenital aplasia of the abducens nucleus where muscle is innervated by cranial nerve III), myasthenia gravis, and thyroid disease all may mimic sixth nerve palsies and should be ruled out with a comprehensive preoperative history and physical exam.

The trigeminal nerve may be damaged during a transtemporal approach to the clivus, acoustic neuroma surgery, or temporal bone resection. In addition, portions of the nerve may be injured by a variety of procedures in the anterior skull base. Disruption of the ophthalmic division of this nerve is a grave injury since it puts the patient at risk of an insensate cornea. This can cause corneal tearing and neurotrophic keratitis, both of which may lead to blindness. Damage to the ophthalmic trigeminal division is especially dangerous if there is concurrent injury to the facial nerve. In this situation, both the motor and sensory arms of the corneal reflex are lost. Primary anastomosis and cable grafting of the ophthalmic nerve have produced highly variable results. But since any recovery of sensation is desirable, steps should be taken to achieve it with either of these mechanisms. In any case of ophthalmic nerve paralysis, the patient should be fitted with protective glasses and should be warned against using contact lenses.

The mandibular or third division of the trigeminal nerve is at risk of injury in surgery of craniopharyngiomas and meningiomas that involve the floor of the middle fossa. The hypesthesia from these cranial neuropathies can be troublesome. If the deficit is unilateral, patients can usually accommodate. The loss of the motor division of V3 can create functional problems with chewing that can be lessened with temporomandibular joint (TMJ) splints and bite retraining therapy.

Cranial Nerve VII

Facial paralysis is a readily apparent and disabling condition for patients following cranial base surgery. The most important principle is avoidance of facial nerve injury if possible. However, if it occurs, measures at the time of surgery can be quite helpful in long-term rehabilitation for the patient. Specifically, if the nerve is transected at the time of surgery, the optimal results occur with direct reanastomosis of the severed ends or, if necessary, an interposition nerve graft. In the postoperative period, the principal concern in a patient with facial paralysis is appropriate care of the eye. If the paralysis is thought to be of a transient nature, aggressive lubrication with methyl-cellulose drops during the day, ointment at night, and use of a moisture chamber will protect the cornea from abrasion or ulceration. If this injury is also coupled with trigeminal injury, the situation is potentially serious as the patient will not feel damage to the cornea. In these patients, the surgical care of the eye even including tarsorrhaphy needs to be considered. If it is expected that there will be several months of complete paralysis, procedures such as gold weight augmentation of the upper lid are helpful to protect the cornea from ulceration.

For patients in whom anatomic integrity of the nerve is lost at the time of surgery but there is not sufficient nerve to perform a reanastomosis, nerve substitution procedures are ideal. The facial to hypoglossal end-to-end anastomosis is currently the technique of choice. If the reanastomosis will be performed early after nerve injury, then the facial to split hypoglossal anastomosis is ideal. In this procedure, the main trunk of the seventh nerve is anastomosed end to side to the hypoglossal nerve. This provides adequate mimetic function for the face, but limits any morbidity from the hypoglossal nerve. However, if the procedure is delayed for a year, at that time there is sufficient fibrosis within the tubules of the distal facial nerve that additional hypoglossal function would be necessary. In this situation, we recommend the full hypoglossal to facial anastomosis. Reanimation procedures usually require approximately 9 months to a year to show the initial benefit, and the maximum result is usually not apparent until 18 to 24 months postoperatively. With the House-Brackmann scale, the best result is a grade III or IV recovery.

For patients in whom reinnervation is not possible because of the duration of time prior to evaluation or the extent of distal facial fiber disruption, facial tone augmentation and partial facial reanimation procedures such as the temporalis sling procedure can be a useful adjunct. Detailed discussion of facial reanimation following skull base surgery is provided elsewhere (Surgical Rejuvenation of the Face, 2nd ed. Baker TJ, Gordon AL, eds. Mosby, 1996).

Cranial Nerve VIII

A loss from damage to the acoustic nerve in skull base surgery is usually noted immediately following the surgery. Particularly in acoustic tumors, patients are well aware of the risk to hearing. However, even in surgeries remote from the eighth nerve, hearing can be jeopardized in posterior fossa surgery because of muscular effects or retraction injuries. If unilateral hearing loss occurs, auditory rehabilitation can be achieved with a contralateral routing of signal (CROS) type of hearing aid, which as its name implies reroutes auditory signals from the uninvolved ear to the contralateral side. Cochlear implants are also an option, even if the translabyrinthine approach is used, if the patient has bilateral peripheral hearing loss.

Vertigo associated with removal of the vestibular division is usually transient, and near normal function can be expected in a matter of weeks. If the patient is especially debilitated, vestibular suppressants may be used on a short-term basis, but the mainstay of rehabilitation requires vestibulo-ocular reflex exercises. However, if the nerve is transected incompletely, severe, potentially intractable vertigo may develop. This could necessitate a second surgical procedure or selectively induced toxicity with aminoglycoside injection.

Cranial Nerves IX and X

The glossopharyngeal and vagus nerves travel together throughout most of their course in the skull base and therefore are often injured simultaneously. Paralysis of these nerves is potentially one of the most deadly complications encountered in skull base surgery. This is due to the fact that simultaneous paralysis of the vagus and glossopharyngeal nerves causes vocal cord paralysis; an inability to elevate the larynx and palate to protect the airway and prevent aspiration and regurgitation; failure to relax the cricopharyngeus muscle to facilitate swallowing; as well as pharyngeal and laryngeal anesthesia, which obliterates the cough and gag reflexes. This can result in dysphagia, aspiration, and an inability to detect and clear harmful stimuli from within the throat, and it often compromises the patient's airway. If concurrent hypoglossal nerve paralysis is also present, dysphagia is even more pronounced, making oral feeding hazardous.

Despite the impact of acute loss, if the function of the lower cranial nerves is lost insidiously (e.g., from compression by a skull base tumor) patients are able to compensate and tend to do quite well. However, if the loss is acute, such as due to surgical trauma, these patients usually experience significant problems with swallowing and aspiration. The aforementioned problems are especially dangerous in the elderly patient with impaired pulmonary function who is unable to clear aspirated secretions.

The glossopharyngeal and vagus nerves are injured most often as a result of tumors in the posterior fossa, clivus, jugular foramen, and foramen magnum. An exceedingly grave situation results when large tumors in the vicinity of the foramen magnum cross the midline, causing bilateral vagal and glossopharyngeal nerve paralysis. This is a potentially life-threatening emergency that requires immediate intubation of the patient to prevent imminent asphyxia. Also in this situation, or in the case of unilateral paralysis that compromises the patient's airway, treatment with both tracheotomy and gastrostomy should be considered. Tracheotomy ensures a patent airway and allows suctioning to improve the pulmonary toilet. Similarly, gastrostomy, which is better tolerated than a nasogastric tube, will allow the patient to be given adequate nutrition without the risk of aspiration. If a compromised airway and significant dysphagia are anticipated preoperatively, gastrostomy may even be done at the time of surgery.

If paralysis of cranial nerves IX and X does occur, there are a variety of techniques that have been developed to deal with many of the ensuing complications. Specifically, in the presence of vocal cord paralysis, vocal cord augmentation by injecting Gelfoam, fat, or collagen will improve the quality of the patient's voice as well as reducing his or her risk of aspiration. If this paralysis is anticipated to be short-lived, treatment with Gelfoam is often indicated, since this substance is resorbed in 6 to 8 weeks.

Formerly, if the injury was anticipated to be of longer duration, vocal cord augmentation was performed using Teflon. However, Teflon has fallen out of favor since it is permanent and is difficult if not impossible to remove once a tissue reaction has occurred. Therefore, we recommend injection of more biocompatible substances such as autogenous fat, which is traditionally harvested from the patient's abdomen, or micronized AlloDerm (Life Cell Technologies), which is a solution of architecturally intact processed human cadaver dermis.

While vocal cord augmentation will result in improved voice and decreased aspiration with high vagal nerve injury, as is usually encountered in skull base surgery, patients lose the function of both the superior laryngeal and recurrent laryngeal nerves. This results in complete vocal cord paralysis, causing the denervated cord to lie in the intermediate position rather than the paramedian position that is seen following isolated recurrent laryngeal nerve injury. In this situation, it is not possible to achieve complete medialization of the membranous portion of the cords. Therefore, even after augmentation the patient may still have a breathy voice and be at risk for aspiration. Thus, many surgeons maintain that the cord should instead be repaired using thyroplasty (10). In this procedure, cartilage or a Silastic wedge is implanted between the thyroid cartilage and thyroarytenoid fascia causing complete medialization of the cord. This can result in superior voice quality and vast improvements in pulmonary toilet. In addition, if loss of vagal function is anticipated preoperatively, the thyroplasty may even be performed several weeks prior to the skull base procedure to eradicate the risk of postoperative aspiration. The main drawback of this procedure is that it is much more invasive than augmentation by injectable substances and may not be tolerated by some patients.

If vagal nerve paralysis is potentially permanent, the patient may be a candidate for the modified Lindeman procedure for laryngotracheal separation (11). In this procedure, which is described in detail elsewhere, the trachea is cut at the second tracheal ring, the proximal portion is oversewn, while the distal portion is sewn to a hole made in the skin. Laryngotracheal separation provides the desired improvements in airway and relief of aspiration while offering the option of reversal if neurologic function is restored. Unfortunately, this is a highly invasive procedure that causes complete loss of speech.

Treatment of dysphagia and pharyngeal incoordination caused by lower cranial nerve palsies usually consists of a barium swallow test and evaluation by a speech therapist trained in rehabilitation of swallowing disorders. Dysphagia is often treated surgically by cricopharyngeal myotomy, which has proven to be highly effective in facilitating swallowing.

Cranial Nerve XI

The spinal accessory nerve, like the glossopharyngeal and vagus nerves, is injured most often as a result of tumors in the posterior fossa, clivus, jugular foramen, and foramen magnum. Many surgeons do not address accessory nerve injury as its sacrifice is considered standard in many head and neck oncologic procedures. However, long-term loss of accessory function can result in atrophy of the sternocleidomastoid and trapezius muscles. This will result in a winged scapula if the arm is abducted past 90 degrees, and also may cause deep shoulder pain and arthropathy. Therefore, if possible, a primary anastomosis should be attempted. Physical therapy is often helpful in rehabilitating these patients.

Cranial Nerve XII

Unilateral hypoglossal paralysis has a relatively good prognosis, since patients learn to speak almost normally after therapy. In contrast, bilateral injury, usually caused by large skull base tumors around the foramen magnum, can cause significant functional impairment. In this situation patients experience significant dysphagia and loss of speech. As is the case with severe vagal and glossopharyngeal nerve palsies, these patients require tracheotomy and gastrostomy to prevent aspiration and to allow administration of adequate nutrition. In addition, consultation with a speech therapist trained in treatment of swallowing disorders should be sought to facilitate reestablishment of oral feeding and speech.

CEREBRAL EDEMA

Cerebral edema, which is inevitable following brain manipulation, is a potentially life-threatening complication that usually occurs several hours after surgery, but has been noted to occur as long as several days postoperatively (8). The degree of edema is most directly related to the degree and duration of intraoperative retraction. Therefore, surgical approaches that minimize this type of manipulation are highly desirable. This can be facilitated most effectively by removal of adequate bone removal during the initial craniotomy. Although achieving adequate visualization has a tendency to increase operative time, the avoidance of edema is well worth this investment.

In addition to adequate visualization, accurate preoperative localization of the tumor using CT and MRI scans is of paramount importance. This will enable the surgeons to choose approaches that will keep brain retraction to a minimum. Similarly, the venous anatomy of the region should be well understood and visualized with arteriogram including small venous anastomoses. This is important because if it is necessary to sacrifice major veins draining a particular brain region, it is essential to preserve collateral circulation to ensure adequate drainage. A technique that may be used during removal of extradural tumors is insertion of a lumbar drain during induction to lower intracranial pressure if needed during the procedure.

Temporal lobe swelling is a serious complication that must be avoided at all costs. This condition is precipitated by inadvertent coagulation of, or damage to, the basilar or occipital veins and especially the vein of Labbé. These veins should be identified and preserved.

The hallmark of cerebral edema is a lateralizing or focal neurologic deficit or altered mental status. Any change in the patient's level of consciousness in the immediate postoperative period should raise suspicions of this condition. A CT scan may be performed routinely within the first 24 hours postoperatively to screen for edema and other complications such as pneumocephalus and hematoma. Once edema is detected, treatment should not be delayed, since the intracranial cavity has a very limited capacity for expansion and edema can quickly compromise blood supply. Treatment of edema once it develops can include hyperventilation, mannitol, or other osmotic agents, or fluid restriction (up to 1,000 mL per day). Corticosteroids may also be used, but they should be reserved for episodes of severe edema since these agents impede wound repair. Life-threatening edema may be treated with a temporary barbiturate coma.

FLUID AND METABOLIC DISTURBANCES

The pituitary gland and hypothalamus, which are structures of vital importance to survival of any patient, may be jeopardized in a variety of skull base procedures. The most commonly encountered skull base lesions that risk injuring these structures are pituitary tumors, craniopharyngiomas, and meningiomas located in the region of the sella turcica. In addition, severe head trauma and surgical manipulation causing ischemia of vital arterial perforators can also result in damage to either the pituitary or hypothalamus. Specifically, following surgery for pituitary tumors, neurogenic hyperthermia may cause coma and death. In addition, permanent hypernatremia with loss of the normal thirst mechanism may occur after extensive damage to the hypothalamus during skull base surgery.

While the above complications (Table 8-2) are serious and potentially life threatening and should be appreciated, by far the most common sequelae of pituitary and hypothalamic manipulation are transient diabetes insipidus (DI) and the syndrome of inappropriate antidiuretic hormone secretion (SIADH). DI, which results from an inadequate secretion of antidiuretic hormone (ADH), limits the ability of the patient to retain free water, causing polyuria, polydipsia, dehydration, and hypovolemia. This condition may be suspected when urine output exceeds 250 mL per hour for 2 hours. In such a situation serum electrolytes will show an osmolarity greater than 290 mOsm/L, a serum sodium in excess of 140 mg/dL, and a urine specific gravity approaching 100. Since these findings may be erroneously confused with postoperative fluid mobilization, efforts must be made to confirm the presence of DI. Because DI is usually self-limited in duration, treatment is usually temporary and often consists only of fluid replacement. In more severe manifestations a course of vasopressin or desmopressin may be considered (Table 8-2).

SIADH, which is clinically the opposite of DI, is also a common manifestation following surgery around the sella turcica. This condition may also result from strokes, systemic metabolic disturbances, or intracranial bleeding, or may originate from an ectopic site, often from small cell carcinoma of the lung. The laboratory criteria for SIADH are a serum osmolarity below 280 mOsm/kg, serum sodium less than 135 mEq/L, an elevated urine sodium of >25 mEq/L, and an inappropriately high urine osmolarity (>300 mEg/L). Like DI, SIADH is self-limited and treatment usually consists of fluid restriction to a maximum of 1,000 mL per day. Severe cases may be treated with a hypertonic saline solution, diuretics, and a competitive inhibitor of ADH such as demeclocycline.

TABLE 8–2. *Possible electrolyte disturbances after cranial-base surgery*[a]

Laboratory parameter	Diabetes insipidus	SIADH
Serum osmolality	Increased	<280 mOsm/kg
Urine osmolality	<150 mOsm/kg	Increased
Serum sodium	>150 mEq/L	<135 mEq/L
Urine sodium	Decreased	>25 mEq/L
Urine specific gravity	<1.005	>1.015
Circulating free water	Decreased	Increased
Volume of urine output	>250 mL/hr for over 2 hr	<30 mL/hr

SIADH, syndrome of inappropriate antidiuretic hormone secretion.

[a] The onset of diabetes insipidus is usually heralded by urine output exceeding 250 mL/hr for 2 consecutive hours; the first sign of SIADH is usually a serum sodium less than 135 mEq/L.

From ref. 8, with permission.

VASCULAR PROBLEMS

Hematomas

Hematomas, which can potentially be fatal, are occasionally encountered following skull base surgery, and most often develop from inadequately coagulated vessels. In intradural hematomas the source of bleeding is usually vessels from the tumor itself, while extradural hematomas are often the result of improper middle meningeal ligation (3). Extradural hematomas may also arise subacutely with leakage of vessels from large craniotomy sites. In any case of a hematoma, one must always consider the possibility that a coagulopathy is present. Most often, a good preoperative history and exam will detect prior coagulopathies and thrombocytopenia. However, these problems may also be iatrogenically induced through excessive transfusion. This problem may be avoided by concurrent infusion of fresh frozen plasma when packed red cells are given. The usual recommendation is one or two units of fresh frozen plasma for every four units of packed red cells. A rare but serious complication that should always be on the differential is disseminated intravascular coagulation, which should always be considered if bleeding cannot be controlled.

Most causes of hematoma can be prevented by meticulous maintenance of hemostasis and proper ligation of exposed vessels. In addition, tumor vessels should be addressed only when they are in direct view, and should not be attacked from a blinded position. All bridging veins under tension and branches of the middle meningeal artery should be carefully coagulated. Dural margins may be tacked to the craniotomy site to obliterate dead space and reduce the risk of epidural seepage.

To lower the risk of bleeding, many tumors, especially highly vascular tumors like meningiomas, jugular and vagal paragangliomas, and nasopharyngeal angiofibromas, are candidates for embolization. A patient's neurologic status and the surgical objective are also factors if this is to be considered. Once deciding the patient is a good candidate for embolization, prior to the surgeon's performing the procedure, the tumor should be evaluated with a highly selective angiogram. This will depict the angioarchitecture of the tumor as well as identify numerous small anastomoses that may be present.

The patient may also be given provocative testing with sodium amytal or lidocaine; if a palsy is induced, the patient is not a candidate for embolization. When properly performed, embolization can significantly reduce postoperative bleeding (12). This risk can also be reduced by employment of proper surgical techniques. These include using sharp dissection in the vicinity of the tumor bed, removing only well-visualized structures, and performing dissection in a plane parallel to visible arteries.

As stated earlier, all patients should have their first postoperative CT scan 24 hours after surgery. If a collection of blood is found, treatment is usually reoperation and evacuation. If arteries are inadvertently lacerated intraoperatively, the proximal carotid artery should be occluded temporarily and the injury should be repaired using simple 6-0 monofilament suture. If primary anastomosis is not feasible, a saphenous vein graft may be interposed between a larger lacerated segment. It is important to recognize that saphenous vein grafts may themselves be the site of hemorrhage if blood pressure is not properly controlled postoperatively.

Stroke and Embolism

Vascular occlusion is a significant source of morbidity and mortality in skull base surgery and most often is related to management of the major blood vessels supplying the brain. Postoperative stroke can be either embolic or thrombotic, or can be related to arterial spasm or significantly increased intracranial pressure caused by uncontrolled cerebral edema. Removal of tumors in the vicinity of the cavernous sinus is especially hazardous since the internal carotid artery (ICA) may be compromised easily.

All patients, especially those who may require carotid sacrifice, should undergo a preoperative cerebrovascular evaluation. This includes the temporary balloon occlusion (TBO) test in which a catheter is advanced into the ICA and inflated. If neurologic signs develop within 10 to 20 minutes of occlusion, the patient is not a candidate for carotid resection. Patients who fail this test outright are at especially high risk of thrombotic occlusion and may be candidates for prophylactic carotid bypass. This will allow anticoagulants to be used until the graft matures without risk of intracranial bleeding, and will forgo the risk of stroke if the carotid artery is sacrificed. Bypass usually consists of either a middle cerebral to superficial temporal arterial anastomosis or interposition of a saphenous vein graft from the extracranial segment to the petrous portion of the carotid artery.

Because 10% to 15% of candidates who pass the TBO test later develop ischemia, we recommend performing a second test, the xenon-enhanced CT scan (XeCT). In XeCT, xenon, which is radiodense, is infused into the ICA, a CT scan is then done to generate digital data. Widespread use of the XeCT has led to the development of criteria that can be used as a prognostic indicator of morbidity if the carotid is sacrificed (13). According to this criteria, if the patient passes the TBO but demonstrates XeCT of ≤30 mL/100 g/min, short-term occlusion is relatively safe, but if carotid resection is necessary a bypass should be done. Patients who pass both exams are considered candidates for carotid resection if it is unavoidable (Table 8-3).

Approximately 2% of patients who pass both the TBO and XeCT will still experience cerebrovascular complications (8). Despite extensive preoperative workup and new imaging modalities, no currently available test can accurately predict the risk of stroke with carotid occlusion.

Unfortunately, the predictive value of tests of the vertebral circulation have proven even less reliable. The standard method is the four-vessel angiogram, but this is of variable

TABLE 8–3. *Cerebrovascular evaluation and treatment options: balloon occlusion test of internal carotid artery*

		No neurologic deficit (xenon CT-CBF study)	
	Neurologic deficit	Reduction of CBF (15–35 mL/100 g/min)	No reduction of CBF (>35 mL/100 g/min)
Hemodynamic stroke risk			
Brief temporary occlusion (<2 hours)	Mild-moderate	None	None
Prolonged temporary occlusion (>2 hrs)	High	Mild	Mild
Permanent	High	Moderate-high	None
Management options if artery must be occluded	ST-MCA bypass	ST-MCA bypass	ICA-ICA short vein graft (benign tumors)
	ST-MCA and direct vein graft ECA-MCA long vein graft	ICA-ICA vein graft	No reconstruction (malignant tumors)

ST-MCA, superficial temporal artery–middle cerebral artery; ICA–ICA, Internal carotid artery–internal carotid artery; ECA-MCA, external carotid artery–middle cerebral artery.
From ref. 8, with permission.

accuracy. Well-known syndromes caused by compromised posterior cerebral circulation, such as the lateral medullary syndrome [due to occlusion of the posterior inferior cerebellar artery (PICA)], have been well documented and are sources of significant morbidity. Surgeons should always be prepared to recognize and deal with cerebrovascular insufficiency whether it occurs in the intra- or postoperative period.

Vasospasm

While vasospasm is most often associated with subarachnoid hemorrhage, fatal vasospasm complications may occur with resection of skull base tumors (14). Hypotheses of the cause of vasospasm have included manipulation and dissection along an artery, mechanical disruption of the arterial wall, release of chemical substances during resection, and damage to the hypothalamus. It has also been hypothesized that since most vasospasm occurs after suprasellar resection in areas supplied by the anterior cerebral artery, a vessel often implicated in aneurysm formation, that a similar pathogenetic mechanism exists—clotted blood in the subarachnoid cistern.

Traditionally, vasospasm has been detected and confirmed by angiography, but recently other methods such as xenon inhalation studies and transcranial Doppler flow velocity have been implemented. Reports of successful treatment for vasospasm have been somewhat limited, although calcium channel blockers and hypertensive hypervolemia hemodilution reportedly have been effective. Intraoperative vasospasm may still be treated with topical papaverine.

PAIN

Although pain frequently follows skull base surgery, this postoperative sequela has received surprisingly little attention in the literature. Pain in the postoperative period can range from a temporary annoyance to chronic and debilitating. This postoperative pain has been associated with the manipulation of almost every major structure in the head, neck, and skull base. Therefore, some degree of postoperative pain is to be expected.

The most common structures of the skull base that have been implicated in pain include the muscles of mastication as well as the trapezius and posterior cervical muscles. Pain from the structures can occur as a result of nerve manipulation, division of the muscles themselves, and removal of their points of insertion from the perimeter of the skull base. In addition, nerve injury and compression have also been implicated in extreme pain and paraesthesias.

In acoustic neuroma surgery, several studies have been undertaken to examine the degree of postoperative pain based on the surgical approach employed. The most common manifestation of pain reported following this type of surgery has been headache. Overall, authors who have examined risk factors for pain after acoustic neuroma removal have found the suboccipital and retrosigmoid approaches, especially when combined with a craniectomy, are associated with more severe postoperative pain than the translabyrinthine and middle fossa approaches (15).

The best results seem to occur in situations combining nonsteroidal antiinflammatories, judicial use of nerve blocks, and behavioral medicines sometimes including biofeedback in a full pain clinic approach. Occasionally, entrapped nerves in scars can be released surgically, although this is certainly not the first line of therapy for postoperative pain in skull base surgery.

SEIZURES

Postoperative seizures are a risk of any procedure that manipulates the temporal lobe, a particularly epileptogenic region of the brain. Usually antiseizure prophylaxis is indicated postoperatively. The postoperative management of seizures requires prompt control to avoid increases of intracranial pressure that could exacerbate cerebral edema and damage brain substance. The medications for postoperative seizure treatment are outlined in Table 8-4. Once the seizure has been controlled, CT and metabolic evaluations are necessary to identify treatable causes. Oral prophylactic antiseizure therapy may be started.

TABLE 8–4. *Treatment postoperative seizure*

	Indication	Dose
Diazepam	Ongoing seizure activity or status epilepticus—may cause respiratory depression; will stop seizures, but will not prevent them; need to follow with loading dose of Dilantin or phenobarbital	10 mg IV q 20 min × 3 if needed
Dilantin	Ongoing seizure activity, status epilepticus, or oral seizure prophylaxis—does not depress respiration; can cause hypotension; do not give faster than 50 mg/min; therapeutic blood levels; 10–20 μg/mL; causes nystagmus on lateral gaze at therapeutic levels	Treatment: 15 mg/kg IV over 30–45 min Prophylaxis: 300 mg/day IV/po
Phenobarbital	Seizure prophylaxis—significant sedative effect in adults; therapeutic blood levels (adult): 20–40 μg/mL	60 mg IV/po b.i.d.
Tegretol	Seizure prophylaxis—can cause blood dyscrasias, leukopenia, and liver dysfunction; can also be used to treat trigeminal neuralgia; therapeutic blood levels: 3–12 μg/mL	100–200 mg IV/po 2 to 3 times/day

From ref. 8, with permission.

CONCLUSION

The ideal management of complications in cranial base surgeries is prevention. The patient should be adequately counseled about the possibility of these difficulties and the plan of action if they were to occur. Advances in tissue transfer, prosthetic materials, and a better understanding of management of postoperative complications continue to improve the care of patients with skull base lesions.

REFERENCES

1. Ketchum AS, Wilkins RH, VanBuren JM, Smith RR. A combined intracranial facial approach to the paranasal sinuses. *Am J Surg* 1966; 106:698.
2. Linskey ME, Lunsford LD, Flickinger JC. Radiosurgery for acoustic neuromas, neurinomas: early experience. *Neurosurgery* 1990;26: 736–745.
3. Sen C, Snyderman CH, Sekhar LN. Complications of skull base operations. In: Sekhar LN, Janecka I, eds. *Surgery of cranial base tumors.* New York: Raven Press, 831–839, 1993.
4. Hoffman RA. Cerebrospinal fluid leak of temporal bone origin. In: Jackler RK, Brackmann DE, eds. *Neurotology*. St. Louis: Mosby, 1994: 919–928.
5. Rodgers GK, Luxford WM. Factors affecting the development of cerebrospinal fluid leaks after translabyrinthine acoustic tumor surgery. *Laryngoscope* 1993;103:959–962.
6. Rueton JF, Friedman CD, Costantino PD. Indications for hydroxyapatite cement reconstruction in lateral skull base surgery. *Am J Otol* 1995; 16(4):465–469.
7. Shetty PG, Shroff MM, Sahanic DR, et al. Evaluation of high resolution CT and MR cisternography in the diagnosis of cerebrospinal fluid fistula. *Am J Neuroradiol* 1998;19(4):633–639.
8. Costantino PD, Janecka IP. Cranial base surgery. In: Baily BJ, ed. *Head and neck surgery: otolaryngology*, 2nd ed. Philadelphia: Lippincott-Raven, 1998:1831–1853.
9. Ing E, Kennerdale JS. Evaluation and treatment of extraocular motility deficits. In: Syms C, Arriaga MA, eds. *Rehabilitations of neurotologic deficits. Otolaryngology Clinics of North America* 1997;30(5): 877–892.
10. Netterville JD, Civantos FJ. Rehabilitation of cranial nerve deficits after neurotologic skull base surgery. *Laryngoscope* 1993;103(2, part 2):45–54.
11. Sekhar LN, Janecka IP: Rehabilitation of swallowing. In: Synderman CH, Johnson JT. *Surgery of cranial base tumors*. New York: Raven Press, 1993:819–824.
12. Murphy TP, Brackmann DE. Effects of preoperative embolization on glomus jugulare tumors. *Laryngoscope* 1989;99:1244–1247.
13. DeVries EJ, Sekhar LN, Janecka IP, et al. Elective resection of the internal carotid artery without reconstruction. *Laryngoscope* 1988;98: 960.
14. Sekhar LN, Janecka IP. Complications of skull base operations. In: Sen C, Snyderman CH, Sekhar LN, eds. *Surgery of cranial base tumors*. New York: Raven Press, 1993:831–840.
15. Driscoll CL, Beatty CW. Pain after acoustic neuroma surgery. In: Syms CA, Arriaga MA, eds. *Rehabilitation of neurotologic disease. Otolaryngology Clinics of North America* 1997;30(5)893–903.

Neurosurgical Issues in Otolaryngology: Principles and Practice of Collaboration,
edited by Moisés A. Arriaga and J. Diaz Day.
Lippincott Williams & Wilkins, Philadelphia © 1999.

CHAPTER 9

Neuroradiology

Bolivia T. Davis and Robert C. Platenberg

Neuroimaging procedures play a vital role in the evaluation and management of patients cared for by neurosurgeons and otolaryngologists. Cross-sectional techniques using computed tomography (CT) and magnetic resonance imaging (MRI) form the foundation of analysis of individuals with cerebellopontine angle (CPA) lesions, jugular foramen lesions, encephaloceles, pituitary abnormalities, cervical spine, facial trauma, and skull base lesions. MRI and CT angiography also play a role in the evaluation of aneurysms. This chapter highlights basic anatomy and cross-sectional imaging techniques of the skull base, temporal bone, and sellar region in regard to neurosurgical issues in otolaryngology. Various pathologic entities of the aforementioned areas with an emphasis on diagnosis, classic appearances, and new techniques are also discussed.

GENERAL TECHNIQUES

Prior to the invention of CT, plain film, film tomography, and angiography were the methods used to evaluate patients with lesions of the skull base, face, and spine. The plain film and film tomographic evaluation of the patient has essentially been replaced by CT. Diagnostic angiography has a role in the preoperative evaluation of some tumors and in patients with small aneurysms; however, the majority of neuroangiographic examinations in many academic centers are performed as neurointerventional procedures using endovascular treatment for therapeutic intervention rather than diagnosis. Endovascular treatment options and techniques are discussed elsewhere.

The basic principles for CT evaluation include high-resolution, thin-slice, small field of view imaging performed with or without intravenous or intrathecal contrast administration. The latest generation, present-day CT machines have postprocessing algorithms capable of edge enhancement of bone window settings and optimizing soft tissue settings. The smallest slice thickness of 1 mm and a field of view of 12 cm are essential for imaging the temporal bones but may not be necessary for the analysis of facial trauma, where a 3- to 5-mm slice thickness with a 22-cm field of view provides images of diagnostic quality. A tailored approach for lesions depending on their location is necessary (Table 9-1).

Intravenous contrast enhancement helps define the size, shape, and contour of tumors and abscesses. With rapid bolusing of contrast and spiral CT scanning of the circle of Willis, generation of CT angiographic images is possible. Postprocessing of the data obtained in this manner provides maximum intensity images similar to MRI angiography.

Intrathecal contrast administration is used to localize the site of cerebrospinal fluid (CSF) leakage and to perform myelography. Metrizamide was the first available, ionic, water-soluble contrast material. It has been replaced by nonionic contrast agents such as Isovue® (Bracco Diagnostics) and Omnipaque® (NYCOMED). Contrast is administered usually through a lumbar puncture and subsequently manipulated through gravitational positioning into the area of interest. The patient is scanned with the area of suspected leak in the dependent position, using high-resolution technique. Nuclear medicine cisternography using indium 111 may be performed to document whether or not a patient has a CSF leak but does not precisely localize the site of leakage. CT cisternography for CSF leak has the advantage of being able to localize the site of CSF leak, but the patient must have an active leak during the performance of the examination for the offending site to be detected.

MRI has revolutionized patient evaluation and management in many areas of medicine. In patients with CPA, skull base lesions, encephaloceles, jugular foramen lesions, and pituitary lesions, MRI plays a predominant imaging role or complementary role to CT. MRI has importance in evaluating cervical spine trauma and in the diagnosis of complica-

B. T. Davis: Department of Radiology, Georgetown University Medical Center, Washington, DC 20007.
R. C. Platenberg: Medical Director, MedTel International Corporation, McLean, Virginia 22102.

TABLE 9–1. *Computed tomography (CT) techniques*

	Slice thickness	FOV	Projections
Temporal bones	1–1.5 mm	18 cm	Axial, coronal
Facial bones	3–5 mm	20–22 cm	Axial, coronal
Cervical spine	1–3 mm	16–18 cm	Axial w/ sagittal/coronal reconstructions
Sella	1–1.5 mm	16–18 cm	Axial, coronal

FOV, field of view.

tions from facial trauma. High-resolution, thin-slice, and small field of view images are desirable. Routine anatomic two-dimensional (2D) imaging has a minimum slice thickness of 3 mm. Volumetric techniques exist that allow the performance of three-dimensional (3D) imaging with slices of 0.8 mm. Time constraints limit the number and types of studies performed. New 3D fast spin echo (FSE) techniques with ultralong echo train lengths and half-Fourier imaging may allow for the evaluation of the internal auditory canal to rule out acoustic schwannoma without the use of intravenous contrast material.

There have been many advancements in coil as well as gradient technology and in the development of new sequences. FSE techniques allow very heavily T2-weighted images to be performed in a reasonably short time. FSE imaging provides higher resolution, better signal to noise capability, and improved image quality. Fluid-attenuated inversion recovery (FLAIR) is a T2 sequence that generates heavily T2-weighted images with suppression of signal from CSF in the ventricles and subarachnoid space. These sequences initially suffered from long scan times, but with fast techniques have become integral sequences for the evaluation of cortical lesions, multiple sclerosis (MS), intracranial infections, and lesions near the ventricular surface (1–3). FLAIR sequences are a routine part of every brain examination in our institution. The use of these imaging techniques may have limitations in the detection of MS plaques in the infratentorial region (1,4), and as a result the evaluation of the postoperative patient with an abnormality in the posterior fossa may require additional routine conventional spin echo imaging if no FLAIR lesion is noted.

MRI is also capable of performing imaging that provides information on flow and physiology. MR angiography (MRA) is capable of visualization of the arterial and venous anatomy of the central nervous system (CNS). MRA, however, may not be a sensitive enough technique to evaluate small dural fistula, slow flow arteriovenous malformations (AVMs), or other vascular abnormalities. MRI phase contrast sequences that are sensitized to moving fluid and slow flow may assist in the detection of CSF leak, hydrocephalus, and shunt malfunction (5). CSF flow waveforms may be generated to assess CSF dynamics (6). MR cisternography is becoming a helpful tool in the evaluation of CSF fistula (see below). Continued research in this area will only improve our understanding of CSF flow.

Diffusion weighted studies assist in the early detection of brain ischemia and infarction (7–9). During the initial hours of cerebral infarction, routine imaging may not detect areas of damaged brain. FLAIR imaging may also underrepresent areas of brain injury and ischemia. Diffusion weighted images allow for the early detection of cytotoxic edema caused by cerebral energy depletion. Hardware and software requirements may limit these techniques to research centers or newer MRI systems. Severe distortion of posterior fossa anatomy may also be problematic. The efficacy of these techniques in the early detection of posterior fossa pathology in the postoperative or trauma patient holds exciting promise, but remains to be proven.

Echo-planar imaging (EPI) allows for obtaining images in as little as 40 msec and plays an important role in functional MRI (fMRI). Using blood oxygen level dependent (BOLD) techniques, research has been performed to evaluate brain activity related to blood flow changes for motor activity, speech, vision, olfaction, and higher cortical functions. Three principles are involved in BOLD imaging: (a) Roy and Sherrington (10) demonstrated that blood flow and brain activity are linked. (b) Thulborn et al. (11) and Brooks and Di Chiro (12) demonstrated that deoxygenated blood acted like contrast material. (c) Fox and Raichle (13), using positron emission tomography (PET), demonstrated a mismatch between oxygen delivery and glucose utilization in areas of brain activation. When a task is performed, more oxygenated blood is delivered to the tissue performing the task than is needed. There is a change in the ratio of oxygenated to deoxygenated blood that can now be measured with clinical-strength magnets and mapped onto anatomic images of the brain. The study of the brain using these techniques has the potential to expand our understanding of brain function in many clinical situations. The relevance of fMRI to the neuro-otologist and skull base neurosurgeon will undoubtedly become defined as more research is performed in these areas.

NORMAL ANATOMY AND VARIATIONS

High-resolution CT (HRCT) demonstrates exquisite intrinsic anatomy of the temporal bones. Although in-depth discussion of normal anatomy is beyond the scope of this chapter, an overview of temporal bone anatomy will be highlighted. Commencing from the outer to inner ear, the external auditory canal (EAC) is approximately 2.5 cm in length and mildly undulating (14). It consists of fibrocartilage in its outer third segment and of bone in the medial two-thirds. The surrounding bone of this air-filled structure provides great contrast for visualization on HRCT in both the axial and coronal planes. The EAC and middle ear are separated by the tympanic membrane. The tympanic membrane, a hairline structure seen on HRCT, is divided into an upper pars flaccida and a lower pars tensa. From superior to inferior, the middle ear is divided into epitympanum, mesotympanum, and hypotympanum. The ossicles reside within the mesotympanum, with the exception of the malleus head and incus body, which lie in the epitympanum. Both axial and coronal HRCT sections are a necessity for complete evaluation of the ossicular chain (15). The aditus ad antrum connects the epitympanum to the mastoid antrum, the largest cells of the mastoid. The mastoid is further subdivided into a central mastoid tract and peripheral mastoid area. Although pneumatization of the temporal bones may be variable, it is often symmetrical (16). The bony labyrinth of the inner ear structures consists of the vestibule, semicircular canals, cochlea, vestibular, and cochlear aqueducts. The bony internal auditory canal (IAC), although not considered a part of the labyrinth, is pertinent in the evaluation of retrocochlear pathology. All of these inner ear structures are well visualized on HRCT.

The two main vascular foramina intimately associated with the temporal bones are the paired jugular foramina and carotid canals. The jugular foramen is formed by both the petrous and occipital bones. It is divided by a fibrous or osseous septum, the jugular spine, into the pars nervosa anteromedially and the pars vascularis posteromedially. There are several variations of the jugular bulb foramen, some of which may cause pulsatile tinnitus and present as a vascular tympanic mass. The most common variation is the asymmetric jugular bulb foramen. Variation in not only symmetry, but size is frequently found. Often, the jugular bulb and associated draining tributaries are larger on the right compared to the left. The surrounding soft tissue and osseous structures are preserved without destruction (Fig. 9-1). The high-riding jugular bulb with or without dehiscence occurs in about 7% of the population (17). With dehiscence of the jugular bulb, the lateral bony plate of the jugular foramen is absent, allowing this venous structure to simulate a bluish retrotympanic mass (Fig. 9-2). Finally, the jugular bulb diverticulum is a focal superior protrusion of the jugular bulb. In these patients, the jugular bulb may be normal or high and the otoscopic examination is normal (16). All of these variations can be easily diagnosed on HRCT. Only in the presence of bony or soft tissue destruction should further workup including MRI or arteriography be considered. The internal carotid arteries traverse the petrous bone, first ascending vertically and then turning horizontally lying on the fibrocartilaginous foramen lacerum. The arteries continue cephalad as the precavernous carotid arteries in the carotid canal.

On MRI, the air-filled spaces of both the EAC and middle ear are invisible. Likewise, the dense bone of the ossicular chain produces no MR signal. Thus, MRI is not the imaging modality of choice to exclude subtle abnormalities of the osseous structures and ossicles. MR imaging is preferred, however, in evaluating intracranial extension, large lesions, and invasion of adjacent soft tissue structures. MRI has also supplanted CT in imaging the CPA, IAC, and membranous labyrinth. Thin gradient echo sequences provide high-contrast images of the fluid-containing membranous and peri-

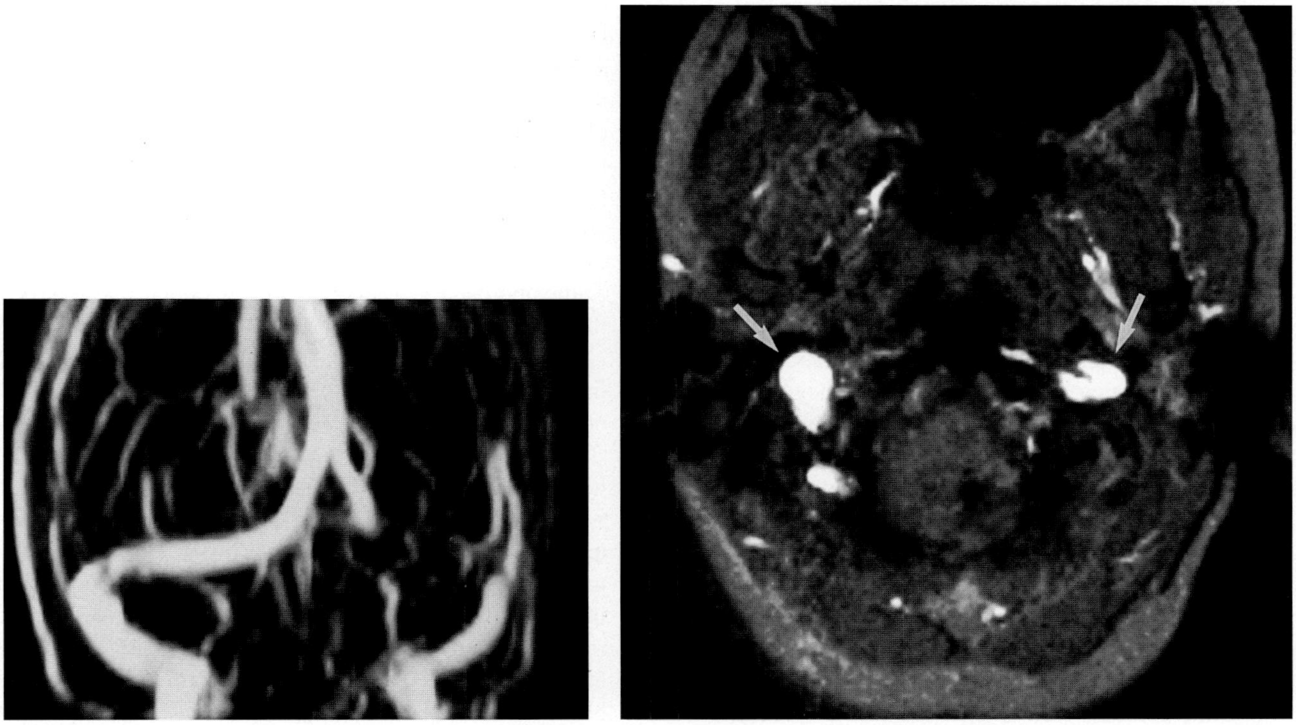

A B

FIG. 9-1. Normal magnetic resonance (MR) venogram maximal intensity **(A)** and source images **(B)** of the dural venous sinuses and jugular bulbs with preferential drainage into the right transverse sinus. Note asymmetry of the jugular bulbs, larger on the right than left (*arrows*).

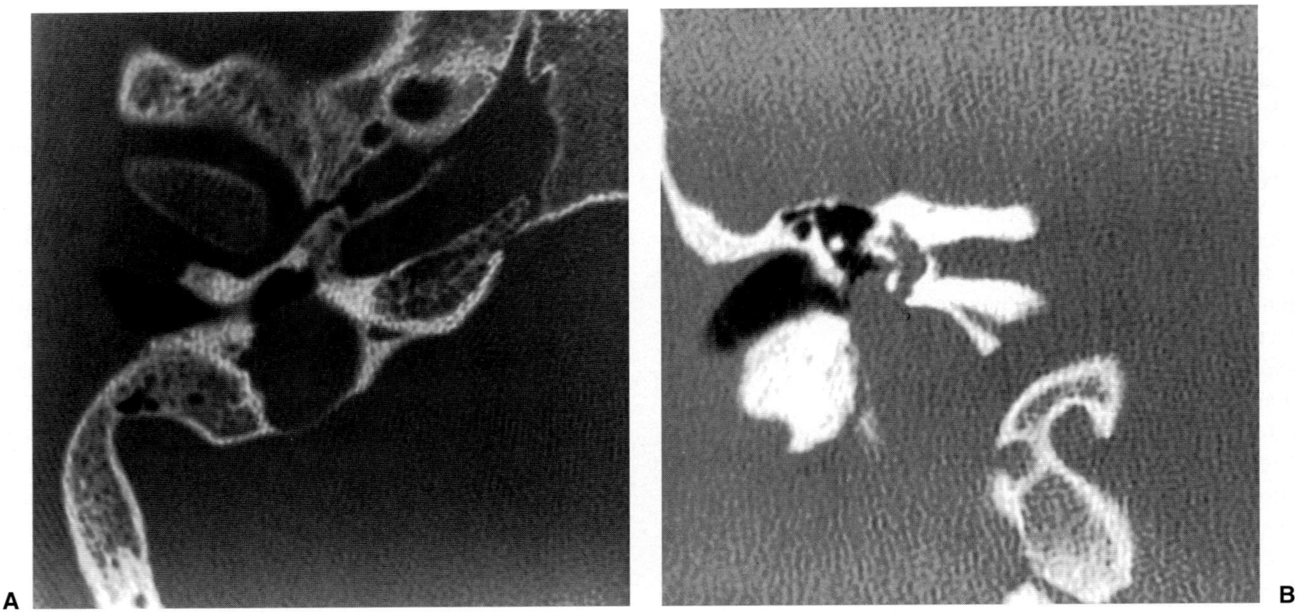

FIG. 9-2. A 16-year-old with a right pulsatile retrotympanic mass. Axial **(A)** and coronal **(B)** noncontrast computed tomography (CT) scans show enlargement of the right jugular foramen with a soft tissue mass protruding into the hypotympanum. High riding jugular bulb with dehiscence.

lymphatic labyrinth, as well as divisions of the facial and vestibulocochlear nerves (18). For this reason, MRI has gained acceptance in imaging patients with sensorineural hearing loss (SNHL) or vertigo (19).

TRAUMA

Temporal bone fractures have been classified into two basic types—longitudinal and transverse—depending on the orientation of the fracture line to the long axis of the petrous pyramid. Often these fractures contain components of both types and are termed complex or mixed. While longitudinal fractures usually result from direct trauma to the temporoparietal region, horizontal fractures result from indirect trauma due to frontal or occipital impact (20). Both types of fractures are seen well on high-resolution thin (1-mm) CT images, especially in the axial projection.

Longitudinal fractures are at least three times more common (70%–90%) than transverse fractures. They have a horizontal orientation passing through the squamous portion of the temporal bone, EAC, middle ear, tegmen tympani, and between the cochlea and semicircular canals. Because of involvement of these structures, perforation of the tympanic membrane, hemotympanum, and conductive hearing loss (CHL) are often present. Ossicular dislocation may also occur, commonly involving the incudostapedial joint because of its weak support. Facial nerve paralysis is seen in 10% to 20% of cases. Occurring as a result of nerve edema distal to the geniculate ganglion, paralysis is often delayed and incomplete, resolving spontaneously.

Transverse fractures are less common (10%–30%) than longitudinal fractures. These fractures have a vertical orientation occurring perpendicular to the long axis of the petrous bone. The inferior to superior extent of the fracture is from the foramen magnum to the middle cranial fossa, often passing through the bony labyrinth or IAC. The involvement of these later structures is the cause of the higher frequency of SNHL than CHL. Injury to the cochlea or the cochlear nerve is the usual cause of this deficit. Facial nerve paralysis is far more common in transverse fractures with reports as high as 50% (20,21). Injury of the facial nerve is likely to involve the labyrinthine segment proximal to the geniculate ganglion. The resultant facial paralysis due to this injury is often immediate and complete. To prevent permanent damage, most authors agree that surgical repair should be performed within a 72-hour period (22). Hearing preservation surgery involves a middle cranial fossa approach, while a translabyrinthe approach is reserved for those patients who have lost their hearing (16).

The resultant intracranial complications of temporal bone fractures are of the greatest clinical concern to the neuro-otologist and neurosurgeon. These abnormalities include CSF leak, meningitis, extraaxial collections and intracranial hemorrhage. CSF otorrhea is due to a defect in the tegmen tympani, usually due to a longitudinal fracture of the temporal bone. There is also perforation of the tympanic membrane, which is common with this type of fracture. CT imaging, especially in the coronal plane with sagittal reformations, is most useful for delineating the site of the fistula. MRI has the added advantage of discerning CSF fluid from blood based on the signal characteristics. Newer techniques are becoming available to assist in determining the site of the actual fistula (see Pituitary Adenoma, below). CSF rhinorrhea, in contrast, occurs in the presence of an intact tympanic membrane with egress of CSF via the eustachian tube into the nasopharynx and nasal cavity. Transverse fractures are the usual cause in this situation. With both CSF otorrhea and rhinorrhea, a CT cisternogram with the introduction of non-ionic contrast via a lumbar puncture is another useful modality for evaluating the site of the fistula that is not readily apparent on routine CT imaging. A persistent CSF leak, pneumocephalus, or the presence of a cephalocele may lead to the subsequent development of meningitis. On both CT and MRI, the findings are usually underwhelming and often normal in early or mild disease. In severe cases, however, exudate within the basilar cisterns with enhancement of the leptomeninges maybe seen. Cephaloceles associated with temporal bone fractures result in the herniation of intracranial contents through the fracture defect if sufficient in size. MRI with its multiplanar capabilities allows ease in making the diagnosis. Hemorrhages of the brain parenchyma and subdural and epidural spaces are readily apparent with the cost-effectiveness and efficiency of CT. MRI, however, becomes useful when these abnormalities are subtle and partially obscured by artifact from the adjacent bone. On MRI from the acute to the late subacute stage, hemorrhage evolves from a predominant hypointense signal on T2-weighted images to a hyperintense signal on both T1- and T2-weighted images.

TUMOR AND TUMOR-LIKE LESIONS

While it is beyond the scope of this chapter to describe all the neoplasms and tumor-like masses within and adjacent to the temporal bone and skull base, the most common lesions of the CPA, jugular foramen, and petrous apex will be discussed.

Schwannomas

Schwannomas are benign tumors of Schwann cell origin that arise from the nerve sheath. Over the years, various terms have been used to describe this tumor, including neurinoma, neurilemoma, and neuroma. *Schwannoma* is the terminology often accepted. The cousin neoplasm of these tumors is the neurofibroma, which on occasion can be difficult to distinguish from schwannomas pathologically. The neurofibroma is also a benign tumor that is composed of both Schwann cells and neural tissue. Both of these tumors contain varying amounts of Antoni A (compact cellular) and Antoni B (loose mxyomatous) tissue. The predominant tissue type reflects the signal characteristic seen on T2-weighted images (T2WIs) (23,24). A predominance of Antoni A tissue because of its higher nuclear-cytoplasmic ratio results in a hypointense signal on T2WI, and, conversely, predominance of Antoni B tissue produces a hyperintense signal.

The vast majority of intracranial schwannomas arise from the superior and inferior vestibular and cochlear nerves in descending order of frequency (24,25). Acoustic schwannomas are also the most common tumor occurring in the CPA and accounts for 75% to 90% of tumors arising in this region (Table 9-2). In adults, they typically appear between the 5th and 7th decades of life and are slightly more common in females. In children and young adults, these tumors tend to occur bilaterally in association with neurofibromatosis 2; however, isolated lesions have been reported (26). These tumors typically produce symptoms of SNHL, tinnitus, and vertigo caused by pressure effects on the vestibular and cochlear nerves.

TABLE 9–2. *Cerebellopontine angle masses*

Acoustic schwannoma
Meningioma
Epidermoid
Arachnoid cyst
Nonacoustic schwannoma
Aneurysm
Paraganglioma
Metastasis

MRI has supplanted conventional CT and air or contrast CT cisternography in the evaluation of these tumors. On T1-weighted images (T1WIs), they are iso- to hypointense, while on T2WI they are relatively hyperintense. After gadolinium administration, small tumors enhance homogeneously. Large tumors tend to demonstrate heterogeneous enhancement representing cyst formation, xanthomatous change, or varying degrees of cellularity (27). Most of the tumors in the CPA have both intracanalicular and cisternal components producing an "ice cream cone" appearance on contrast MR images (Fig. 9-3). Less than 20% are solely intracanalicular or cisternal (25). By far the most common intracanalicular mass is an acoustic schwannoma, followed by postoperative scar (Fig. 9-4) (28). Other intracanalicular enhancing lesions include hemangioma, meningioma, Bell's palsy, and Ramsay Hunt syndrome (herpes zoster otitis) (Fig. 9-5 and Table 9-3). The interface of these tumors with the temporal bone produces an acute angle, in contrast with meningiomas, which form an obtuse angle. The association of peritumoral edema and arachnoid cysts is not uncommon (29). In general on angiography, the majority of these tumors are hypo- or avascular, producing mass effect on surrounding vessels.

Nonacoustic schwannomas resemble acoustic schwannomas and account for less than 5% of all intracranial schwannomas (30). Symptoms produced by these tumors are related to the cranial nerve affected. Trigeminal schwannomas are the second most common schwannoma after those involving the acoustic nerve. These tumors may arise intradurally from the CPA and Meckel's cave or extradurally from the gasserian ganglion in the middle cranial fossa (31). These tumors in comparison to acoustic schwannomas have a more cystic appearance (32). Facial schwannomas are the next most common site of cranial nerve involvement. The geniculate ganglion is the most frequent site; however, any

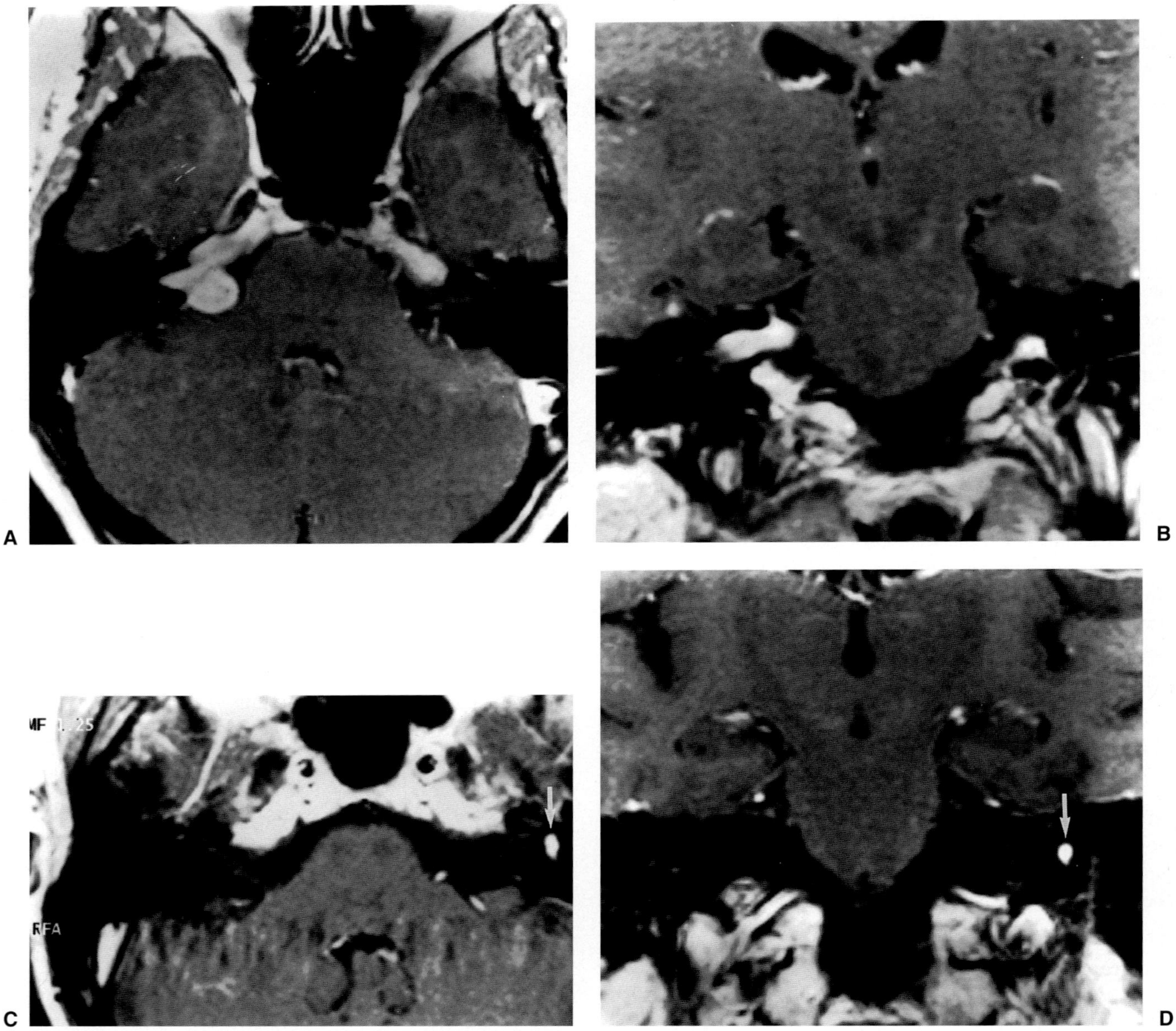

FIG. 9-3. A 59-year-old woman with right hearing loss and acoustic schwannoma. Axial **(A)** and coronal **(B)** postcontrast T1-weighted MR images (T1WIs) demonstrate an enhancing cerebellopontine angle (CPA) and intracanalicular mass on the right. Axial **(C)** and coronal **(D)** postcontrast T1WIs of a vestibular schwannoma isolated to the vestibule.

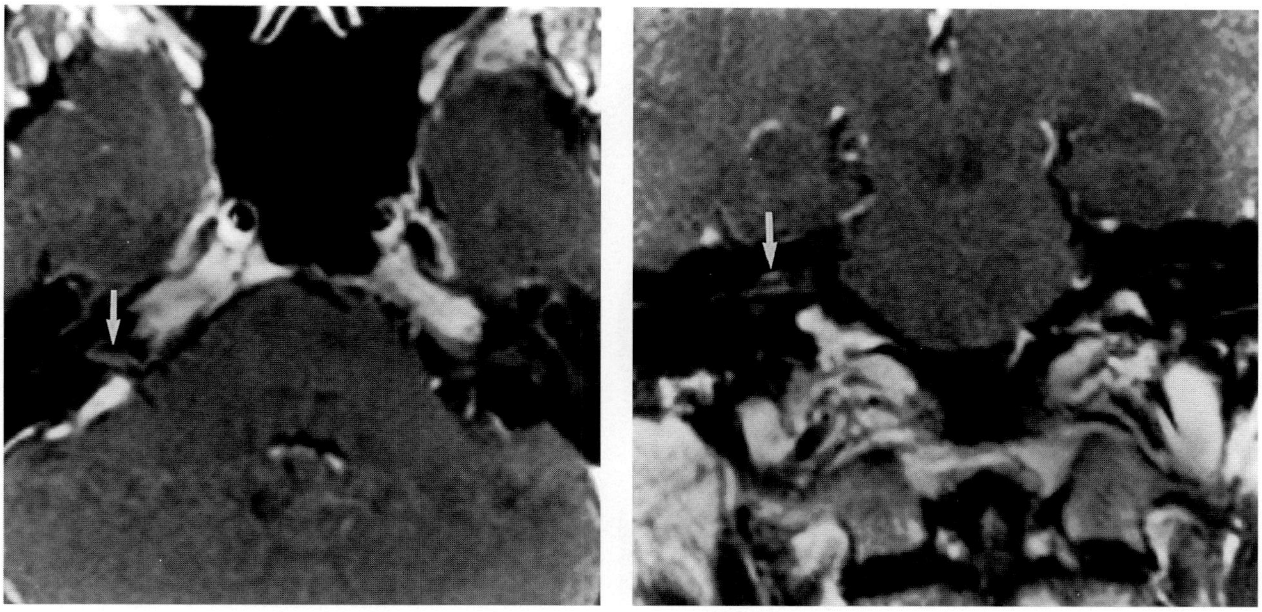

A B

FIG. 9-4. A,B: Same patient as in Fig. 3 following surgery. Postcontrast T1WIs demonstrate enhancing scar tissue in the right internal auditory canal (IAC) (*arrows*).

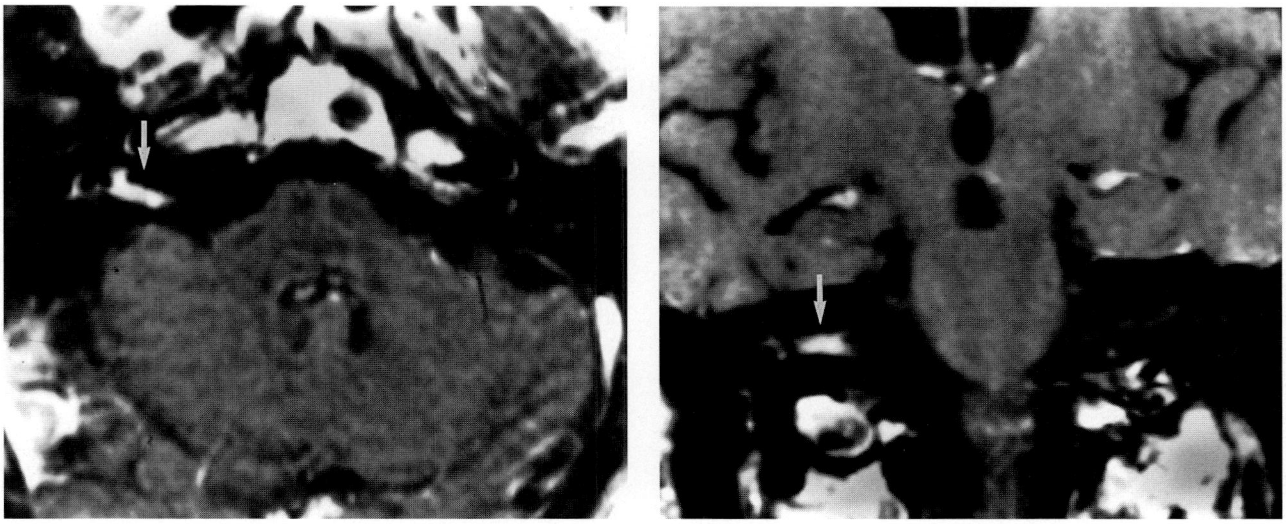

A B

FIG. 9-5. A 67-year-old man with right ear pain and vesicles of the right tympanic membrane. Postcontrast axial **(A)** and coronal **(B)** T1WIs demonstrate linear enhancement within the right IAC and along the 7th nerve (*arrows*). Ramsay-Hunt syndrome. *(Continued.)*

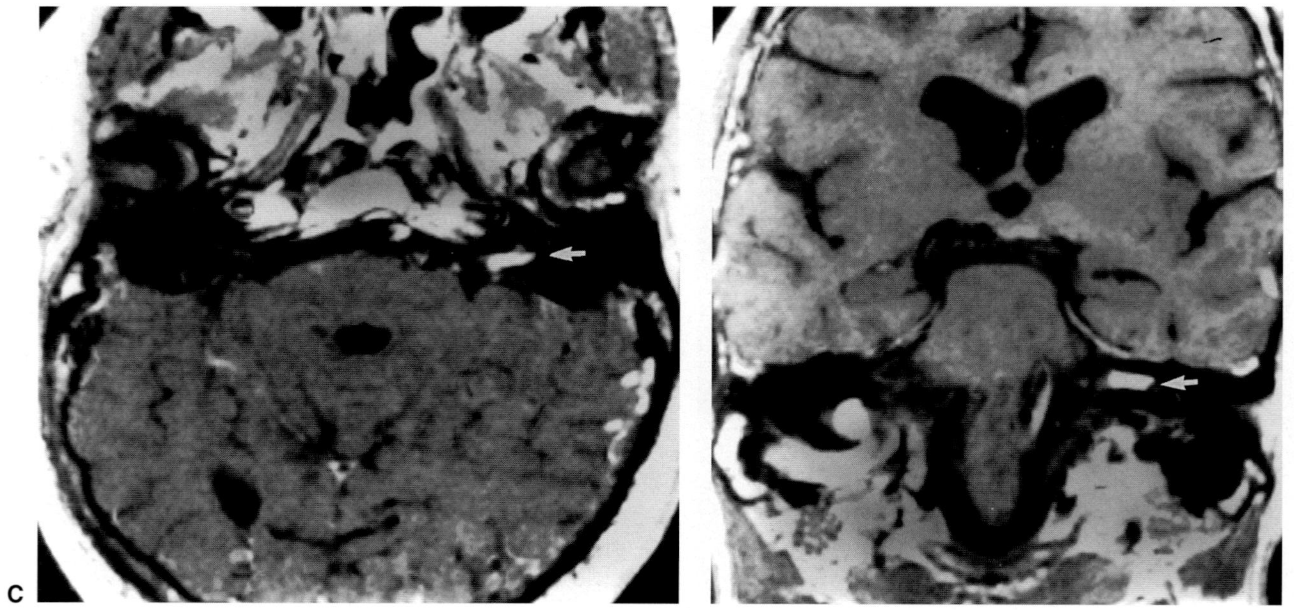

FIG. 9-5. *Continued.* In contrast to Ramsay-Hunt syndrome an intracanalicular schwannoma is seen in the left IAC on post-gadolineum T1W axial **(C)** and T1W coronal **(D)** MR images.

portion of the intratemporal facial nerve may be involved and with contiguous segments (Fig. 9-6) (33). When these tumors arise within the IAC, they can be clinically and radiographically indistinguishable from acoustic schwannomas (30). Schwannomas arising from the jugular foramen of cranial nerves IX, X, and XI are uncommon. Tumors that are large may extend superiorly from the jugular foramen and produce mass effect on the brainstem, simulating an acoustic schwannoma (Fig. 9-7). Cranial nerve involvement of the oculomotor, abducens, and trochlear nerves have been reported, but are rare. And finally, there is the rare intralabyrinthine schwannoma. They arise from Schwann cells of the acoustic nerve within the vestibule or cochlea. MRI with gadolinium is the most sensitive imaging modality in evaluating and differentiating these tumors from other lesions of the labyrinth (34,35). On MRI, they are sharply marginated tumors with intense enhancement confined to a portion of the labyrinth, apposed to the poorly marginated diffuse enhancement seen with inflammatory lesions (35).

Meningiomas

Meningioma is the most common nonglial primary brain tumor of the CNS (36). The majority of these tumors originate from the arachnoid cap cell, a meningoepithelial cell, most numerous in the region of the arachnoid villi along the dural venous sinuses. Any meningoepithelial cell, whether intracranial, intradiploic, spinal, or ectopic, can potentially result in the formation of this tumor (37). Some tumors, however, arise from dural fibroblasts and arachnoid associated with cranial nerves and choroid plexus (38).

TABLE 9–3. *Intracanalicular masses*

Acoustic schwannoma
Neuritis
Facial schwannoma
Meningioma
Hemangioma
Metastasis

Within the posterior fossa, meningiomas may arise from the tentorium cerebelli, cerebellar convexities, CPA clivus, and foramen magnum. Within the CPA, meningioma is the second most common tumor, representing less than 5% of all intracranial meningiomas (39). The acoustic schwannoma, the most common lesion at this site, must be differentiated from meningioma. There are several characteristics found on imaging that are useful in distinguishing these tumors. The meningioma is a dural-based, well-circumscribed mass that usually forms an obtuse angle with the adjacent temporal bone. Homogeneous contrast enhancement is usually seen on both MRI and CT; however, 10% to 15% have an atypical pattern suggesting hemorrhage, cyst formation, or metaplasia (38). The so-called dural tail seen on contrast MR images is the adjacent linear enhancement extending from the tumor along the dural surface (Fig. 9-8). Although originally described in association with meningiomas, the dural tail has been found with other tumors such as acoustic schwannoma (40,41). Other findings that may be detected in association with these tumors are calcifications (25%), hyperostosis, bone erosion, and enlarged vascular channels. Meningiomas within the posterior fossa may derive their vascular supply from several arterial trunks including the internal carotid, middle meningeal, occipital, ascending pharyngeal, vertebral, and cerebellar arteries (42). Although these tumors have varying degrees of vascularity,

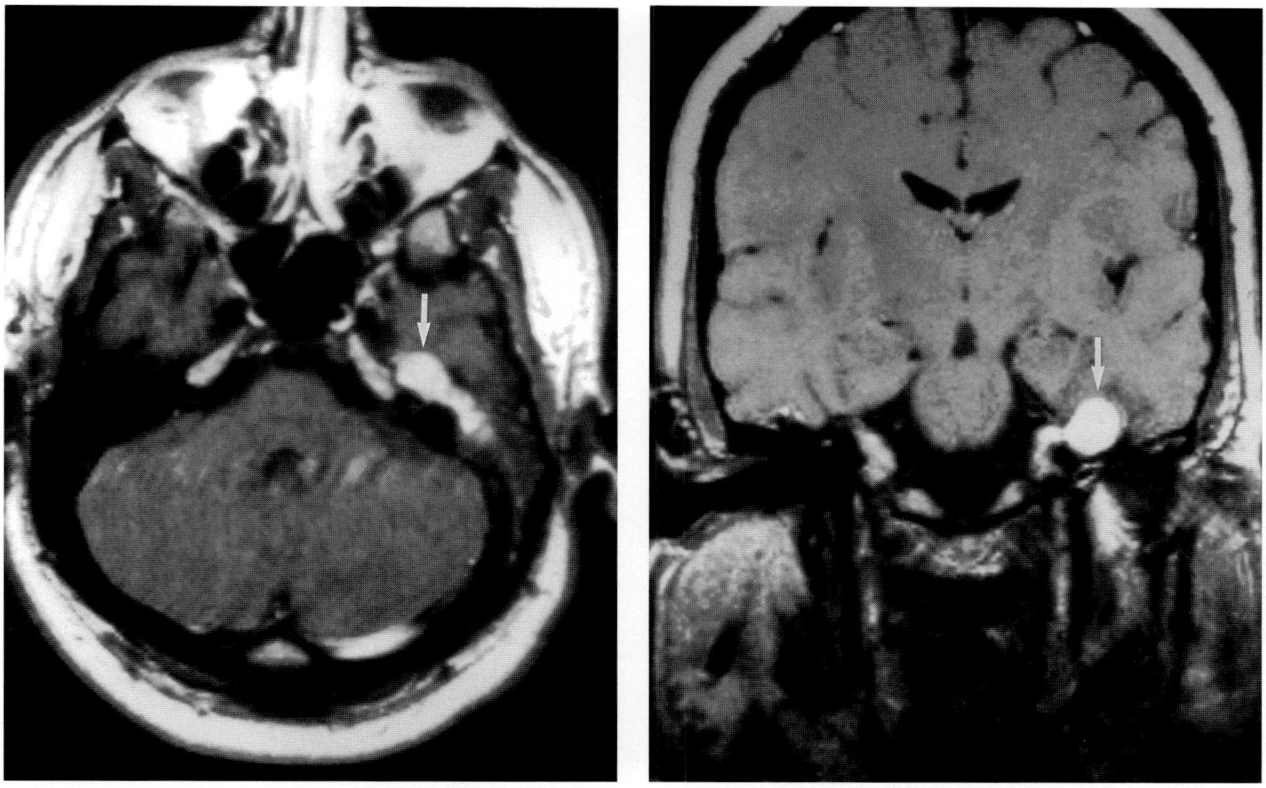

A B

FIG. 9-6. Axial **(A)** and coronal **(B)** postcontrast T1WIs of a facial schwannoma of the facial nerve with the largest component of the mass seen at the geniculate ganglion (*arrows*).

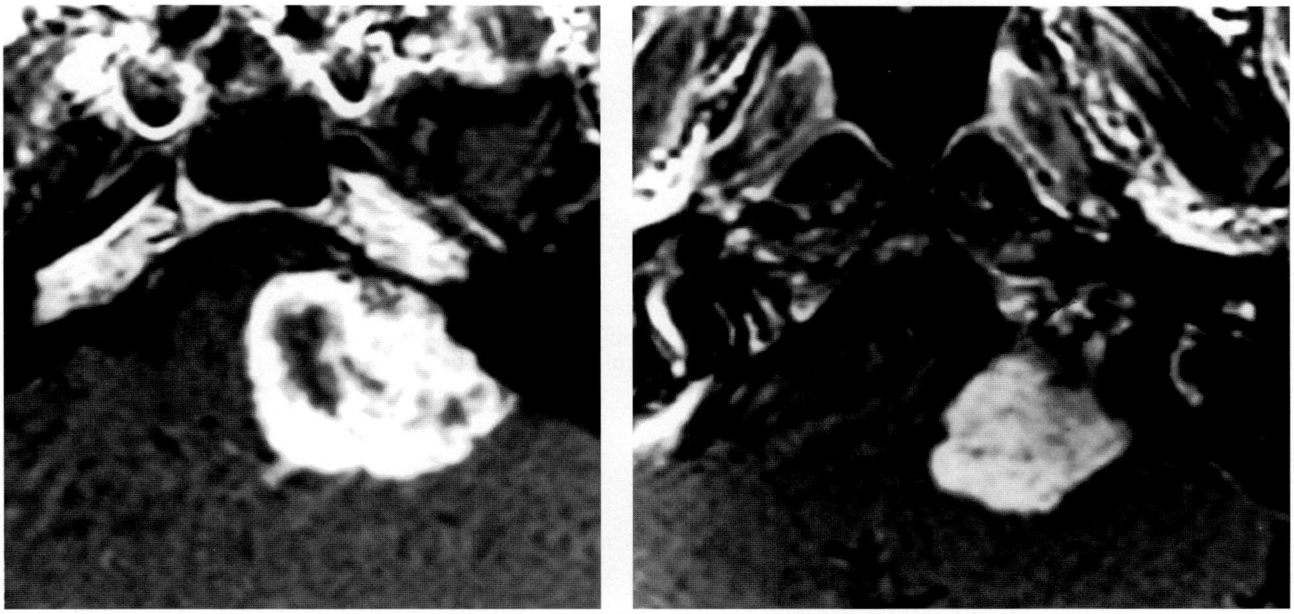

A B

FIG. 9-7. Axial **(A)** and coronal **(B)** postcontrast T1WIs of a large heterogeneous enhancing left glosso-pharyngeal schwannoma. An inferior axial image **(C)** demonstrates the tumor arising from the left jugular foramen.

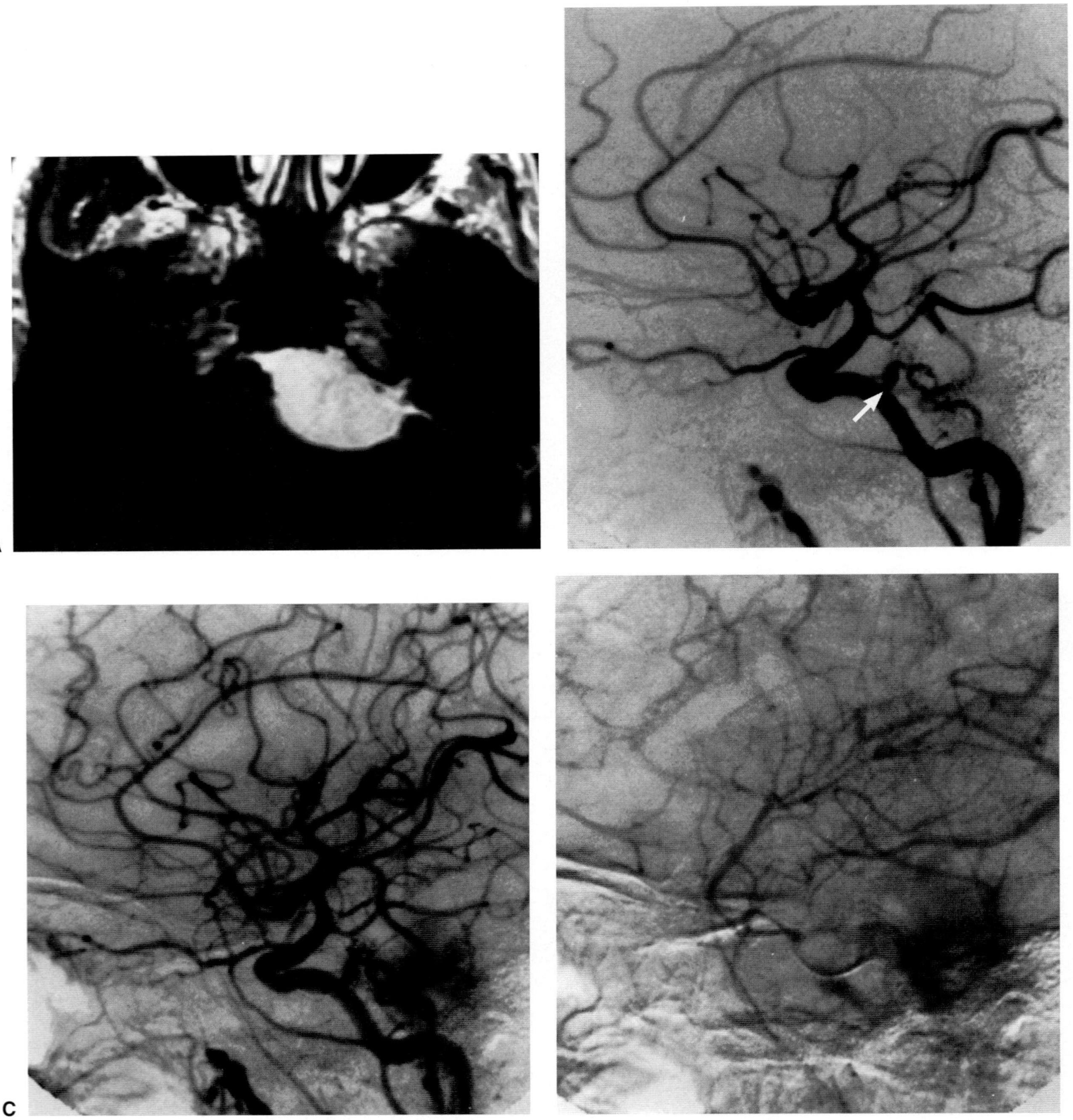

FIG. 9-8. Axial T1WI **(A)** shows an enhancing left extraaxial meningioma with associated dural enhancement. Angiography from a left common carotid artery injection **(B–D)** demonstrates a blush that persists from the arterial to venous phase. Note hypertrophy of the meningohypophyseal trunk (*arrow*).

on angiography most of these tumors demonstrate homogeneous dense tumor stain that persists into the venous phase. This angiographic finding was described by Buetow et al. (Armed Forces Institute of Pathology) as the ''mother-in-law sign,'' i.e., it comes early and stays late (Fig. 9-8) (37).

Paragangliomas

Paragangliomas (also called chemodectomas or glomus tumors) are vascular tumors derived from paraganglia cells of neural crest cell origin. The majority of these cells are located along nerves of the carotid artery bifurcation, vagus nerve, jugular bulb, and middle ear in the head and neck region (43). Accordingly, these tumors are named from where they arise as follows: carotid body tumor, glomus vagale, glomus jugulare, and glomus tympanicum. Of these sites, the carotid artery bifurcation is the most frequent location; however, these tumors are the most common primary neoplasms involving the middle ear and jugular foramen (Table 9-4). When the tumor is extensive, involving both

TABLE 9–4. *Jugular foramen masses*

Paraganglioma
Schwannoma
Meningioma
Metastasis
Chondroma
Chondrosarcomas

the jugular fossa and middle ear cavity, the term *glomus jugulotympanicum* is used. Tumors found in this location follow the course of Jacobson's nerve (tympanic branch of the glossopharyngeal nerve) and Arnold's nerve (mastoid branch of the vagus nerve).

When these tumors arise within the temporal bone or skull base, presenting symptoms may include pulsatile tinnitus, CHL or SNHL, and cranial nerve deficits. Middle-aged adults are commonly affected, with a female to male preponderance of 3:1. Multiple lesions may occur in 3% to 26% of patients; however, the higher incidence has been found when the disorder is familial (44). These tumors may secrete hormones such as epinephrine, norepinephrine, or adrenocorticotropic hormone (ACTH); however, this is unusual in most cases. Likewise, rarely do these tumors metastasize, but rather locally invade surrounding structures. Intracranial extension of these tumors are not uncommon and has been reported as high as 40% (44,45).

The initial evaluation of these lesions involving the temporal bone can be performed utilizing dynamic contrast CT scanning with axial and coronal sections (Fig. 9-9). Paragangliomas demonstrate moderate to marked contrast enhancement (46). The vascular nature of these tumors is the reason for their avid uptake of contrast. CT is also useful in detecting subtle bone erosion that is often difficult to detect on MRI. MRI, however, has the added advantages of defining tumor extension, characterizing tumor vascularity, and determining the relationship of tumor with adjacent vascular structures more easily than CT. Smaller tumors may demonstrate homogeneous enhancement, making the differentiation from a schwannoma or meningioma difficult. Tumors that are 2 cm or larger have a characteristic "salt and pepper" appearance on postcontrast T1-weighted MR images, a distinguishing feature from other lesions (Fig. 9-10). Enlarged feeding arteries, early draining veins, and a dense arterial blush can be seen on angiography. While angiography is usually not necessary for tympanicum tumors (41), it is most essential for tumors involving the jugular foramen. Angiography provides the surgeon with a vascular plot of arterial feeders and collaterals that usually involves tributaries of the ascending pharyngeal artery. Assessment of patency of the internal jugular vein is important especially with large tumors of the jugular foramen. Lastly, preoperative embolization, presently a common therapeutic procedure for vascular tumors, may dramatically reduce intraoperative blood loss during surgery (47).

Hemangiopericytoma

Hemangiopericytoma is a rare tumor of the CNS and arising even less often in the posterior fossa. This tumor arises from pericytes of Zimmermann surrounding the capillaries. Although originally classified by the World Health Organization (WHO) as a tumor of uncertain origin, the WHO has eliminated the term *angioblastic meningioma* in favor of *hemangiopericytoma* (48). Unlike meningioma, this tumor has a slight male preponderance occurring between the

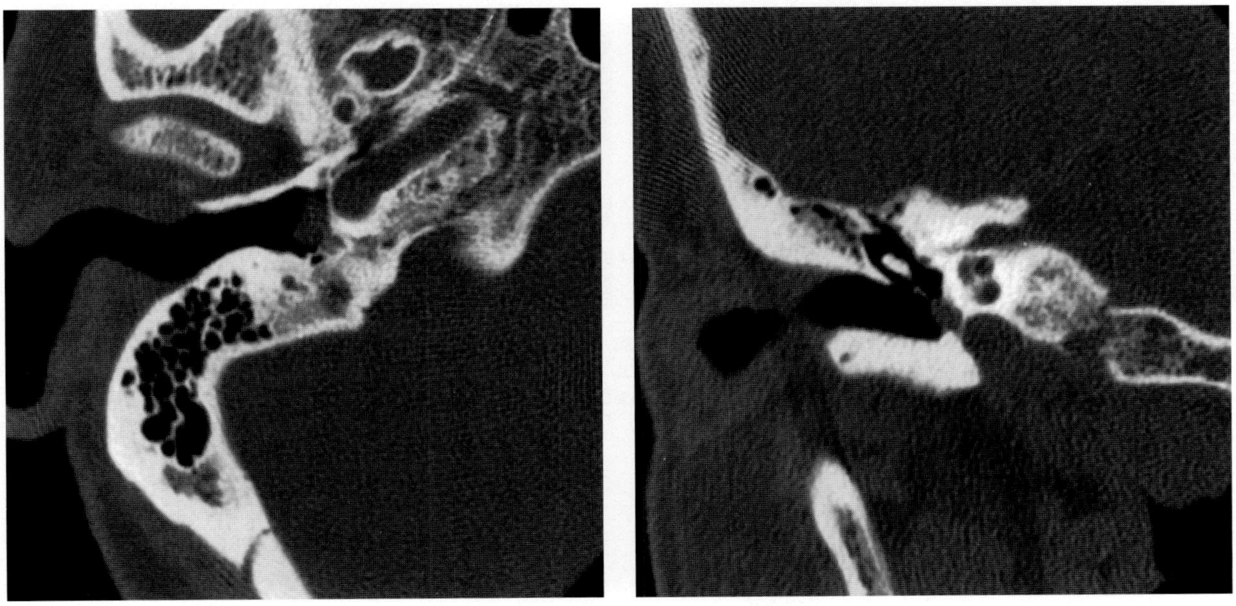

FIG. 9-9. Axial **(A)** and coronal **(B)** CT images of the temporal bones show a soft tissue mass along the cochlear promontory and isolated within the hypotympanum. Glomus tympanicum.

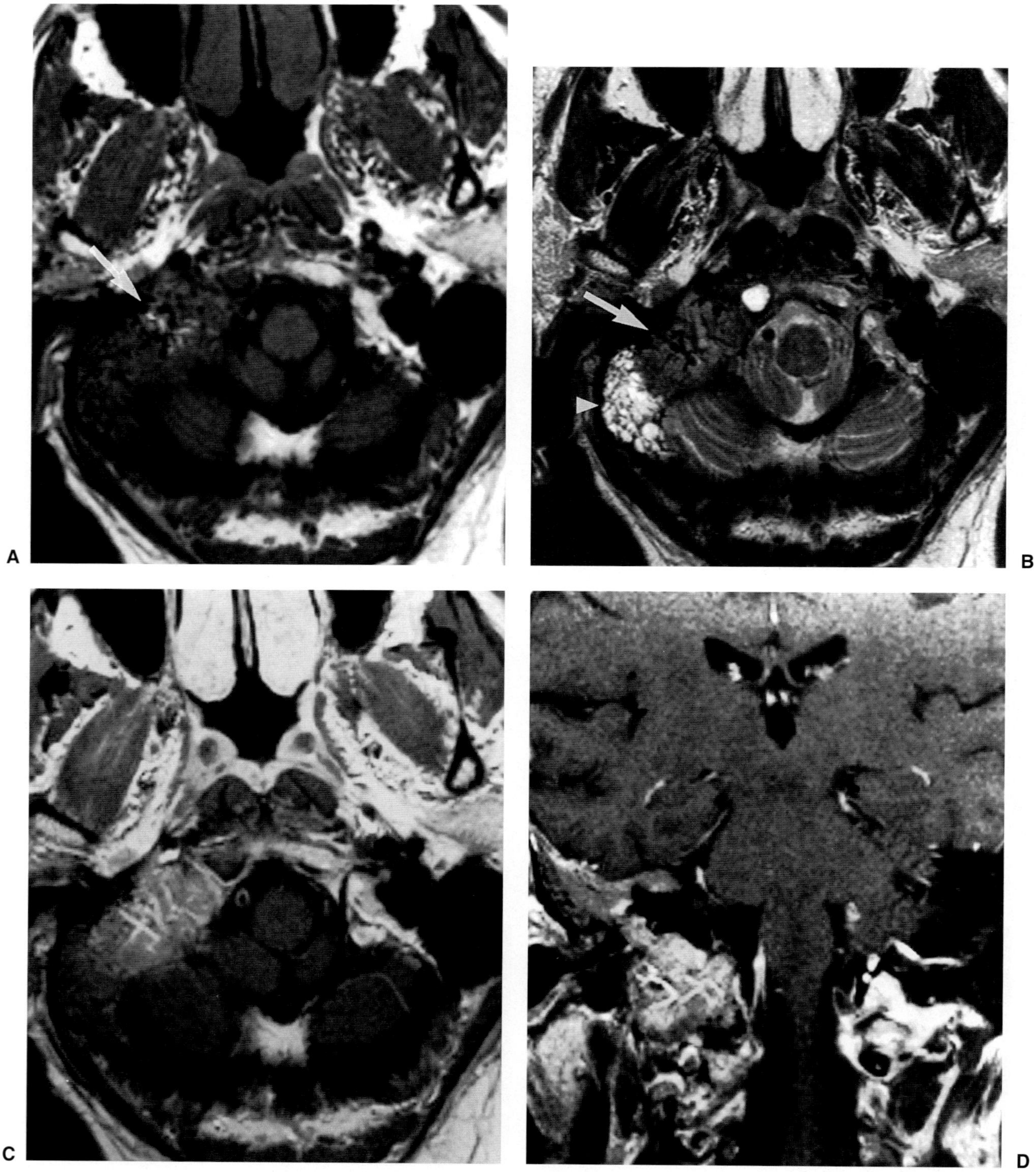

FIG. 9-10. A 67-year-old man with pulsatile tinnitus, otalgia, and decreased hearing of the right ear. Precontrast axial T1WI **(A)** and T2WI **(B)** show a lobulated right jugular foramen mass with central "flow voids" (*arrows*). Note the hyperintense mastoid effusion on the T2WI due to bone erosion of the mastoid (*arrowhead*). Postcontrast axial **(C)** and coronal **(D)**. T1WIs demonstrate strong contrast enhancement. Glomus jugulare.

fourth and sixth decades (49). However, a recent report by Chiechi et al. (48) found a slightly higher prevalence in females. Also in contrast to meningiomas, these tumors tend to have an aggressive behavior with an earlier age at presentation and a higher incidence of both metastasis and local recurrence.

On CT and MRI, these tumors are heterogeneous, but with strong enhancement due to tumor hypervascularity. Angiography confirms the hypervascularity of these tumors with the demonstration of a dense tumor stain. Within the jugular fossa, hemangiopericytomas may mimic glomus tumors with the radiographic findings of a markedly enhancing mass with lytic and expansile destruction of the jugular foramen (50).

Chondrosarcomas

Chondrosarcoma is an uncommon, slowly growing, locally invasive primary bone neoplasm. While the most common locations for these tumors to arise are the pelvis and femur, 5% to 12% may occur in the head and neck region (51). The primary cranial site is the cartilaginous synchondroses of the skull base. In a report by Myers et al. (52), the majority of these lesions occurred at or near the petro-occipital synchondrosis. Other less common sites included the spheno-occipital and sphenoethmoid synchondroses.

MRI with its multiplanar capabilities and superior contrast resolution is superior to CT in the evaluation of skull base neoplasms. On MRI, chondrosarcomas have a low to intermediate signal on T1WIs and high signal on T2WIs, and demonstrate marked enhancement after contrast (Fig. 9-11) (51,52). Heterogeneity can be seen in some tumors due to calcifications that are often readily apparent on CT. CT is also useful in determining the extent of bone destruction. The primary differential diagnosis of the skull base chondrosarcoma is the chordoma. However, unlike the chordoma, the majority of chondrosarcomas tend to arise off the midline (Fig. 9-12). Most previous reports suggest it may be difficult to reliably differentiate these tumors on both clinical and radiographic findings. Other common tumors to be included for diagnostic consideration are meningioma and metastatic lesions. Since complete resection is the most effective treatment for these tumors, it is critical that imaging adequately defines tumor extent.

Epidermoid Cyst

Epidermoid cysts are inclusions cysts that may be either congenital or acquired. The congenital variety is the result of inclusion of ectodermal elements at the time of neural tube closure, which may occur within the temporal bone, calvarium, brain, meninges, or other parts of the body (53). The acquired type, usually the result of trauma or surgery, is secondary to implantation of epidermis into the deeper underlying tissues, with the formation of a cyst that continues to desquamate keratin (38). Pathologically, the two types are similar.

Intracranially, these tumors are found in the CPA, sellar region, and the middle cranial fossa. Between 40% and 50% of epidermoid tumors are found in the CPA cistern, making this tumor the third most common CPA mass (after

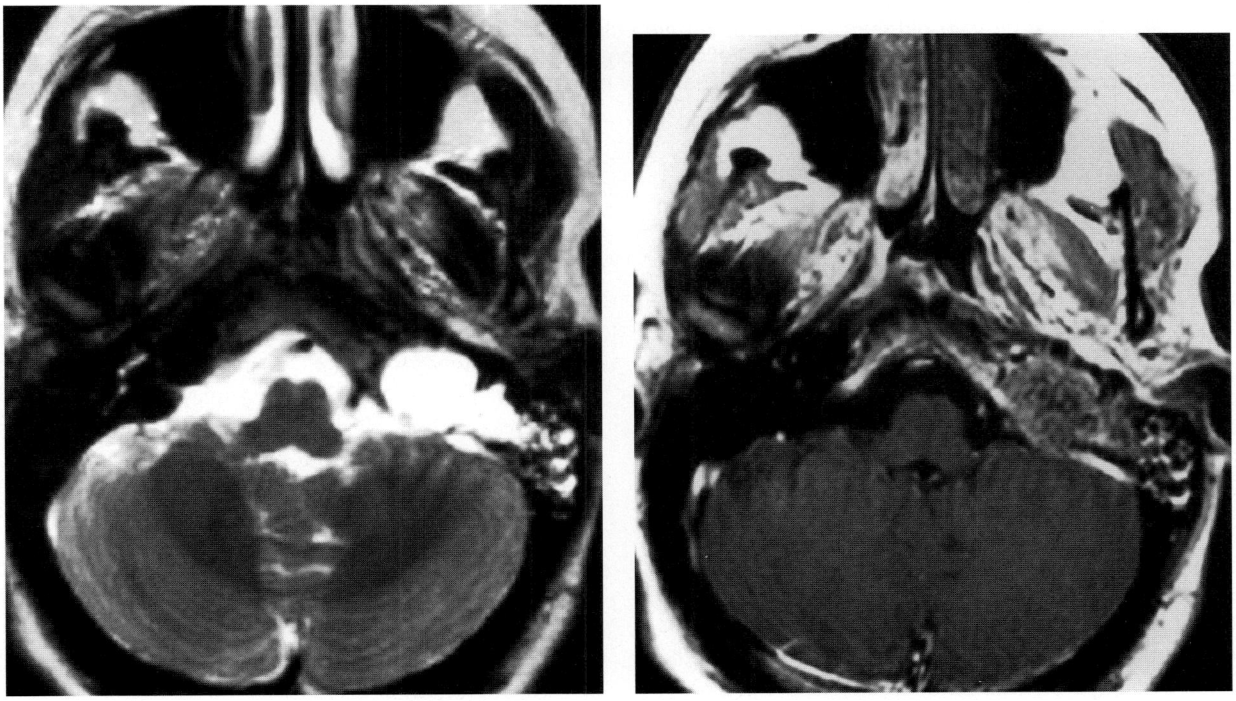

A B

FIG. 9-11. A 29-year-old woman presents with left ear pain. Axial T2WI **(A)** and axial postcontrast T1WI **(B)** demonstrate a hyperintense and enhancing mass of the left mastoid. Chondrosarcoma.

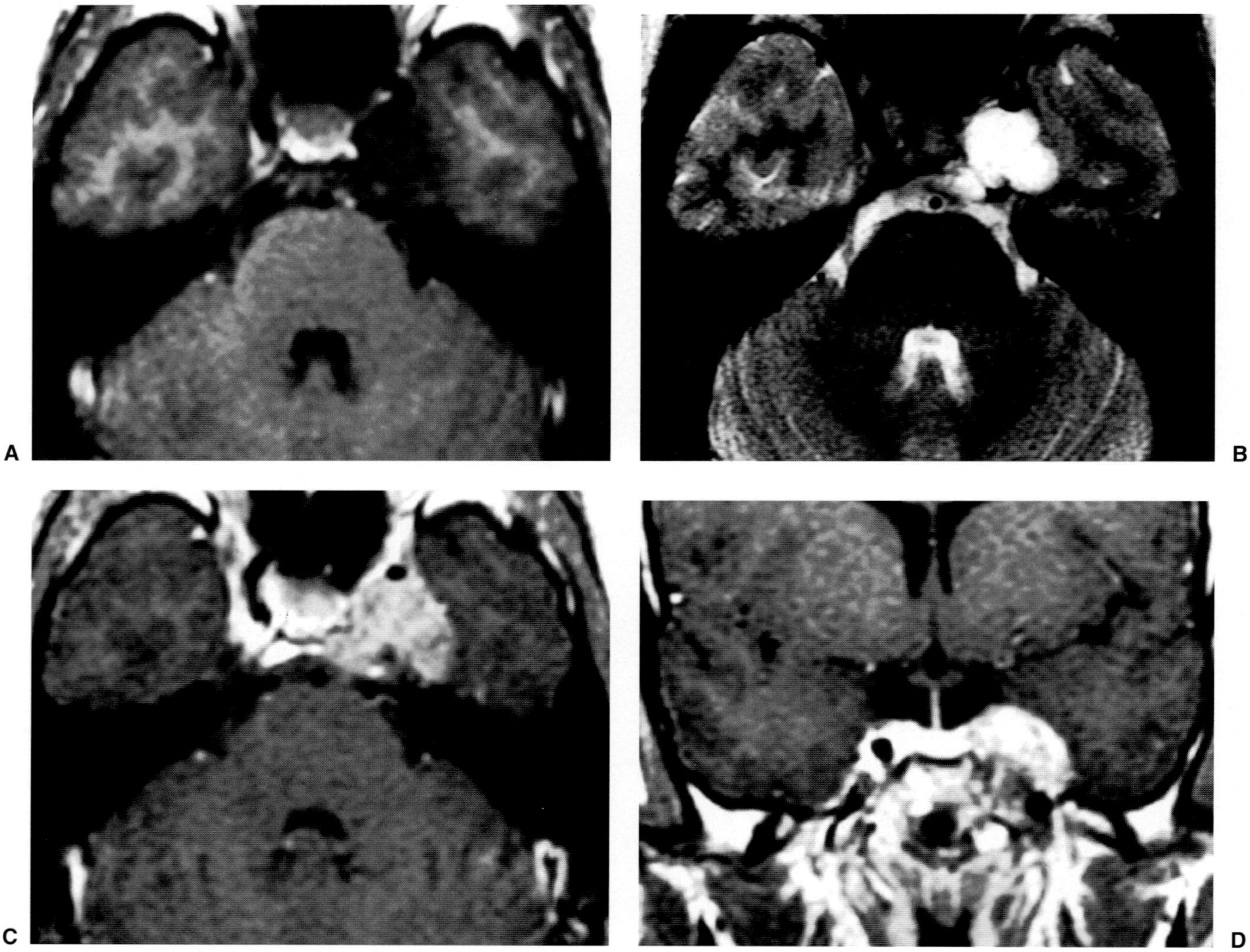

FIG. 9-12. A 26-year-old man with left 5th nerve palsy. Precontrast axial T1WI **(A)** and T2WI **(B)** MR scans show a lobulated mass within Meckel's cave on the left of hypo- and hyperintensities, respectively. Postcontrast axial **(C)** and coronal **(D)** T1WIs show moderate contrast enhancement. Chordoma.

schwannoma and meningioma) (38). On unenhanced CT scans, epidermoids are lobulated masses with attenuation similar to that of CSF. Enhancement is usually absent on both CT and MRI after contrast, although enhancement at the tumor margin has been observed (54). On MRI, these tumors typically have signal ranging from isointense to slightly hyperintense to CSF on all spin echo sequences. Recent advances of MRI technique with the development of FLAIR and CISS (constructive interference in steady state) sequences have depicted epidermoid tumors in the subarachnoid space better than conventional spin echo images (55). Since these tumors generally do not enhance, the major differential diagnostic consideration is the arachnoid cyst. Diffusion-weighted MR imaging, introduced in the late 1980s, can be useful in distinguishing between these tumors. This technique is based on molecular brownian motion with the generation of an apparent diffusion coefficient (ADC) MR image. Tsuruda et al. (56) found the ADC of arachnoid cysts were similar to stationary water, whereas the ADC of epidermoid tumors were similar to brain parenchyma, indicating the solid nature and the slower diffusion rate of epidermoid tumors.

Within the temporal bone, epidermoids may occur in the petrous apex, mastoid, middle ear, middle ear and mastoid, external ear canal, and within the squamous portion of the temporal bone (53). The intraosseous petrous apex epidermoid is a slow-growing expansile lesion, oval to spherical in shape, with slightly scalloped margins on CT. The lack of aggressive bone destruction of these tumors is a useful differentiating feature from other lesions that can occur in the petrous apex (Table 9-5). On MRI, they have long T1

TABLE 9–5. *Petrous apex*

Epidermoid (primary cholesteatoma)
Cholesterol granuloma
Mucocele
Neuroma
Metastatic disease
Histiocytosis X
Carotid aneurysm

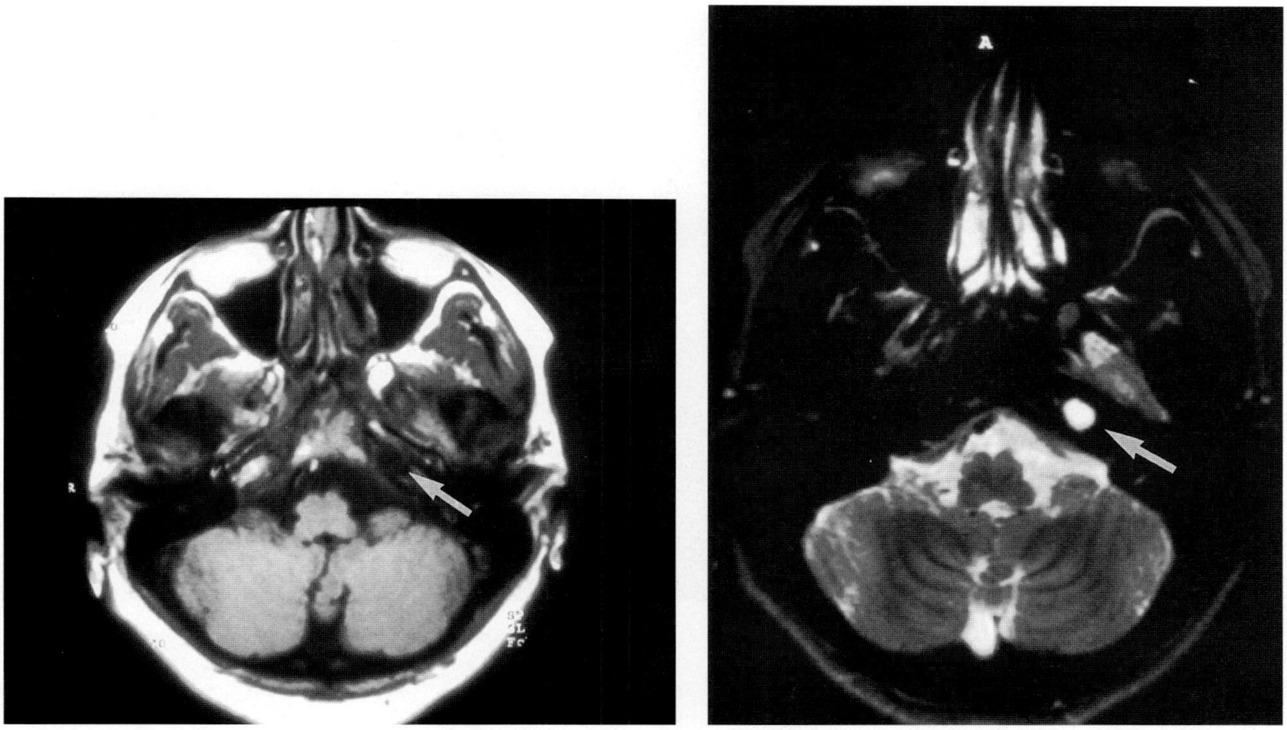

A B

FIG. 9-13. A round mass of hypointensity is seen on T1WI **(A)** and hyperintensity on axial T2WI **(B)**. Epidermoid.

(iso- to hypointense) and T2 (hyperintense) relaxation times (Fig. 9-13). Noninfected epidermoid cysts demonstrate no enhancement following intravenous administration of gadolinium–diethylenetriamine pentaacetic acid (Gd-DTPA) (53).

Cholesterol Granuloma

Cholesterol granuloma is an inflammatory mass of tissue thought to be initiated by chronic obstruction to ventilation and drainage of pneumatized spaces (57). This obstruction causes negative pressure buildup, which ultimately produces mucosal edema and bleeding. The breakdown of hemorrhagic by-products leads to cholesterol crystal formation, which in turn incites an irreversible granulomatous reaction (58). These lesions may occur in the middle ear, mastoid, or petrous apex. Since there is usually associated ear disease, lesions involving the middle ear and mastoid tend to be smaller and are detected earlier (58).

Cholesterol granulomas of the petrous apex, however, are slow-growing expansile lesions that are typically clinically silent until reaching a critical size that may lead to compressive effects on the temporal lobe or CPA region. It is estimated that one symptomatic cholesterol granuloma of the petrous apex occurs for every 30 acoustic neuromas, making it the most common benign lesion of the petrous apex (52). The so-called giant cholesterol cyst is thought by some authors to represent a different lesion because of its histopathologically characteristics, while other authors disagree. Mafee et al. (53) propose that the giant cholesterol cyst of the petrous apex is probably a variant of the more commonly seen cholesterol granuloma.

On CT, cholesterol granulomas of the petrous apex are well-circumscribed, lytic and expansile lesions. Scalloping, if present, favors an epidermoid rather than cholesterol granuloma (53). Erosive changes may extend to involve the clivus, jugular tubercle, anterior carotid canal, and IAC (59). While the CT findings are nonspecific, other lesions should be considered in the differential diagnosis specifically the epidermoid (primary cholesteatoma). On MR images, however, cholesterol granulomas have a characteristic appearance (Fig. 9-14). They typically demonstrate increased signal on both T1- and T2-weighted sequences and do not enhance after the administration of Gd-DTPA (53,58,59). This is in contrast to the epidermoid, which is of low signal on T1WIs and high signal on T2WIs.

SELLAR AND PARASELLAR LESIONS

Both CT and MRI play important roles in the diagnostic workup of patients with sellar and parasellar pathologies. While CT has largely been replaced by MR as the initial imaging modality, its utility cannot be underscored. No other modality exquisitely displays the osseous structures in 2D fine detail other than CT. This is particularly important in evaluating lesions involving the skull base. In evaluating the sellar region, CT accurately determines the presence of sellar floor erosion and adjacent bone destruction, the septum of the sphenoid sinus, and the bony covering of the cavernous carotid arteries. These are all important structures to evaluate

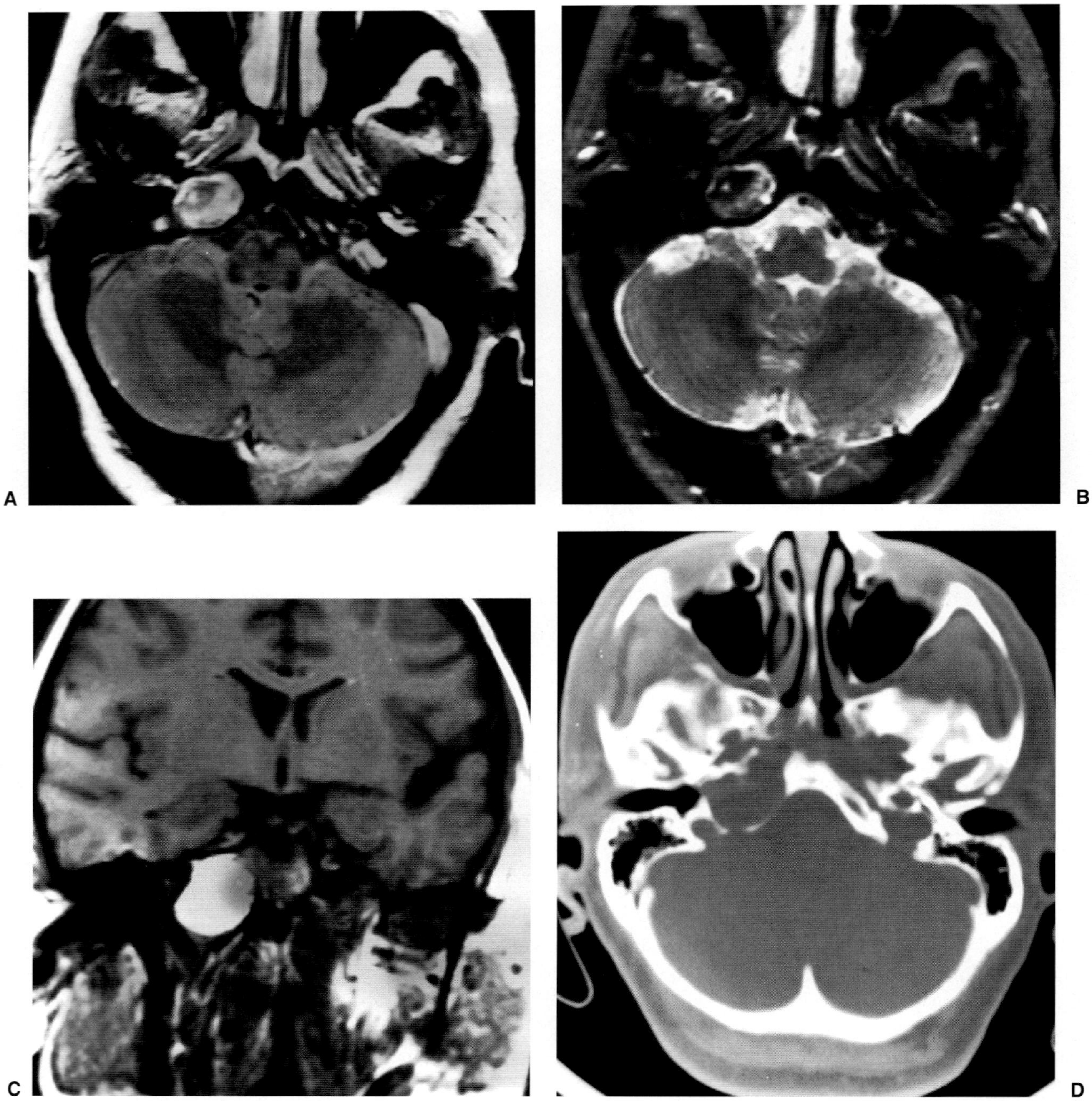

FIG. 9-14. A heterogeneous predominantly hyperintense mass is noted in the right petrous apex on axial T2WI **(A,B)** and coronal T1WI **(C,D)**. CT also demonstrates this expansile lytic lesion. Cholesterol granuloma.

prior to transsphenoidal surgery. In contrast with CT, MRI with its multiplanar capabilities has the advantage of providing high-contrast resolution images in orthogonal planes free of streak artifacts produced by neighboring bone structures and dental amalgam. MRI allows better soft tissue characterization of lesions, thus leading to a more accurate diagnosis.

In general, MRI of the sella includes the acquisition of 3-mm coronal and sagittal T1WIs with Gd-DTPA. At least one plane, usually the coronal projection, is obtained before contrast. Previous reports have found that precontrast images have a high detection rate for the diagnosis of microadenomas that is enhanced by the administration of contrast (60). Gradient echo postcontrast or dynamic postcontrast images may also be obtained to enhance the conspicuity of these small lesions. In evaluating lesions of the skull base, the additional fat suppression techniques with contrast quell the background of the hyperintense fatty marrow, allowing better contrast resolution of enhancing lesions.

Anatomy

The sellar and parasellar anatomy primarily involves the entire sphenoid bone, clivus, and the adjacent surrounding soft tissue structures. The saddle-shaped sella turcica is the central depression of the basisphenoid bone, which houses the pituitary gland. The anterior and posterior aspects of the sella are the tuberculum and dorsum sella, respectively. The anterior clinoids arise from the lesser wings of the sphenoid, while the posterior clinoids arise from the dorsum sella. The inferior extension of the dorsum sella is the clivus, which is formed from the union of the basisphenoid of the sphenoid bone to the basiocciput of the occipital bone.

The pituitary gland is composed of two lobes, the adenohypophysis or anterior lobe and the neurohypophysis or posterior lobe. The anterior lobe is derived from Rathke's pouch, whereas the posterior lobe, median eminence, and pituitary stalk are derivations of extensions of the hypothalamus. Some reports, however, suggest the anterior lobe may be of neuroectodermal origin (61). Superior to the pituitary gland is a dural reflection, the diaphragma sella, through which the pituitary stalk passes via a central opening. The suprasellar cistern, a five-point star-shaped subarachnoid space above the diaphragma sella, contains the circle of Willis, optic chiasm and nerves, and the proximal pituitary stalk. Just superior to the pituitary stalk are the supraoptic recess of the third ventricle and hypothalamus.

Lateral to the pituitary fossa are the cavernous sinuses bounded by two layers of dura. These paired septated venous channels contain the cavernous internal carotid arteries and cranial nerves III, IV, VI, V1, and V2. They also connect with other venous channels including the contralateral sinus via the intercavernous venous network, superior ophthalmic, and superior and inferior petrosal veins.

Pituitary Adenoma

In adults, pituitary adenomas are the most common intrasellar neoplasms. Based on size criteria, these tumors are divided into two types: microadenomas measuring smaller than 10 mm in diameter and macroadenomas larger than 10 mm in diameter. The majority of the tumors produce symptoms related to the production of excess hormones, of which prolactin is the most common. The remaining nonfunctional tumors are either detected incidentally or due to mass effect on the surrounding structures, primarily the optic chiasm.

While there is no general consensus of the single best imaging modality in the evaluation of these lesions, MRI is generally preferred over CT. However, for those clinicians who would treat a clinically suspected prolactinoma, CT is an efficient, sensitive, and inexpensive study for excluding macroadenomas or other tumors in this region. On CT and MRI, microadenomas are relatively nonenhancing lesions that are well delineated by normal surrounding pituitary tissue. An important caveat to remember is that these tumors will become isointense with the normal pituitary tissue with delayed imaging. However, macroadenomas typically demonstrate homogeneous contrast enhancement, although 37% of these tumors may have heterogeneous signal on MRI due to cystic or hemorrhagic changes (62). While suprasellar extension of these tumors may be diagnosed with ease on MRI, the ability to detect cavernous sinus invasion remains challenging (Fig. 9-15). The most specific finding to date is the presence of carotid artery encasement (63).

Meningiomas

Meningiomas are the second most common tumor in adults to arise in the suprasellar region. However, of all meningiomas, only 5% to 10% occur in this region (38). Like meningiomas that occur elsewhere in the neurospinal axis, they are more common in middle-aged women. The majority of these tumors arise from the cavernous sinus dura, sphenoid ridge, diaphragma, dorsum, or tuberculum sellae (64). On imaging, hyperostosis of the adjacent bone may be seen. In the era prior to CT, this finding on plain film was felt to be pathognomonic for meningioma. Meningiomas range from isodense to hyperdense on precontrast CT scans and demonstrate avid contrast enhancement on postcontrast images. The finding of compressed cortex and buckling of the white matter supports the extraaxial location of these lesions. The dural tail sign, which represents either dural reactive change or dural extension of tumor, is suggestive of the diagnosis of meningioma.

Craniopharyngioma

Craniopharyngiomas are nonglial tumors that arise from squamous epithelial remnants of the involuted hypophyseal pharyngeal duct (Fig. 9-16) (65). While more than half of these tumors occur within the first two decades of life, a bimodal distribution of craniopharyngiomas is seen. The second peak is seen in adults ranging from 40 to 60 years of age. Males and females are equally affected.

On imaging, craniopharyngiomas may have a variable appearance. On MRI and CT, these lesions can be solid and/or cystic, resulting in a heterogeneous suprasellar mass. On MRI, the cystic component of the lesion often follows signal of CSF, i.e., hypointense on T1WIs and hyperintense on T2WIs. However, in some tumors a hyperintense signal can be seen on T1WIs within the cystic component of the lesion due to either increased protein content or blood degradation products of the fluid. In addition, calcium, which is readily identified on CT and often present within these tumors, may produce a hypointense MR signal as well. On postcontrast images, avid but often heterogeneous enhancement is seen.

PITFALLS AND DIAGNOSTIC PROBLEMS

Patients with tumors, accidental trauma, or surgical intervention to the skull base, mid-face, and parasellar area fre-

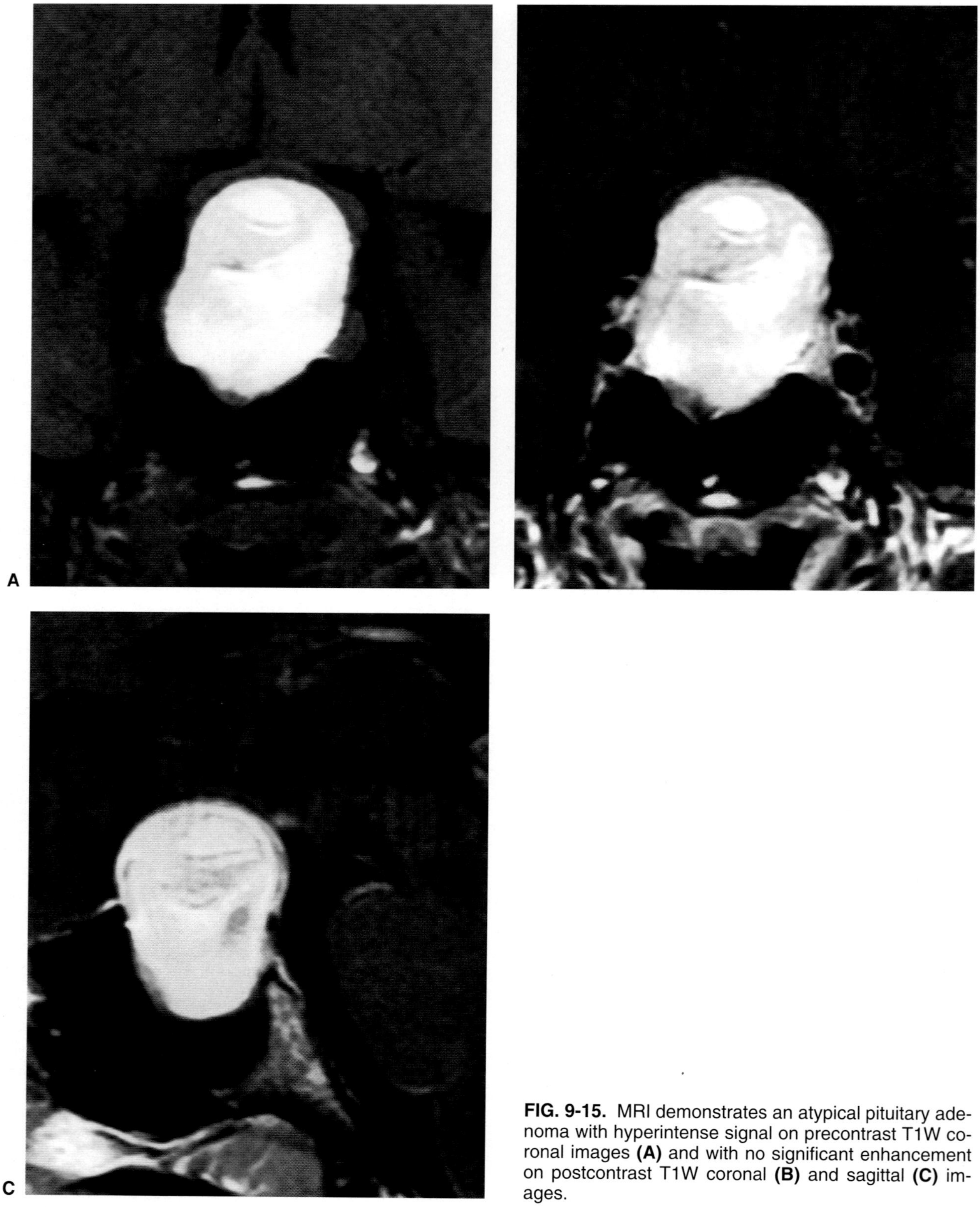

FIG. 9-15. MRI demonstrates an atypical pituitary adenoma with hyperintense signal on precontrast T1W coronal images **(A)** and with no significant enhancement on postcontrast T1W coronal **(B)** and sagittal **(C)** images.

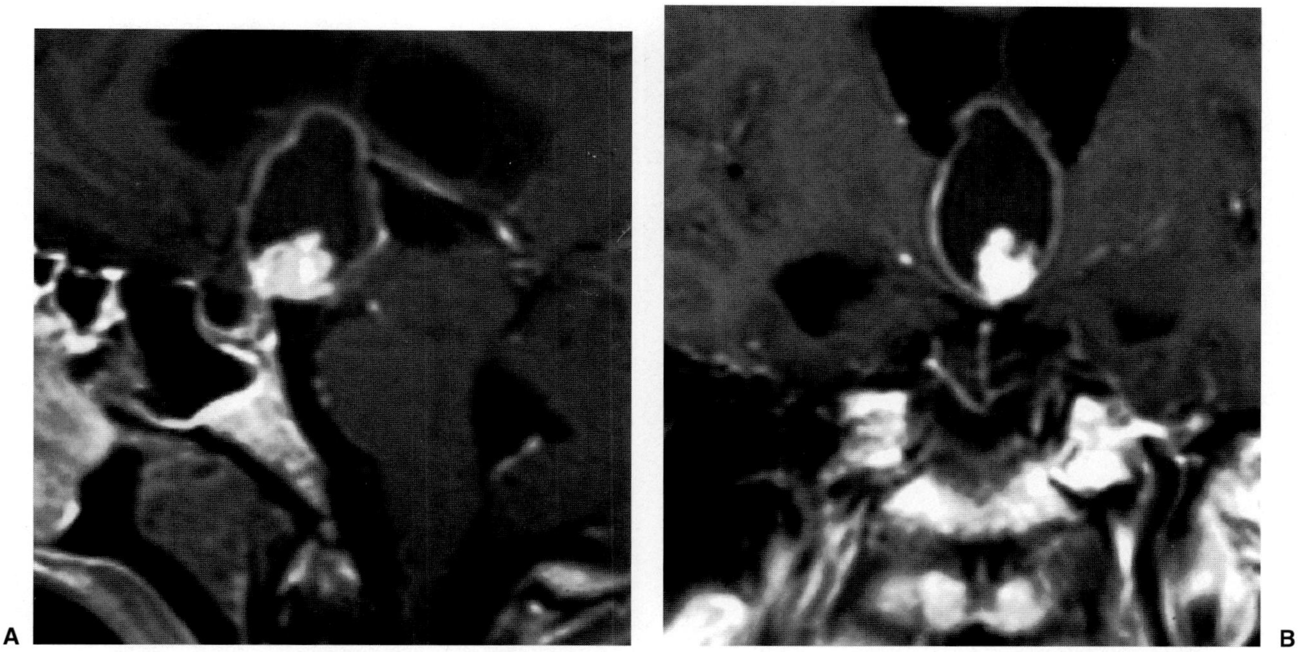

FIG. 9-16. Sagittal **(A)** and coronal **(B)** postcontrast T1WIs demonstrate a rim enhancing cystic mass with an enhancing mural nodule. Craniopharyngioma.

quently require diagnostic imaging for the evaluation of their condition and treatment planning. The preceding sections focused on imaging parameters and disease entities that are frequently encountered in neuro-otolgic practice. This section covers associated conditions, pitfalls, and potential management problems from an imaging standpoint.

Cervical Spine Injury

Individuals who undergo high-speed, rapid deceleration injury to the head and neck often present with multiple-system injury. An organized approach to the assessment and stabilization of the patient is crucial to survival. An organized approach to the imaging of the patient is just as important. The evaluation of injury to the mid-face, for instance, does not take precedence over evaluation of the spinal column or brain. In a study by Lewis et al. (66), in 982 cases of cervical spine injury, there was a 19.3% incidence of facial injury. If one were to focus only on the facial injury in these patients, serious errors could be made regarding patient stabilization and safety. Eliminating the possibility of an unstable neck fracture may be difficult but must be performed before imaging of facial and orbital trauma is performed. Plain films of the spine play a critical role in the initial evaluation of the traumatized patient. The screening series at most institutions includes a cross-table lateral, anteroposterior (AP), and open mouth odontoid view. Bilateral oblique views and a Swimmer's view complete the more standard trauma series. The *Advanced Trauma Life Support Manual* recommends that in severe injury, a cross-table lateral film be obtained and resuscitation of the patient be completed prior to obtaining other plain film views (67). There have been some reports that a significant number of fractures have been missed on plain film examinations (68,69). If there is a high suspicion of spinal column injury or instability, CT and MRI may assist in evaluating the stability of the spine and integrity of the spinal canal and spinal cord. Quencer et al. (70) recommend the use of routine CT examination in patients who are at high risk for spine injury if they meet certain clinical criteria based on the mechanism of injury, associated injuries, and/or diminished mental status. These studies may be performed after clinical stabilization of life-threatening injury to the brain, chest, and abdomen have been addressed, and may be performed at the same time that CT studies are performed of the head, chest, and abdomen. High-resolution thin-cut CT with multiplanar reconstruction may be obtained quickly using spiral scanning techniques (Fig. 9-17). The use of plain film and CT together demonstrated 100% of injuries according to work done by Borock et al. (71); however, it is interesting to note that CT alone demonstrated 98% of these injuries.

The MRI evaluation of trauma patients may provide significant information regarding the evaluation of the cord, extent of vertebral fracture, associated disc herniations, and vascular integrity (Fig. 9-18). The performance of MRI studies, however, is more involved and the MRI environment is potentially hostile to the multiple instrumented patient, and as a result the MRI exam must be planned properly to minimize risk to the patient. With new fast techniques, information regarding cord contusion, cord hematoma, or cord compression may be obtained relatively quickly. At our institution, MRI of the injured cord, unless contraindicated, is preferable to CT myelography.

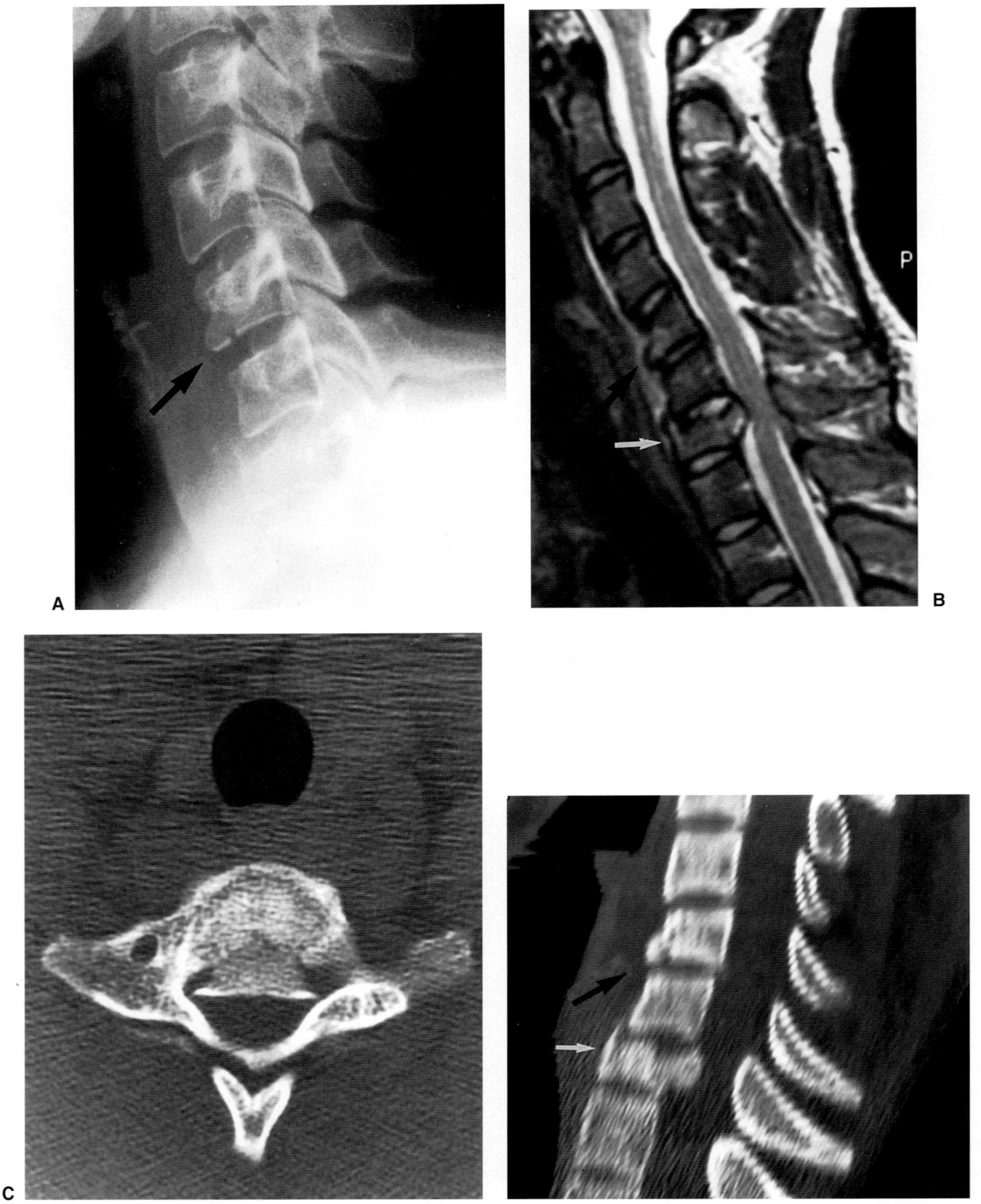

FIG. 9-17. A teenage boy involved in a fight sustained an anterior inferior avulsion fracture of C5 (*black arrows*) and burst fracture of C7 with cord impingement (*white arrows*) demonstrated on lateral plain film **(A)** and sagittal T2WI **(B)**. CT axial **(C)** and sagittal CT reformation **(D)** eloquently demonstrate the large retropulsed fracture fragment.

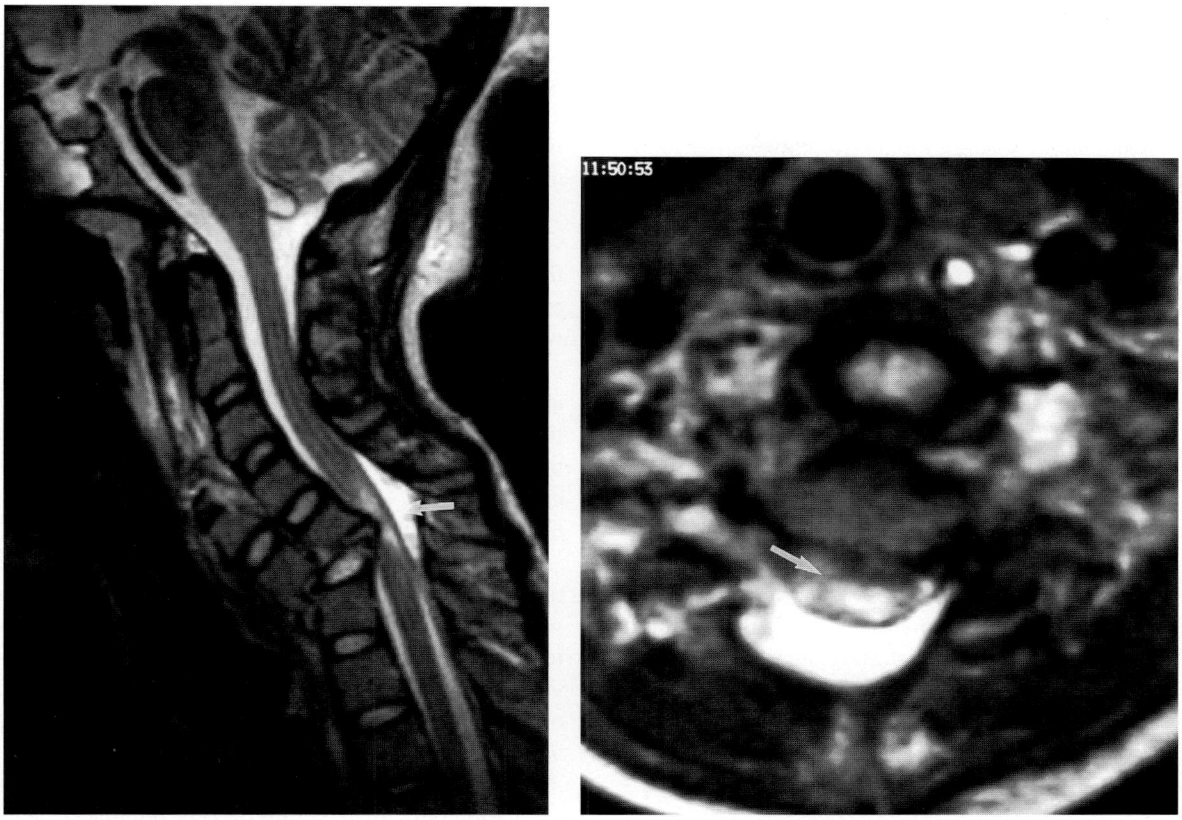

A B

FIG. 9-18. MR sagittal **(A)** and axial **(B)** T2WIs demonstrate a checkerboard fracture/dislocation of C5 and C6 producing cord edema (*arrows*) in a 15-year-old girl involved in a motor vehicle accident. (Courtesy of Faser Henderson, M.D.)

Related Brain Injury

Evaluation of the brain in the trauma setting must not interfere with patient stabilizing procedures or other lifesaving measures. Fulton et al. (72) examined 462 consecutive patients with blunt trauma and noted that only 5% of these patients required neurosurgical intervention. When imaging evaluation is needed, the CT examination of the patient with head trauma remains the initial examination in virtually every institution. MRI may miss blood in the subarachnoid space due to the increased oxygen tension of the CSF, and obtaining a CT in the patient with multiple trauma is not as complicated an ordeal for the trauma team and the patient as the performance of an MRI. However, in a blinded comparison of CT and low-field MRI of the brain following closed head injury, Orrison and Gentry's group (73,74) found MRI significantly more sensitive than CT for the detection of contusion, subdural/epidural hematoma, white matter shear injury, and sinus involvement. CT was more sensitive than MRI in the detection of fracture, and the modalities were equivalent in the detection of superficial soft tissue injury (73). CT remains the initial imaging study in patients with cranial trauma; however, a normal CT scan is not sufficient to exclude intracranial pathology. Diffuse axonal shear injury may be detected after mild head injury using MRI techniques in the face of a normal CT examination (75). MRI examination is also superior when evaluating intraparenchymal and extraaxial collections in the posterior fossa (76), for the evaluation of traumatic brainstem injury (77), and for the evaluation of secondary forms of injury such as arterial infarction, cerebral herniation, and brain injury from increased intracranial pressure (74). Newer imaging techniques may have a role in the evaluation of patients who suffer from trauma. Smith et al. (78) found that diffusion-weighted imaging may demonstrate regions of focal contusion more accurately and earlier than conventional MRI sequences. Blatter et al. (79) used MRI-based volumetric quantification of brain and CSF space volumes to predict eventual cognitive outcome in brain injured patients. They found a particularly strong correlation between the volume of the left temporal horn of the lateral ventricle and verbal IQ scores.

CSF Fluid Fistula

Determining the site of a CSF fistula may be a very difficult imaging challenge. Multiple modalities have been used to evaluate the site and extent of CSF leak. Radionuclide cisternography has largely been replaced by anatomic imaging studies such as CT cisternography and MRI cisternography. Initial studies with intrathecal administration of the water-soluble contrast, metrizamide, into the CSF, subsequent gravity manipulation into the area of suspected leak, and CT imaging provided very useful diagnostic information (80–82). Non-ionic water-soluble contrast agents have replaced metrizamide and are safer compounds for instillation into the subarachnoid space. Frequently, however, if there is no active leak during the performance of the CT examination, the site of leak may not be identified. High-resolution CT (HRCT) examinations without the use of contrast material have also proven valuable (83,84). Gammal et al. (85) performed MR cisternography with very heavily T2-weighted fast spin echo images (TR 10,000, TE eff 200) and found that MR cisternography proved to be an accurate diagnostic technique with an 87% sensitivity and a 78% accuracy. Shetty et al. (86) evaluated high-resolution thin-cut CT in the prone position with slice thickness of 1 to 3 mm and MR cisternography using heavy T2 weighting and found that together the combination of HRCT and MR cisternography were accurate in 96% of patients. They propose an imaging algorithm that starts with HRCT, once a CSF leak is suspected or confirmed by laboratory tests. If the findings on CT are uncertain, then MR cisternography may be performed. CT cisternography with water-soluble contrast material is reserved for those patients who have CSF fistula not detected by the previous performed modalities.

Miscellaneous Conditions

Cephaloceles are uncommon protrusions of intracranial contents through a congenital defect in the cranial vault. Detailed discussion is beyond the scope of this chapter; however, these defects may occur anywhere in the skull, are usually midline in location, and occur in the skull base 10% of the time (87). Meningoceles involve the meninges and subarachnoid space, while encephaloceles involve brain tissue as well. Meningoceles have been reported to occur in the middle ear spontaneously (88–91) and have also been reported as a result of trauma with recurrent bacterial meningitis (Fig. 9-19) (92). HRCT imaging and MRI techniques with heavily T2-weighted sequences help define the anatomic extent of these abnormalities.

Posttraumatic vascular injury is potentially devastating. Carotid and vertebral artery dissection, carotid-cavernous fistula, and traumatic aneurysms are conditions that are best evaluated with catheter angiography and are discussed elsewhere in this text. MR angiographic techniques may have a role in follow-up examinations to assess vascular patency and the effects of endovascular treatment of fistula or dissection. MR angiography may overestimate vascular stenosis, may miss slow flow in dural fistulas, and may serve as a complementary test to conventional angiography in the post-traumatic patient.

The evaluation of cranial nerve dysfunction using functional MRI techniques is rapidly progressing as the hardware, software, image registration, and data manipulation techniques improve. Pilot studies and refereed abstracts of vestibular function and olfaction to include patients with olfactory dysfunction are in the MRI, neurophysiology, and neuroscience literature.

Neuroradiologic procedures play an important role in the evaluation of patients with lesions or trauma to the temporal bone, skull base, mid-face, cervical spine, and sellar regions. To provide the most accurate neuroradiologic diagnosis, HRCT and MRI studies can be utilized to define lesion extent and involvement of adjacent or related structures. New techniques, improvements in both software and hardware, as well as continuing research into brain function, CSF flow, brain ischemia, and injury will assist the otolaryngologist and neurosurgeon in patient management. This brief discus-

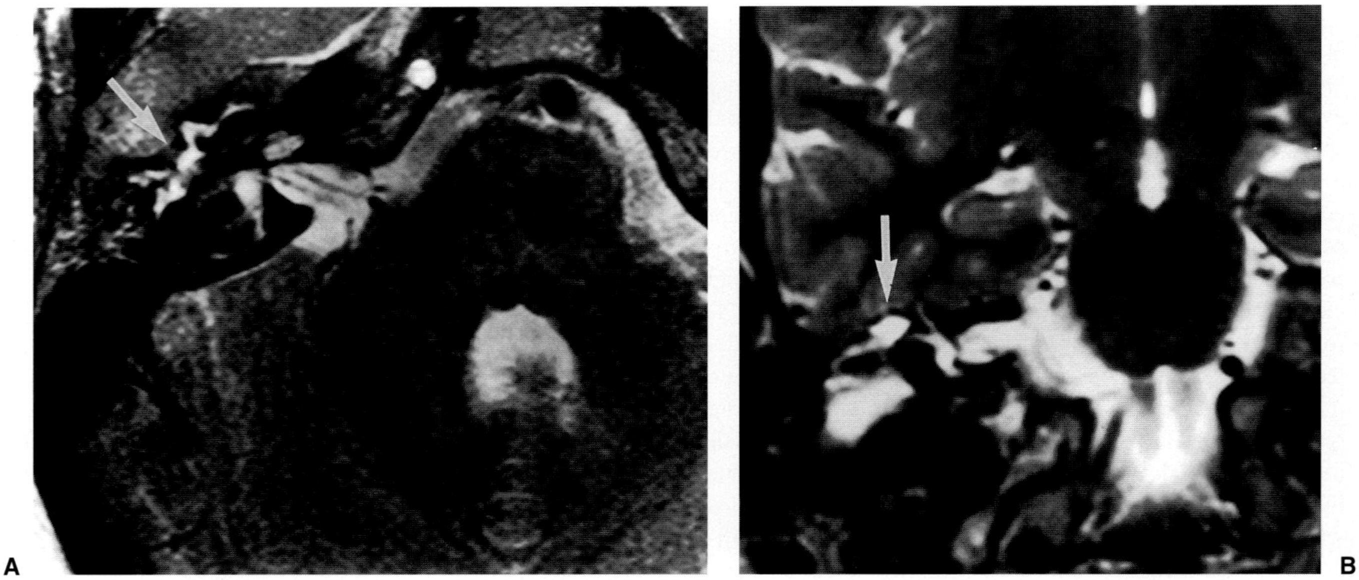

FIG. 9-19. MR axial **(A)** and coronal **(B)** T2WIs of a meningocele of the right temporal bone (*arrows*) in a patient who presented with recurrent meningitis and otorrhea.

sion of techniques, common lesions, and potential pitfalls can aid clinicians in their day-to-day practice.

REFERENCES

1. Bastianell S, Bozzao A, Paolillo A, et al. Fast spin echo and fast fluid-attenuated inversion-recovery versus convention spin-echo sequences for MR quantification of multiple sclerosis lesions. *Am J Neuroradiol* 1997;18:699–704.
2. Tsurushima H, Meguro K, Wada M, et al. FLAIR images of patients with head injuries. *No Shinkei Geka* 1996;24(10):891–895(abst).
3. Tsuchiya K, Inaoka S, Mizutani Y, Hachiya J. Fast fluid-attenuated inversion-recovery MR of intracranial infections. *Am J Neuroradiol* 1997;18:909–913.
4. Filippi M, Yousry T, Baratti C, et al. Quantitative assessment of MRI lesion load in multiple sclerosis; a comparison of conventional spin-echo with fast-fluid attenuated inversion recovery. *Brain* 1996;2: 1349–1355.
5. Levy L, Di Chiro G. MR phase imaging and cerebrospinal fluid flow in the head and spine. *Neuroradiology* 1990;32:399–340.
6. Bhadelia R, Bogdan AR, Wolpert SM. Analysis of cerebrospinal fluid flow waveforms with gated phase-contrast MR velocity measurements. *Am J Neuroradiol* 1995;16:389–400.
7. Mosely ME, Cohen J, Mintrovitch J, et al. Early detection of regional cerebral ischemia in cats: comparison of diffusion and T2-weighted MRI and spectroscopy. *Magn Reson Med* 1990;14:330–346.
8. Mosely ME, Kucharczyk J, Mintorovitch J, et al. Diffusion weighted MR imaging of acute stroke: correlation with T2-weighted and magnetic susceptibility-enhance MR imaging in cats. *Am J Neuroradiol* 1990;11:423–429.
9. Le Bihan DL, Breton E, Lallemand D, Aubin ML, Vignaud J, Laval-Jeantet M. Separation of diffusion and perfusion in intravoxel incoherent motion MR imaging. *Radiology* 1988;168:497–505.
10. Roy CS, Sherrington CS. On the regulation of the blood supply of the brain. *J Physiol* 1980;11:85–108.
11. Thulborn KR, Waterton JC, Matthews PM, Radda GK. Oxygenation dependence of the transverse relaxation time of water protons in whole blood at high field. *Biochem Biophys Acta* 1982;714:265–270.
12. Brooks RA, Di Chiro G. Magnetic resonance imaging of stationary blood: a review. *Med Phys* 1987;14:903–913.
13. Fox PT, Raichle ME. Focal physiological uncoupling of cerebral blood flow and oxidative metabolism during somatosensory stimulation in human subjects. *Proc Natl Acad Sci USA* 1986;83:1140–1144.
14. Hermans R, Marchal G, Feenstra L, et al. Spiral CT of the temporal bone: value of image reconstruction at submillimeter table increments. *Neuroradiology* 1995;37:150–154.
15. Donaldson JA, Miller JM. Anatomy of the ear. In: Paprella MM, Shumrick DA, eds. *Otolaryngology, vol 1, basic sciences and related disciplines.* Philadelphia: WB Saunders, 1980:26–62.
16. Swartz JD, Harnsberger HR. *Imaging of the temporal bones,* 2nd ed. New York: Thieme, 1992.
17. Nager G, Levin LF. Congenital aural atresia: embryology, pathology, genetics, classification and surgical management In: Paparella MM, Shumrick DA, eds. *Otolaryngology, vol 2. The ear.* Philadelphia: WB Saunders, 1980:1303–1344.
18. Virapongse C, Sarwar M, Bhimani S, et al. Computed tomography of temporal bone pneumatization: normal pattern and morphology. *AJNR* 1985;6:551–559.
19. Casselman JW, Kuhweide R, Deimling M, et al. Constructive interference in steady state (CISS)-3DFT MR imaging of the inner ear and cerebellopontine angle. *AJNR* 1993;14:47–57.
20. Lindeman RC. Temporal bone trauma and facial paralysis. *Otolaryngol Clin North Am* 1979;12:403.
21. Aguilar EA, Yeakley JW, Ghorayeb BY, et al. High resolution computed tomography of temporal bone fractures: association of facial nerve paralysis. *Head Neck Surg* 1987;9:162–166.
22. Coker NJ, Kendall KA, Jenkins HA, Alford BR. Traumatic intratemporal facial nerve injury: management rationale for preservation of function. *Otolaryngol Head Neck Surg* 1989;97:26–29.
23. Grossman RI, Yousem DM. *Neuroradiogy: the requisites.* St. Louis: Mosby, 1994.
24. Goldberg HI, Lavi E, Atlas SW. Extraaxial brain tumors. In: Atlas SW, ed. *Magnetic resonance imaging of the brain and spine,* 2nd ed. Philadelphia: Lippincott-Raven Press, 1996:423–487.
25. Brogan M, Chakeres DW. Gd-DTPA-enhanced MR imaging of cochlear schwannoma. *AJNR* 1990;11:407–408.
26. Krause CJ, McCabe BF. Acoustic neuroma in a 7-year-old girl: report of a case. *Arch Otolaryngol* 1971;94:359.
27. Cohen LM, Schwartz AM, Rockoff SD. Benign schwannomas: pathologic basis for CT inhomogeneities. *AJR* 1986;147:141–143.
28. Mueller DP, Gantz BJ, Dolan KD. Gadolinium-enhanced MR of the postoperative internal auditory canal following acoustic neuroma resection via the middle fossa approach. *AJNR* 1992;13:197–200.
29. Mulkens TH, Parizel PM, Martin J-J, et al. Acoustic schwannoma: MR findings in 84 tumors. *AJR* 1993;160:395–398.
30. Lo WWM, Solti-Bohman LG. Tumors of the temporal bone and the cerebellopontine angle. In: Som PM, Curtin H, eds. *Head and neck imaging,* 3rd ed. St. Louis: Mosby, 1996:1449–1534.
31. McCormick PC, Bello JJA, Post KD. Trigeminal schwannoma: surgical series of 14 cases with review of the literature. *J Neurosurg* 1988;69: 850–860.
32. Goldberg R, et al. Varied appearance of trigeminal neuroma on CT. *AJR* 1980:134:57.
33. Martin N, Sterkers O, Mompoint D, et al. Facial nerve neuromas: MR imaging. *Neuroradiology* 1992;34:62–67.
34. Maffee MF, Lachenauer CS, Kumar A, et al. CT and MR imaging of intralabyrinthine schwannoma: report of two cases and review of the literature. *Radiology* 1990;174:395–400.
35. Wilson DF, Talbot M, Hodgson RS. Magnetic resonance imaging-enhancing lesions of the labyrinth and facial nerve. *Arch Otolaryngol Head Neck Surg* 1994;120:560–564.
36. Russell DS, Rubinstein LJ. *Pathology of tumors of the nervous system,* 5th ed. Baltimore: Williams & Wilkins, 1989.
37. Buetow MP, Burton PC, Smirniotopoulos JG. Typical atypical, and misleading features in meningioma. *Radiographics* 1991;11: 1087–1100.
38. Osborne AG. *Diagnostic neuroradiology.* St. Louis: Mosby-Year Book, 1994.
39. Mikhael MA, Ciric IS, Wolff AP. Differentiation of cerebellopontine angle neuromas and meningiomas with MR imaging. *J Comput Assist Tomogr* 1985;9:852–856.
40. Sze G. Diseases of the intracranial meninges: MR imaging features. *AJR* 1993;160:727–733.
41. Goldsher D, Litt AW, Pinto RS, Bannon KR, et al. Dural "tail" associated with meningiomas on Gd-DTPA-enhanced MR images: characteristics, differential diagnostic value, and possible implications for treatment. *Radiology* 1990;176:447–450.
42. Zanella FE, Valavanis A. Interventional neuroradiology of lesions of the skull base. In: Drayer BP, Weber AL, eds. *Neuroimaging Clinics of North Am* 1994;4(3):619–637.
43. Olsen WL, Dillon WP, Kelly WM, et al. MR imaging of paragangliomas. *AJNR* 1986;7:1039–1042.
44. Batakis JG. *Tumors of the head and neck: clinical and pathological considerations.* Baltimore: Williams & Wilkins, 1979:369–379.
45. Myers EM. *Head and neck oncology: diagnosis, treatment and rehabilitation.* Boston: Little, Brown, 1991:100.
46. Chakeres MD, LaMasters DL. Paragangliomas of the temporal bone: high resolution CT studies. *Radiology* 1984;150:749–753.
47. Simpson GT II, et al. Immediate post embolization excision of glomus jugulare tumors: advantages of new combined techniques. *Arch Otolaryngol* 1979;105:639.
48. Chiechi MV, Smirniotopoulos JG, Mena H. Intracranial hemangiopericytomas: MR and CT features. *AJNR* 1996;17:1365–1371.
49. Guthrie BL, Ebersold MJ, Scheithauer BW, Shaw EG. Meningeal hemangiopericytoma: histopathologic features treatment and long term followup of 44 cases. *Neurosurgery* 1989;25:514–522.
50. Weber AL, McKenna MJ. Radiologic evaluation of the jugular foramen: anatomy, vascular variants, anomalies and tumors. In: Drayer BP, Weber AL, eds. *Neuroimaging Clinics of North Am* 1994;4(3): 579–598.
51. Brown E, Hug EB, Weber AL. Chondrosarcoma of the skull base. In: Drayer BP, Weber AL, eds. *Neuroimaging Clinics of North Am* 1994; 4(3):529–541.
52. Myers SP, Hirsh WL, Curtin HD, et al. Chondrosarcomas of the skull base: MR imaging features. *Radiology* 1992;184:103–108.
53. Mafee MF, Kumar A, Heffner DK. Epidermoid cyst (cholesteatoma)

and cholesterol granuloma of the temporal bone and epidermoid cysts affecting the brain. In: Drayer BP, Weber AL, eds. *Neuroimaging Clinics of North Am* 1994;4(3):561–578.
54. Gao P-Y, Osborn AG, Smirniotopoulos JG, Harris CP. Epidermoid tumor of the cerebellopontine angle. *AJNR* 1992;13:863–872.
55. Ikushima I, Korogi Y, Hirai T, Sugahara T, et al. MR of epidermoids with a variety of pulse sequences. *AJNR* 1997;18:1359–1363.
56. Tsuruda JS, Chew WM, Mosley ME, Norman D. Diffusion-weighted MR imaging of the brain: value of differentiating between extraaxial cysts and epidermoid tumors. *AJNR* 1990;11:925–931.
57. Plester D, Steinbach E. Cholesterol granuloma. *Otolaryngol Clin North Am* 1982;15:665–672.
58. Lo WWM, Solti-Bohman LG, Brackmann DE, Gruskin P. Cholesterol granuloma of the petrous apex: CT diagnosis. *Radiology* 1984;153:705–711.
59. Greenberg JJ, Oot RF, Wismer GL, et al. Cholesterol granuloma of the petrous apex: MR and CT evaluation. *AJNR* 1988;9:1205–1214.
60. Wolpert SM, Davis BT. Pituitary imaging. In: Moore WT, Eastman RC, eds. *Diagnostic endocrinology,* 2nd ed. St. Louis: Mosby-Year Book, 1996:95–124.
61. Elster AD. Modern imaging of the pituitary. *Radiology* 1993;187:1–14.
62. Lundin P, Nyman R, Burman P, et al. MRI of pituitary macroadenomas with reference to hormonal activity. *Neuroradiology* 1992;34:43–51.
63. Scotti G, Chin-Yin Y, Dillon WP, et al. MR imaging of cavernous sinus involvement by pituitary adenomas. *AJNR* 1988;9:657–664.
64. Chong BW, Newton TH. Hypothalamic and pituitary pathology. *Radiol Clin North Am* 1993;31:1147.
65. Rutka JT, Hoffman HJ, Drake JM, et al. Suprasellar and sellar tumors in childhood and adolescence. *Neurosurg Clin North Am* 1992;3:803.
66. Lewis VL, Manson PN, Morgan RF, Cerullo LJ, Meyer PR Jr. Facial injuries associated with cervical fractures: recognition, patterns and management. *J Trauma* 1985;25(1):90–93.
67. Committee on Trauma of the American College of Surgeons. Hospital and prehospital resources for optimal care of the injured patient. *Bull Am Coll Surg* 1986;71:4–12.
68. Ahmad AA, Coin CG, Becerra JL, Nunez DB Jr, Soto RF, LeBlang SD. Plain films versus spiral CT in the evaluation of cervical spine injuries. *Radiology* 1993;189:325(abst).
69. Blacksin MF, Lee HJ. Frequency and significance of fractures of the upper cervical spine detected by CT in patients with severe neck trauma. *AJR* 1995;196:741–745.
70. Quencer RM, Nunez D, Green BA. Controversies in imaging acute cervical spine trauma. *Am J Neuroradiol* 1997;18:1866–1868.
71. Borock EC, Gabram SGA, Jacobs LM, Murphy MA. A prospective analysis of a two year experience using computed tomography as an adjunct for cervical spine clearance. *J Trauma* 1991;31:1001–1006.
72. Fulton RL, Everman D, Mancino M, Raque G. Ritual head computed tomography may unnecessarily delay lifesaving trauma care. *Surg Gynecol Obstet* 1993;176(4):327–332.
73. Orrison WW, Gentry LR, Stimac GK, Tarrel RM, Espinosa MC, Cobb LC. Blinded comparison of cranial CT and MR in closed head injury evaluation. *Am J Neuroradiol* 1994;15(2):351–356.
74. Gentry LR, Godersky JC, Thompson B. MR imaging of head trauma: review of the distribution and radiopathologic features of traumatic lesion. *Am J Roentgenol* 1988;150(3):663–672.
75. Mittl RL, Grossman RI, Hiehle JF, et al. Prevalence of MR evidence of diffuse axonal injury in patients with mild head injury and normal head CT findings. *Am J Neuroradiol* 1994;15(8):1583–1589.
76. Zimmerman RA, Bilaniuk LT, Hackney DB, Goldberg HI, Grossman RI. Magnetic resonance imaging in temporal bone fracture. *Neuroradiology* 1987;29(3):246–251.
77. Gentry LR, Godersky JC, Thompson BH. Traumatic brain stem injury: MR imaging. *Radiology* 1989;171(1):177–187.
78. Smith DH, Meaney DF, Lenkinski RE, et al. New magnetic resonance imaging techniques for the evaluation of traumatic brain injury. *J Neurotrauma* 1995;12(4):573–577.
79. Blatter DD, Bigler DG, Sterling CJ, et al. MR-based brain and cerebrospinal fluid measurement after traumatic brain injury: Correlation with neuropsychological outcome. *Am J Neuroradiol* 1997;18:1–10.
80. Drayer BP, Wilkins RH, Boehnke MJA, Rosenbaum AE. Cerebrospinal fluid rhinorrhea demonstrated by metrizamide CT cisternography. *Am J Roentgenol* 1977;129:149–151.
81. Manelfe C, Cellerier P, Sobel D, Prevost C, Bonafe A. Cerebrospinal fluid rhinorrhea: evaluation with metrizamide cisternography. *Am J Roentgenol* 1982;138:471–476.
82. Chow JM, Goodman D, Mafee MF. Evaluation of CSF rhinorrhea by computerized tomography with metrizamide. *Otolaryngol Head Neck Surg* 1989;100:99–105.
83. Tolley NS, Lloyd GA, Williams HO. Radiological study of primary spontaneous CSF rhinorrhea. *J Laryngol Otol* 1991;105:274–277.
84. Creamer MJ, Blendonohy P, Katz R, Russell E. Coronal computerized tomography and cerebrospinal rhinorrhea. *Arch Phys Med Rehabil* 1992;73:599–602.
85. Gammal TE, Sobol W, Wadlington VR, et al. Cerebrospinal fluid fistula: detection with MR cisternography. *Am J Neuroradiol* 1998;19:627–631.
86. Shetty P, Shroff MM, Sahani DV, Kirtane MV. Evaluation of high-resolution CT and MR cisternography in the diagnosis of cerebrospinal fluid fistula. *Am J Neuroradiol* 1998;19:633–639.
87. Curtin HD, Som PM, Braun IF, Nadel L. Skull Base. In: Som PM, Curtin H, eds. *Head and neck imaging,* 3rd ed. St. Louis: Mosby, 1996:1233–1299.
88. Kaseff LG, Seidenwurm DJ, Nieberding PH, Nissen AJ, Remley KR, Dillon W. Magnetic resonance imaging of brain herniation into the middle ear. *Am J Otol* 1992;13:74–77.
89. Gavilan J, Trujillo M, Gavilan C. Spontaneous encephalocele of the middle ear. *Arch Otolaryngol* 1984;110:206–207.
90. Kemink JL, Graham MD, Kartush JM. Spontaneous encephalocele of the temporal bone. *Arch Otolaryngol Head Neck Surg* 1986;112:558–561.
91. Gray BG, Willinsky RA, Rutka JA, Tator CH. Spontaneous meningocele, a rare middle ear mass. *Am J of Neuroradiol* 1995;16:203–207.
92. Giunta G, Piazza I. Recurrent bacterial meningitis occurring five years after closed head injury and caused by an post-traumatic meningoencephalocele. *Postgrad Med J* 1991;67(786):377–379.

Neurosurgical Issues in Otolaryngology: Principles and Practice of Collaboration, edited by Moisés A. Arriaga and J. Diaz Day. Lippincott Williams & Wilkins, Philadelphia © 1999.

CHAPTER 10

Miscellaneous Neurosurgical Techniques Relevant to the Otolaryngologist

D. Kyle Kim

This chapter provides an overview of practical techniques that are usually performed by neurosurgeons. However, a basic understanding of these techniques by the otolaryngologist is helpful in collaborative surgery.

INTRACRANIAL PRESSURE MONITORING

The indications for intracranial pressure (ICP) monitoring include trauma, intracranial hemorrhage, neoplasms, as well as postoperative management—in short, all those situations in which there exists either the likelihood or the potential for raised ICP. The value of ICP monitoring has been debated in some circles; however, it is an established modality for many neurosurgeons. It is most commonly accepted for use in the management of patients with traumatic brain injury.

Some neurosurgeons would argue that ventricular catheters provide the most faithful rendering of ICPs. In addition, ventricular catheters provide the additional benefit of allowing the neurosurgeon to use cerebrospinal fluid (CSF) drainage to help treat raised ICP. The disadvantages of ventricular catheters are that they are the most invasive form of monitoring of ICP, and they're associated with a 10% chance of infection rate for extended monitoring. They also are associated with a 3% risk of development of seizures and a lesser risk of development of symptomatic intracerebral hematoma. If they are placed in the operating room as they are in some centers out of concern for infection risk, then they can be a disruption to the operating room schedule in that they are usually performed as emergencies.

For these reasons, other ICP monitoring solutions have been developed in the past two decades. These include the now superseded subdural monitoring devices, the so-called Richman bolts, which are also placed in the operating room. They provide a measurement of subdural pressures through a fluid catheter device. A more recent development, the fiber-optic ICP monitoring device (Camino) and the strain gauge pressure device (Codman), have proven to be efficacious, safe, and convenient. These devices are placed at the bedside through a twist drill. They need not be placed at Kocher's point but on the side of interest just behind the hairline if possible. They require the placement of a fiber-optic or a strain gauge device into the parenchyma but just below the surface. They have been associated with a low risk of seizures, hematoma, or infections. One disadvantage of these alternatives to ventricular catheters is that CSF drainage cannot be used to assist in the control of elevated ICPs.

PLACEMENT OF VENTRICULOSTOMY CATHETERS

The first monitors of ICPs were ventricular catheters, which are still widely used today. These are placed either at the bedside or in the operating room. Most commonly, the nondominant side, i.e., the right side, is used. Either a twist drill or a bur hole can be placed at Kocher's point 2 to 3 cm lateral to the midline or just anterior to the coronal suture. Ideally, the dura is visualized and incised under direct vision with a fine scalpel. The dural edges are coagulated and a ventriculostomy catheter is placed using a stylet initially. Once the frontal horn has been cannulated, usually at about 3 cm, the catheter is then passed without the stylet to a depth of $5\frac{1}{2}$ to 6 cm. It is advisable to mark the $5\frac{1}{2}$ cm mark with a silk tie secured with a surgeon's knot. (Even when the catheters are marked with indicators by the manufacturers, it is often all too easy to forget which mark is intended.) The ventriculostomy catheter may be inserted freehand or with the use of a commercial tripod device. It is critical that the ventriculostomy catheter is inserted at an angle perpendicular to the surface of the brain. The tripod device attempts to ensure a perpendicular approach.

D. K. Kim: Allegheny General Hospital, Pittsburgh, Pennsylvania 15212.

Once the stylet is removed, one can tell with certainty whether or not the ventricular system has been entered. If raised ICP is present, CSF will shoot out of the catheter with considerable force. In the presence of low ICP, it may sometimes be difficult to ascertain if one has entered the ventricular system. If CSF pulsations can be demonstrated, by filling the catheter with saline, then this is good evidence that the catheter tip is in the frontal horn. Sometimes an airlock may be sufficient to retard the emission of CSF.

Once it is determined that the catheter is indeed in the frontal horn, the distal end of the catheter is then passed through a separate stab incision to form a tunnel underneath the galea. This tunneling technique has been shown to reduce the incidence of infections. CSF is collected for routine laboratory analysis. If the ventricular catheter is placed in patients with subarachnoid hemorrhage from a ruptured aneurysm, it is highly advisable not to drain more than a few milliliters of CSF; sudden changes in subarachnoid pressure may precipitate rerupture of the aneurysm. Once the tunneling has been performed, the catheter is then connected to a drainage bag and the wound is irrigated and closed in standard fashion. CSF testing for routine surveillance of ventriculitis is performed on a regular basis. CSF is tested for glucose and protein, cell count, as well as Gram stain and culture and sensitivities. Maintenance of the catheter system and the reservoir system in an aseptic matter is critical to preventing catheter infections.

LUMBAR DRAIN PLACEMENT

Indications for placement of lumbar drains can be varied. They are useful in the management of CSF leaks, for treatment of hydrocephalus under certain conditions, and as a trial when considering placement of a permanent CSF shunt. Lumbar drains are placed with the patient in the lateral decubitus position preferably or with the patient sitting as necessary. The catheter is placed ideally in the lumbar 4th to 5th inner space in the midline. However, it is sometimes necessary to use the L3-4 space. It is advisable not to use the L2-3 space unless it has been demonstrated that a low-lying conus is not present. While the spinal cord usually ends at the L1-2 level, on occasion it can descend to as low as L2-3.

The Silastic catheter is placed through a Touhy needle, which is a 14-gauge introducer needle with a slightly bent tip. The catheter is introduced only when there is a rush of CSF through the Touhy needle. The catheter is passed to a depth of perhaps 25 or 30 cm before the needle is then removed over the catheter. It is advisable not to use a wire stylet unless passage of the catheter on its own proves difficult. If the CSF flow is not robust, then it may be difficult to pass the catheter even with a stylet.

The presence of diffuse degenerative lumbar disease may hinder the placement of the Touhy needle in the ideal spot. It is often very difficult to pass the Touhy needle into the thecal sac in the acromegalic patient who commonly has ankylosed lamina. With some patients, it may be necessary to perform lumbar drain placement under fluoroscopic guidance or even following a small laminotomy in the operating room.

Occasionally, lumbar CSF drainage can prove dangerous. For example, in those patients with surgical or traumatic disruption of the anterior cranial fossa, if there has been less than perfect dural repair at the anterior cranial fossa, lumbar CSF drainage may result in the passage of entrapped air via a ball valve mechanism through the anterior cranial fossa. This may result in cerebellar tonsillar herniation.

Upon completion of lumbar CSF drainage, the catheter must be removed with the patient in the position used to place the drain, i.e., either in the lateral decubitus position with the hips flexed and the knees bent or sitting up with the same. As with routine management of ventricular catheters, it is some matter of controversy whether or not prophylactic antibiotics are used either for placement of the catheter itself or during prolonged CSF drainage.

LUMBOPERITONEAL VERSUS VENTRICULOPERITONEAL SHUNTING

Ventriculoperitoneal shunting, either through the use of the Frazier's point or Kocher's point, is the most commonly used permanent CSF shunt system currently. However, certain circumstances may favor placement of a lumboperitoneal (LP) shunt, although this point itself may be in dispute. LP shunting has proven not to be as efficacious on a long-term basis as a ventriculoperitoneal shunting. LP shunts appear to fail more routinely; in addition, they have been associated with the development of chronic tonsillar herniation, as shown in a number of pediatric cases. Thus, on a routine basis, LP shunting is not advocated. However, in certain better-grade patients following subarachnoid hemorrhage who manifest hydrocephalus, LP shunts may be useful. Their utility with these patients lies in their increased tendency to fail. With this group of good-grade subarachnoid hemorrhage patients, the hydrocephalus may be a short-term problem. Thus the LP shunt, which may be expected to fail in the long term, may be useful in these patients for whom a long-term shunt may not be necessary.

The LP shunt is an amalgam of techniques used for lumbar drain placement and for ventriculoperitoneal shunt placement. The patient is placed in a lateral decubitus position with both the lumbar region, the flank, and the abdomen exposed and prepped. The peritoneal cavity then is exposed as with ventriculoperitoneal shunt placement. In the lumbar region, a small skin incision is placed ideally in the L4-5 inner space. The Touhy needle is then placed through the soft tissue and fascia into the thecal sac. A catheter is then placed through the needle into the thecal sac and, following the removal of the Touhy needle, the distal catheter is then tunneled subcutaneously to the abdominal incision. All connections are secured with silk ties. CSF again is collected from the tip of the catheter, prior to placement of the catheter into the peritoneal cavity. Some neurosurgeons advocate placement of a flushing reservoir to be located in the subcutaneous tissue of the flank, perhaps over a lower rib, to serve as an access to diagnose shunt infection or shunt failure.

DURAL OPENING AND CLOSURE

Dural openings should be planned ahead of time, as with scalp flaps and bony openings. The type of flap may vary according to the site of the lesion being exposed as well as the location of the procedure. For example, in the midline cerebellar exposure, the classic opening is a Y-shaped opening with linear midline portion inferiorly and the limbs extending diagonally along the cerebellar hemispheres (Fig. 10-1). In general, dural flaps are based toward the midline, where the draining veins are located, or toward the aspect of the brain that may be most difficult to close.

The dura is opened by elevating it with a sharp hook (Fig. 10-2) or with fine forceps with tips, and lightly making an incision with a fine scalpel. Once the dura has been nicked, one edge of the incised dura is then elevated and fine scissors with rounded tips are used to extend the opening. Care must be taken if raised ICP is present in that dural opening may injure the underlying cortex. The use of fine patties to protect the brain is then valuable.

Linear openings are advantageous in that they are easier to close. However, linear incisions tend to limit the exposure. Cruciate incisions, while appealing in concept, may be limited in that they are difficult to close and again suffer from often inadequate exposure. Dural openings should not be made near the bone flap as this would make the closure more difficult; a safe margin, moreover, should be allowed for dural openings toward the various draining sinuses, e.g., those made in the suboccipital region near the sigmoid sinus (Fig. 10-3).

With conditions of raised ICP, for example with certain tumors or subdural hematoma, it is often advisable to initially limit the opening until a partial decompression has

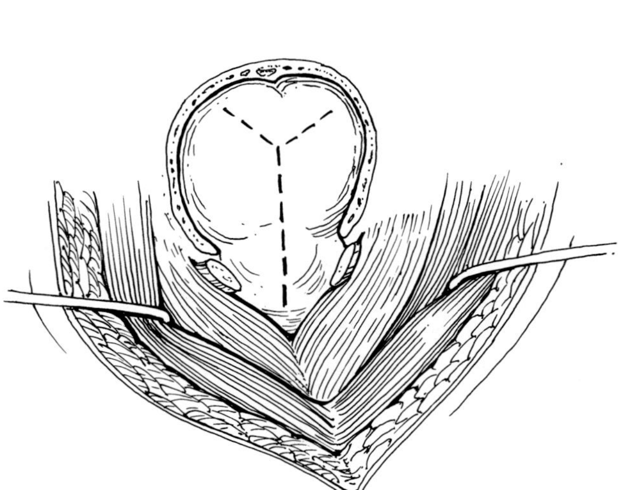

FIG. 10-1. Y-shaped dural flap for exposing the cerebellum.

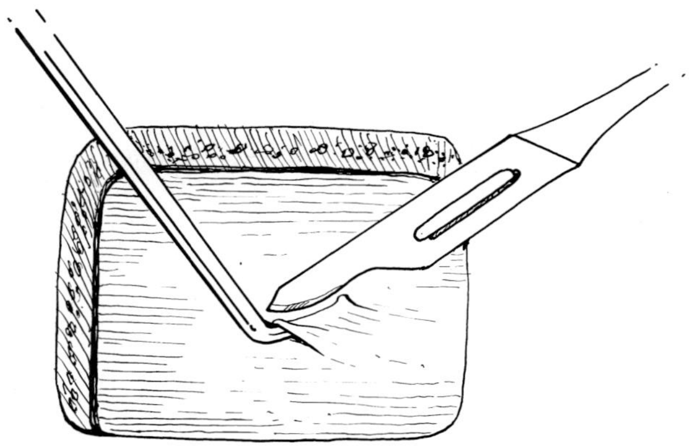

FIG. 10-2. Elevation of the dura with a hook before making an incision.

been accomplished before completing the dural flap. Bleeding from dural edges may be stopped by bipolar coagulation; however, one should keep in mind that the diathermy can result in shrinkage of the dura and may hinder closure later. An alternative to coagulation is either hemostatic clips or compression of the meningeal vessels with hemostats. Once open, the dura may be retracted with sutures either tied down to a local anchor or placed on tension using hemostats. During the procedure, it is advisable to wrap the dural flap with a moist Telfa strip or patty to minimize shrinkage from desiccation.

Prior to dural closure, it is advisable to ensure absolute hemostasis by a variety of techniques. Dural closure may be initiated by one or more anchoring sutures placed at intervals. These anchoring sutures help to prevent "dog ears" as well as help to bring the dural edges together. The dura then may be closed with a variety of techniques. The dura may be safely approximated using either interrupted or running suture technique. If one is using a running suture, then the technique may be a locking stitch. While it may appear that a running suture, which after all is the technique used to close carotid endarterectomy incisions, may be considered the technique that best provides watertight closure, the running lock technique has the advantage of providing help in approximating and bringing the dural edges together with each locking stitch. The interrupted technique also has its advocates for dural closure. Again, the type of suture appears not to be critical other than that it should be a nonabsorbable suture. Due to close quarters involved in many instances of dural closure, a 4-0 suture with a small, fine needle is recommended. Once dural closure is completed, one or more sutures can be used to hold up the dura next to the bone flap through small openings placed through the bone flap (Fig. 10-4). In addition, either at the beginning of the procedure or at the end, sutures to tack up the dura against the bone flap at the edges is recommended. These techniques are performed to minimize the chance of formation of an epidural hematoma postoperatively. If the dural tack-up sutures are performed at the beginning of the procedure, any potential

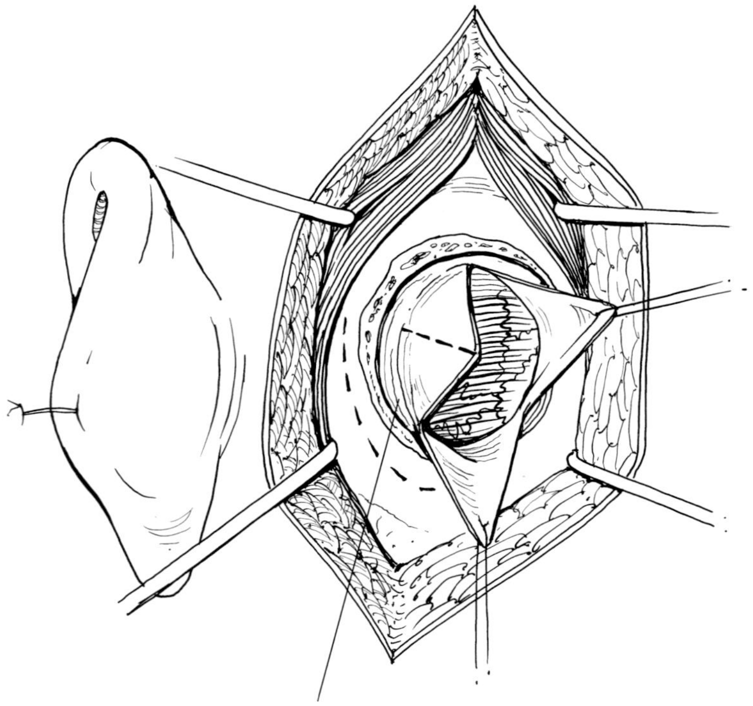

FIG. 10-3. Dural opening near the sigmoid sinus.

subdural hematoma that may have formed from an inadvertent tear of a cortical vessel is more likely to be recognized as the case is performed than if the tack-up sutures are placed at the end of the case. Once the dura is closed, any bleeding meningeal vessels can now be more aggressively coagulated with undue fear of shrinkage of the dura itself. Finally, some surgeons would now cover the dura with a layer of Surgicel again to minimize the chance of formation of postoperative epidural hematoma.

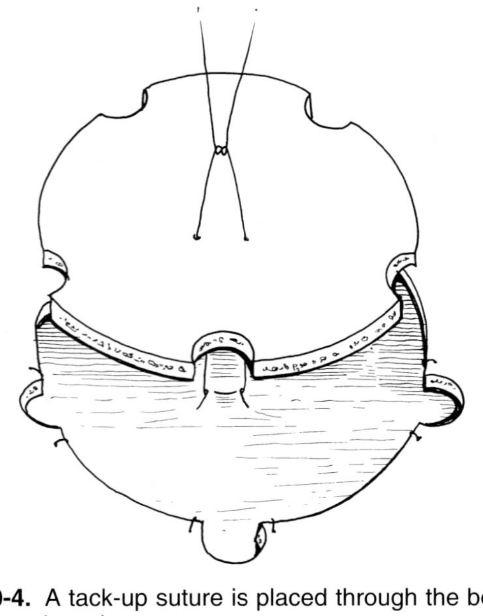

FIG. 10-4. A tack-up suture is placed through the bone flap and along the edges.

TURNING A FREE (OSTEOCLASTIC) BONE FLAP

Air-powered craniotomes with disposable perforator bits are extremely useful for placement of burr holes either for ventricular access or in the design of the bone flap. The air-powered drills are much preferred to the Hudson-Brace type of hand drills, which can also perform bur holes (Fig. 10-5). Making a bur hole with the latter and a dull bit can take as long as 10 minutes. In contrast, a bur hole placed with air-powered craniotome should take only a few seconds. Once the bur holes are placed, the inner table is removed either with cervical curettes or a Penfield no. 1 or a similar dural dissector. Following the placement of multiple bur holes, the dura may be separated from the skull using the Penfield no. 3 elevator or a Gigli saw passer.

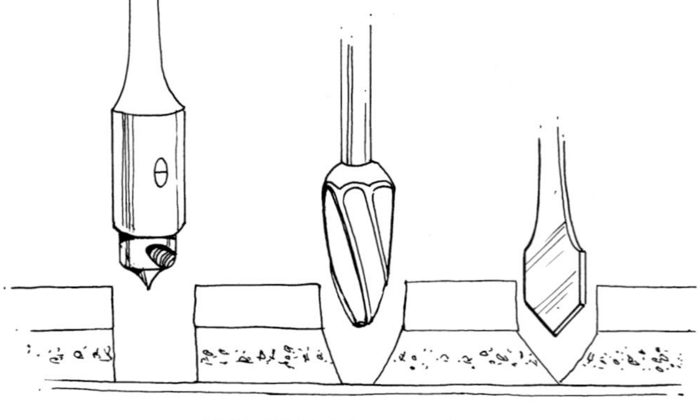

FIG. 10-5. Types of burs.

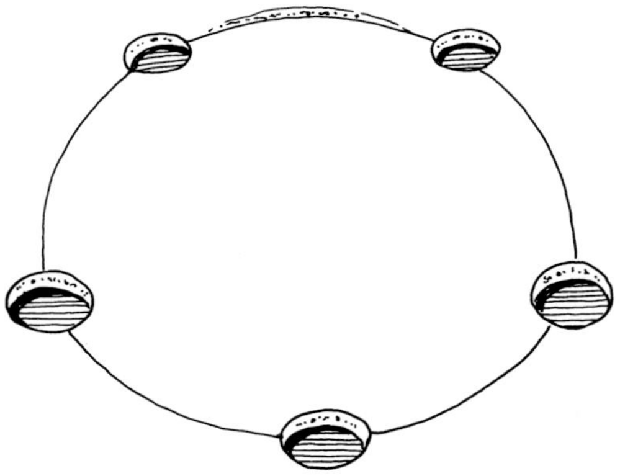

FIG. 10-6. Multiple bur holes for bone flaps are recommended in many situations.

For general purposes, a power saw with a footed attachment is recommended for turning a bone flap. It has been suggested that the advantage of the footed attachment is that a bone flap may be elevated using a single burr hole or with a small opening created with a power drill and a small burr. In the very young or the very old patient, however, multiple bur holes are recommended (Fig. 10-6); with patients of extremes of age, the dura can be quite adherent to the skull; a cavalier approach to the elevation of the bone flap can result in an unintended dural flap being created with the footed attachment. Thus, while performing a craniotomy through a single burr hole may appear to save time, it may actually create more work; more importantly, in the event of a tight brain, this may result in parenchymal injury.

One disadvantage of multiple burr holes may be the cosmetic result. However, this is now obviated with multiple ways to repair cranial defects using various titanium plates and screws; alternatively, even split-thickness bone grafts may be used to repair any number of cosmetic problems.

Power saws with the footed attachments do create a prominent footprint. This may be an issue particularly on the forehead or around the supraorbital region. For an optimal cosmetic result, a Gigli saw is preferred (Fig. 10-7). This device, used for limb amputations, leaves a small footprint, can be highly flexible with angles, and can be surprisingly swift in experienced hands.

While the power saws with footed attachments can be used for nearly any type of bone flap, the surgeon should be aware that the footed attachment can cut across dural sinuses if the dura has not been sufficiently stripped from the skull (Fig. 10-8). If one desires maximum safety, one may wish to cross dural sinuses by thinning either with a cutting burr or a diamond burr and removing the thinned bone with Kerison's rongeurs.

The above-described techniques are used for performing an osteoclastic (free) bone flap. An alternative to free flaps for frontal and temporal exposures is the osteoplastic bone flap in which the bone flap is left attached to the temporalis muscle. The techniques described above can be used for this flap as well.

EPIDURAL HEMATOMAS

Traumatic intracranial hematoma is a common indication for emergency craniotomy. The location and size of the hematoma guides the treatment. The invention of the computed tomography (CT) scanner revolutionized the management of traumatic brain injuries.

Epidural hematomas can be evacuated through a smaller scalp flap and bone flap than subdural hematomas. As the source of the hemorrhages are the meningeal artery or veins, the scalp flaps and bone flaps are directed toward the temporal region or the convexity. Typically a smaller reverse question mark (trauma-type) scalp flap is the most versatile; however, a linear type scalp incision may occasionally suffice. Once the scalp flap has been fashioned, a single bur hole is then placed using a craniotome and perforator bit or a power drill with either a cutting or diamond burr. A single bur hole is usually all that is required in that the hematoma itself has performed much of the dissection of the dura away from the skull. Then a bone flap situated to match the location and size of the hematoma is elevated. The hematoma is scooped out using dural elevators or cup forceps with the residual removed using irrigation and aspiration. Once the removal of the hematoma has been completed, multiple tack-up sutures through the edges of the bone are critical to prevent recurrence. The speed with which the diagnosis is made, the patient is taken to the operating room, and the bone flap is elevated is all-important in that epidural hematomas represent a traumatic intracranial lesion from which patients can be readily salvaged.

SUBDURAL HEMATOMAS

Unlike patients harboring epidural hematomas, patients with subdural hematomas commonly have underlying parenchymal injuries. Nonetheless, a prompt decompression can result in many instances in good recovery. With patients who are deteriorating from herniation syndrome, immediate decompression is indicated. In contrast, there may be other patients who are awake with a thin subdural clot that need not be evacuated. Between these extremes, other criteria such as extent of mass effect, measurement of ICP, and neurologic and medical status may all influence whether or not an operation is mandated.

Should the decision be made that the hematoma requires evacuation, then a large reverse question mark (trauma-type) scalp flap is fashioned. A large bone flap with multiple bur holes is elevated. The brain and the hematoma will be full against the skull. The large bone flap is recommended to assure complete evacuation of hematoma, which tends to spread over a large surface of the brain; also, in some centers, decompressive craniectomy is performed in conjunction with evacuation of the hematoma with craniectomies. With craniectomies, a large decompression is better than a small one. The dura is then opened hastily with one small comfort—that the hematoma will likely be found between the

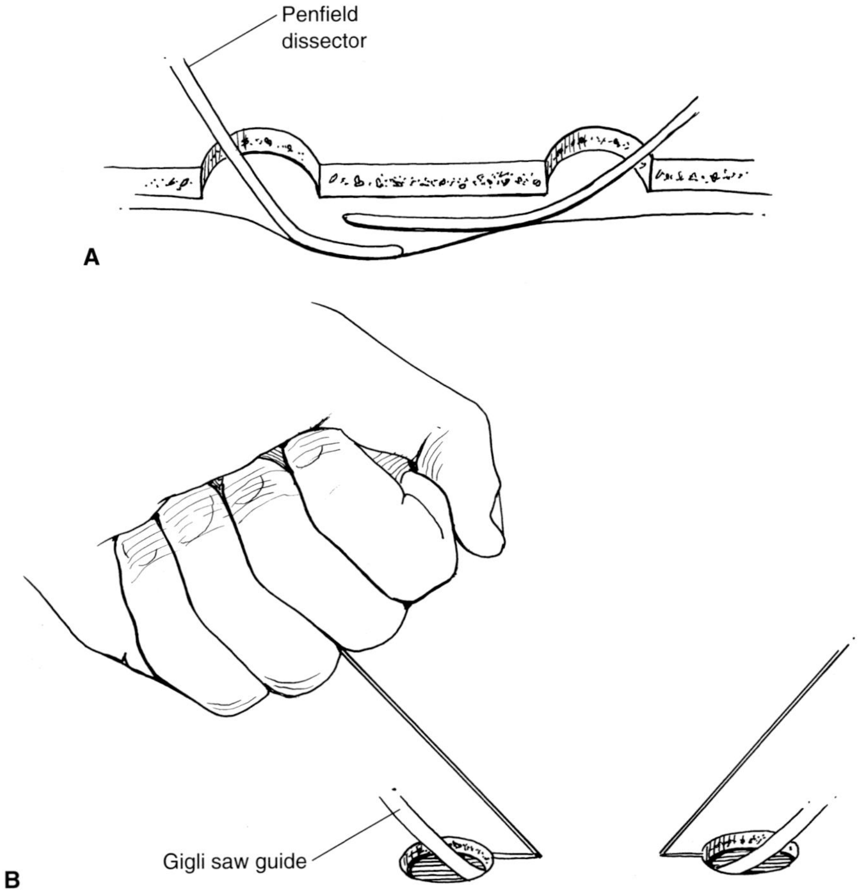

FIG. 10-7. A: Passing the Gigli saw guide. **B:** Using the Gigli saw.

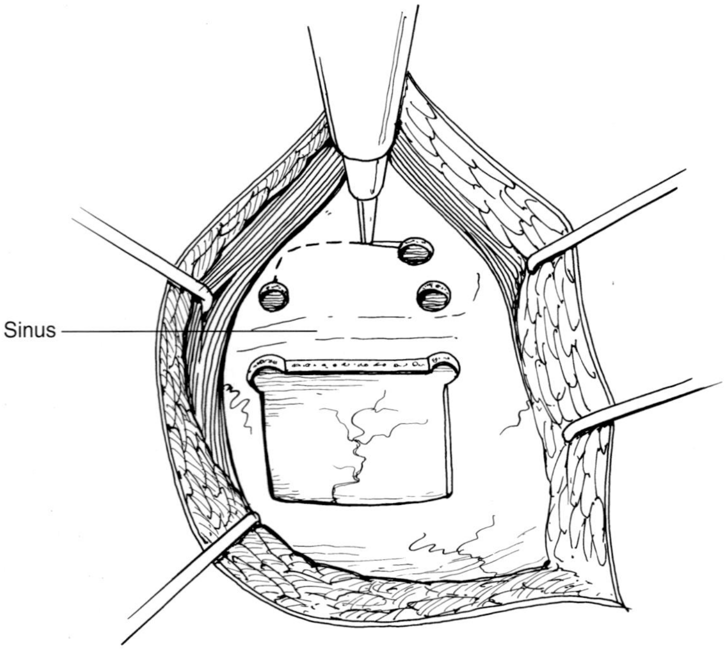

FIG. 10-8. Craniotomy across a dural sinus.

until 1961 (10). Dandy and Cushing did not work well together and parted ways while independently pursuing common goals of advancing the field of neurosurgery.

Dandy's operative mortality continued to decrease, and it was recognized that smaller tumors had decreased mortality. Dandy liberally clipped or cauterized blood vessels surrounding the tumor, and some suggest that this accounted for significant morbidity and mortality. Atkinson (11) in 1949 discovered that occlusion of the anterior-inferior cerebellar artery is the cause of much operative mortality in acoustic neuroma surgery. Before this study, brainstem infarction and cerebellar edema noted at autopsy were believed to be secondary to excessive intraoperative manipulation. Atkinson found thrombosis or surgical division of the anterior-inferior cerebellar artery in six cases of postoperative death. He described necrosis of the pons and cerebellar peduncle in each case. The surgeons made no attempt to change their procedure for fear that the patients would surely die from intraoperative or postoperative hemorrhage. Also, no attempt was made to save the facial nerve, and all patients had a complete facial paralysis postoperatively.

In the 1930s and 1940s, audiometric equipment improved dramatically, and unilateral hearing loss was readily detected by otolaryngologists looking for otosclerosis, especially since Lempert had developed the fenestration operation for otosclerotics. X-rays and vestibular testing improved as well. Otolaryngologists recognized that a unilateral hearing loss and unilateral facial numbness was an acoustic tumor until proven otherwise. They referred the patients to their neurosurgical colleagues and, because the tumors were detected earlier and the surgical morbidity and mortality so high, some neurosurgeons suggested that the patient should wait and enjoy normal facial function despite the increased risk of surgery at a later time (12). Others, including Cushing believed that the patient should have the operation sooner rather than later, recognizing the increased morbidity and mortality of operating on larger tumors.

Operative experience on morbidity and mortality became clear during this period. Dandy's lifetime mortality was 22.1% but it had decreased to 5% toward the end of his career. Significant reasons for this decrease were multifactorial and include, among others, earlier detection, better instrumentation, and improved anesthesia but certainly experience accounted for some of the improvement. Olivecrona (13) operated on 415 acoustic tumors between 1931 and 1960. His overall mortality was 19.7% with 22.5% for large tumors and 4.5% for small tumors. The Mount Sinai Hospital series had an overall mortality of 31% (14). Ricks Hospital in Copenhagen reported on their morbidity that included 100% facial paralysis and 18% severe ataxia (15). Surgeons continued to search for new diagnostic and surgical techniques to advance the treatment of acoustic neuromas.

1961–Present

The microsurgical techniques developed by House revolutionized the surgical management of acoustic neuromas. In 1956, early in his career as an otolaryngologist, House diagnosed an acoustic neuroma in a young fireman who complained of only hearing loss and tinnitus (16). He referred the patient to a neurosurgeon who chose to follow the patient until he developed trigeminal nerve dysfunction, papilledema, and headaches 1 year later. The patient underwent a suboccipital, retrosigmoid craniotomy and died on postoperative day three. House diagnosed and referred two more tumors in the next year; both patients survived the surgery but had significant neurologic sequelae including total facial paralysis and cerebellar ataxia. House was then developing the middle fossa, subtemporal craniotomy approach to the IAC and realized that the facial nerve could be reliably identified near the lateral end of the IAC in its labyrinthine portion (17). House first worked with John B. Doyle, a Los Angeles neurosurgeon, in developing these new techniques. They, in consultation with Jack Urban, made modification to the Zeiss operating microscope and developed a surgeon's chair on which the operator could rest his arms for increased stability.

On August 1, 1958, the first intracranial procedure, a middle fossa decompression, was accomplished with the use of a microscope (18). On February 15, 1961, the first use of microsurgical techniques in neurosurgery and acoustic neuroma surgery was accomplished. This was the first team approach to an acoustic neuroma. Between February 1961 and May 1962, the first eight cases of acoustic neuroma excision using an operating microscope and the middle fossa, subtemporal craniotomy were carried out by House and Doyle (19). They removed a great deal of labyrinthine bone and never accomplished total tumor removal. House then performed a series of cadaver dissections using the translabyrinthine approach while preserving the posterior wall of the external auditory canal (EAC), mesotympanum, and facial nerve. He postulated that the preservation of the EAC and tympanic membrane and ring should decrease the incidence of CSF leak. He used a microscope and, because of his background as a dentist, used a dental drill and a suction-irrigation unit. The first translabyrinthine craniotomy and excision of an acoustic neuroma with the aid of an operating microscope were accomplished by House in 1962. Doyle had grave concerns on the translabyrinthine approach and refused to participate in the operation. In July 1963, William E. Hitselberger, a recently trained neurosurgeon, began to work with House and they developed a team that lasted almost 30 years. Hitselberger learned temporal bone anatomy, drilling techniques, and microscopic skills. This surgical team was closely scrutinized by the medical staff and other members of the Los Angeles medical community. Early in his career, Hitselberger was ostracized by his neurosurgical colleagues. On the national level, neurosurgeons voiced grave concerns over the translabyrinthine approach and the use of an operating microscope. Despite these concerns, the team members continued with this approach, reported their results, held symposiums, and educated others on their ideas, slowly gaining credibility.

In December 1964, the *Archives of Otolaryngology* devoted an issue to a monograph on acoustic neuromas (19). House modeled the monograph after Cushing's 1917 monograph (4). House carefully and painstakingly stepped through each case in exquisite detail. In June 1964, the team had operated on 54 patients: three by the retrosigmoid approach, ten by the middle fossa approach, and 41 by the translabyrinthine approach. The number of deaths for the middle fossa, retrosigmoid, and translabyrinthine approaches were two, one, and zero, respectively. Dandy's overall mortality was 22.1% but it was 2.4% for his last 41 cases. The two middle fossa deaths were due to pulmonary embolism in one patient and presumed infection and hemorrhage in the second patient. Anterior-inferior cerebellar artery thrombosis was the cause of death in the retrosigmoid patient. The California tumor registry documented 85 cases of acoustic neuromas operated on between 1942 and 1962 (10). It reported a 36.5% mortality at 1 month and a 43.5% mortality at 1 year.

The House series had three cases of meningitis, two cases of postoperative hemorrhage requiring surgical exploration, and five cases of CSF leak requiring surgical repair. The team used a temporalis muscle plug to close the mastoid defect rather than abdominal wall fat. One middle fossa patient had significant cerebellar ataxia postoperatively. No translabyrinthine patients had cerebellar symptoms. Facial nerve disorder was evaluated as a function of approach. In the ten middle fossa patients, one patient showed no return of function, and three showed decreased movement with the ability to close their eye. In the three retrosigmoid patients, one had a total facial paralysis and one had decreased movement without the ability to close the eye. In the 41 translabyrinthine patients, 36 had normal function, and five had only partial return of facial function including one patient who had a total transection of the facial nerve and then a primary anastomosis. These were the first cases where facial function was consistently preserved after acoustic neuroma surgery. Hitselberger and Raney, in the same monograph, discussed in the suboccipital, retrosigmoid approach how the facial nerve is on the anterior aspect of the tumor: "Because the facial nerve is not under direct visualization, it is injured or destroyed unknowingly in many cases during dissection by section of the nerve as it arches over the tumor" (19). They also discuss the potentially higher recurrence rates of the retrosigmoid approach in tumors impacted into the lateral end of the IAC. The translabyrinthine approach reliably identified the facial nerve in its labyrinthine segment independent of tumor size.

The team encouraged visitors, fellows, and students to learn these techniques and to decide for themselves which approach and technique was the best. Soon, the operating microscope became the standard in posterior fossa surgery and the translabyrinthine craniotomy the approach of choice for acoustic neuromas surgery. The team set the standard for facial nerve preservation and cerebellar complications. Hitselberger recognized that the judicious use of the cautery in the posterior fossa decreased morbidity and mortality. He suggests that this is one of the main reasons surgical complications have decreased over the last 40 years.

The *Archives of Otolaryngology* in 1968 devoted an issue to monograph II on acoustic neuromas (20). This work reported on the team's first 200 cases of acoustic neuroma excision. The monograph thoroughly and systematically reported on the auditory testing, vestibular findings, imaging studies, anesthetic considerations, and complications for each patient. It confirmed the importance of auditory findings, showing that 54% of tumors presented with zero discrimination and only 25% had discrimination scores greater than 62%. It observed the trend that the greater the tumor size, the poorer the hearing. Of the 32 dead ears at presentation, 13 were large and 19 were of medium size. No small tumor presented with a dead ear. The monograph noted that 82% of patients with acoustic neuromas have a reduced vestibular response in the affected ear.

As the team's experience increased, the number of total tumor removals increased. In its first 50 cases, total tumor removal was accomplished in 56% of cases. In its last 50 cases, total tumor removal was accomplished in 86% of cases. The team described two indications for partial tumor removal: (a) vital sign changes during surgery, and (b) an elderly patient or poor surgical risk. The team generally agreed with Dandy's concept that it is more advantageous to remove the tumor totally the first time despite some increased mortality rather than undergo a risky second operation.

The fatality rate was 7% (14 of 200 patients). There were 11 fatalities in the primary operation and three fatalities in 12 revision operations. There were no fatalities in five small tumors, three fatalities in 131 medium tumors (2.2%), and 11 fatalities in 64 large tumors (17%). The deaths were scrutinized and classified by cause: four postoperative hemorrhage, three postoperative edema, three anterior-inferior cerebellar artery infarction, two pulmonary embolism, one extradural hematoma, and one gastrointestinal hemorrhage and myocardial infarction.

Facial nerve function was evaluated in all patients who had at least 1 year follow-up. Therefore, only 150 cases were available. In 102 cases (68%), there was no facial dysfunction at 1 year. In 32 cases (23%), there was facial weakness at 1 year. In seven cases (5%), there was complete loss of facial function. The postoperative CSF leak rate was 10%, and 12 of 200 cases (6%) had a postoperative hemorrhage requiring surgical intervention.

House and Hitselberger's work continued to gain respect. They emphasized the team approach to these lesions and taught several courses and seminars on the translabyrinthine approach and the use of the microscope.

Facial Nerve Preservation

In the era prior to 1961, facial nerve preservation rates were essentially zero. Dandy's dictum that facial paralysis is a small price to pay for the removal of this serious tumor was the prevailing theory. Tumors during Cushing's time were detected when they were large, microscopes were not available, and surgical mortality was so high that consideration was not given to preserving the facial nerve. House and Hitselberger began preserving facial nerves in acoustic neuroma surgery in the 1960s. In 1988, the first commercial facial nerve monitor was available and it is now used in most neurotologic procedures. Arriaga et al. (21) examined long-term facial function in 515 who underwent acoustic neuroma surgery between 1982 and 1989. The long-term follow-up (minimum 1 year) showed 74.8% House-Brackmann grades I and II, 19% House-Brackmann III and IV, and 6.2% House-Brackmann V and VI (22). Of these 515 cases, 92.8% were performed translabyrinthine and 7.2% through the middle fossa. Previous studies have shown that facial nerve function postoperatively is better with smaller tumors (23).

Diagnostic Considerations

The ability to detect smaller acoustic tumors continues to improve. Cushing's patients presented near death with severe ataxia, multiple cranial neuropathies, and, often, respiratory compromise. The 1960s brought more advances in behavioral audiometry with more accurate measurement of asymmetric hearing, speech discrimination, and discrimination rollover. Auditory brainstem evoked potentials became a useful tool to diagnose retrocochlear pathology (24). Asymmetry of greater than 0.2 msec in the latency of wave V alerted otolaryngologists and audiologists of potential retrocochlear pathology. Electronystagmography continued advancing and for the first time was used as a clinical tool on which to base therapy.

Imaging studies of the IAC including x-rays and polytomography facilitated the detection of smaller tumors. Posterior fossa myelography combined with x-rays and polytomography further advanced the detection of smaller tumors (25,26). Computed axial tomography (CAT) scanning revolutionized neuroradiology and allowed the detection of intracranial masses with more definition than previous studies. Improvements in hardware and software, as well as contrast administration, enhanced the CAT scan's ability to detect tumors in the posterior fossa. Magnetic resonance imaging (MRI) further improved the imaging of the CPA (27). The administration of contrast mediums improved MRI's sensitivity and specificity for detecting acoustic neuromas (28). Now, tumors just a few millimeters in diameter are readily detected by MRI. These advances in earlier detection certainly contributed to the decreased morbidity and mortality because the tumors are smaller.

The otolaryngology community educated its colleagues about the importance of evaluating a unilateral hearing loss. The workup of an asymmetric sensorineural hearing loss patient and a unilateral tinnitus patient are commonplace in an otolaryngology practice. All of these advancements contribute to the earlier detection of acoustic neuromas so that appropriate therapy can be initiated.

Cushing removed tumors with his finger. Continued advancements in medical instrumentation have changed the surgical management of these lesions. Medical instrument companies were founded and were eager to design and manufacture new tools to add to the surgeons armamentarium. House and Hitselberger worked closely with Jack Urban, an engineer, who helped them develop new instrumentation including the House-Urban dissector for the intracapsular removal of tumor and the middle fossa retractor for holding the temporal lobe superiorly.

Improvement in optics and light sources permitted wider fields of vision, better light, and improved depth perception. Cameras were attached to the microscope to enable visitors to watch the surgery live outside of the operating room and videotapes soon followed that enable one to review the surgery. Dental drills, first used by House, were replaced by stronger and faster electric and pneumatic drills.

All of these advances facilitated earlier detection of acoustic neuromas and increased the surgical armamentarium for the physician to expeditiously and safely remove the tumor.

ADVANTAGES OF TEAM SURGERY

The concept of team surgery, developed in the early 1960s, implies two different specialties working together inside and outside of the operating room for the joint goal of performing the best procedure for alleviating the patient's symptomatology and disease while minimizing morbidity and mortality. Otolaryngologists did not have the expertise to manage intracranial problems as well as neurosurgeons, and neurosurgeons did not have the same level of expertise with issues pertaining to hearing, vestibular dysfunction, and temporal bone anatomy. Consequently, the concept of working together, each discipline bringing its particular expertise, arose with respect to acoustic neuroma management.

Each specialty not only must strive for expertise in its own field, but also must learn as much as possible about the other specialty. This facilitates a relationship of mutual respect and allows the team members to discuss the diagnostic and operative issues together, combining their individual expertise synergistically. They hold each other accountable and frequently discuss how they could have altered their approach to improve outcome.

There is no discrete distinction between which part of the operation each team member performs, but some loose guidelines are generally followed. In the translabyrinthine approach, the otologist starts the operation by developing the skin and periosteal flap, drilling out the mastoid, labyrinth, and IAC, identifying Bill's bar and the facial nerve, and avulsing the superior vestibular nerve in the lateral IAC. The neurosurgeon proceeds with intracranial facial nerve dissection, tumor removal, hemostasis, and packing the eustachian tube, middle ear, and temporal bone defect. It is critical for each team member to understand the surgical goal and to have a working knowledge of the other's role to facilitate mutual respect and permit the other team member to start or assume the surgery in case of sickness, difficulty, or fatigue. Each step of the operation impacts the remainder of the operation. Inadequate exposure on a large tumor adversely affects safe tumor removal later or a poorly developed periosteal flap will increase the chances of a CSF leak. Frequently, both surgeons will discuss their findings and change their plans intraoperatively. The otologist should not view himself as just performing the approach, with no responsibility or interest in the CPA anatomy, intracranial complications, or facial nerve outcome. In a similar manner, the neurosurgeon must be interested in hearing and balance issues including audiometry, speech discrimination, auditory brainstem evoked potentials, facial nerve evoked electromyography, temporal bone anatomy, etc.

Most of this discussion involves the roles of the otologist and neurosurgeon. However, there are other critical team members involved in diagnosis and management. Internists evaluate patients preoperatively and follow them in the hospital and after discharge. These internists become intimately familiar with the course of these craniotomy patients and they are the experts in dealing with hypertension, diabetes insipidus, diabetes mellitus, and other medical disorders. A neuroradiologist evaluates the imaging studies. More than once the neuroradiologist has correctly suggested that the CPA tumor was not an acoustic neuroma but actually a meningioma, chondrosarcoma, lipoma, metastatic melanoma, cholesteatoma, or other disorder, changing the operative plan. An audiologist performs preoperative tests of hearing, facial nerve function, and balance. These tests often determine the approach to tumor removal, and most physicians are more confident making decisions based on their own evaluation. Audiologists monitor intraoperative facial nerve function and, where applicable, auditory brainstem evoked potentials. Their experience facilitates informing the surgeon of valuable intraoperative data, culling out artifact and other nonessential information. The anesthesia team is familiar with issues such as cranial nerve monitoring, fluid management, and deep venous thrombosis. Nursing personnel are trained in the management of postoperative craniotomies. All of these factors breed a degree of familiarity and expertise in all aspects of acoustic neuroma surgery.

SURGICAL TECHNIQUE

The surgical technique described here is the method of Brackmann and Hitselberger. We do not suggest that this is the only or the best method, but it is the method currently preferred by the senior authors.

The patient is placed in the supine position on the operating table and general anesthesia is administered by intravenous agents and endotracheal intubation. Pneumatic compression boots are placed before anesthesia is administered. An intraarterial catheter is placed depending on the size of the tumor and the anesthesiologist's preference. A Foley catheter is placed. Skeletal muscle relaxants are used only for induction because a facial nerve monitor, evaluating the orbicularis oris and the orbicularis oculi on different channels, is used. The operated ear is placed up and a generous postauricular and supraauricular shave is made. The left lower quadrant is shaved and prepped for fat harvest. The ipsilateral neck is prepped down to the clavicle in the same field in case a greater auricular nerve graft is needed. The skin is washed with a povidone-iodine solution and a plastic drape coated with an iodine solution is placed over the prepped areas. The postauricular area is injected with 10 cc of 1% lidocaine with a 1 to 100,000 epinephrine solution for hemostasis.

An incision is made approximately 4 cm posterior to the auricular crease from the mastoid tip to 2 to 3 cm superior to the auricle. The soft tissue is dissected anteriorly, the ear reflected anteriorly, and held in place with a self-retaining retractor. It is important not to lacerate the skin of the EAC. The mastoid periosteum is incised in a T or L fashion. The skin incision and mastoid periosteal incision are not superimposed to minimize CSF leak. A Lempert periosteal elevator is used to elevate the mastoid periosteum anteriorly to the EAC and 3 cm posterior to the sigmoid sinus. The spine of Henle, root of the zygoma, temporal line, and mastoid tip to the insertion at the sternocleidomastoid muscle are identified. It is again important to keep the skin of the EAC intact medially to the mastoid periosteum to prevent CSF leak.

The bony dissection is divided into three parts: mastoidectomy, labyrinthectomy, and IAC dissection. A pneumatic, high-speed drill with suction-irrigation is used to perform a cortical mastoidectomy. All bone is completely removed over the posterior fossa dura and sigmoid sinus from 2 cm posterior to the posterior border of the sigmoid sinus to the posterior semicircular canal. The middle fossa dura is skeletonized from the sinodural angle to the labyrinth. The lateral bone is saucerized to permit the instruments to enter the wound freely. The mastoid antrum is opened to expose the short process of the incus and lateral semicircular canal. Do not violate the bone of the posterior EAC to decrease the chance of a CSF leak. Some authors suggest leaving an island of bone over the sigmoid sinus (Bill's island) to protect it from potential tears and lacerations, especially from the drill shaft. The extensive lateral bony dissection is not always necessary for smaller tumors, but it is helpful to decompress the dura for increased exposure and instrument maneuverability. Also, the larger lateral exposure allows more light into the wound. This completes part one of the bony dissection.

Some surgeons stop operating at this point and review the MRI and audiogram to confirm tumor location, hearing status, and laterality. The labyrinthectomy begins by drilling medially in the sinodural angle. The dissection proceeds anteriorly with the side of the burr, and the posterior semicircu-

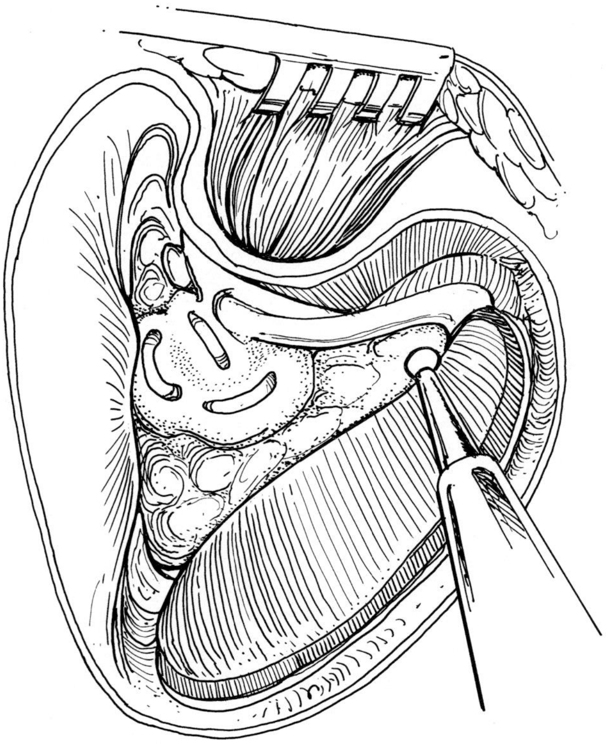

FIG. 11-1. Facial nerve skeletonized in its descending portion with the semicircular canals opened. Note the thinned external auditory canal and extensive bone removal.

lar canal, lateral semicircular canal, and superior semicircular canal are removed. The canals are not isolated and followed individually. The facial nerve is identified anterior to the lateral semicircular canal and then skeletonized, keeping just a thin layer of bone over its posterior margin to increase exposure (Fig. 11-1). The ampullated end of each semicircular canal is identified and the bone over the posterior and middle fossa dura is removed. The vestibule is entered anteriorly and the labyrinthectomy is complete (Fig. 11-2).

The IAC dissection starts inferiorly by drilling a trough between the jugular bulb and the inferior border of the IAC. This trough is developed from posteriorly at the posterior fossa dura to anterior, inferiorly at the jugular bulb, and superiorly at the inferior border of the IAC. The dissection in this trough continues medially throughout the width and length of the trough until the cochlear aqueduct is identified. The location of the glossopharyngeal, vagus, and spinal accessory nerves is reliably identified by their relationship to the cochlear aqueduct. The dissection continues superior to the cochlear aqueduct to prevent neural injury. The bone is completely removed from the inferolateral border of the IAC and at least 30 degrees from the inferomedial quadrant of the IAC. A similar trough is developed between the middle fossa dura and the superior border of the IAC, with its posterior border of the trough at the posterior fossa dura and the anterior border at the lateral end of the IAC (Fig. 11-3). It is critical that all of the bone is removed from the posterior fossa dura and at least 240 degrees around the IAC, with only its medial portion intact. In the anterior aspect of the superior trough at the lateral end of the IAC, the facial nerve is identified in its labyrinthine portion. In the lateral IAC, a crest of bone (Bill's bar) separates the facial nerve from the superior vestibular nerve.

The dissection proceeds to the facial recess where the incus is removed and the facial recess opening is extended

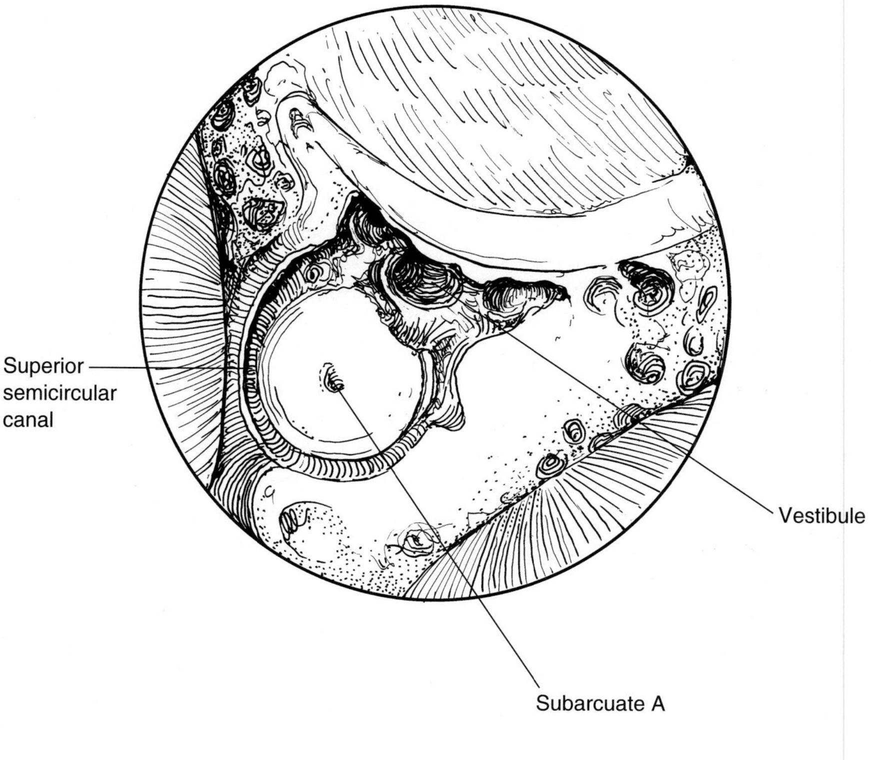

FIG. 11-2. The completed labyrinthectomy with the ampullated ends of the superior and inferior semicircular canals seen. The medial wall of the superior semicircular canal remains for orientation.

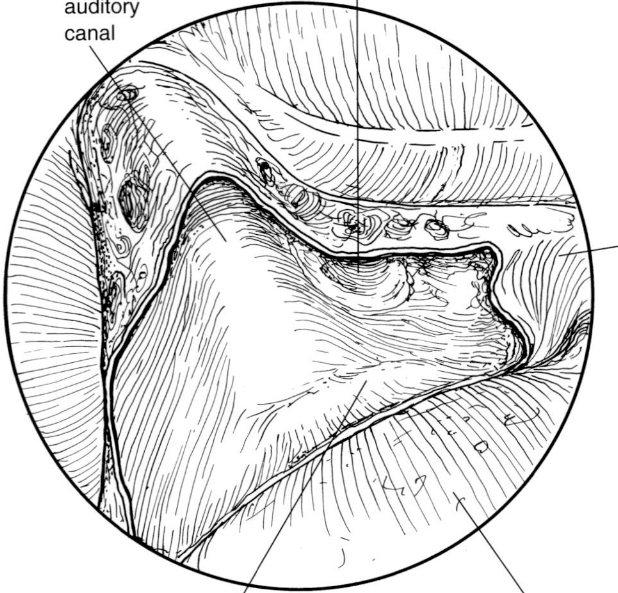

FIG. 11-3. The internal auditory canal (IAC) is visible after bone removal.

inferiorly. The operation, thus far, is completely extradural and the surgical field is copiously irrigated with antibiotic solution.

The dura is opened by making an incision over the posterior fossa dura and extending it anteriorly over the IAC. Generally, the larger the tumor, the larger the incision. The dura is retracted laterally during the incision to avoid injuring vessels immediately under the dura. A sharp hook is placed against Bill's bar and the superior vestibular nerve is avulsed from its lateral attachment (Fig. 11-4). The tumor capsule is opened by sharp dissection and the intracapsular tumor is debulked using the House-Urban dissector. Blood vessels are rarely cauterized and often dissected sharply off of the tumor and out of the field. The facial nerve is followed from laterally to medially while the tumor is dissected free. The inferior vestibular and cochlear nerves are cut laterally and the tumor/nerve complex is dissected free laterally. The facial nerve is inspected and stimulated at the brainstem. The tumor is removed after the trigeminal nerve, glossopharyngeal nerve, and anterior-inferior cerebellar artery are identified. Any significant bleeding is controlled with a bipolar cautery. The wound is inspected for bleeding and then copiously irrigated with an antibiotic solution.

A large plug of fat is obtained from the abdominal wall. The incision is usually made in the left lower quadrant so as to not get mistaken for a previous appendectomy incision. The wound is closed with 3-0 and 4-0 absorbable sutures in a subcuticular fashion after placing a Penrose drain. The fat is then cut into strips about 3 to 4 cm long and 1 cm wide.

The dura is closed with a 4-0 nonabsorbable suture. There is a defect laterally in the canal where the dura does not reach to form a watertight seal. The suture is still placed, creating a trellis of suture bridging across the adjacent dura. Small pieces of fat are dumbbelled into the trellis defects. The eustachian tube is packed with Surgicel and the middle ear and facial recess are packed with fat (29). Care is taken to avoid lacerating the tympanic membrane. Bone wax is packed over the opening of the vestibule. These actions try to prevent CSF from entering the middle ear and leaking into the eustachian tube. The strips of abdominal wall fat are placed into the wound. A bayonet forceps is used to place the tip of the fat strip medially into the wound to the level of the dura. A suction holds the fat inferiorly and another piece is placed superiorly down to the level of the dura, pushed inferiorly, held in place with a suction, and the process is repeated until the mastoid defect is packed tightly. The fat is not pushed medially directly into the CPA because it could tear the dura and herniate into the angle. Consequently, it is packed inferior against the bone.

The wound is copiously irrigated and the mastoid periosteum is closed with 0 chromic suture. The subcutaneous tissue is closed with 0 chromic and 3-0 absorbable sutures.

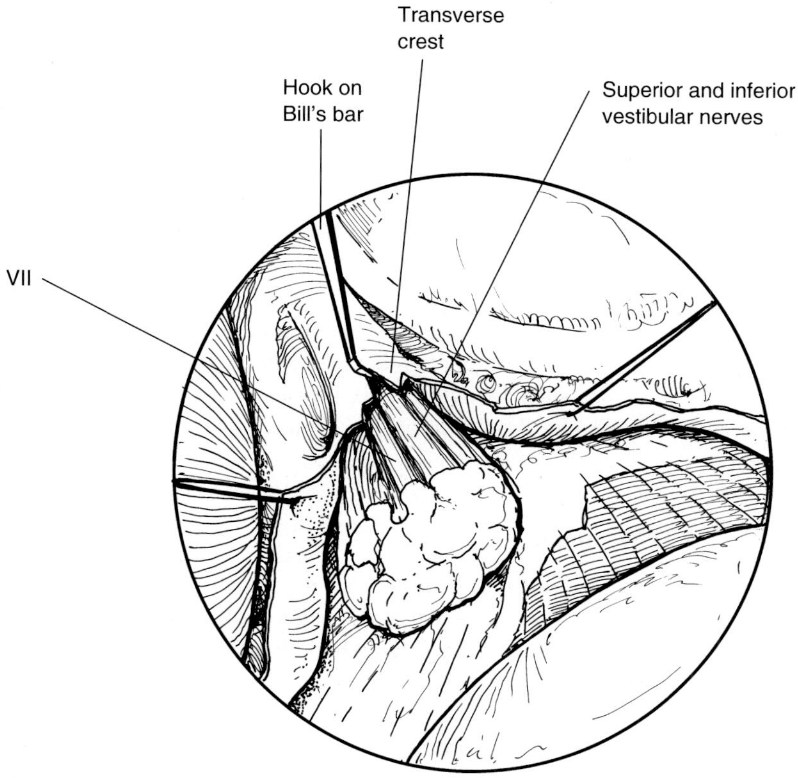

FIG. 11-4. The dura and the lateral IAC are opened to show the relationship of the nerves.

The skin is closed with a 4-0 absorbable suture, a 4-0 nylon, and/or staples. The wound is not drained. A sterile mastoid dressing is placed and kept in placed for 4 days and changed when soiled.

POTENTIAL PITFALLS

Preoperative Pitfalls

1. Misdiagnosis. All information including the history, physical examination, audiologic studies and imaging studies form the basis for the differential diagnosis. Not all CPA tumors are acoustic neuromas, and the index of suspicion must be high so as not to be misled by an unusual lesion. Meningiomas, facial neuromas, lipomas, chondrosarcomas, cholesteatomas, metastatic breast carcinoma, metastatic melanomas, and gliomas are known to occur in the CPA. Consequently, reviewing the history, physical examination, and studies, especially the MRI with and without gadolinium, help alert the team to the likelihood of an unusual lesion.
2. Inaccurate audiometric testing. The basis for choosing the translabyrinthine approach relates to tumor size, location, and hearing status. Recent accurate audiograms, auditory brainstem evoked potentials, and electronystagmography are often necessary to make informed decisions about the best approach for tumor removal. An increased number of patients are referred with previous audiometric testing. Look carefully for any inconsistencies, and if there is any questions, it is best to do one's own preoperative evaluation to ensure repeatable, accurate data for decision making.
3. Medical risk. Knowledge of complicated medical problems is often outside the realm of otologists and neurosurgeons. Consequently, all patients are evaluated preoperatively and followed in the hospital by the team's internist and anesthesiologist. There is a clear advantage to this team approach because these colleagues have followed most of the previous patients and they are familiar with the risks and complications. Knowledge of life expectancy and the natural history of acoustic neuromas is essential because a large number of tumors do not grow and the patient is followed with serial MRIs, obviating potentially risky surgery (30,31).
4. Previous stereotactic radiation. Studies show obscured tissue planes, fibrosis, and an increased risk of facial paralysis in patients undergoing surgery after stereotactic radiation (32).

Intraoperative Pitfalls

1. Contracted mastoid. A sclerotic, contracted mastoid with an inferior middle fossa plate and an anterolateral sigmoid sinus makes the approach considerably more difficult (33). All bone over the middle fossa dura, sigmoid sinus, and 3 to 4 cm posterior to the sigmoid sinus allows compression and retraction of the dural sinuses and dura. The bony labyrinth is the same size in all individuals and, if lateral exposure is maximized, the

labyrinthectomy and IAC dissection proceeds without incident.

2. Dural sinus injury. The dural sinuses are low-pressure vessels that are controlled with intraluminal and extraluminal packing. Usually Surgicel is used to gently pack the injured area. Care is taken to avoid the packing from going into the vessel and creating an embolus. Also, an air embolism is possible with larger venous injuries. In rare instances, the sigmoid sinus is suture ligated to control bleeding.
3. External auditory canal injury. An injury of the EAC, tympanic membrane, or in a previous canal-wall-down mastoidectomy prevents effectively packing the mastoid defect to prevent a CSF leak. Minor soft tissue injuries to the skin of the EAC lateral to the mastoid periosteum or over the bone of the EAC can often be repaired with fascia and /or suture. However, significant bony defects or tears greatly predispose the patient to a CSF leak through the EAC or the eustachian tube. These cases are managed by suturing closed the EAC, removing all squamous tissue medial to the closure, and ablating the middle ear space. It is critical to completely remove all of the squamous epithelium medial to the closure or a cholesteatoma may form.
4. Facial nerve injury. Any known injury to the facial nerve is repaired during the same operation. The ipsilateral neck is prepared and draped in every case to facilitate harvesting the greater auricular nerve without preparing another site. An injury in the CPA is repaired with a primary anastomosis or an interposition graft using the greater auricular nerve (34,35).

Postoperative Pitfalls

See Management of Complications, below.

MANAGEMENT OF COMPLICATIONS

Cerebrospinal Fluid Leak

Cerebrospinal fluid rhinorrhea is the primary symptom of a CSF leak (36). The fluid travels into the middle ear space, down the eustachian tube, and into the nasal cavity. Leaks rarely occur through the wound or the ear canal. Initially, these leaks are treated with a head dressing, bed rest, stool softeners, and acetazolamide. If the leak does not stop, a lumbar-subarachnoid drain is placed and spinal fluid is drained at 8 to 10 cc per hour for 3 to 5 days, with a tight head dressing in place. If the lumbar drain is removed and the leak continues or recurs, the patient is taken back to the operating room for the repair of the leak. The wound is opened, the fat removed, and the wound is methodically repacked in the manner described above (see Surgical Technique). Often, new fat is harvested from a different abdominal incision, or leftover fat from the original surgery is taken from the freezer and used. Postoperatively, a lumbar-subarachnoid drain is placed at a different level and kept in place for 3 to 5 days.

If the leak occurs through the EAC, packing is placed in the canal and the head dressing is replaced. If the leak continues, the EAC is inspected for defects. If the canal or tympanic membrane is lacerated and the leak is through this defect, the patient is taken to the operating room and the ear canal is closed in a two-layer fashion (37). A lumbar-subarachnoid drain is placed for 3 to 5 days to allow adequate healing.

If the wound edges are leaking CSF, the skin edges are oversewn in a running, locked fashion with a nonabsorbable suture such as nylon. This is usually done at the bedside under local anesthesia. A lumbar-subarachnoid drain is rarely necessary.

Meningitis

Postoperative patients do not routinely get antibiotics or steroids. We believe that this helps clarify postoperative scenarios of fever, increased white blood cell counts, and meningismus. The routine use of antibiotics and steroids can mask meningitis, cause leukocytosis, immunosuppress, select out resistant organisms, and generally confuse the clinical issues. Some describe a relationship between meningitis and CSF leak (38).

The key to preventing the complications of meningitis are a high index of suspicion, early lumbar puncture, and aggressive antimicrobial therapy. Consequently, vigilant questioning and thorough physical examination are conducted at least once daily in search of the symptoms and signs of meningitis. If the patient exhibits symptoms and signs, a lumbar puncture is performed and antimicrobial therapy is initiated. If the cultures show no growth after 5 days and the patient is afebrile with no leukocytosis, the antimicrobial therapy is terminated and the patient observed. If the cultures are positive, intravenous antimicrobial therapy is continued for 7 to 10 days and oral antibiotics are given on an outpatient basis for an additional 10 to 14 days. All patients are given an instruction sheet that educates them about the signs and symptoms of meningitis. Patients are instructed to take their temperature several times a day and to call immediately if it is elevated.

Facial Nerve Dysfunction

Anatomic preservation of the facial nerve in acoustic neuroma surgery is greater than 90% in most reported series. Functional results vary widely, with most patients with unsatisfactory outcomes having larger tumors (23,39). Exposure keratitis is the main early complication of facial nerve dysfunction. Lacrimation is usually impaired due to disruption of parasympathetic input to the lacrimal gland. Eye closure problems are treated early with drops, ointment, a moisture chamber, and evening patching and taping. A trigeminal nerve injury leads to impaired corneal sensation and exacerbates the injury. An ophthalmologist is consulted early and, in cases where long-term facial nerve dysfunction is expected, definitive surgical therapy is performed before the patient leaves the hospital. Some patients get considerable relief and protection from a contact lens. Patients are warned of a delayed facial palsy after hospital discharge and instructed to call and seek treatment immediately. Long-term issues related to facial reanimation reserved for long-standing facial paralysis are beyond the scope of this chapter.

Cranial Nerve Injury

Cranial nerve injuries other than the facial nerve or the cochleovestibular nerve are very rare, but the glossopharyngeal nerve, vagus nerve, or the spinal accessory nerve may be involved. The hypoglossal nerve is rarely injured, even with large tumors. Dysphagia, odynophagia, hoarseness, and aspiration are the primary symptoms and signs of such injuries. Aspiration has the greatest potential for complications because it can cause pneumonia and lung abscess. An insensate larynx, poor laryngeal elevation, poor vocal fold adduction, and an ineffective cough make the patient most susceptible to these complications. A simultaneous hypoglossal nerve injury adds significantly to the dysfunction because of the patient's ability to propel the food bolus posteriorly. Consultation with a laryngologist and speech therapist are often helpful. These patients often benefit from a gastrostomy tube and sometimes a vocal fold medialization procedure and/or a cricopharyngeal myotomy. The patient's medical condition, nutritional status, and expected duration of dysfunction dictate treatment.

Intracranial Vascular Compromise

An acute postoperative posterior fossa hemorrhage is a true neurosurgical emergency that is best treated by opening the wound to allow decompression of the brainstem. This is performed at the bedside and the patient is then taken to the operating room for wound exploration, evacuation of clot, and control of hemorrhage. The anterior-inferior cerebellar artery often travels near the porus acousticus. An interruption of this artery often leads to pontine infarction, respiratory compromise, and death. It is more common to get a partial anterior-inferior cerebellar artery syndrome due to interruption of an end branch of this artery. Rehabilitation is the best treatment for this syndrome.

Edema

Postoperative edema is generally treated with high-dose corticosteroids. If obstructive hydrocephalus ensues, a ventriculoperitoneal shunt is placed. Fluid restriction, head elevation, and mechanical ventilation are other tools useful in treating brain edema. The suspected etiology is brainstem manipulation and acute venous insufficiency. Occasionally blood clots will block the aqueducts, and shunting is necessary.

Cerebellar Ataxia

Cerebellar ataxia is a rare complication of the translabyrinthine approach. The cerebellum is not retracted and its assumed etiology is vascular compromise. It is treated supportively with physical and occupational therapy. The ataxia frequently improves over time and no surgical therapy is indicated.

Recurrence

Recurrence is thought to occur from residual tumor lateral in the IAC. Because the translabyrinthine approach dissects the most lateral portion of the canal, recurrences are fewer than 10 in over 3,000 cases performed at the House Ear Clinic.

SUMMARY

The concept of collaborative surgery implies different specialties working together inside and outside of the operating room for the common goal of treating the patient while minimizing morbidity and mortality. This has been practiced at the House Ear Clinic in the treatment of neurotologic disorders for the last 35 years. Empirically, we believe that this concept is applicable to translabyrinthine excision of acoustic neuromas and, ultimately, benefits the patient significantly.

REFERENCES

1. Bell C. *The nervous system of the human body: embracing the papers delivered to the Royal Society on the subject of nerves.* London: Longman, Reese, Orme, Brown, and Green, 1830.
2. Cruveilhier J. *Anatomie pathologique du corps humain.* Paris: Chez J. B. Baillère, 1842.
3. Ballance CA. *Some points in the surgery of the brain and its membranes.* London: Macmillan, 1907.
4. Cushing H. *Tumors of the nervus acusticus and the syndrome of the cerebellopontile angle.* Philadelphia: Hafner, 1917.
5. Panse R. Ein glioms des akustikus. *Arch Ohrenh* 1904;61:251–255.
6. Zange J. Translabyrinthäre operationen von acusticus und kleinhirnbrückenwink—eltumoren. *Berl Klin Wochenschr* 1915;52:1334.
7. Schmiegelow E. Bietrag zur translabyrinthären entfernung der akustikustumoren. *Z Ohrenheilkd* 1915;73:1.
8. House WF. A history of acoustic tumor surgery 1900–1917, the Cushing era. In: House WF, Luetje CM, eds. *Acoustic tumors, vol 1: diagnosis.* Los Angeles: House Ear Institute, 1985:9–21.
9. Henschen F. Die akustikustumoren, eine neue gruppe radiographisch darstellbarer hirntumorer. *Fortschr Geb Röntgenstr* 1912;18:207–216.
10. House WF. A history of acoustic tumor surgery 1917–1961, the Dandy era. In: House WF, Luetje CM, eds. *Acoustic tumors, vol 1: diagnosis.* Los Angeles: House Ear Institute, 1985:25–31.
11. Atkinson WJ. Anterior-inferior cerebellar artery. *J Neurol Neurosurg Psychiatry* 1949;12:137–151.
12. Pennybacker JB, Cairnes H. Results in 130 cases of acoustic neurinoma. *J Neurol Neurosurg Psychiatry* 1950;13:272–277.
13. Olivecrona H. Acoustic tumors. *J Neurosurg* 1967;26:6–13.
14. Bloch JM, Nathanson M. Results in acoustic neuroma surgery. *J Mt Sinai Hosp NY* 1963;30:217–227.

15. Thomsen J. Suboccipital removal of acoustic neuromas: results of 125 operations. *Acta Otolaryngol* 1976;81:406–414.
16. Glasscock ME, Steenerson RL. A history of acoustic neuroma surgery 1961–present. In: House WF, Luetje CM, eds. *Acoustic tumors, vol 1: diagnosis*. Los Angeles: House Ear Institute, 1985:33–41.
17. House WF. Surgical exposure of the internal auditory canal and its contents through the middle, cranial fossa. *Laryngoscope* 1961;71: 1363–1385.
18. House WF. Forward. In: Jackler RK, Brackmann DE, eds. *Neurotology*. St. Louis: Mosby, 1994:xxi–xxv.
19. House WF. Report of cases: monograph, transtemporal bone microsurgical removal of acoustic neuromas. *Arch Otolaryngol* 1964;80: 617–667.
20. House WF. Acoustic neuroma monograph II. *Arch Otolaryngol* 1968; 88:575–715.
21. Arriaga MA, Luxford WM, Atkins JS Jr, Kwartler JA. Predicting long-term facial nerve outcome after acoustic neuroma surgery. *Otolaryngol Head Neck Surg* 1993;108:220–224.
22. House JW, Brackmann DE. Facial nerve grading system. *Otolaryngol Head Neck Surg* 1985;93:146–147.
23. Kartush JM, Lundy LB. Facial nerve outcome in acoustic neuroma surgery. *Otolaryngol Clin North Am* 1992;25:623–647.
24. MacKay A, Hosobuchi Y, Williston JS, Jewett D. Auditory evoked brainstem potentials in acute posterior fossa mass lesions. *Surg Forum* 1978;29:523–525.
25. Scanlan RL. Positive contrast medium (iophendylate) in diagnosis of acoustic neuroma. *Arch Otolaryngol* 1964;80:698–706.
26. Glasscock ME 3rd, Overfield RE, Miller GW. Polytomography in an otologic practice. *South Med J* 1976,69:1433–1437.
27. Valvassori GE, Marates FG, Placios E, et al. MR of the normal and abnormal internal auditory canal. *AJNR* 1988;9:115–119.
28. Haughton VM, Rimm AA, Czervionke LF, et al. Sensitivity of Gd-DTPA-enhanced MR imaging of benign extraaxial tumors. *Radiology* 1988;166:829–833.
29. Pulec JL. Technique to avoid cerebrospinal fluid otorhinorrhea with translabyrinthine removal of acoustic neuroma. *Laryngoscope* 1994; 104:382–386.
30. Thomsen J, Tos M. Acoustic neuroma: clinical aspects, audiovestibular assessment, diagnostic delay, and growth rate. *Am J Otol* 1990;11: 12–19.
31. Charabi S, Thomsen J, Mantoni M, et al. Acoustic neuroma (vestibular schwannoma): growth and surgical and nonsurgical consequences of the wait-and-see policy. *Otolaryngol Head Neck Surg* 1995;113:5–14.
32. Slattery WH 3rd, Brackmann DE. Results of surgery following stereotactic irradiation for acoustic neuromas. *Am J Otol* 1995;16:315–319, discussion 319–321.
33. Friedman RA, Brackmann DE, van Loveren HR, Hitselberger WE. Management of the contracted mastoid in the translabyrinthine removal of acoustic neuroma. *Arch Otolaryngol Head Neck Surg* 1997;123: 342–344.
34. Brackmann DE, Hitselberger WE, Robinson JV. Facial nerve repair in cerebellopontine angle surgery. *Ann Otol Rhinol Laryngol* 1978;87: 772–777.
35. Luetje CM, Whittaker CK. The benefits of VII-VII neuroanastomosis in acoustic tumor surgery. *Laryngoscope* 1991;101:1273–1275.
36. Giddings NA, Brackmann DE. Surgical treatment of difficult cerebrospinal fluid otorhinorrhea. *Am J Otol* 1994;15:781–784.
37. Brackmann DE, Rodgers GK. Management of postoperative cerebrospinal fluid leaks. In: Brackmann DE, Shelton C, Arriaga MA, eds. *Otologic surgery*. Philadelphia: WB Saunders, 1994:709–715.
38. Bryce GE, Nedzelski JM, Rowed DW, Rappaport JM. Cerebrospinal fluid leaks and meningitis in acoustic neuroma surgery. *Otolaryngol Head Neck Surg* 1991;104:81–87.
39. Jackler RK. Acoustic neuroma (vestibular schwannoma). In: Jackler RK, Brackmann DE, eds. *Neurotology*. St. Louis: Mosby, 1994: 729–785.

Neurosurgical Issues in Otolaryngology: Principles and Practice of Collaboration,
edited by Moisés A. Arriaga and J. Diaz Day.
Lippincott Williams & Wilkins, Philadelphia © 1999.

CHAPTER 12

Hearing Preservation in Acoustic Neuroma Surgery

Moisés A. Arriaga and Takanori Fukushima

OVERVIEW

The principal objective of acoustic neuroma surgery is safe, total removal of the tumor. Recent advances in patient outcomes including very low mortality (less than 1%), routine anatomic preservation of the facial nerve (more than 90%), and excellent rates of functional preservation of the facial nerve have encouraged further attempts at functional preservation in acoustic neuroma surgery (1–3). Hearing preservation is now a realistic goal for many patients with acoustic neuroma (4). The opportunity to focus on hearing preservation as a viable goal of acoustic tumor surgery is the result of significant multidisciplinary collaboration. This chapter provides a brief historical overview of the objectives of acoustic neuroma surgery, proposes principles of collaboration for this surgery, and discusses specific surgical techniques for hearing preservation acoustic neuroma surgery. Surgical outcomes, potential pitfalls, and the management of complications of various techniques are discussed.

HISTORICAL MANAGEMENT

Harvey Cushing's meticulous clinical record of patients and surgeries with acoustic neuroma provided the first insight into the clinical progression of acoustic tumor symptoms (5). He described six clinical stages: (a) labyrinthine symptoms (auditory and vestibular); (b) occipitofrontal pains with suboccipital discomforts; (c) cerebellar incoordination and instability; (d) involvement of adjacent cranial nerves; (e) intracranial hypertension with papilledema; and (f) dysarthria, dysphagia, cerebellar crises, and respiratory difficulties, culminating in obtundation and death (6). Despite improved imaging and diagnosis, through the first half of the 20th century surgical techniques lagged far behind diagnostic techniques. Because of the high morbidity in the management of these tumors, surgical intervention was delayed until the tumors had reached a significant size to produce symptoms of brainstem compression. The advent of microsurgical techniques, especially beginning with the reintroduction of the translabyrinthine approach by William House, produced a dramatic decrease in mortality following acoustic neuroma surgery. This allowed a focus on functional outcomes. The preservation of the facial nerve was facilitated by understanding of the microsurgical temporal bone anatomy. This was further augmented by the application of intraoperative electromyogram (EMG) facial nerve monitoring. These developments have evolved to the state that the facial nerve can anatomically be preserved in over 90% of patients undergoing acoustic neuroma surgery with generally excellent functional outcomes regardless of the surgical approach. Intraoperative facial nerve monitoring can safely be described as the standard of care in acoustic neuroma surgery.

As facial nerve results improved, the next category of attempted functional preservation became hearing. The middle fossa approach had been an infrequently used technique for acoustic neuroma limited to hearing preservation attempts in small intracanalicular acoustic tumors (7). The principal limitation to its application was diagnosis of these lesions at a small size when the middle fossa approach was applicable. With the advent of gadolinium-enhanced magnetic resonance imaging (MRI), there has been a significant increase in the reported cases of middle fossa surgery as well as an improvement in the outcomes with this technique. Posterior fossa acoustic neuroma surgery has generally evolved from the suboccipital exposure, which avoided entry

M. A. Arriaga: Allegheny General Hospital, Pittsburgh, Pennsylvania 15212.

T. Fukushima: Carolina Skull Base Surgery Center, Carolina Neuroscience and Ear Research Institute, Raleigh/Durham, North Carolina 27609.

into any mastoid air cells, to the modern retrosigmoid technique, which extends the surgical exposure to the sigmoid sinus and mastoid (8). Simultaneously there have been developments in auditory monitoring including audiometric brainstem response, electrocochleography, otoacoustic emissions, and direct 8th nerve action potential monitoring. Microsurgery, as with the rest of medicine, is focusing increasingly on outcomes including objective measurement parameters as well as patient reporting. In fact, patient advocacy organizations such as the Acoustic Neuroma Association are increasingly influencing the information provided to patients and the medical emphasis on short- and long-term functional outcomes (9,10).

PRINCIPLES OF COLLABORATION: GENERAL CONCEPTS

The current high degree of collaboration in acoustic neuroma surgery is in sharp contrast to the tremendous degree of confrontation and animosity in the early days of multispecialty management of acoustic tumor patients. Historically, acoustic neuroma surgery was the sole province of neurosurgeons. Through the pioneering efforts and perseverance of William House (an otologist) and William Hitselberger (a neurosurgeon), otolaryngology and neurosurgery collaborative management of acoustic tumor patients is generally accepted, although the nature of the collaboration varies from institution to institution (11). The expertise of the two specialties lends itself to a synergistic benefit for patients with acoustic neuroma. The neuro-otologists' background with measurements of auditory and vestibular function, management of hearing loss and middle ear conditions, as well as surgical manipulation of the temporal bone from every approach is critical. Similarly, the neurosurgeon deals with the central nervous system (CNS) effects of intracranial tumors regularly in addition to management of cerebrovascular pathology, brainstem compression, cerebrospinal fluid (CSF) shunting, and seizure issues. The training of both specialties allows substantial overlap so that either specialist can manage patients with acoustic neuromas independently, although collaboration allows these two specialties' expertise to benefit the patient, particularly in hearing preservation cases.

Maximum temporal bone exposure of the internal auditory canal (IAC) without violating the labyrinth is a necessary first step to accomplish the first goal of tumor surgery—total tumor removal. Similarly, appropriate and gentle use of retraction is required for adequate exposure to accomplish tumor removal in addition to facial nerve and cochlear nerve preservation.

In general, the neuro-otologist and neurosurgeon should work on these procedures as co-surgeons. Each specialist must have an intimate familiarity with the other's expertise to the point of being able to perform the other's usual role. In this manner, a true collaboration can develop. Interestingly, even within our own institution, roles of the different specialists vary depending on who the constituent members of the team are for that particular case. Collaboration is a dynamic process that evolves and improves with time.

SURGICAL TECHNIQUE

Middle Fossa (MF)

Middle fossa acoustic neuroma surgery is offered to patients with useful hearing and intracanalicular acoustic tumors with up to 0.5 cm extension into the cerebellopontine angle (CPA). The definition of useful hearing is subject to debate and interpretation. In general, we would recommend the approach for patients with speech reception threshold (SRT) at 30 dB and 70% speech discrimination (SD), and offer it as an option for patients with 50-dB SRT and 50% SD. However, multiple factors are involved (4). The principal criterion is how useful the patient finds his/her hearing. This is often based on the status of the contralateral ear. In general, greater than a 30-dB difference in SRT between the two ears is a significant impediment to normal binaural hearing. Nonetheless, some patients with hearing even poorer than the standard described above still are interested in hearing preservation. In addition, because of the increased fragility of the dura, we avoid middle fossa surgery in patients over 70 years of age.

In borderline cases, electrophysiologic data provide useful information for patient selection for hearing preservation approaches. Auditory brainstem response (ABR) waveform morphology that remains robust despite interaural latency delays is a positive prognostic factor. In contrast, we have not found presence or absence of caloric weakness on electronystagmogram (ENG) a useful prognostic factor for hearing preservation. Although there is a small possibility of hearing improvement after tumor removal, we generally counsel patients to expect their current level of hearing as the best possible outcome following acoustic tumor surgery.

Prior to surgery, a coronal thin-cut computed tomography (CT) scan is useful for identifying middle fossa landmarks and the extent of pneumatization of the petrous bone above the IAC.

Prior to induction, the patient is administered 10 mg of Decadron IV and 1 g of cefazolin. In addition, mannitol 0.5 to 1 g/kg is administered as well as furosemide (Lasix) (20 mg) during the initial craniotomy opening. The patient is positioned supine on the operating table with the head turned with the operative side upward. We generally use head pins with the Mayfield head holder (Ohio Medical Instrument Co., Cincinnati, OH) to facilitate positioning of our preferred retractor system. However, the patient can be placed directly on the table, and the retractors can be anchored to the brace alongside the table (which is often used for anchoring ear speculum holders and other instruments). Following general anesthesia, EMG electrodes are placed for continuous facial nerve monitoring. In addition, the ground electrodes for ABR monitoring are placed. Finally, the foam microphone is placed in the ear canal and the ear is draped with adhesive plastic drapes to secure the earphone in the ear and prevent moisture from entering the electrode. Shaving and preparation is performed by shaving a vertical strip extending from the preauricular region toward the vertex approximately 3 cm wide. The hair is held back with stapled, plastic adhesive drapes. The preauricular region is treated with 1% lidocaine with epinephrine (1:100,000) and the ear is prepared with povidone-iodine skin solution. The abdomen is also prepared and draped for a small abdominal fat graft (Fig. 12-1).

A vertical preauricular incision is made extending approximately 6 cm superior to the pinna. The temporalis muscle is split longitudinally and retracted with blunt skin hooks (Elekta Instruments, Atlanta, GA). The temporal squama is exposed and a temporal craniotomy is fashioned with high-speed drill or a footplate attachment. The craniotomy flap is centered over the root of the zygoma approximately 5 × 5 cm. Following removal of the craniotomy flap, rongeurs and drills are used to bring the inferior extent of the craniotomy down to the floor of the middle fossa to avoid any overhanging bone. Dural elevation then proceeds from a posterior to anterior direction. The preoperative CT scan at this point is useful to identify the position of the arcuate eminence and the position of the superior semicircular canal. The proximity of the arcuate eminence and the superior canal varies from patient to patient. The preoperative scan allows aggressive removal of supralabyrinthine air cells without concern of fenestrating the otic capsule. The posterior to anterior direction of dural elevation prevents inadvertent damage to the greater superficial petrosal nerve (GSPN) and geniculate ganglion. We have found antidromic stimulation of the GSPN useful for confirming its position to facilitate identification of landmarks on the floor of the middle fossa.

Following identification of the GSPN, attention is focused more anteriorly to the region of the foramen spinosum (12). Troublesome bleeding in this region is controlled with bipolar cautery and absorbable packing. To minimize the retraction force on the dura, the middle meningeal artery may be cauterized and transected. At this point, the dural elevation is continued further medially in a posterior to anterior direction with the limit being the true petrous ridge. If force is necessary to keep the dura retracted to expose the petrous ridge, then additional anterior dural elevation is accomplished by identifying V3 at the foramen ovale and elevating the dura propria from the gasserian ganglion by sharply dividing the connective tissue bands (13). It should be noted that this region represents the posterior lateral limit of the cavernous sinus. Occasionally bridging veins from the temporal lobe can extend directly to the cavernous sinus across the posterolateral surface of the cavernous sinus. Troublesome oozing from this region is controlled with judicious bipolar cautery and small pledgettes of Surgicel.

Once the petrous ridge is clearly identified, just posterior to the arcuate eminence and anteriorly to approximately the level of the facial hiatus, the retractors can be placed. We have found the single-blade rigid middle fossa retractor systems (such as House-Urban) troublesome because the posterior aspect of the blade can interfere with instrumentation and visualization (Fig. 12-2). Our preferred retractor system utilizes two adjustable, multijointed, "snake" retractors (Fukushima System, Elekta Instruments), which are anchored to the Mayfield headrest or the side rail of the operative table by a multidirectional C-clamp. This clamp permits positioning of the retractors from any direction. Thin-blade, malleable, spatula dural retractors are connected to the multijointed arms for precise positioning. This system does not provide the same force of retraction provided by the rigid single-blade retractors. Accordingly, additional dural eleva-

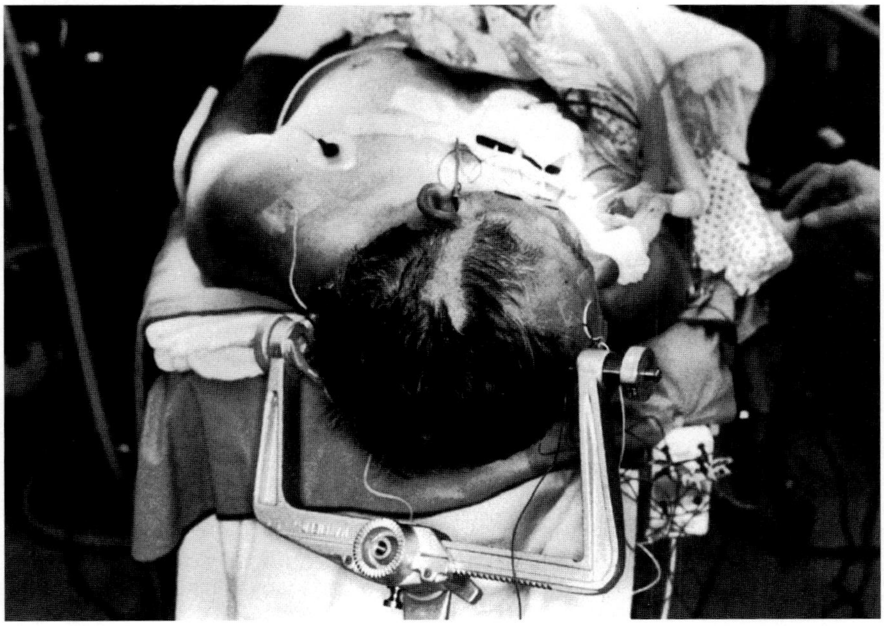

FIG. 12-1. Patient prepared for middle fossa acoustic neuroma surgery. The operative ear is upward with the patient supine on the table. A minimal hair shave permits adequate incisional exposure. Head pins may be utilized as illustrated; however, depending on the surgeon's preference, the patient's head may rest on the table itself. Facial nerve monitoring and auditory brainstem response (ABR) electrodes are in place.

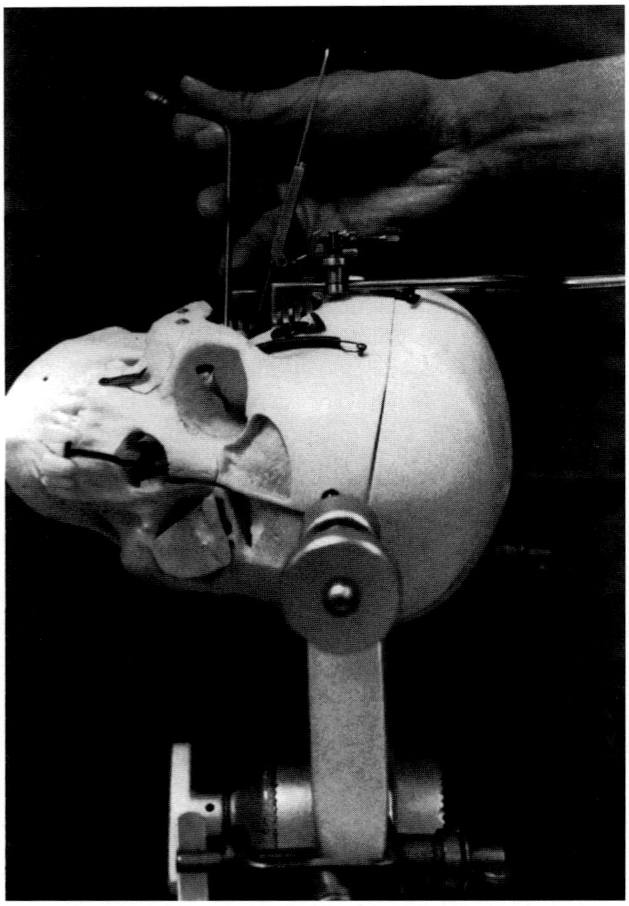

FIG. 12-2. House-Urban middle fossa retractor positioned on a dry cadaver skull. The posterior aspect of the retractor blade can interfere with visualization and instrumentation in the operative field.

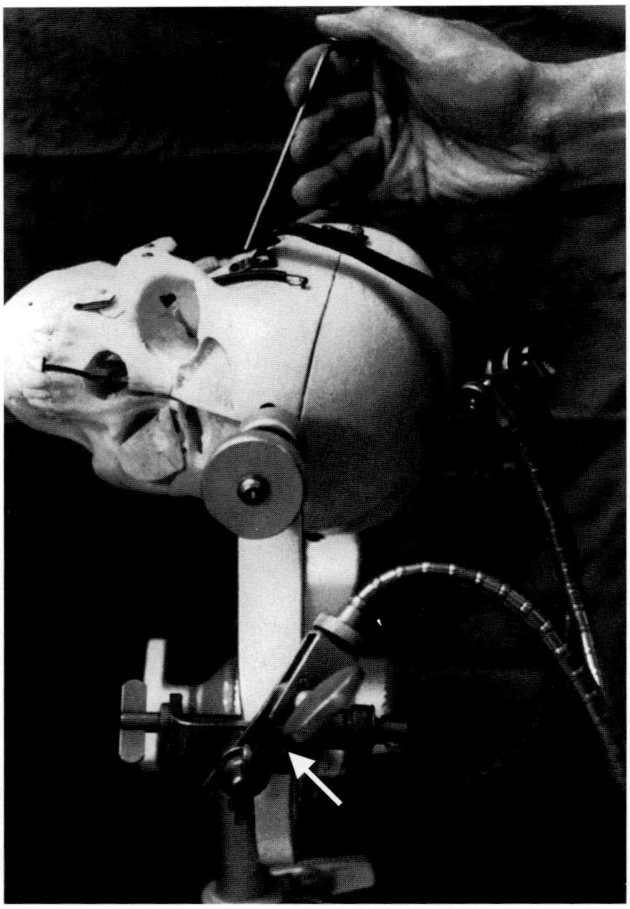

FIG. 12-3. Fukushima retractor system positioned on a dry cadaver skull. The spatula blades may be contoured to a low profile to enhance visualization and instrumentation. The C-clamp (*arrow*) permits use of the retractor system on the head pins or operative table brace.

tion is necessary for their successful use. However, we feel this is an advantage as less force is being placed on the temporal lobe. In addition, as these retractors are adjustable and the blade itself is malleable, it can be contoured to a low profile to prevent interference with visualization and instrumentation through the incision (Fig. 12-3). The tip of the retractor blade is braced on the petrous ridge, which prevents movement of the retractor and exposure during the drilling or tumor removal. Generally, we use two of the malleable retractors to allow adequate exposure of the drilling area (Fig. 12-4).

Our preferred technique for surgical exposure of the IAC is medially near the porous acousticus. Drilling begins along an imaginary line that bisects the angle formed by the GSPN and the arcuate eminence. However, by drilling medially, the surgeon is a safe distance away from the cochlea and superior canal prior to definitive identification of the dura of the porus acousticus. Once the dura of the porous acousticus is defined, the IAC is skeletonized 270 degrees medially. Alternative techniques to identify the IAC include retrograde exposure from the GSPN to the geniculate ganglion, to the labryrinthine segment of the facial nerve, and to the

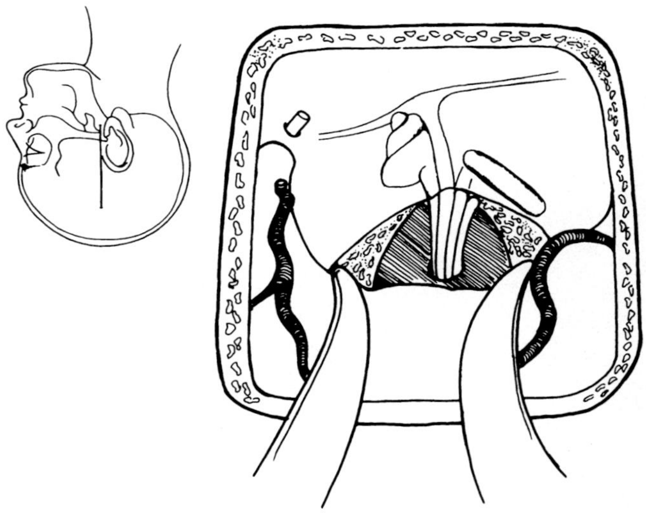

FIG. 12-4. Right middle fossa exposure illustrating transected middle meningeal artery with two spatula retractors braced between the petrous ridge and the temporal lobe. Complete exposure of the internal auditory canal (IAC) fundus is accomplished by following the labyrinthine segment of the facial nerve to the geniculate ganglion.

IAC as originally described by House (13). Another alternative exposure of the IAC described by Ugo Fisch first exposes the blue line of the superior semicircular canal. A 60-degree angle anterior to this blue line defines a safe drilling area for the IAC termed the *meatal plane.* Extensive exposure is necessary anteriorly near the petrous apex as well as posteriorly medial to the level of the superior canal to allow for adequate tumor manipulation and exposure of the more lateral contents. Once the IAC dura is completely exposed, the dura is opened along the posterior aspect of the IAC as the facial nerve lies anteriorly. The dural flap is reflected forward. The first step in tumor dissection is to separate the facial nerve from the tumor. The facial nerve is just under the anterior aspect of the IAC dura. The tumor adhesions are divided sharply under high magnification. The tumor can then be dissected in a medial to lateral direction. A series of micropicks and curettes are useful for internal tumor debulking and assure tumor removal from beneath any bone ledges. Minimal bipolar cautery is used to avoid damage to the blood supply to the cochlear nerve. A particularly useful technique has been the positioning of thin cottonoids to protect the nerve when cautery is necessary within the IAC. While auditory brainstem response is monitored throughout the procedure, we have recently begun utilizing direct 8th nerve monitoring with small, flat, plate metal electrodes (Adtech Medical, Racine, WI) on the 8th nerve, which gives more immediate feedback because fewer repetitions are necessary with this near-field technique. However, we are not yet convinced that this has truly affected our hearing outcomes. Nonetheless, as experience is gained with this technique, intraoperative management of the cochlear nerve and its blood supply may be enhanced.

Once tumor removal is complete, abdominal fat is placed within the IAC. The craniotomy flap is repositioned and may be secured with microplates, and the wound closed in layers.

Retrosigmoid Approach (RS)

The retrosigmoid approach is offered to patients with useful hearing and tumors that extend beyond the IAC into the CPA over 0.5 cm from the porous acoustics. Our guidelines for useful hearing are the same with the retrosigmoid approach as with the middle fossa approach. We encourage hearing preservation in patients with 30-dB SRT, 70% speech understanding, and a subjective sense of useful hearing in that ear. Patients with less acute hearing, up to 50-dB SRT and 50% speech discrimination, are offered but not encouraged to undergo hearing preservation acoustic neuroma surgery (4).

The principal advantage of the retrosigmoid approach for hearing preservation is wide posterior fossa exposure with access to the IAC while still preserving the otic capsule (14). The principal limitation is that the fundus of the IAC usually cannot be exposed with the RS approach without violating the labyrinth. Although the RS approach may be performed in a supine head turned position, we find the ipsilateral shoulder can obstruct visualization and placement of surgical instruments. In those situations we prefer positioning for the RS approach in the modified park bench position—to rotate the shoulder away from the path of visualization and instrument placement. The head is secured with pins in the Mayfield head holder.

A wide area of hair above and behind the pinna (6 cm) is shaved. In addition to EMG facial muscle electrodes, an ABR foam ear canal insert is placed and the pinna is sealed with an occlusive plastic dressing. The ipsilateral lower quadrant of the abdomen is also prepared with sterile drapes. Following a postauricular incision, a separate myofascial flap is incised in a staggered fashion from the skin incision. The mastoid cortex and suboccipute are exposed. A mastoidectomy is performed for complete skeletonization of the sigmoid sinus. Next, a retrosigmoid craniotomy is accomplished, extending from the transverse sinus superiorly to the most inferior extent of the sigmoid sinus inferiorly. This posterior craniotomy flap is approximately 3.5 × 3.5 cm. Bone is removed completely from the sigmoid sinus and transverse junction with a diamond burr. This exposure will allow maximum rotation of the retrosigmoid dura anteriorly and minimize the need for cerebellar retraction. Inferiorly toward the area of the foramen magnum, rongeurs are helpful to assure complete bone removal.

The retrosigmoid dura is incised as an anteriorly based C-shaped flap beginning inferiorly. The inferior dura is opened for approximately 1.5 cm to permit placement of small cottonoids and allow drainage of CSF from the foramen magnum and CPA cistern. This fluid drainage is critical to minimize the need for cerebellar retraction. If this drainage is not accomplished, the CSF pulsations will herniate the cerebellum through the dural opening. Once this drainage has been accomplished, the remainder of this C-shaped dural incision is accomplished, extending anteriorly up to the sigmoid transverse junction. The dura is held forward with multiple 4-0 braided nylon sutures. Multiple sutures are placed through the dural flap to maximize exposure. In this fashion, the sigmoid sinus itself is held forward from its usual position to facilitate full visualization of the posterior aspect of the petrous bone (Fig. 12-5).

The initial step in tumor removal is placement of microthin cottonoids around the tumor capsule. Arteries and veins adherent to but not penetrating the capsule are carefully separated. Facial nerve stimulation along the posterior aspect of the tumor rules out an unusual positioning of the facial nerve. Debulking begins by sharp incision into the tumor on the posterior aspect and a combination of scissors, bipolar cautery, and CUSA (Cavitron ultrasonic surgical aspirator), or rotary suction dissection device. In general, the lower pole is dissected first, assuring that the lower cranial nerves are freed from the tumor and the intracapsular debulking is accomplished. Next, the superior pole is dissected, with specific attention to free the tumor from adhesions to the trigeminal nerve. At this point, the tumor is rolled anteriorly. The cochlear nerve is identified extending usually along the infe-

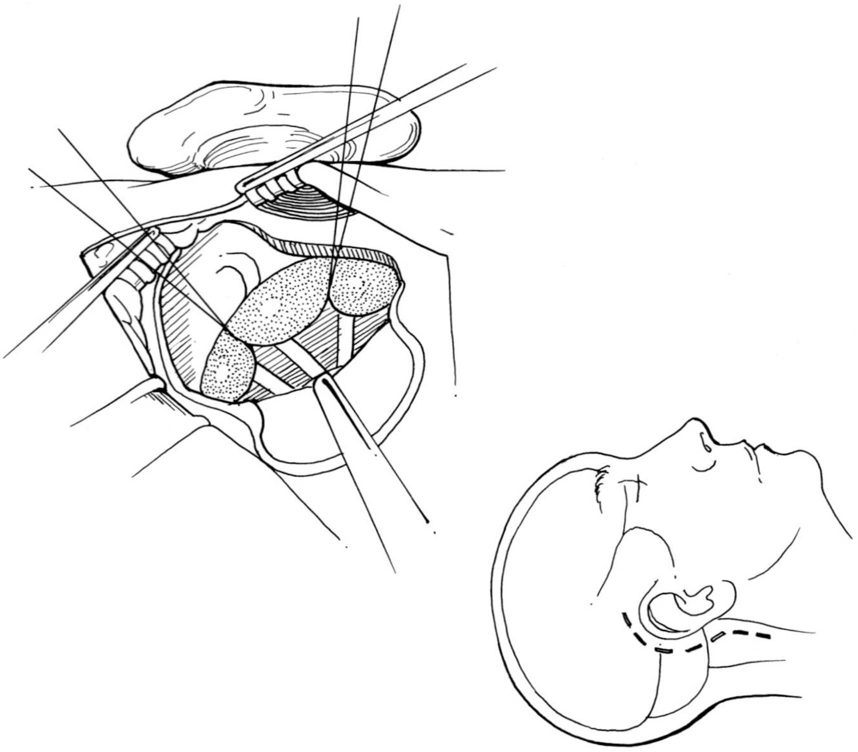

FIG. 12-5. Retrosigmoid dural opening. Mastoid exposure allows complete decompression of the sigmoid sinus, which facilitates anterior retraction with the retrosigmoid sutures. Anterior dural retraction sutures and cerebrospinal fluid release from the foramen magnum cistern minimize the need for cerebellar retraction in this approach. The endolymphatic duct represents the lateral limit for safe retrosigmoid drilling of the IAC.

rior aspect of the tumor. In our experience, the intraoperative finding of a distinct cochlear nerve is a good prognosis for postoperative hearing. However, significant attenuation of those nerve fibers usually results in serious postoperative hearing loss. Once the tumor is adequately debulked, dissection of the IAC can be accomplished.

The first step in the dissection of the bone of the posterior aspect of the IAC is to remove the dura from the posterior face of the petrous bone overlying the IAC. In general, a safe dissection can usually be accomplished up to 7 mm laterally from the porous acoustics medially. However, a patient-specific landmark is the position of the endolymphatic sac and duct. Bone exposure can be safely accomplished medial to that level (Fig. 12-6). Drilling lateral to this landmark risks injury to the overlying posterior semicircular canal and vestibule. The bone is removed under magnification with continuous suction irrigation and high power diamond and rough diamond drills. Gelfoam (Johnson & Johnson, Kalamazoo, MI) is placed surrounding the IAC and adjacent CPA to prevent dispersion of bone dust into the posterior fossa and subarachnoid space. There is some evidence that suggests that this is the cause of postoperative headaches in acoustic neuroma surgery (15). Cottonoids should not be used adjacent to an area being drilled because the fibers can become attached to the spinning drill, converting the cottonoid into a spinning blade with a wide swathe that can damage the adjacent brain, nerves, and blood vessels.

Particular care is necessary in exposing the inferior aspect of the IAC as a high riding jugular bulb can be adjacent to the IAC. Inadvertent injury of the bulb is controlled with Surgicel and Gelfoam. Packing of an injured jugular bulb must be performed carefully to prevent embolization of packing material to the lung. The authors prefer to place the hemostatic material on the surface of the injured jugular bulb and cover the area with bone wax to permit continued drilling adjacent to the area. Drilling begins medially at the porus acoustics. The dura of the IAC is identified and followed from medial to lateral. Superior and inferior troughs parallel to the IAC provide space for tumor manipulation during microsurgical tumor dissection (16). The lateral limit of IAC drilling if hearing preservation is attempted is the endolymphatic duct. However, if this limitation does not permit full exposure of the tumor, complete exposure of the IAC regardless of the effect on hearing should be accomplished if complete tumor removal cannot be accomplished otherwise.

Once the IAC is exposed to the apex of the tumor, dissection can proceed in a medial to lateral direction, identifying the facial nerve at the brainstem, anterior and superior to the position of the eighth nerve. The cochlear nerve and seventh nerve are followed in a medial to lateral direction. Care is necessary to continue to debulk large remnants of tumor before trying to excise the remaining tumor and capsule as a single block. We have found microcurettes (Elekta Instruments) helpful for tumor debulking especially when small portions of the tumor are adherent to the capsule. Our objective is to thin the capsule as much as possible prior to dissecting the capsule from the brainstem and the cranial nerves. Traction and potential injury of the acoustic and facial nerves are minimized by debulking as much as possible

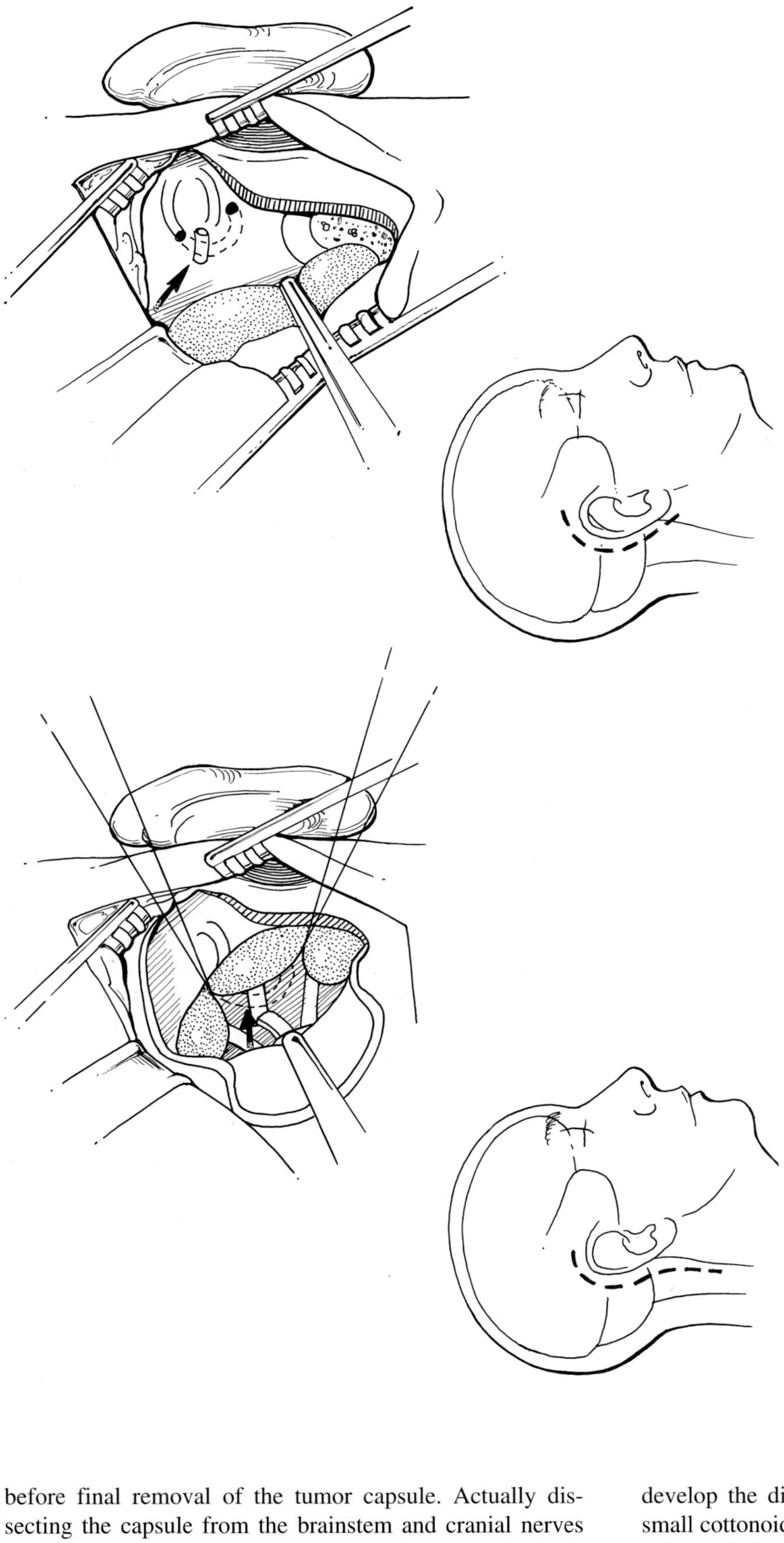

FIG. 12-6. Top: Full mastoidectomy permits identification of the semicircular canals, occlusion of the membranous labyrinth, and resection of the posterior semicircular canal. Dotted line indicates previous position of posterior semicircular canal prior to plugging the lumen (*black dots*) and resection. Without the intervening labyrinth, the IAC can be skeletonized in the presigmoid exposure. **Bottom:** Retrosigmoid exposure after controlled posterior semicircular canal resection permits hearing preservation exposure of the lateral IAC. Dotted line indicates the position previously occupied by the posterior semicircular canal. Identification of the IAC before retrosigmoid dural opening permits exposure of the lateral IAC and hearing preseveration.

before final removal of the tumor capsule. Actually dissecting the capsule from the brainstem and cranial nerves is accomplished under high-power magnification with both sharp and blunt dissection. Using the suction to keep the capsule on stretch, thin-blade microscissors are useful to develop the dissection plane. If this plane is not distinct, small cottonoids are useful to help develop the dissection in a blunt fashion. If the nerves have already been partially dissected, we often find cottonoids placed behind the nerves as useful dissection aids by providing a firmer base upon which to dissect without having to place excessive traction on the nerves that are entering the cochlear modiolus and fallopian canal. Sharp, flat microdissectors are also useful for removal of small capsular adhesions to the facial and cochlear nerves.

Once the cranial nerves have been partially dissected, they are particularly vulnerable to cautery injury. If bleeding occurs adjacent to the facial or cochlear nerves, we avoid cautery and use hemostatic material such as Surgicel and Gelfoam with light pressure and suction over a cottonoid. If this is not successful, the nerves are protected with small cottonoids, and bipolar cautery of the bleeding vessel is performed with fine-tipped bayonet forceps and current applied in short bursts.

The suction instrumentation is also important in these hearing preservation cases. Although we generally find the fenestrated (Brackmann) suctions useful to suction adjacent to a nerve without damaging the nerve, the fenestrations limit the usefulness of the suction for holding the tumor and capsule with countertraction for dissection. In posterior fossa dissection we utilize suction instruments with a tear-drop shaped suction hole (Ruggles, Elekta Instruments). This design permits the surgeon to adjust the intensity of suction from minimal to strong with movement of the thumb over the teardrop-shaped opening. This device permits delicate use of the suction adjacent to cranial nerves and more aggressive use of the suction as a tumor holder with countertraction.

Once tumor removal is complete, a systematic inspection for exposed air cells is undertaken to place bone wax to prevent CSF leakage. Abdominal fat is secured in the IAC and the mastoid. The craniotomy flap is secured and the wound is closed in layers.

SURGICAL OUTCOMES AND POTENTIAL PITFALLS

An important obstacle to comparing the outcomes of hearing preservation acoustic neuroma surgery techniques is the method of reporting results. Various criteria for success have been used for reporting results. The American Academy of Otolaryngology–Head and Neck Surgery (AAO-HNS) has recently developed a staging system for reporting hearing outcomes in acoustic neuroma surgery. This method will be useful for comparing results of groups of patients. However, the success for an individual patient depends on many factors. Saving any hearing in a patient with neurofibromatosis II or an only-hearing ear is a success. In contrast, saving only sound recognition without speech discrimination in one ear with a normal contralateral ear is of marginal benefit.

We recently reported a retrospective series of 330 consecutive acoustic neuroma surgeries performed between 1989 and 1996 (4). During this interval 60 of the 330 surgeries were hearing preservation attempts (34 middle fossa and 26 retrosigmoid).

Measurable postoperative hearing was present in 77% of cases (middle fossa 85% and retrosigmoid 65%). Table 12-1 lists hearing results according to the classification of the AAO-HNS. Useful hearing (class A, B, or C) was preserved in 67% (middle fossa 74%, retrosigmoid 58%). The difference in hearing preservation between middle fossa and retrosigmoid cases was not statistically significant despite significantly smaller mean tumor diameter for the middle fossa cases (0.72 ± 0.34 cm) versus the retrosigmoid cases (1.66 ± 0.76 cm).

The authors feel that surgical approaches for hearing preservation acoustic neuroma surgery should be individualized to patient and tumor characteristics. In general, the effectiveness of hearing preservation surgery has been related to tumor size. Interestingly, in our series there was not a statistically different rate of hearing preservation for middle fossa and retrosigmoid surgery despite a significant difference in tumor diameter for lesions operated by those approaches. We feel that this comparable success despite tumor diameter difference supports the contention that individualizing the hearing preservation surgical approach is helpful for improving the rates of successful hearing preservation in acoustic neuroma surgery.

Overall, there were few complications in this series. There was one case of bacterial meningitis (2%) and four cases of CSF leakage requiring reoperation (7%). Postoperative facial function at the last postoperative visit was excellent with 90% grade I and II (House-Brackmann scale).

Does hearing preservation acoustic neuroma surgery pose a greater risk to the facial nerve? Intuitively it would appear that the translabyrinthine approach has an advantage in facial nerve preservation because the nerve can be identified laterally (at Bill's bar) and medially (at the CPA) (17). For the middle fossa approach, a specific comparison study for similar size tumors did not reveal a difference in facial nerve preservation and function when middle fossa cases were compared with translabyrinthine cases (18). Similarly, for retrosigmoid surgery, there is no evidence of poorer facial nerve outcomes than for the translabyrinthine approach (19). The widespread applications of continuous facial nerve monitoring is the most likely explanation for comparable facial nerve outcomes in translabyrinthine surgery and hearing preservation surgery (20). While some authors feel that comparable facial nerve rates justify attempts at hearing preservation regardless of tumor size and preoperative hearing, we generally offer hearing preservation to patients with serviceable hearing and CPA tumor of 2 cm or less. We feel results of hearing preservation should include full audiometric data including speech discrimination or categorization according to the AAO-HNS method (21). Nonetheless, patients' wishes should be respected. Our team has on occasion preserved hearing in patients with CPA tumor diameters of 4.0 cm and 3.5 cm who insisted on attempts at hearing preservation (Table 12-1) (14). Usually, however, hearing cannot be preserved in tumors of that size.

Often patients who are suitable candidates for hearing preservation surgery elect translabyrinthine surgery when they realize that hearing improvement is very unlikely. Pa-

TABLE 12–1. *Consecutive hearing preservation cases*

Case no.	Year of surgery	Surgical approach	Maximum tumor diameter (cm)	Preoperative Classification[a]	Preoperative SRT	Preoperative SDS	Postoperative Classification[a]	Postoperative SRT	Postoperative SDS	Facial nerve grade[b]
1	1989	Retrosigmoid	1.5	B	46	62	D	NR	NR	1
2	1990	Retrosigmoid	1.5	A	10	100	D	45	76	1
3	1991	Retrosigmoid	1	A	10	100	D	NR	NR	1
4	1991	Retrosigmoid	2	B	35	75	D	NR	NR	1
5	1992	Retrosigmoid	0.6	A	0	100	D	NR	NR	1
6	1992	Retrosigmoid	1	B	45	72	B	45	80	1
7	1992	Retrosigmoid	1	A	20	96	A	20	88	1
8	1992	Retrosigmoid	1	A	30	76	D	NR	NR	1
9	1993	Retrosigmoid	2	C	65	52	D	NR	NR	1
10	1994	Retrosigmoid	1.5	B	50	76	C	60	64	1
11	1994	Retrosigmoid	1.5	A	30	64	D	NR	NR	1
12	1994	Retrosigmoid	1.5	C	60	80	B	50	60	1
13	1994	Retrosigmoid	1.5	A	30	88	B	45	80	1
14	1994	Retrosigmoid	2.5	B	35	84	A	50	68	1
15	1994	Retrosigmoid	3.5	D	45	28	D	65	4	1
16	1995	Retrosigmoid	1	A	20	100	A	30	96	1
17	1995	Retrosigmoid	1.5	A	5	96	A	0	100	1
18	1995	Retrosigmoid	1.5	B	35	68	A	30	92	1
19	1995	Retrosigmoid	1.5	A	30	84	B	45	80	1
20	1995	Retrosigmoid	2	A	20	100	A	30	92	1
21	1995	Retrosigmoid	2.5	C	30	52	D	NR	NR	4
22	1996	Retrosigmoid	1	A	20	88	A	25	84	1
23	1996	Retrosigmoid	1	B	45	68	D	NR	NR	1
24	1996	Retrosigmoid	1.5	A	25	80	B	40	88	1
25	1996	Retrosigmoid	2	B	30	60	D	85	NR	5
26	1996	Retrosigmoid	4	A	0	100	A	10	100	1
27	1989	Middle fossa	1	A	10	100	A	25	80	3
28	1989	Middle fossa	1	D	25	40	A	25	72	1
29	1990	Middle fossa	1	A	20	100	D	65	NR	3
30	1991	Middle fossa	0.5	A	20	92	A	15	92	1
31	1991	Middle fossa	0.5	A	28	96	B	45	84	1
32	1991	Middle fossa	0.5	A	10	100	A	10	100	2
33	1992	Middle fossa	0.5	A	20	100	A	30	100	1
34	1992	Middle fossa	0.5	B	41	76	B	40	72	1
35	1992	Middle fossa	0.5	A	10	96	D	NR	NR	1
36	1992	Middle fossa	1	A	30	80	A	16	80	3
37	1993	Middle fossa	0.4	B	40	96	B	48	100	1
38	1993	Middle fossa	0.4	B	35	96	B	40	96	1
39	1993	Middle fossa	0.5	B	35	60	D	NR	NR	4
40	1993	Middle fossa	1.5	A	25	72	A	20	100	1
41	1994	Middle fossa	0.3	A	10	96	A	20	100	1
42	1994	Middle fossa	0.4	A	5	100	A	12	100	1
43	1994	Middle fossa	0.4	A	15	84	B	35	100	1
44	1994	Middle fossa	0.5	A	20	86	D	NR	NR	1
45	1994	Middle fossa	0.5	A	10	100	A	30	80	1
46	1994	Middle fossa	0.6	B	30	68	B	50	84	1
47	1994	Middle fossa	1.4	A	10	100	A	30	92	1
48	1995	Middle fossa	0.3	A	10	92	D	55	24	4
49	1995	Middle fossa	0.4	C	50	64	C	50	60	1
50	1995	Middle fossa	0.4	A	5	96	A	10	96	1
51	1995	Middle fossa	0.4	A	10	96	D	NR	NR	1
52	1995	Middle fossa	0.8	A	10	100	D	85	NR	1
53	1995	Middle fossa	1	D	25	44	C	60	60	1
54	1995	Middle fossa	1	B	35	80	B	40	80	1
55	1995	Middle fossa	1	B	50	36	B	40	60	1
56	1995	Middle fossa	1	A	15	96	A	25	96	1
57	1995	Middle fossa	1	A	15	100	A	20	100	1
58	1995	Middle fossa	1.5	A	25	88	D	NR	NR	1
59	1996	Middle fossa	0.5	C	50	60	D	60	44	2
60	1996	Middle fossa	1	A	0	96	A	20	92	1

[a] American Academy of Otolaryngology hearing classification.
[b] Long-term House-Brackmann facial nerve grade.
SDS, speech discrimination score; SRT, speech reception threshold; NR, no response.

tients are counseled that their preoperative hearing level is the best they can hope for postoperatively. However, our recent experience demonstrates a small chance of postoperative hearing improvement (8 of 60 patients in our series had 10-dB improved SRT or 10-dB improved speech discrimination).

A nagging concern with the popularity of hearing preservation surgery is the possibility of tumor recurrence. Neely's (22) study of en bloc acoustic tumor resection demonstrated histopathologic evidence of cochlear nerve involvement by acoustic neuromas. So, despite the surgical report of total tumor removal, microscopic foci of tumor may remain. Thus far, this theoretical concern has not translated into a higher incidence of recurrent tumors in hearing preservation surgery. A formal evaluation of the recurrence rate in hearing preservation surgery is needed to answer this question.

EXPERIMENTAL APPROACHES

Investigation of new approaches for hearing preservation acoustic neuroma surgery is proceeding. Historically, through experiences with fenestration procedures for otosclerosis, otologists have recognized that opening of the semicircular canals can be a routine component of hearing preservation procedures. In the modern era, posterior semicircular canal occlusion procedures are performed for recalcitrant positional vertigo with high rates of hearing preservation (23). These experiences prompted McElveen et al. (24) to report a modification of the translabyrinthine procedure with sealing of the vestibule after removing the semicircular canals with successful hearing preservation. Similarly, we have recently reported a modification of the retrosigmoid procedure with planned systematic opening and sealing of the posterior semicircular canal prior to retrosigmoid exposure of the lateral extent of the IAC (Fig. 12-6) (25). These procedures are encouraging developments for operations that in the future may combine the benefits of translabyrinthine surgery with the opportunity for hearing preservation.

MANAGEMENT OF COMPLICATIONS

As in all of skull base surgery, the ideal management of complications is avoiding having them. The principal complications requiring distinct management procedures are facial nerve paralysis, CSF leakage, and meningitis (see Chapter 8).

A crucial step in dealing with complications is patient education. We provide our patients with a detailed form listing the complications prior to the surgery. In addition to the medicolegal relevance, this allows the patients and family to know the possible difficulties associated with the surgery.

Facial Nerve

Injury or transection of the facial nerve is best managed intraoperatively. Facial nerve transection is ideally managed with end-to-end anastomosis (26). In middle fossa surgery, the injury occurs in the IAC, and facial nerve rerouting will not provide additional length. In those cases, an interposition graft can be placed. The minimal number of sutures necessary for reapposition are placed (usually two or three separate 9-0 or 10-0 monofilament sutures). In retrosigmoid cases the injury is usually at the level of the porus acoustics or CPA. Repair at the CPA or brainstem level is more difficult since the nerve does not have a distinct epineural layer and the suture can pull through easily. In addition, the CSF pulsations produce significant motion in the nerve endings. Although our preferred repair is suture anastomosis, apposition of the nerve ends with Surgicel or similar absorbable, hemostatic collagen material has comparable success rates. Again, CPA repair usually requires an interposition graft that can be harvested from the greater auricle nerve or sural nerve. If direct repair is not possible, then nerve substitution procedure such as the facial hypoglossal anastomosis procedure is employed. We prefer to perform nerve substitution procedures at a separate time after recovery from the CPA tumor procedure. Physiologically the best functional outcome following facial nerve grafting is a House-Brackmann grade III/VI. This is because synkinesis will inevitably occur as axons growing through the interposed segment will not all grow into the corresponding motor end plates for that cell body.

Cerebrospinal Fluid Leak

Avoidance again is the preferred management of this complication. In middle fossa surgery, air cells to the mastoid and middle ear can be waxed and occluded with fat, fascia, or muscle. The IAC is packed with abdominal fat or temporalis muscle. If leakage develops, lumbar drainage of spinal fluid is usually sufficient (27). In rare cases where the leakage persists and hearing has been preserved, the eustachian tube can be occluded through a transmastoid, facial recess route. In retrosigmoid surgery, the same conservative measures are employed as in middle fossa surgery. A watertight dural closure is attempted in these cases, and fat is placed in the mastoid as well as over the dural closure. In cases of leakage, a pressure dressing may be placed to help tamponade the leakage in addition to use of a lumbar drain. In rare cases where this does not succeed, the wound can be reexplored and the offending air cell sealed. Simple resuturing of the wound with locking sutures is an option if leakage occurs through the incision itself.

CONCLUSION

Hearing preservation in acoustic neuroma surgery is becoming a realistic possibility for patients due to improved diagnostic and surgical techniques. The fundamental priorities of the acoustic neuroma surgery—safe total tumor removal and facial function preservation—must be kept in mind. However, for patients who are good audiometric and medical candidates, hearing preservation is a worthwhile goal if surgical approaches are individualized to patient- and tumor-specific issues. We feel that patient outcomes are maximized when hearing preservation acoustic neuroma surgery is performed as a collaboration between otolaryngology and neurosurgery.

REFERENCES

1. Arriaga M, Brackmann D. Surgical approaches for posterior fossa skull base neoplasm. In: Cummings CW, Fredrickson C, Krause C, et al., eds. *Otolaryngol head and neck surgery,* 2nd ed. St. Louis: Mosby, 1992:3338–3352.
2. Friedman RA, House JW. Facial nerve result. In: House WF, Luetje CM, Doyle KJ, eds. *Acoustic tumors, diagnosis and management.* San Diego: Singular, 1997:255.
3. House WF. Preface. In: House WF, Luetje CM, Doyle KJ, eds. *Acoustic tumors, diagnosis and management.* San Diego: Singular, 1997:xi.
4. Arriaga MA, Chen DA, Fukushima T. Individualizing hearing preservation in acoustic neuroma surgery. *Laryngoscope* 1997;107: 1043–1047.
5. Cushing H. *Tumors of the nervous acousticus and the syndrome of cerebellopontine angle,* 2nd ed. New York: Hafner, 1917. (Reprinted 1967 by WB Saunders, Philadelphia.)
6. House WF. A history of acoustic tumor surgery: 1800–1961. In: House WF, Luetje CM, Doyle KJ, eds. *Acoustic tumors, diagnosis and management.* San Diego: Singular, 1997:11.
7. Shelton C, Brackmann D, House WF, et al. Middle fossa acoustic tumor surgery: results in 106 cases. *Laryngoscope* 1989;99(4):405–408.
8. Arriaga M. Anatomy of transtemporal surgery. In: Janecka IP, Tiedemann K, eds. *Skull base: anatomy, biology, and technology.* New York: Lippincott-Raven, 1997.
9. Wiegand DA, Ogemann RG, Fickel V. Surgical treatment of acoustic neuroma (vestibular schwannoma) in the United States: a report from the acoustic neuroma registry. *Laryngoscope* 1996;106(1 pt 1):58–66.
10. Yu KCY, Arriaga MA, Chen DA. Cerebellopontine angle tumor outcomes in patients with hazardous occupations. *Laryngoscope* 1997; 107:1610–1613.
11. Glasscock MF, Bohrer PS, Steenerson RL. A history of acoustic tumor surgery: 1961–present. In: House WF, Luetje CM, Doyle KJ, eds. *Acoustic tumors, diagnosis and management.* San Diego: Singular, 1997:23.
12. Arriaga MA, Haid RM, Massel DM. Antidromic stimulation of the greater superficial petrosal nerve (GSPN) in middle fossa surgery. *Laryngoscope* 1995;105(1):102–105.
13. Chen DA, Arriaga MA, Fukushima T. Technical refinements in retraction for middle fossa surgery. *Am J Otol* 1998;19:208–211.
14. Glasscock MF, Bohrer PS. Suboccipital approach. In: House WF, Luetje CM, Doyle RJ, eds. *Acoustic tumors, diagnosis and management.* San Diego: Singular, 1997:189.
15. Catalno PJ, Jacobowitz O, Post KD. Prevention of headaches after retrosigmoid removal of acoustic tumors. *Am J Otol* 1996;17(6): 904–908.
16. Jackler RK. Overview of surgical neurotology. In: Jackler RK, Brackmann DE, eds. *Neurotology.* St. Louis: Mosby-Yearbook, 1994:660.
17. House JW. Translabyrinthine Approach in Otologic Surgery. Brackmann DE, Shelton C, Arriaga MA, eds. Philadelphia: WB Saunders, 1994:605.
18. Arriaga MA, Berliner K, Luxford WM. Facial nerve function following middle fossa and translabyrinthine acoustic neuroma surgery. *Am J Otol* 1994;15(5):620–624.
19. Samii M, Matthies C. Management of 1,000 vestibular schwannomas (acoustic neuromas): the facial nerve—preservation and restitution of function. *Neurosurgery* 1997;40(40):684–695.
20. Beck DL, Atkins JS, Benecke J, et al. Intraoperative facial nerve monitoring: prognostic aspects during acoustic tumor removal. *Arch Otolaryngol Head Neck Surg* 1991;104:780–782.
21. Committee on hearing and equilibrium. Guidelines for the evaluation of hearing preservation in acoustic neuroma (vestibular schwannoma). *Otolaryngol Head Neck Surg* 1995;113(3):179–180.
22. Neely JG. Is it possible to totally resect an acoustic tumor and conserve hearing? *Otolaryngol Head Neck Surg* 1984;92(2):162–167.
23. Parnes LS, McClure JA. Posterior semicircular canal occlusion in the normal hearing ear. *Otolaryngol Head Neck Surg* 1991;104:52–57.
24. McElveen JT, Wilkins RH, Erwin A, et al. Modifying the translabyrinthine approach to preserve hearing during acoustic tumor surgery. *J Laryngol Otol* 1991;105:34–37.
25. Arriaga MA, Gorum M. Enhanced retrosigmoid exposure with posterior semicircular canal resection. *Otolaryngol Head Neck Surg* 1996; 115(1):46–48.
26. Arriaga M, Brackmann D. Technique and outcome of facial nerve repair in cerebellopontine angle tumor surgery. *Am J Otol* 13(4):356–359.
27. Rodgers GK, Luxford WM. Factors affecting the development of cerebrospinal fluid leak and meningitis after translabyrinthine surgery. *Laryngoscope* 1993;103(9):959–962.

Neurosurgical Issues in Otolaryngology: Principles and Practice of Collaboration,
edited by Moisés A. Arriaga and J. Diaz Day.
Lippincott Williams & Wilkins, Philadelphia © 1999.

CHAPTER 13

Nonacoustic Cerebellopontine Angle Lesions

C. Phillip Daspit, Robert F. Spetzler, and A. Giancarlo Vishteh

Historically, pathologies arising in the posterior fossa, including those in the cerebellopontine angle (CPA), were formidable challenges for the surgeon. Mortality rates as high as 50% were reported in early operative series (1). In approaching lesions of the CPA, the working space is limited by local bony structures on the one hand and vital neural structures on the other. Early neurosurgical attempts at extirpation of lesions in this area entailed undue retraction on vital neural tissues; hence, the high mortality rates. Advances in the fields of microneurosurgery as well as neuro-otology, especially temporal bone surgery, revolutionized approaches not only to acoustic neuromas but also to other lesions of the CPA.

''Skull base'' teams composed of neurosurgeons, neuro-otologists, otorhinolaryngologists, plastic surgeons, and endovascular interventionalists evolved in the early 1980s in response to the multidisciplinary efforts to minimize patient morbidity and mortality rates in approaching extensive lesions of the CPA and cranial base. A close cooperation between neurosurgeons and neuro-otologists became especially crucial when tackling these formidable lesions. Experience on the part of both specialists was and remains vital. The neurosurgeon must be versed not only in brainstem and cranial nerve surgery but, to some degree, in vascular neurosurgery as well. The neuro-otologist must be a specialist dedicated to the anatomy and surgery of the temporal bone. If such surgeries are not routinely performed by either specialist, dissections must be practiced on cadaveric specimens to keep these skills honed.

Most lesions in the CPA are neoplastic. Tumors of the CPA account for approximately 5% to 10% of all intracranial tumors (2). Most of these tumors (76–92%) are acoustic neuromas (2–13). The most common types of nonacoustic lesions in the area are CPA meningiomas (3–13%) followed by CPA epidermoids (2–6%) (2,4,6,9,11,12). A small number of other rare lesions (neoplastic or nonneoplastic) that can also arise or extend into this area are discussed briefly. Surgery for vestibular schwannomas (acoustic neuromas) is discussed elsewhere in this text. This chapter focuses on the retro- and presigmoid (transpetrosal) as well as combined petrosal approaches to nonacoustic lesions of the CPA and on those extending beyond the CPA, respectively. The indications, techniques, and complications associated with each approach are presented.

C. P. Daspit, R. F. Spetzler, and A. G. Vishteh: Barrow Neurological Institute, Phoenix, Arizona 85013-4496.

ANATOMY

The CPA cistern, or alternatively the CP cistern (14), refers to the pyramidal space that has as its apex the union of the cerebellum and the pons. The posterior ridge of the petrous bone forms the slanted base of the pyramid. The four sides of the pyramid are formed by the lateral pons anteriorly, the cerebellar hemisphere posteriorly, the tentorium superiorly, and the roof of the cerebellomedullary cistern inferiorly. The fifth, seventh, and eighth cranial nerves, along with the anterior inferior cerebellar artery (AICA), the superior cerebellar artery (SCA), and the superior petrosal veins, course within this space. Posteromedially, the flocculus of the cerebellum also indents the arachnoid of the cistern.

Superiorly, the fifth cranial nerve courses anteriorly in a superolateral direction from the pons to Meckel's cave. The seventh and eighth cranial nerves arise at the pontomedullary junction and enter the internal auditory canal (IAC) laterally. At the level of the IAC, this bundle is composed of the seventh cranial nerve (anterosuperiorly), the eighth cranial nerve (anteroinferiorly), the superior vestibular nerve (posterosuperiorly), and the inferior vestibular nerve (posteroinferiorly). Furthermore, the transverse osseous crest separates the seventh cranial nerve and the superior vestibular nerves from the eighth cranial nerve and the inferior vestibular nerve in a horizontal plane. The vertical osseous crest (Bill's bar) separates the seventh cranial and the superior vestibular nerves in a coronal plane. The sixth cranial nerve, which lies just beyond the medial aspect of the CP cistern, exits the pontomedullary junction ventromedially and courses anteriorly to enter the cavernous sinus via Dorello's canal.

Although the lower cranial nerves (IX, X, and XI) are not within the CP cistern, knowledge of their anatomy is important. Cranial nerve IX exits the medulla dorsal to the olive and enters the jugular foramen (pars nervosa) usually as a single nerve bundle. Rarely, this cranial nerve may exit the skull via its own separate foramen (15,16). Cranial nerve X likewise courses from the medulla laterally toward the jugular foramen (pars venosa) as multiple nerve filaments. Cranial nerve XI is composed of both spinal and brainstem rootlets and enters the jugular foramen (pars venosa) as well. Cranial nerve XII exits the medulla ventral to the olive and enters the hypoglossal canal of the occipital condyle.

Venous structures of note include the superior petrosal vein, which courses as single or multiple channels from the cerebellum to the superior petrosal sinus. The AICA, or rarely an AICA–posterior-inferior cerebellar artery (PICA) trunk, branches from the basilar artery at variable locations. Usually, however, the AICA branches from the basilar artery at or near the level of the seventh and eighth cranial nerve complex. This vessel gives rise to the labyrinthine artery. The premeatal, meatal, and the postmeatal segments of the labyrinthine artery often can be appreciated encircling the seventh and eighth cranial nerve complex in normal anatomic specimens (17–19). Dolichoectatic basilar and vertebral arteries (and/or their respective branches) may also reach the CPA cistern.

PATHOLOGY

Lesions of the CPA can arise directly from the neurovascular structures within this space, or they may indirectly extend into the cistern from surrounding neural tissue or osseous structures. These lesions may be intra- or extraaxial or intra- or extradural. Excluding vestibular schwannomas (acoustic neuromas), the most common lesions in this cistern are the CPA meningiomas (posterior petrous ridge meningioma) followed by epidermoid tumors. Dermoid tumors and lipomas are rare (20–22). Arachnoid cysts are benign entities that arise in the CPA; however, they may lead to brainstem or cranial nerve symptoms as the result of mass effect. Neuroepithelial cysts of the CPA have also been reported (23–25).

Lesions that can extend into the CPA include trigeminal schwannomas, the rare seventh cranial nerve schwannoma or malignant nerve sheath tumor, as well as rostral extensions of lower cranial nerve schwannomas (2,3,11,26–37). Primary brainstem tumors that can extend into the CPA include ependymomas and brainstem gliomas (6,9,11,12,38). A rare medulloblastoma involving the CPA has also been reported (38). Choroid plexus papillomas can grow in a fungate fashion through the lateral aperture(s) of the fourth ventricle (foramen of Luschka) and into the CPA superiorly (9,39). Hemangioblastomas rarely involve the CPA.

Vascular lesions can project into or involve the blood vessels that traverse this cistern and include large or giant aneurysms (of the AICA, SCA, or midbasilar artery). Brainstem arteriovenous malformations (AVMs) and dural fistulas can also be fed or drained by vessels of the CP cistern. Although extraaxial (cranial nerve) cavernous malformations are extremely rare (40,41), the more frequently encountered brainstem cavernous malformations originating in the brainstem may reach a pial surface along the CPA.

Primary tumors of the osteocartilaginous skull base can extend into and compress the CPA and its neurovascular structures epidurally (sometimes subdurally as well). Petroclival chondrosarcoma (42) is one such tumor. Clivus chordomas usually arise in the midline but may extend laterally into the CPA as can the rare osteosarcoma of the lateral skull base.

Nonosseous tumors arising within the petrous bone can also extend into the CPA. These lesions include cholesteatomas (intraosseous epidermoids) and cholesterol granulomas (3,9,11,42–44). Tumors arising from the structures that are housed in the petrous temporal bone include paragangliomas (glomus jugulare, glomus tympanicum) and endolymphatic sac carcinomas. Depending on their individual size, these lesions can also extend to the CPA (3,9,11). Metastatic tumors can reach the CPA by hematogenous spread or direct extension (e.g., nasopharyngeal carcinoma, adenoid cystic carcinoma). Granulomatous inflammatory masses rarely involve the CPA (45).

Meningiomas and Epidermoids

The two most common nonacoustic lesions in the CPA are meningiomas (2–6,9–13,44,46–54) and epidermoids (2–5,9,11,22,43,46,48,54–57). The clinical features and microsurgical strategies for the resection of both of these tumors warrant further discussion. In the case of CPA meningiomas, unlike vestibular schwannomas, hearing loss (4,9,33) may be a late manifestation, while symptoms related to the fifth cranial nerve (e.g., trigeminal neuralgia, diminished corneal response) or paresis of the seventh cranial nerve may be early findings (53). Patients can also present with obstructive hydrocephalus and/or symptoms of brainstem compression. The surgical objectives for CPA meningiomas include gross total tumor resection (if possible), protection of local neurovascular structures, and minimization of blood loss.

Depending on the size of the tumor, the dural base (vascular supply) should be carefully devascularized first. Next, the tumor is debulked internally (similar to acoustic neuromas). Depending on the consistency of the tumor, resection may proceed piecemeal with microinstruments using sharp dissectors (e.g., round knife), suction/bipolar technique, or an ultrasonic aspirator. The ''hollowed shell'' can then be diligently dissected from surrounding structures. Larger sphenopetroclival meningiomas frequently encase blood vessels (e.g., internal carotid artery, basilar artery) and nerves. If complete resection is the goal, preoperative angiography to determine the patency of the parent vessel and collateral circulation and possible embolization are important. At present, we do not advocate revascularization for gross total meningioma resection. Instead, we recommend preservation of the parent vessel. Furthermore, because we are skeptical of the predictive value of the balloon occlusion test, especially in the case of tumors (58), we are not strong advocates of using this test to determine the safety of sacrificing the parent vessel. Nevertheless, gross total resections may be attempted by using the arachnoidal plane around these vessels in dissecting of tumor. Proximal and distal vascular control is essential in such cases, and the resection proceeds forward from the segment of vessel uninvolved by tumor. If the tumor cannot be easily resected from these vital structures, despite meticulous arachnoid plane dissection, we recommend that tumor be left behind. Patients with small tumor residuals may be candidates for stereotactic radiosurgery.

In the case of epidermoids of the CPA, patients may present with cranial nerve or cerebellar dysfunction that develops over a number of years (33,59). Hemifacial spasm has also been reported as the initial presentation of CPA epidermoids (3,55,56). Furthermore, microsurgical goals tend to be a bit different in the case of epidermoids. These lesions frequently develop multiple finger-like projections that interdigitate between cranial nerves and brainstem fissures and sulci. Because of the local inflammatory reaction caused by the epidermoid, ''stripping'' its capsule may lead to undue injury of the cranial nerves or brainstem. On the other hand, leaving an epidermoid capsule behind may lead to recurrence. If, however, the capsule is adherent and not easily resected, it is best to leave it behind. Postoperatively, patients are kept on a moderate dose of steroids and are weaned slowly to prevent sequelae of chemical meningitis. Thereafter, patients are followed with brain magnetic resonance imaging (MRI) at appropriate intervals to rule out a recurrence. All things considered, it is potentially less dangerous to return to resect the epidermoid at a later date than to strip adherent capsules (59).

DIAGNOSTIC IMAGING

Brain MRI with gadolinium is the gold standard for the evaluation of patients with nonvascular CPA lesions. MRI, MR angiography, and venography are noninvasive tests that help identify some pathologies with vascular origins (e.g., cavernous malformations and giant aneurysms) and screen for other pathologies (e.g., aneurysms, AVMs), while also disclosing the patency of the venous sinus. A formal cerebral angiogram should be performed to permit more detailed anatomic evaluation of aneurysms and AVMs. In cases where pathology is identified on MRI (e.g., AVM, paraganglioma), both angiography and embolization (where indicated) can be performed in the same setting. In the case of more extensive tumors with vascular ''encasement,'' angiography discloses information about the patency of the parent vessel and collateral circulation. A head computed tomography bone algorithm is of value in determining the degree of bony involvement by the tumor, especially in the case of osteocartilaginous petrous tumors. This modality also can help determine the location of the jugular bulb (especially two-dimensional coronal temporal bone reconstructions). The specific neuroradiologic appearances of the lesions of this region are discussed elsewhere in this text.

Preoperative audiometry is widely used in acoustic neuroma surgery. It may also have some utility in the management of nonacoustic CPA lesions by determining the degree of hearing loss and the efficacy of sacrificing residual hearing if a more complete petrosectomy is needed.

APPROACHES AND INDICATIONS

When discussing approaches to the CPA, it is helpful to categorize the techniques based on their anatomic relationship to the sigmoid sinus. Approaches that are posterior to the sigmoid sinus are known as retrosigmoid, while those anterior to the sigmoid sinus are known collectively as presigmoid approaches. The presigmoid approaches are otherwise known as posterior transpetrosal approaches and are further subdivided into the retrolabyrinthine, translabyrinthine, and transcochlear approaches depending on the degree of petrosectomy. Lesions that extend above or below the CPA may require a combination approach. Such combinations usually include a presigmoid approach with a posterior subtemporal (combined supra- and infratentorial), a far-lateral (combined-combined), or a subtemporal and pterional orbitozygomatic approach (orbitozygomatic combined).

For a small subset of intraaxial lesions that reach the pial surface along the CPA (especially cavernous malformations), a simple method we have devised, termed the *two-point method,* can help select the appropriate approach. This method fulfills important surgical objectives: It avoids a brainstem incision while allowing optimal resection of a lesion. Using MRI (preferably axial), one point is placed in the center of the lesion and the second point is placed in the area where the lesion reaches the pial surface. The line connecting these two points represents the axis of approach to the lesion. For example, a cavernous malformation originating in the pons and abutting the pial surface at the CPA, but slightly inferior to the seventh and eighth cranial nerve complex, may be approached via a retrolabyrinthine approach.

Intraoperative localization of the area where these minuscule lesions reach the brainstem surface, however, is cumbersome. The precision of frameless stereotactic navigation (e.g., ISG Wand, Mississauga, Ontario, Canada) in such cases, therefore, is indispensable. Another important intraoperative adjunct in CPA surgery is neurophysiologic monitoring of the cranial nerves. We routinely monitor the seventh (electromyography) and eighth cranial nerves (brainstem auditory evoked potentials) during approaches to lesions of the CPA. Cranial nerve stimulators are also available and allow identification of the facial nerve in cases where the anatomy is distorted by the pathology.

In addition to the choice of approach (based on lesion location), other surgical goals must be established preoperatively. The amount of exposure is based on the type of lesion being approached (e.g., proximal and distal vascular control for aneurysms), its extension, and other objectives (e.g., debulking versus gross total resection of a tumor). In the subset of patients with obstructive hydrocephalus, preoperative placement of a ventriculostomy catheter and the potential need for permanent diversion of the cerebrospinal fluid (CSF) postoperatively are also considerations.

Retrosigmoid Approach

Indications

The retrosigmoid approach is a versatile technique, helpful in the extirpation of lesions restricted to the CPA and in line with the axis of the posterior petrous ridge. Because the petrous bone is not really drilled in this approach, lesions ventral to the brainstem are not visualized from this angle of approach without undue retraction. This technique, however, may be used in combination with the far-lateral approach to gain access to the inferior portion of lesions that extend toward the foramen magnum anteriorly.

Technique

The patient is positioned supine with a roll under the ipsilateral shoulder, and the head is rotated 90 degrees so that the axis of the head is parallel with the floor (alternatively, the lateral park bench or sitting bench can be used). A linear incision approximately 1 cm medial to the posterior margin of the mastoid and extending from the level of the superior nuchal line to the mastoid tip is made. Instead of a making a burr hole at the transverse sigmoid junction, we routinely expose the sigmoid sinus with cutting and diamond burrs of various sizes (we prefer a MedNext drill, MedNext, Riviera Beach, FL). The sigmoid sinus is skeletonized from its junction with the transverse sinus down to the level of the jugular bulb. All entered mastoid air cells are waxed. Next, after the retrosigmoid dura has been separated from suboccipital bone, a Midas Rex drill (Midas Rex Pneumatic Tools, Inc., Fort Worth, TX) with a footplate attachment is used to turn a retrosigmoid craniotomy. Before the dura is opened, Decadron® and mannitol along with hyperventilation are administered to relax the cerebellar tissue. The dura is opened along the sigmoid sinus and T'd-up toward the transverse sigmoid junction, as well as more inferiorly toward the jugular bulb. Once the durotomies have been completed, the cerebellum is relaxed further by fenestrating the cerebellomedullary cistern anteromedially or the cisterna magna posteriorly.

Once the cerebellum is relaxed, telfa strips are placed along the lateral margin of the cerebellar hemisphere, and the CPA is approached with gentle retraction. "Key hole" retraction is afforded by a sucker in the surgeon's nondominant hand and a dissecting microinstrument in the dominant hand (the shaft of the sucker rests on a telfa pad on the lateral cerebellar hemisphere while the sucker tip remains in the area of dissection). Traditional retractors are not needed routinely. Microscopic dissection and resection can now proceed. The petrosal vein is not routinely sacrificed unless additional exposure is needed. At the end of the case, the mastoid area is reexamined, and residual air cells are obliterated with bone wax. The dura is closed in a watertight fashion using a pericranial graft (if needed). The posterior fossa bone flap is reaffixed to the skull at the end of the case using titanium microplates.

Potential intraoperative complications of this approach include injury to the sigmoid sinus during bone resection. The cerebellum, brainstem, and cranial nerves, especially the seventh and eighth cranial nerves, can be layered during the intradural portion of the procedure.

Postoperatively, CSF leakage is the most common complication and usually results from improperly waxed mastoid air cells or a nonwatertight dural closure. Chemical meningitis, also common postoperatively, is responsive to a short course of steroids (if the patient is not on steroids already). In patients with larger CPA tumors and coexistent obstructive hydrocephalus at presentation, postoperative ventriculoperitoneal shunting may also be needed. Postoperative hemorrhage in the dissection bed can be a potentially devastating complication and can occur with any of the petrosal approaches as well. Wound infections are also possible after any of the approaches to the CPA.

Presigmoid Approaches

Posterior petrosectomy is classified into three subtypes: retrolabyrinthine, translabyrinthine, and transcochlear based on the degree of bony resection. In the retrolabyrinthine approach, after the sigmoid sinus has been skeletonized, bone is removed between this structure and the semicircular canals laterally. To provide maximal working space without sacrificing hearing, the semicircular canals are skeletonized but not perforated. In the translabyrinthine approach, the semicircular canals are drilled out (ipsilateral hearing is sacrificed) (8,46,60–62). This maneuver provides increased exposure to the ventral brainstem. In the transcochlear approach, the seventh cranial nerve is skeletonized out of its bony canal and the cochlea is removed (8,46,60,61,63). With the sequential increase in petrosectomy, a wider corridor is opened toward the CPA and the ventral brainstem. This exposure, however, carries a heavy price, namely, sacrifice of hearing and temporary dysfunction of the seventh cranial nerve.

Extended Retrolabyrinthine Approach

Indications

The retrolabyrinthine approach preserves hearing. Therefore, the CPA is exposed along a narrow corridor between the semicircular canals and the sigmoid sinus (Fig. 13-1). This approach is frequently combined with the posterior subtemporal craniotomy as a combined approach. Other than complications related to the intradural resection of the lesion, postoperative CSF leakage is the most common associated complication.

Technique

The patient is positioned similarly to the retrosigmoid approach with minimal inclination of the vertex of the head downward so that the mastoid tip is the highest point of the operative field. The incision starts at the level of the zygoma 1 cm anterior to the tragus. It then curves above and around the ear and inferiorly to the mastoid tip. The flap is retracted effectively with the aid of a Leyla bar (Aesculap, San Francisco, CA) and fishhooks rubberbanded.

The dissection of the petrous bone starts with a superficial mastoidectomy under microscopic magnification. We routinely use the MedNext drill with a suction irrigator. Drilling starts posterior to the zygomatic bone along the temporal line. This cut is essentially along and slightly inferior to the tegmen (floor) of the middle fossa. The second cut is made perpendicular to the first cut and extends from the tegmen to the posterior wall of the ear canal down to the mastoid tip. A generous superficial cortical mastoidectomy is key in allowing appropriate visualization (and prevention of injuries) to deeper structures in the petrous bone. Superficially, the bone is resected with a large burr. A large diamond burr (not rough-cut or supercut) is used as the sigmoid sinus is approached to prevent inadvertent puncture of the sinus, which can occur with a small diamond bit. Frequently, a thin transparent rim of bone (Bill's island) is left on top of the sigmoid sinus as added protection to prevent injury during other portions of the mastoidectomy. The deeper portion of the mastoidectomy includes removal of the bone along the sinodural angle and skeletonization of the semicircular canals.

Once the mastoid antrum has been entered, the horizontal semicircular canal is identified. This landmark subsequently leads the surgeon to the external genu of the seventh cranial nerve medially and inferiorly, the posterior semicircular canal posteriorly, and the epitympanum and the superior semicircular canal anteriorly. The posterior and superior semicircular canals are skeletonized, drilling as far anteriorly as possible. Resection of bone under the common crus of the posterior and superior semicircular canals is important because it provides an additional 2 to 3 mm of exposure. Bony resection above and below the otic capsule exposes

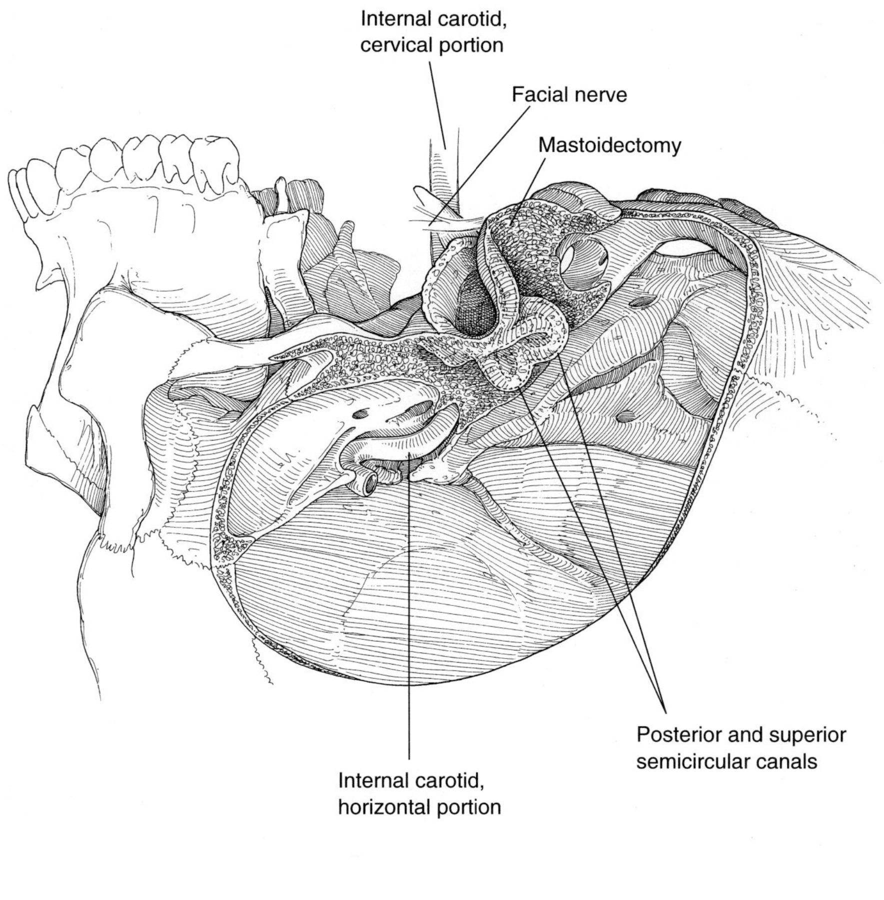

FIG. 13-1. Extended retrolabyrinthine approach. (Reprinted with permission from Barrow Neurological Institute.)

the middle fossa dura, superior petrosal sinus, and the jugular bulb.

When the bone resection is complete, a large dural surface is exposed. The dura must be opened carefully to prevent injury to the endolymphatic sac and its aqueduct at the end of the case. Once the intradural portion of the surgery is completed, every attempt is made to obtain a watertight dural closure. The bone defect is further reinforced with fat harvested from the abdomen. Overall, this approach provides a narrow corridor to the CPA and in isolation is inappropriate for more extensive lesions with large portions that are ventral to the brainstem.

Translabyrinthine Approach

Indications

The translabyrinthine approach sacrifices hearing by resecting the semicircular canals, but it provides a more anterior angle of approach to lesions of the CPA (Fig. 13-2). In comparison to the retrolabyrinthine approach, the amount of working space is also increased. Complications are otherwise similar to those associated with other petrosal approaches and include postoperative CSF leakage as well as potential injury to the seventh cranial nerve during drilling of the petrous bone.

Technique

The positioning, incision, and superficial mastoidectomy are similar to those used in the retrolabyrinthine approach. In the translabyrinthine approach, however, the neuro-otologist further resects the three semicircular canals and skeletonizes the posterior half to two-thirds of the IAC. The lateral wall of the internal auditory canal fundus is made by the medial wall of the vestibule and the ampulla of the superior semicircular canal. Next, the IAC is unroofed using a diamond burr. The superior vestibular nerve, which is encountered first, lies posteriorly and superiorly. In the coronal plane, the seventh cranial nerve is situated anteriorly and superiorly and is separated from the superior vestibular nerve by the vertical crest or Bill's bar. The superior vestibular nerve, therefore, is an important landmark in identifying the seventh cranial nerve, which is ultimately partially skeletonized but kept in a thinned bony canal. Inferiorly, the jugular bulb is also unroofed to maximize exposure below the IAC.

Once the intradural portion of the procedure is completed, all air cells previously not obliterated are waxed, and the eustachian tube is obliterated. To obtain optimal obliteration of the eustachian tube, the mucosa is exenterated, followed by sequential packing of the tube with bone wax. The eustachian tube orifice may subsequently be covered with pericranium or fascia lata. The bone defect is once again packed with harvested abdominal fat.

This graduated petrous bone resection affords a more anterior angle approach to the CPA and the clival area. More ventral lesions, however, require yet more aggressive petrous bone resection.

Transcochlear Approach

Indications

The transcochlear approach entails a complete petrosectomy and is a forward extension of the translabyrinthine

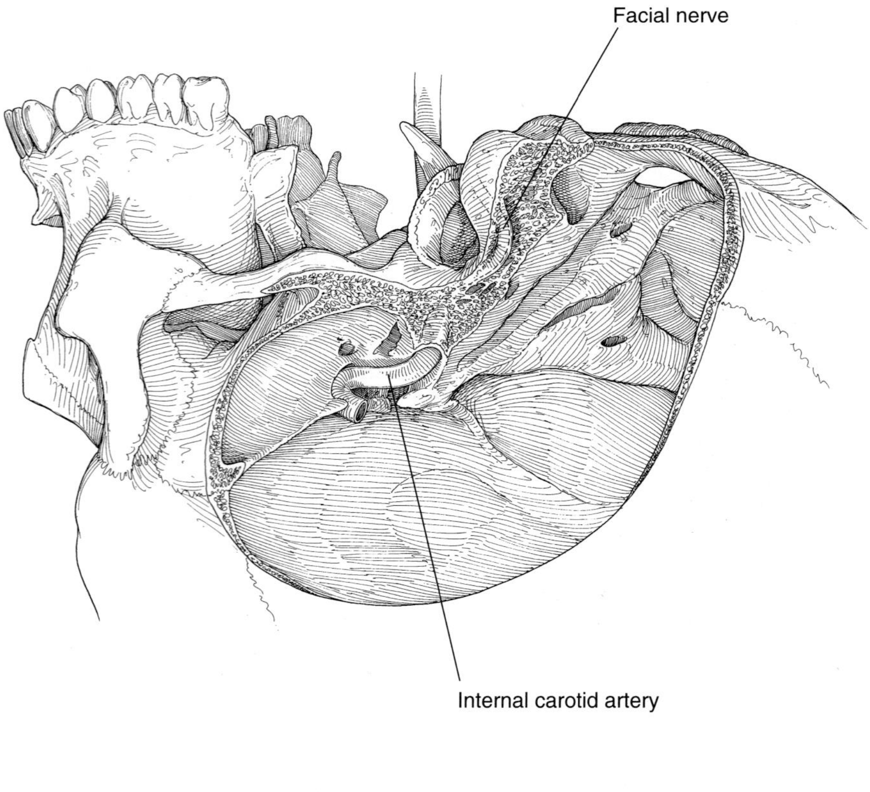

FIG. 13-2. Translabyrinthine approach. (Reprinted with permission from Barrow Neurological Institute.)

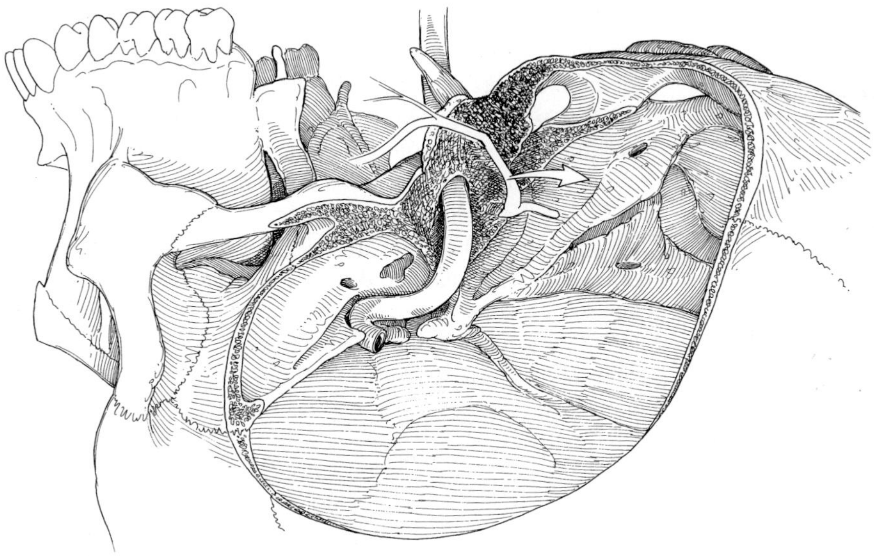

FIG. 13-3. Transcochlear approach. (Reprinted with permission from Barrow Neurological Institute.)

approach with additional resection of the cochlea along with the ear canal, tympanic membrane, and the middle ear ossicles. The facial nerve is unroofed completely and transposed from its bony canal (Fig. 13-3). This approach permits exposure of lesions of the CPA with extension ventrally to the brainstem. Complications inherent to this approach include the sacrifice of hearing and transient paresis of the seventh cranial nerve because it must be manipulated. Another postoperative complication is the cosmetic deformity created at the petrosectomy site.

Technique

The initial portion of this procedure, including patient positioning, is similar to that of the translabyrinthine approach. While the scalp flap is reflected forward, the external auditory canal is encountered, transected, and oversewn in two layers. The flap is next retracted more anteriorly. The mastoidectomy and labyrinthinectomy are performed as in the translabyrinthine approach.

To reroute the seventh cranial nerve, it is completely drilled out of its canal from its entry at the IAC to its exit at the stylomastoid foramen. To complete this task, the facial recess first must be drilled out. The facial recess itself is composed of air cells and is bound laterally by the chorda tympani, medially by the mastoid segment of the seventh cranial nerve, and superiorly by the fossa incudis. Opening the facial recess allows exposure of the middle ear and its bony ossicles (the incus and the stapes), the cochlear promontory, the horizontal portion of the seventh cranial nerve, and Jacobson's nerve.

Once the epitympanum has been entered, the ossicles are removed. Next, in order to transpose the seventh cranial nerve, it must be released at its tethering points, which include the takeoff points of the chorda tympani nerve to the stapedius and the greater superficial petrosal nerve (GSPN). The chorda tympani is sectioned inferiorly at its point of origin from the descending portion of the seventh cranial nerve while the GSPN is sectioned anteriorly at its point of origin from the geniculate ganglion. Once the seventh cranial nerve is released, it is freed from the fallopian canal and rerouted posteriorly.

The next step, resection of the cochlea, starts at the promontory, which houses the basal turn of the cochlea. Drilling continues forward until the septum between the basal turn of the cochlea and internal carotid artery is encountered. The jugulocarotid bony septum is also drilled out to expose the jugular bulb completely. Thorough knowledge of the anatomy of cranial nerves IX, X, and XI is also imperative to avoid injuring them inadvertently, especially near the region of the jugular foramen. The dura overlying the IAC is kept intact during the petrous drilling to provide an additional layer of protection between the drill and this portion of the seventh cranial nerve.

Once drilling has been completed, the superior petrosal sinus is visualized from the sinodural angle to Meckel's cave superiorly. Inferior exposure includes the jugular bulb and the inferior petrosal sinus. Anteriorly, the internal carotid artery and the orifice of the eustachian tube are exposed, as is the periosteum of the temporomandibular joint. More medially, the clivus is visualized.

As in the translabyrinthine approach, occlusion of residual air cells with bone wax and meticulous obliteration of the eustachian tube are crucial to prevent CSF leaks. To repair the petrosectomy defect, numerous techniques have been devised, but the split bone graft technique (64) for covering the petrosectomy sites may be the easiest. Covering the site with titanium mesh or hydroxyapatite carries an additional risk of infection, especially if CSF leakage is present.

The transcochlear approach offers the widest possible petrosal approach to the ventral brainstem via a complete petrosectomy.

Combination Approaches

Combined Supra- and Infratentorial Approach

For lesions with rostral and/or caudal extensions beyond exposure of the transpetrosal or retrosigmoid approaches, a variety of combination approaches can be used. The combined approach connects the supra- and infratentorial compartments via one of the petrosal approaches. A supra- and infratentorial craniotomy is followed by the division of the tentorium (Fig. 13-4) (46–48,54,61,65,66). This approach offers a wide exposure of the medial petrous and clival regions.

Technique

After the neuro-otologist has completed the petrosal drilling, the posterior fossa dura is visualized posterior to the petrosectomy, and the middle fossa dura is seen superior to the petrosectomy. Using the exposed dura along the petrosectomy borders, an L-shaped craniotomy is turned. The craniotomy is performed by drilling posterior to the sigmoid sinus to the suboccipital area. The drilling then proceeds cephalad and crosses the transverse sinus, where the drilling is oriented anteriorly and caudally toward the lateral and inferior temporal lobe dura. Next, the drill is turned posteriorly along the floor of the middle fossa, and the bone overlying the transverse sinus is crossed again anterior to the previous crossing point at the junction of the transverse and sigmoid sinuses. The bone flap is elevated after the dura has been dissected meticulously from its underside. When this portion of the procedure is completed, the transverse, sigmoid, and superior petrosal sinuses are all visualized.

Before the dura is opened, the brain is relaxed with mannitol and hyperventilation. In the posterior fossa, the dura is opened in the presigmoid area up to the superior petrosal sinus. The supratentorial dural incision curves posteriorly along the inferior temporal lobe toward the superior petrosal sinus, stopping just short of its entry into the junction of the transverse and sigmoid sinuses. Extreme caution must be exercised during this portion of the procedure (connecting the supra- and infratentorial durotomies) to ascertain that the veins(s) of Labbé is not low-lying or draining into the superior petrosal sinus. If such aberrant venous drainage is not encountered, the superior petrosal sinus can be coagulated or doubly clip-ligated.

Previously, we used angiographic information about the patency of the contralateral sigmoid sinus as well as test measurements of intraoperative occlusion pressure as criteria to determine the safety of sacrificing the sigmoid sinus. This sacrifice was mainly to gain additional exposure. We no longer advocate routine sacrifice of the sigmoid sinus, even if the contralateral sinus is patent and intraoperative test occlusion pressures are acceptable (e.g., an increase of no greater than 7 mm Hg above baseline pressures). There have been case reports of the delayed formation of dural

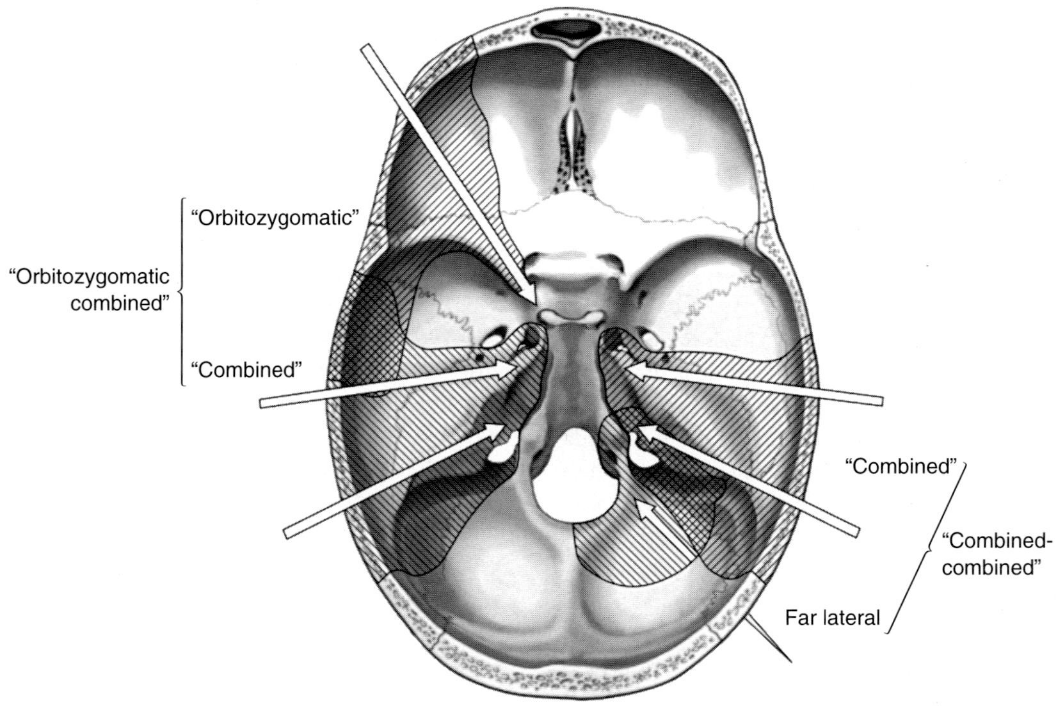

FIG. 13-4. Diagrammatic representation of the combination approaches. (Reprinted with permission from Barrow Neurological Institute.)

arteriovenous fistulae in patients who had previously undergone ligation of the sigmoid sinus during surgical approaches (67).

After the dural incision is completed, the tentorium is incised medially toward the tentorial hiatus and parallel to the superior petrosal sinus. As the hiatus is approached and the last tentorial cuts are made, care should be taken to avoid injuring the fourth cranial nerve, which lies just medial to the tentorial edge. Once the tentorial incision is completed with a slight upward retraction of the posterior temporal lobe (caution must be exercised not to place the vein of Labbé under undue tension), the entire petroclival region from the lower brainstem to the upper clivus and posterior cavernous sinus region is exposed.

Far-Lateral Combined Supra- and Infratentorial (Combined-Combined) Approach

Occasionally, CPA lesions extend caudally to the foramen magnum and rostrally to the upper clivus. For such lesions, the combined approach alone may not provide enough exposure to extirpate portions of the tumor at or below the level of the foramen magnum without undue retraction of neural structures. For such extensive lesions, a far-lateral craniotomy (48,65,66,68,69) is added to the *combined* approach (Fig. 13-4). We refer to this approach (combined supra- and infratentorial approach and far-lateral approach) as a *combined-combined* approach (61,65,66,68).

Technique

The far-lateral approach consists of the lateral suboccipital craniotomy with the addition of an ipsilateral posteromedial condylectomy, C1 laminectomy, and bony resection of the lateral foramen magnum. The degree of condylectomy depends on the amount of ventral access needed. Condylar approaches can be divided into the far- and extreme-lateral approaches with graduated condylectomies (similar to petrosal approaches) providing increased ventral access to the upper cervical spine and lower brainstem as well as to the lower cranial nerves and the vertebrobasilar junction.

Patient positioning for the combined-combined approach is essentially the same as for the far-lateral approach. At our institution we routinely use a previously described (61,65,66,68) positioning scheme that maximizes the working space and access to the ventral brainstem for transcondylar cases. The patient is placed in the lateral park-bench position with the lesion side up. The operating table is extended by pulling a ¾-inch plastic board overlaid by a mattress approximately 20 cm beyond the head of the table. Next, the dependent arm is positioned over the extended end of the table. The arm is flexed at the elbow and cradled in a padded sling along the gap between the Mayfield head holder (Codman, Shurtleff, Raynham, MA) and its table attachment.

The position of the head is crucial. A series of three maneuvers positions the head appropriately after application of the Mayfield head holder. With the body in a lateral decubitus position, the head is flexed on the anteroposterior plane with the chin approximately one finger's breadth from the sternum. Next, the head is rotated 45 degrees away from the side of the lesion (down) and flexed laterally 30 degrees toward the contralateral shoulder. This maneuver brings the mastoid process to the highest point of the operating field and opens up the working space not only between the head and upper cervical spine but also the angle between the head and ipsilateral shoulder. At the end of the positioning, the clivus is perpendicular to the floor, allowing the surgeon to look down the axis of the basilar artery between the lower cranial nerves.

We use a "hockey-stick" incision that extends from the midline upper cervical spine (C4) superiorly to the inion. It then curves above the superior nuchal line and the ipsilateral pinna down to the point approximately 1 cm anterior to the tragus at the level of the zygoma. Once the incision is completed, a muscle flap is created, leaving behind a cuff of muscle and fascia (for later reattachment) along the superior nuchal line. After the myocutaneous flap has been retracted inferolaterally, the lateral temporal bone, mastoid, lateral suboccipital cranium, and C1-C2 laminae are exposed. Bony resection includes petrosectomy, C1 laminectomy, partial suboccipital craniotomy, and condylar resection. To facilitate the petrosectomy, the head can be readjusted so that it is parallel to the floor.

Once the neuro-otologist has completed the petrosectomy, a C1 laminectomy is performed using a Midas Rex footplate attachment. The lateral cut of the laminectomy is made along the sulcus arteriosus of the vertebral artery, and additional bone is removed laterally until the transverse foramen is reached. The V_3 segment of the vertebral artery from the transverse foramen of C1 to the site of dural penetration is now exposed. If the need should arise to mobilize the vertebral artery, bone along the dorsal aspect of the transverse foramen of C1 (and C2, if needed) is removed.

The next step consists of the suboccipital and suprainfratentorial craniotomies. The first craniotomy cut connects the foramen magnum and the anterior margin of the petrosectomy overlying the inferior temporal lobe and crosses the transverse sinus. The second cut connects the lateral foramen magnum with the posteroinferior margin of the petrosectomy immediately behind the sigmoid sinus. Once again, before the bone flaps are removed, the dural sinuses are dissected free from the underside of the bone. The lateral bone of the foramen magnum and the jugular tubercle and the posteromedial bone of the occipital condyle are removed using a high-speed drill. The amount of condylar bony resection depends upon the degree of ventral exposure needed. A more extensive condylectomy provides a more direct view of the ventral cervicomedullary region.

After the desired condylectomy is completed, the dura is opened in one of two ways. A single dural opening that extends from the lateral aspect of the C1 dura toward the midline and then to the presigmoid region sacrifices the sigmoid sinus and eventually ends along the dura of the posterolateral temporal lobe. To preserve the sigmoid sinus, an alternate opening consists of two separate dural flaps: a presigmoid suprainfratentorial dural opening and a retrosigmoid dural opening that extends from the transverse sigmoid junction to the dura at the level of C1. Along with the division of the tentorium, these two durotomies expand the view of the clivus and brainstem from the foramen magnum up to and above the tentorial hiatus and to the level of the posterior cavernous sinus. With intradural dissection and arachnoidal release, the third through 12th cranial nerves can be visualized along with the vertebrobasilar system from the extradural V_3 segment of the vertebral artery to the basilar terminus.

Orbitozygomatic-Combined Infratentorial Approach

If an extensive lesion along the foramen magnum, petroclival regions, and cavernous sinus with extensions along the sphenoid or anterior fossa should require resection, a combined suprainfratentorial approach can be supplemented with an orbitozygomatic craniotomy. The latter adds an anterior route to the brainstem, the cavernous sinus blood vessels, and the anterior cranial fossa and sphenoidal wing.

The orbitozygomatic craniotomy consists of a pterional craniotomy with the additional removal of the superior orbital roof and rim, the lateral orbital rim and wall, and the zygomatic arch as a single piece. The *orbitozygomatic-combined* supratentorial-infratentorial approach (51) affords the surgeon a wide exposure of the anterior, middle, and posterior fossae. Lesions encircling vascular structures can be approached from different angles, thus minimizing injury to these critical vessels and their respective branches.

Barrow Neurological Institute Experience

Between 1985 and 1993, 83 patients underwent the combined supra- and infratentorial approach for large lesions involving the CPA and extending above the tentorial hiatus (46,48,54). The initial 46 patients were reported in 1992 with a detailed analysis of outcomes (54). The updated group was further reported in 1993 (48).

Most of the pathologies consisted of meningiomas and schwannomas (fifth, seventh, and eighth cranial nerves). The remainders of the pathologies are shown in Table 13-1. There were no operative mortalities in this series. The complications for these 83 patients included temporary facial nerve paresis (30%), CSF leak (13%), and sixth nerve paresis (7%). Other operative complications included numbness, aphasia, sepsis, hemiparesis, pneumonia, and hematoma (2–4% each). These numbers compare favorably with morbidity and mortality rates from previous operative series. Mortality rates for resection of clival and petrous meningiomas were approximately 50% in early series (70) and between 9% and 11% in more recent series (1,10,52,70).

TABLE 13–1. *Number of patients undergoing combined approach for lesions of petrous and clival regions at the Barrow Neurological Institute from 1985 to 1993*

Lesion type	No. of patients
Meningioma	32
Schwannoma	29
Brainstem cavernous malformations	6
Epidermoid	4
Cerebellopontine arteriovenous malformation	3
Midbasilar aneurysm	2
Glomus tumor	2
Basal-cell carcinoma	1
Mucous epidermoid carcinoma	1
Squamous-cell carcinoma	1
Dermoid cyst	1
Chordoma	1
Total	83

From ref. 48, with permission.

CONCLUSION

With the evolution of multidisciplinary skull base surgical teams and specific advances in neurosurgery and neuro-otology, approaches to extensive lesions of the CPA, including nonacoustic tumors, have evolved greatly during the past two decades. This evolution has led to preferential bone resection over undue neural tissue retraction for the surgical exposure of different pathologies. Advances in the field of temporal bone surgery have been based on the monumental work of William House, who is almost single-handedly responsible for the addition of the radical petrosectomy to the neuro-otologic and neurosurgical armamentarium. With the rapid evolution of such skull base techniques, previously unreachable lesions have become accessible for surgical extirpation. Although the indications for petrosal and combined approaches are limited, if the need for these techniques arises, the surgery carries with it fewer relative risks for morbidity and mortality.

REFERENCES

1. Malis LI. Surgical resection of tumors of the skull base. In: Wilkins RH, Rengachary SS, eds. *Neurosurgery*. New York: McGraw-Hill, 1985: 1011–1021.
2. McElveen JT Jr, Saunders JE. Tumors of the cerebellopontine angle: neuro-otologic aspects of diagnosis. In: Wilkins RH, Rengachary SS, eds. *Neurosurgery*. New York: McGraw-Hill, 1996:1039–1048.
3. Barker FG II, Ojemann RG. Surgical approaches to tumors of the posterior fossa cranial nerves (excluding acoustic neuromas). In: Barrow DL, ed. *Surgery of the cranial nerves of the posterior fossa*. Park Ridge, IL: American Association of Neurological Surgeons, 1993:289–305.
4. Buchheit WA, Getch CC. Tumors of the cerebellopontine angle: clinical features and surgical management via a retrosigmoid approach. In: Wilkins RH, Rengachary SS, eds. *Neurosurgery*. New York: McGraw-Hill, 1996:1085–1094.
5. Buchheit WA, Rosenwasser RH. Tumors of the cerebellopontine angle: clinical features and surgical management. In: Schmiedek HH, Sweet WH, eds. *Operative neurosurgical techniques: indications, methods and results*. Orlando, FL: Grune & Stratton, 1988:673–683.

6. Hitselberger WE, Gardner G Jr. Other tumors of the cerebellopontine angle. *Arch Otolaryngol* 1968;88:164–166.
7. House WF. Monograph I. Transtemporal bone microsurgical removal of acoustic neuromas. *Arch Otolaryngol* 1964;80:597–616.
8. House WF. Transtemporal bone microsurgical removal of acoustic neuromas: report of two cases. *Arch Otolaryngol* 1964;80:617–667.
9. Martuza RL, Parker SW, Nadol JB Jr, Davis KR, Ojemann RG. Diagnosis of cerebellopontine angle tumors. *Clin Neurosurg* 1985;32: 177–213.
10. Samii M, Ammirati M. Cerebellopontine angle meningiomas (posterior pyramid meningiomas). In: Al-Mefty O, ed. *Meningiomas*. New York: Raven, 1991:503–515.
11. Shramek JK, Gray L. Tumors of the cerebellopontine angle: imaging. In: Wilkins RH, Rengachary SS, eds. *Neurosurgery*. New York: McGraw-Hill, 1996:1049–1062.
12. Thomsen J. Cerebellopontine angle tumours, other than acoustic neuromas: a report on 34 cases—a presentation of 7 bilateral acoustic neuromas. *Acta Otolaryngol* 1976;82:106–111.
13. Vogel FS. Tumors of the cerebellopontine angle: pathology. In: Wilkins RH, Rengachary SS, eds. *Neurosurgery*. New York: McGraw-Hill, 1996:1035–1038.
14. Yasargil MG. *Microsurgical anatomy of the basal cisterns and vessels of the brain, diagnostic studies, general operative techniques and pathological considerations of the intracranial aneurysms*. Stuttgart: Georg Thieme Verlag, 1984.
15. Lang J. Anatomy in and on the jugular foramen. In: Frowein RA, Brock M, Klinger M, eds. *Advances in neurosurgery*. Berlin: Springer-Verlag, 1989:125–132.
16. Rhoton AL Jr, Buza R. Microsurgical anatomy of the jugular foramen. *J Neurosurg* 1975;42:541–550.
17. Rhoton AL Jr. Microsurgical anatomy of acoustic neuromas. *Neurol Res* 1984;6:3–21.
18. Rhoton AL Jr. Microsurgical anatomy of cerebellopontine angle. In: Wilkins RH, Rengachary SS, eds. *Neurosurgery*. New York: McGraw-Hill, 1996:1063–1084.
19. Samii M, Sepehrnia A, Mahran A, Bini W. Surgery of the jugular foramen. In: Frowein RA, Brock M, Klinger M, eds. *Advances in neurosurgery*. Berlin: Springer-Verlag, 1989:140–152.
20. Christensen WN, Long DM, Epstein JI. Cerebellopontine angle lipoma. *Hum Pathol* 1986;17:739–743.
21. Graves VB, Schemm GW. Clinical characteristics and CT findings in lipoma of the cerebellopontine angle: case report. *J Neurosurg* 1982; 57:839–841.
22. Truwit CL, Barkovich AJ. Pathogenesis of intracranial lipoma: an MR study in 42 patients. *AJNR* 1990;11:665–674.
23. Ciricillo SF, Davis RL, Wilson CB. Neuroepithelial cysts of the posterior fossa: case report. *J Neurosurg* 1990;72:302–305.
24. Leung SY, Ng THK, Fung CF, Fan YW. An epithelial cyst in the cerebellopontine angle: case report. *J Neurosurg* 1991;74:278–282.
25. Umezu H, Aiba T, Unakami M. Enterogenous cyst of the cerebellopontine angle cistern: case report. *Neurosurgery* 1991;28:462–466.
26. Bordi L, Compton J, Symon L. Trigeminal neuroma: a report of eleven cases. *Surg Neurol* 1989;31:272–276.
27. Bordi L, Symon L, Cheesman AD. Hypoglossal neuroma following excision of a huge recurrent acoustic neuroma and facio-hypoglossal anastomosis: a complex management problem. *Acta Neurochir (Wien)* 1990;104:143–146.
28. Franklin DJ, Moore GF, Fisch U. Jugular foramen peripheral nerve sheath tumors. *Laryngoscope* 1989;99:1081–1087.
29. Horn KL, House WF, Hitselberger WE. Schwannomas of the jugular foramen. *Laryngoscope* 1985;95:761–765.
30. Iwasaki K, Kondo A. Accessory nerve neurinoma manifesting with typical jugular foramen syndrome. *Neurosurgery* 1991;29:455–459.
31. McCormick PC, Bello JA, Post KD. Trigeminal schwannoma: surgical series of 14 cases with review of the literature. *J Neurosurg* 1988;69: 850–860.
32. Muhlbauer MS, Clark WC, Robertson JH, Gardner LG, Dohan FC Jr. Malignant nerve sheath tumor of the facial nerve: case report and discussion. *Neurosurgery* 1987;21:68–73.
33. Odake G. Intracranial hypoglossal neurinoma with extracranial extension: review and case report. *Neurosurgery* 1989;24:583–587.
34. O'Donoghue GM, Brackmann DE, House JW, Jackler RK. Neuromas of the facial nerve. *Am J Otol* 1989;10:49–54.
35. Sweasey TA, Edelstein SR, Hoff JT. Glossopharyngeal schwannoma: review of five cases and the literature. *Surg Neurol* 1991;35:127–130.
36. Tew JM Jr, Yeh H-S, Miller GW, Shahbabian S. Intratemporal schwannoma of the facial nerve. *Neurosurgery* 1983;13:186–188.
37. Yasui T, Hakuba A, Kim SH, Nishimura S. Trigeminal neurinomas: operative approach in eight cases. *J Neurosurg* 1989;71:506–511.
38. House JL, Burt MR. Primary CNS tumors presenting as cerebellopontine angle tumors. *Am J Otol* 1985 Suppl:147–153.
39. Ford WJ, Brooks BS, El Gammal T, Massey CE, Beveridge WD. Adult cerebellopontine angle choroid plexus papilloma: MR evaluation. *AJNR* 1988;9:611.
40. Linskey ME, Jannetta PJ, Martinez AJ. A vascular malformation mimicking an intracanalicular acoustic neurilemoma: case report. *J Neurosurg* 1991;74:516–519.
41. Pappas DG, Schneiderman TS, Brackmann DE, Simpson LC, Chandra-Sekar B, Sofferman RA. Cavernous hemangiomas of the internal auditory canal. *Otolaryngol Head Neck Surg* 1989;101:27–32.
42. Al-Mefty O, Fox JL, Rifai A, Smith RR. A combined infratemporal and posterior fossa approach for the removal of giant glomus tumors and chondrosarcomas. *Surg Neurol* 1987;28:423–431.
43. Altschuler EM, Jungreis CA, Sekhar LN, Jannetta PJ, Sheptak PE. Operative treatment of intracranial epidermoid cysts and cholesterol granulomas: report of 21 cases. *Neurosurgery* 1990;26:606–614.
44. House WF, Hitselberger WE, McElveen JT Jr, Shelton C. The middle cranial fossa approach to lesions of the temporal bone and cerebellopontine angle. In: Wilkins RH, Rengachary SS, eds. *Neurosurgery*. New York: McGraw-Hill, 1996:1101–1106.
45. Mokry M, Flaschka G, Kleinert G, Kleinert R, Fazekas F, Kopp W. Chronic lyme disease with an expansive granulomatous lesion in the cerebellopontine angle. *Neurosurgery* 1990;27:446–451.
46. Daspit CP, Spetzler RF, Pappas CTE. Combined approach for lesions involving the cerebellopontine angle and skull base: experience with 20 cases—preliminary report. *Otolaryngol Head Neck Surg* 1991;105: 788–796.
47. Hakuba A, Nishimura S, Jang BJ. A combined retroauricular and preauricular transpetrosal-transtentorial approach to clivus meningiomas. *Surg Neurol* 1988;30:108–116.
48. Hamilton MG, Spetzler RF, Daspit CP. The combined supra- and infratentorial approach for lesions of the petrous and clival regions. *BNI Quarterly* 1993;9:2–8.
49. Kawase T, Shiobara R, Toya S. Anterior transpetrosal-transtentorial approach for sphenopetroclival meningiomas: surgical method and results in 10 patients. *Neurosurgery* 1991;28:869–876.
50. Langman AW, Jackler RK, Althaus SR. Meningioma of the internal auditory canal. *Am J Otol* 1990;11:201–204.
51. Lawton MT, Daspit CP, Spetzler RF. The orbitozygomatic-combined supra- and infratentorial approach: technical note. *Barrow Neurol Inst Q* 1996;12:4–9.
52. Samii M, Ammirati M, Mahran A, Bini W, Sepehrnia A. Surgery of petroclival meningiomas: report of 24 cases. *Neurosurgery* 1989;24: 12–17.
53. Sekhar LN, Jannetta PJ. Cerebellopontine angle meningiomas: microsurgical excision and follow-up results. *J Neurosurg* 1984;60: 500–505.
54. Spetzler RF, Daspit CP, Pappas CTE. The combined supra- and infratentorial approach for lesions of the petrous and clival regions: experience with 46 cases. *J Neurosurg* 1992;76:588–599.
55. Auger RG, Piepgras DG. Hemifacial spasm associated with epidermoid tumors of the cerebellopontine angle. *Neurology* 1989;39:577–580.
56. Berger MS, Wilson CB. Epidermoid cysts of the posterior fossa. *J Neurosurg* 1985;62:214–219.
57. Yasargil MG, Abernathey CD, Sarioglu AC. Microneurosurgical treatment of intracranial dermoid and epidermoid tumors. *Neurosurgery* 1989;24:561–567.
58. Brackmann DE, Bartels LJ. Rare tumors of the cerebellopontine angle. *Otolaryngol Head Neck Surg* 1980;88:555–559.
59. Samii M, Tatagiba M, Piquer J, Carvalho GA. Surgical treatment of epidermoid cysts of the cerebellopontine angle. *J Neurosurg* 1996;84: 14–19.
60. Daspit CP, Lawton MT. The transpetrosal approaches. In: Dickman CA, Sonntag VKH, Spetzler RF, eds. *Surgery of the craniovertebral junction*. New York: Thieme 1998;483–490.

61. Lawton MT, Daspit CP, Spetzler RF. Presigmoid approaches to skull base lesions. *Adv Tech Stand Neurosurg* 1997;23:189–204.
62. McElveen JT Jr. The translabyrinthine approach to cerebellopontine angle tumors. In: Wilkins RH, Rengachary SS, eds. *Neurosurgery*. New York: McGraw-Hill, 1996:1107–1113.
63. Pellet W, Cannoni M, Pech A. The widened transcochlear approach to jugular foramen tumors. *J Neurosurg* 1988;69:887–894.
64. Nakamura M, Tamaki N, Hara Y, Nagashima T, Tamura S. Use of a split bone graft to correct the cosmetic deformity associated with the transpetrosal-transtentorial surgical approach: technical report. *Neurosurgery* 1997;40:1089–1091.
65. Lawton MT, Daspit CP, Spetzler RF. Transpetrosal and combination approaches to skull base lesions. *Clin Neurosurg* 1995;43:91–112.
66. Lawton MT, Daspit CP, Spetzler RF. Transpetrosal and combination approaches to skull base lesions. In: Friedman M, Horn K, Hankinson HL, eds. *Otolaryngology—head and neck surgery*. Philadelphia: WB Saunders, 1996:159–167.
67. Sakaki T, Morimoto T, Nakase H, Kakizaki T, Nagata K. Dural arteriovenous fistula of the posterior fossa developing after surgical occlusion of the sigmoid sinus: report of five cases. *J Neurosurg* 1996;84:113–118.
68. Baldwin HZ, Miller CG, van Loveren HR, Keller JT, Daspit CP, Spetzler RF. The far lateral/combined supra- and infratentorial approach: a human cadaveric prosection model for routes of access to the petroclival region and ventral brain stem. *J Neurosurg* 1994;81:60–68.
69. Heros RC. Lateral suboccipital approach for vertebral and vertebrobasilar artery lesions. *J Neurosurg* 1986;64:559–562.
70. Mayberg MR, Symon L. Meningiomas of the clivus and apical petrous bone: report of 35 cases. *J Neurosurg* 1986;65:160–167.

Neurosurgical Issues in Otolaryngology: Principles and Practice of Collaboration,
edited by Moisés A. Arriaga and J. Diaz Day.
Lippincott Williams & Wilkins, Philadelphia © 1999.

CHAPTER 14

Jugular Foramen Tumors

Moisés A. Arriaga and Douglas A. Chen

Tumors of the jugular foramen are uncommon lesions of the skull base. They traverse intracranial and extracranial boundaries, presenting unique technical considerations when planning surgical resections, reconstruction, and rehabilitation. The comprehensive skull base team consists of otolaryngologists specializing in neurotology and head and neck surgery, neurosurgeons, critical care specialists, speech therapists, and reconstructive surgeons. Although most tumors of the jugular foramen are benign, they can be massive and destructive. With modern multidisciplinary teams, even large tumors can be resected safely. Glomus jugulare tumors represent the vast majority of benign neoplasms in the jugular foramen; however, schwannomas and meningiomas occur in this region.

HISTORICAL MANAGEMENT

In 1941, Stacy Guild (1) described an anatomic structure in the dome of the jugulare bulb and on the promontory that he called a glomus jugulare tumor. Harry Rosenwasser in 1946 (2) reported a surgical case of vascular tumor of the middle ear. He later became aware of Guild's report and is credited with acknowledging the origin of vascular tumors arising in the middle ear. Through the 1940s and 1950s, there were multiple surgical reports describing vascular tumors of the middle ear. In general, they were treated with radical mastoidectomy. Facial nerve injury and persistent and recurrent tumor complications were high. Radiation therapy became popularized during this period. In 1969, Valvassori (3) demonstrated the pathologic relationship of glomus jugulare tumors in the skull base. Using polytomography, he was able to demonstrate loss of the vascular crest between the carotid canal and the jugular bulb in patients with glomus jugulare tumors.

M. A. Arriaga and D. A. Chen: Allegheny General Hospital, Pittsburgh, Pennsylvania 15212.

In 1960, Alford and Guilford (4) classified glomus tumors into glomus tympanicum lesions, which were tumors limited to the middle ear, and the glomus jugulare tumors, which were lesions involving the jugular bulb in the middle ear as well (4). Fortunately, improved diagnostic techniques now permit accurate preoperative planning. Modern imaging has revealed the actual extent of these tumors and identified why radical mastoidectomy was an inadequate procedure in many cases.

Accurate preoperative imaging required consistent categorization of tumors through standardized classification schemes in order to adequately treat the entire tumor (5–7). As tumors were found to require cross-specialty expertise, the modern era of interdisciplinary skull base surgery developed.

GLOMUS JUGULARE TUMORS

The most common of all the jugular foramen tumors is the glomus jugulare tumor. Other common terminology includes chemodectomas and paragangliomas. Glomus bodies occur along the carotid artery, aortic arch, and several sites in the temporal bone. They occur along the glossopharyngeal nerve, the auricular branch of the vagus, and Arnold's nerve. It is thought that the glomus jugulare tumor arises from the glomus body in the jugular foramen. Regardless of the site of origin, chemodectomas are histologically identical. They produce a characteristic ''zelballen'' formation of epithelioid and sustentacular chief cells. Endocrinologically secreting tumors occur in up to 3% of cases and vasoactive substances such as epinephrine and norepinephrine should be screened preoperatively with vanillylmandelic acid (VMA) in patients with a history of hypertension or cardiac disease.

Most tumors occur in adulthood with a female to male predilection of 6:1 (8). Multiple tumors can occur in 10% of the cases. The most common combination of multiple tumors comprises an ipsilateral glomus tympanicum and a carotid body tumor (9). A familial form of glomus jugulare is thought to arise through an autosomal dominant pattern with incomplete penetrance. The tendency for multicentricity is higher in familial tumors and is reported to be as high as 25% to 50%.

The incidence of metastases is approximately 3% to 4% (10). The most common site of metastasis in decreasing frequency are the lungs, lymph nodes, liver, vertebrae, ribs, and spleen. The chief cells of the glomus tumor are one of the cells of the diffuse neuroendocrine system. Glomus tumors have consequently been associated with secondary malignancy of cells with similar derivation. Thyroid carcinoma, pheochromocytomas, and multiple endocrine neoplasias are all secondary primaries and have been identified in up to 7% of patients with glomus tumors.

The tumors proliferate generally in the direction of the pars nervosa of the jugular foramen. The direction of extension from this point is variable and can involve the carotid canal, petrous apex, and infratemporal fossa anteriorly. Often, however, these tumors will follow the jugular foramen intracranially and can cause extensive brainstem compression. Similarly, the tumors can extend through the skull base into the upper cervical regions with extensive involvement of the neck. This potential for extensive expansion may produce paralysis of the lower cranial nerves, conductive and sensorineural hearing loss, and, occasionally, hypesthesia of the trigeminal nerve.

Preoperative Evaluation

Thorough preoperative evaluation permits surgical planning for complete and safe tumor removal. Advances in imaging technology permit accurate preoperative assessment of tumor involvement within the temporal bone, neck, and intracranial extensions.

Physical Examination

A thorough otolaryngologic examination is critical in the preoperative assessment. Otomicroscopy begins by careful inspection of the tympanic membrane. If a vascular mass is identified, its location is carefully noted. Bluish masses in the inferior aspect of the tympanic membrane may represent dehiscent and prominent jugular bulbs. Similarly, pulsatile masses that are somewhat yellowish-white in appearance in the anterior mesotympanum often represent aberrant internal carotid arteries. In contrast, paragangliomas are often quite reddish in color. Occasionally, insufflation of the ear canal and tympanic membrane with a Siegle speculum will blanch the mass and confirm its vascularity. Complete otolaryngologic evaluation with mirror and possibly flexible nasopharyngoscope is essential to assess the sensitivity of the hypopharynx and larynx and the mobility of the palate and vocal cord.

Routine Hearing Tests

Air, bone, and speech audiometry are performed to assess the degree of conductive and sensorineural hearing impairments.

Cranial Computed Tomography (CT)

The mainstay of assessment of glomus tumors of the temporal bone is thin-section (1 mm) cranial CT using bone algorithm. Tumors confined to the middle ear and mastoid are distinguished from tumors that involve the jugular bulb. The key feature to identify is the caroticojugular spine. The distinguishing feature between glomus jugulare tumors and extensive glomus tympanicum tumors is erosion of the partition between the vertical petrous carotid artery and jugular bulb. In addition, CT is quite useful for identifying aberrant carotid arteries, high jugular bulbs, or dehiscent jugular bulbs. In many cases, cranial CT is the only examination necessary for planning treatment. At this time, retrograde jugular venography in the assessment of glomus jugulare tumors is of historic interest only.

Magnetic Resonance Imaging (MRI)

While CT is the primary imaging modality, MRI provides exquisite detail of soft tissue involvement by the tumor (11). In addition, MRI can indicate occlusion of the jugular bulb and vein through flow sensitive weighting of the image [magnetic resonance angiography (MRA) and magnetic resonance venography (MRV)]. In intradural tumors, MRI can more clearly delineate the tumor–brain interface in the relationship of the lesion to the intradural structures. An important warning regarding interpretation of MRI in glomus tumors is that the T1 image may overestimate the degree of tumor involvement. Marrow-containing bone of the petrous apex is hyperintense and indistinguishable from the enhancing tumor in the petrous apex (12,13).

Arteriography

Four-vessel angiography is indispensable for evaluating the involvement of the glomus tumor with the jugular bulb, carotid artery, or intradural structures. This methodology is particularly critical for indicating the extent of involvement and luminal compression of the internal carotid artery. However, arteriography additionally assures preoperative identification of other glomus lesions, if present.

Brain Perfusion and Flow Studies

For lesions with extensive carotid artery involvement, the adequacy of cerebral cross-perfusion from the contralateral internal carotid artery must be assessed. At this time, the most useful technique for cross-perfusion assessment is angiography with temporary balloon occlusion of the internal carotid artery. The assessment is both clinical and quantitative. Clinical evaluation is performed during 20 minutes of occlusion with careful neurologic examination. In addition, perfusion can be evaluated with xenon blood flow and CT or radioisotope studies with quantification of cerebral perfusion via cross-circulation of the circle of Willis (14,15). In certain cases with extensive invasion of the carotid artery and acceptable results on the perfusion studies of the contralateral artery, the involved carotid artery may be permanently occluded with a detachable balloon. In general, however, we prefer not to perform a permanent occlusion because there still remains a chance of cerebral infarction. Accordingly, in cases with extensive carotid artery involvement, if carotid artery sacrifice is essential, then carotid artery reconstruction with a saphenous vein graft or prosthetic conduit may be performed depending on individual factors including the patient's age, health status, extent of disease, and previous treatment.

Embolization

The hallmark of glomus tumor surgery is significant intraoperative blood loss. Preoperative embolization of feeding vessels is a significant adjunct in surgical removal (16). The embolization is usually performed at the time of the initial diagnostic arteriography and the embolization material is usually Ivalon. The procedure is usually performed 1 or 2 days before the surgery. Waiting longer after embolization for surgery can result in revascularization of the tumor. In addition, only those feeders from the external carotid artery are safe for embolization, as distal propagation of embolic material in the internal carotid artery could produce neurologic defects.

Biopsy

Diagnostic biopsy of potential vascular middle ear masses is strongly discouraged. Clinical and radiographic features of paragangliomas are distinctive enough for definitive management without a tissue diagnosis. In addition, we perform a frozen section biopsy of the tumor early in the surgery prior to irreversible surgical maneuvers to prevent major misdiagnosis or erroneous management. Efforts in obtaining a tissue diagnosis prior to completion of radiologic evaluation can result in injury to an aberrant carotid artery or a high jugular bulb as well as significant bleeding from the tumor itself.

Radiation

The therapy for glomus tumors of the temporal bone continues to be controversial. Because the clinical characteristics and growth rates of these tumors are variable, the full gamut of management has been recommended from observation alone through radiation therapy and surgical management. Although there are isolated cases of prolonged survival without treatment, these lesions can be quite deadly (17). Figure 14-1 is a postmortem photograph of a patient who died from brainstem compression of an extensive glomus jugulare tumor with intracranial extension. The studies of Brown, Spector et al., Rosenwasser (18–21), and others have documented mortality rates from 5% to 13% for glomus jugulare tumors. Glomus tumors (paragangliomas) are true neoplasms. The effect of radiation therapy is essentially a sclerosis of the blood supply. The photomicrograph (Fig. 14-2) illustrates the pretreatment and postradiotherapy appearance histopathologically of a paraganglioma. Of note, in the postradiated lesion, the critical distinction from preoperatively is the obliterative endarteritis of the blood supply. The tumor cells themselves appear histologically viable. In fact, our experience has been that radiation often will produce a 10- to 15-year hiatus in tumor growth. Unfortunately, these lesions begin growth again in most cases with newly recruited blood vessels.

There is additional interest in treating these lesions with

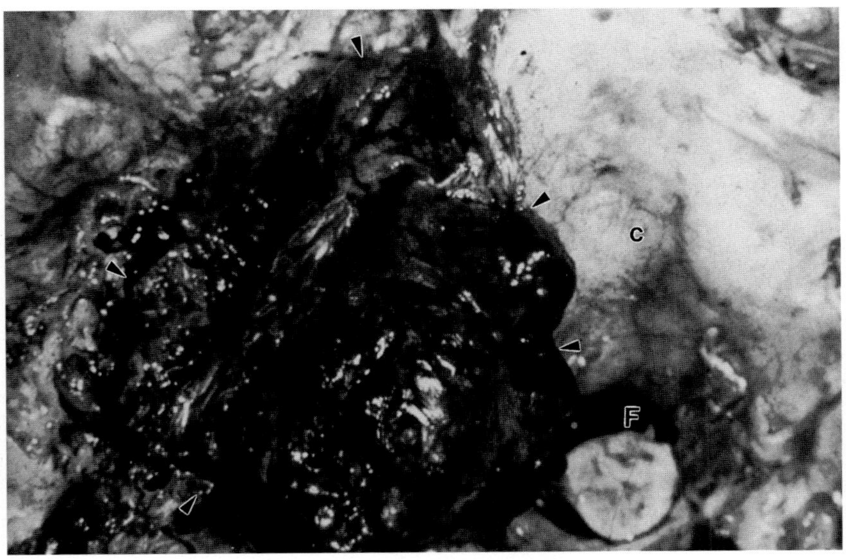

FIG. 14-1. Autopsy photograph of a fatal glomus jugulare tumor (*arrowheads* illustrate tumor eroding intracranially via the jugular foramen) with brainstem compression. C, clivus; F, cervical spinal cord at foramen magnum. (Courtesy of House Ear Institute.)

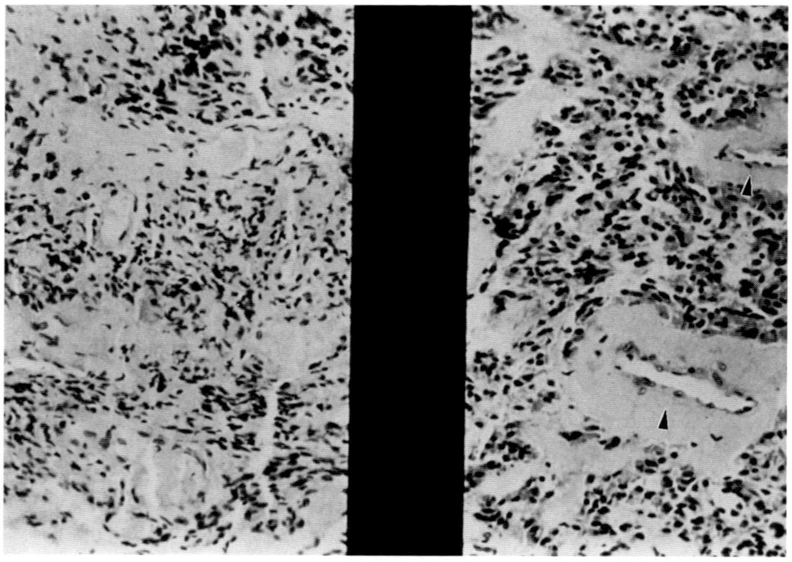

FIG. 14-2. Untreated **(left)** and postradiation **(right)** photomicrograph of glomus jugulare tumor. Tumor cells are viable but there is obliterative endarteritis (*arrowheads*) with fibrosis of the supporting cells. (Courtesy of House Ear Institute.)

more focused radiation such as gamma knife or linear accelerator. These treatments represent focused radiation therapy, which spares the surrounding structures. Nonetheless, the clinical effect is the same. We are unaware of any series with over a 15-year follow-up following treatment with contemporary doses of gamma knife therapy. Although there are some initial reports of efficacy of gamma knife, they all are of short term (less than the 15 years required for regrowth in most cases of conventional external beam radiation). In addition, in an effort to minimize complications, the overall treatment dosage has decreased. Accordingly, follow-up of the contemporary dosages of gamma knife or linear accelerator therapy are vital before recommending this as standard therapy for younger patients. Nonetheless, an older patient who is medically unstable for surgical intervention is a suitable candidate for radiation if the expected life span is less than the 10- to 15-year control effect of the radiation therapy itself.

PATIENT SELECTION

The selection of surgical approach and treatment of a patient with a paraganglioma and the subsequent evaluation, reporting, and comparison treatment results are based on accurate preoperative classification. Two popular classification schemes are those proposed by Ugo Fisch (5) and Gary Jackson/Michael Glassock (6) (Tables 14-1 and 14-2). These classification schemes have been proposed primarily based on tumor origin and anatomic extent of lesion. We find most useful the clinical/surgical classification proposed by Antonio de la Cruz in planning the clinical management of patients with paragangliomas (Table 14-3) (7). This system is particularly helpful because it combines the anatomic location of the tumor with the planned surgical approach. A series of operations that correspond to the extent of tumor is used.

TABLE 14–1. *Glomus tumors: Fisch classification*

Type A	Tumors limited to the middle ear cleft
Type B	Tumors limited to the tympanomastoid area with no infralabyrinthine compartment involvement
Type C	Tumors involving the infralabyrinthine compartment of the temporal bone and extending into the petrous apex
Type D	Tumors with an intracranial extension less than 2 cm in diameter
Type E	Tumors with an intracranial extension greater than 2 cm in diameter

TABLE 14–2. *Glassock-Jackson glomus tumor classification*

Type	Physical findings
Glomus tympanicum	
Type I	Small mass limited to the promontory
Type II	Tumor completely filling middle ear space
Type III	Tumor filling middle ear and extending into mastoid
Type IV	Tumor filling middle ear, extending into mastoid or through tympanic membrane to fill external auditory canal; may also extend anterior to internal carotid artery
Glomus jugulare	
Type I	Small tumor involving jugulare bulb, middle ear, and mastoid
Type II	Tumor extending under the internal auditory canal; may have intracranial extension
Type III	Tumor extending into petrous apex; may have intracranial extension
Type IV	Tumor extending beyond petrous apex into clivus or infratemporal fossa; may have intracranial extension

TABLE 14–3. *Modified De la Cruz glomus tumor classification with associated surgical approach*

Classification	Surgical approach
1. Tympanic	Transcanal
2. Tympanomastoid	Mastoid-extended facial recess
3. Jugular bulb	Mastoid-neck (possible limited facial nerve rerouting)
4. Carotid artery	Infratemporal fossa ± subtemporal
5. Transdural	Infratemporal fossa/intracranial
6. Craniocervical	Transcondylar
7. Vagale	Cervical

Jugular Bulb Tumor

This lesion arises from the glomus body of the dome of the jugular bulb. It may extend into the middle ear and also into the bulb itself. This lesion is limited to involvement of the middle ear, mastoid, and the jugular bulb. By definition, it does not extend onto the carotid artery or medially into the skull base or intracranially.

Carotid Artery Glomus Tumor

This lesion arises from the jugular bulb but extends beyond the confines of the jugular bulb and vein and contacts the carotid artery. Small tumors of this category may involve only the carotid artery at the skull base, whereas larger tumors may extend far medially and may also involve the horizontal portion of the internal carotid artery and the petrous apex.

Transdural Tumor

These lesions arise from the jugular bulb and extend not only to the internal carotid artery but also through the jugular foramen intracranially.

Craniocervical Tumor

These lesions are extensive intracranial extensions of glomus jugulare tumors with compression of the brainstem toward the foramen magnum. However, extensive glomus vagale tumors may also extend superiorly through the foramen magnum to produce brainstem and cervical compression as well.

SCHWANNOMA

Schwannomas of the jugular foramen are extremely rare even though they are the second most frequently occurring tumor of the jugular foramen. They arise from the schwann cells of cranial nerves IX, X, and XI. The most common cranial nerve to be affected is the vagus (22,23). The clinical distinction between glomus vagale tumors and vagal schwannomas is that glomus vagale tumors develop vocal cord paralysis early in their course (24).

Presentation of the jugular foramen schwannoma depends upon the growth pattern. Kaye et al. (25) categorized three different patterns: A, B, and C. Type A tumors present primarily in the posterior fossa. Type A tumors with intracranial extension may present with ninth, tenth, or 11th cranial nerve palsies. However, like most cerebellopontine angle tumors, hearing loss and/or vertigo may be the only significant presenting symptoms. Type B tumors remain confined to the skull base with extension often into the clivus. Type C tumors begin in the jugular foramen and extend inferiorly into the neck. Type B and C tumors present more frequently with lower cranial neuropathies than do type A tumors (25).

Radiologic assessment is performed with MRI and CT. MRI of a jugular foramen schwannoma will demonstrate a smooth contoured mass isodensed on T1; high signal intensity is usually noted on T2, and significant enhancement occurs on T1-weighted gadolinium scans (Fig. 14-3).

CT is helpful in differentiating schwannoma from glomus jugulare tumors. Schwannomas tend to produce a smooth bone erosion of the jugular foramen. Glomus tumors tend to show an irregular bone margin and bone structure of the jugular foramen (Fig. 14-4). Schwannomas also tend to enhance less than glomus jugulare tumors after contrast injection.

Treatment of jugular foramen schwannomas is surgical excision. A consensus on a single surgical approach does not exist. Tumors that present primarily with intracranial extension may be excised through a combined retrolabyrinthine and suboccipital craniotomy. If hearing is poor, a translabyrinthine approach has been described (23). Tumors involving primarily the jugular foramen and skull base should be approached through mastoid-neck or infratemporal fossa approaches. The age of the patient, general medical condition, and size of the tumor may influence other modalities of treatment, such as radiation or observation.

Meningiomas of the jugular foramen may be difficult to distinguish from schwannomas preoperatively. An enhancing "dural tail" on MRI is helpful. The treatment considerations are comparable to schwannoma of the jugular foramen.

PATIENT COUNSELING

Patients with jugular foramen tumors should be informed of the risks inherent in complete removal of their tumors. Specifically, facial nerve transposition may be necessary and carries the attendant risk of facial paresis. Furthermore, these patients should be informed of the risk of lower cranial nerve injury and possible vascular complications as well. Any patient with intradural tumor extension must be informed of the risks of craniotomy, including postoperative hemorrhage, cerebrospinal fluid leakage, meningitis, coma, and even death.

SURGICAL APPROACHES

The following surgical techniques are used for removal of glomus jugulare tumors of the temporal bone. However,

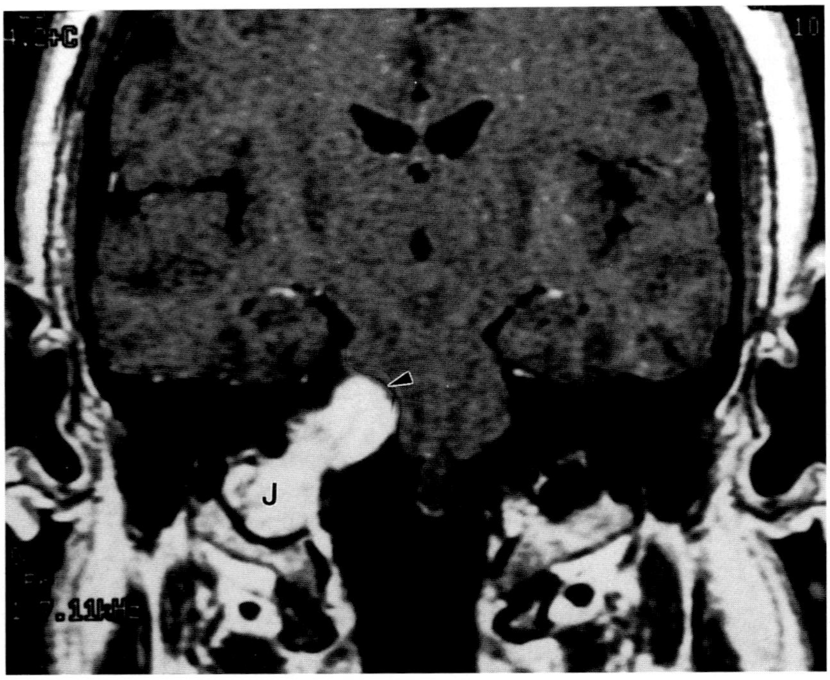

FIG. 14-3. Coronal enhanced T1 magnetic resonance imaging (MRI) of a jugular foramen schwannoma with intradural extension. Note the smooth expansion of the bone of the jugular foramen (J) and brainstem compression (*arrowhead*).

the basic techniques can be used for surgical exposure of schwannomas and meningiomas of the jugular foramen. Notice that the specific approaches described correspond to the tumor classification system described earlier (Table 14-3).

Mastoid and Neck Approach

The mastoid and neck approach is used for small glomus jugulare tumors (Fig. 14-5). These tumors involve the jugular bulb but do not extend onto the internal carotid artery or into the neck or posterior fossa. The preoperative evaluation of these patients may include angiography because involvement of the jugular bulb raises the question of possible carotid artery involvement. Continuous intraoperative facial nerve monitoring is used. Additionally, electromyographic electrodes in the sternocleidomastoid muscle are useful for monitoring cranial nerve XI, electrodes in the lateral pharyngeal wall can monitor cranial nerve IX, and electrodes in the vocalis muscle can monitor cranial nerve X. A recent modification is use of a specially adapted endotracheal tube with imbedded EMG Electroder (Xomed-Treace, Jacksonville, FL) to monitor the tenth nerve. The procedure is performed by initially completing a mastoid-extended facial recess approach, then amputating the mastoid tip. The periosteum of the digastric groove is followed anteriorly until it turns abruptly laterally at the stylomastoid foramen. Drilling laterally along the digastric ridge both anteriorly and posteriorly frees the entire mastoid tip. The incision is then carried into the neck along the anterior border of the sternocleidomastoid muscle. This muscle is freed from the mastoid tip and retracted posteriorly. The mastoid tip can then be removed by grasping it with a Kocher clamp and cutting with a curved Mayo scissors along the bone. The posterior belly of the digastric muscle is identified and freed from the digastric groove and retracted anteriorly to allow exposure of the major neurovascular structures of the neck. Once the internal jugular vein is identified and dissected free from surrounding tissues, it is occluded with multiple 2-0 silk sutures. The jugular vein is followed over the transverse process of the first cervical vertebra into the base of the skull. In this fashion, the 11th cranial nerve is identified (usually lateral to the vein) and preserved.

In limited tumors that do not extend into the neck or skull base, it is usually possible to preserve the ninth, tenth, and 11th cranial nerves. The neck exposure is necessary to permit ligation of the jugular vein.

Exposure of the sigmoid sinus and jugular bulb is then completed with diamond burrs. Although limited tumors do not involve the medial wall of the jugular foramen, the tumor arises from the dome of the jugular bulb, and the bulb must be resected in continuity with the tumor. The proximal sigmoid sinus is controlled with extraluminal packing of oxidized cellulose. Preservation of the bone over the midportion of the sigmoid sinus permits extraluminal packing of this portion of the sigmoid sinus. Because the jugular vein has been tied in the neck, the sigmoid sinus may be opened just distal to the proximal packing. Bleeding occurs at this point from the patent inferior petrosal sinus and condylar vein. Oxidized cellulose is advanced into the jugular bulb to control this bleeding. This packing must not be placed too firmly, as weakness of cranial nerves IX, X, and XI may result.

The tumor is now ready for resection in continuity with the dome of the jugular bulb. Bipolar cautery helps in hemostasis and shrinkage of the tumor bulk. Once the tumor and dome of the jugular bulb are excised, hemostasis is completed with oxidized cellulose packing. Complete tumor resection is accomplished, and if the tympanic membrane or

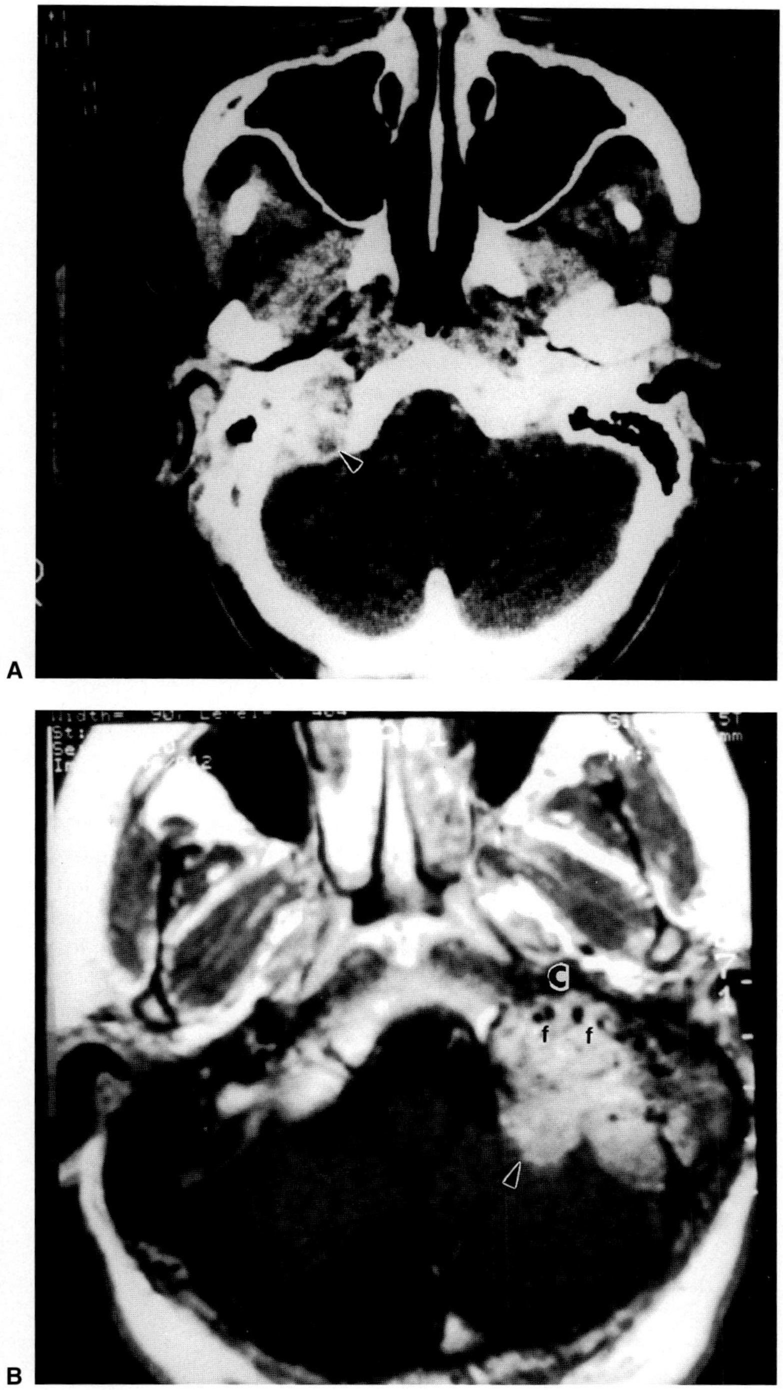

FIG. 14-4. A: Computed tomography (CT) of a jugular bulb glomus tumor. Note the irregular destruction of the jugular foramen (*arrowhead*). **B:** T1-enhanced MRI of glomus jugulare tumor involving carotid (*C*) (carotid artery tumor) with limited intradural extension (*arrowhead*). Note flow voids (*F*).

ossicles are involved, reconstruction may be performed as described earlier. It is usually possible to preserve the ninth, tenth, and 11th cranial nerves with these limited tumors unless there is preoperative involvement of these structures. Postoperatively, these patients are cared for in the intensive care unit because the possibility of an acute lower cranial neuropathy or major postoperative hemorrhage exists. Usually, minimal morbidity is associated with this approach, and patients are stable and may be discharged from the hospital within a few days. The major pitfall associated with this approach is related to inaccurate preoperative assessment of tumor extent. The mastoid-neck approach is too limited if the tumor involves the carotid artery.

Mastoid and Neck with Limited Facial Nerve Rerouting

A useful modification of the mastoid-neck approach adds a limited facial nerve rerouting to the procedure (Fig. 14-5). Additional exposure in the mastoid-neck approach may be achieved by totally decompressing the facial nerve from the second genu throughout the entire vertical segment. The

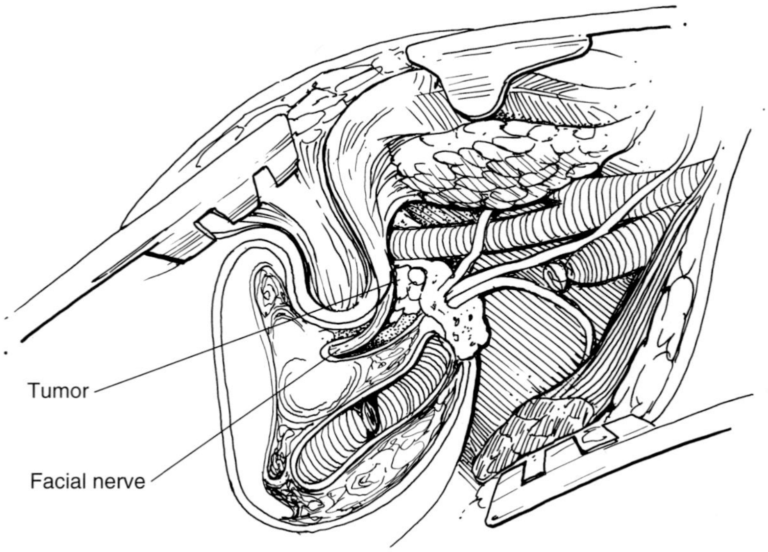

FIG. 14-5. Mastoid and neck approach: a complete mastoidectomy with extended facial recess is combined with exposure of the upper neck. Small glomus jugulare tumors and glomus tympanicum lesions that do not involve the carotid artery may be managed with this approach. The facial nerve may be left in situ or partially mobilized with a limited facial nerve rerouting as illustrated in the diagram.

periosteum of the facial nerve at the stylomastoid foramen is preserved, but the fibrous attachments to the nerve in its vertical portion are sharply transected. The mobilized nerve can be transported laterally along with the periosteum at the stylomastoid foramen and the attached posterior belly of the digastric muscle. A suture through the stylomastoid periosteum can be used to hold the nerve laterally and prevent traction on this structure. Such transposition of the facial nerve will permit further bone removal in the area of the vertical facial canal and retrofacial air cells along the infralabyrinthine air cell tract. This modification of the mastoid and neck approach with limited facial nerve rerouting is ideal for neuromas of the jugular foramen because they are not as intimately involved with the carotid artery as are glomus tumors. The surgeon should be cautious about applying this approach for glomus tumors that involve the carotid artery. The tympanic annulus and posterior wall still limit the surgeon's view of the vertical portion of the carotid artery if extensive manipulation is necessary in this area.

Infratemporal Fossa Approach (Posterior)

The development of the infratemporal fossa approach by Fisch (26) has been a significant advance in our ability to totally remove large glomus jugulare tumors (Fig. 14-6). Previous approaches that did not remove the external auditory canal or reroute the facial nerve did not allow adequate exposure of the tumor or internal carotid artery. There are eight distinct steps in the infratemporal fossa exposure:

1. Patient preparation
2. Management of the ear canal and tympanic ring
3. Mastoidectomy
4. Initial preparation of the jugular vein and neck exposure
5. Transposition of the facial nerve
6. Completion of the neck exposure and identification of the lower cranial nerves and skull base carotid artery
7. Tumor removal and intracranial extension
8. Wound closure

Continuous facial nerve monitoring and electromyographic monitoring of the lower cranial nerves are employed as previously described. A wide shave is performed, and a large postauricular incision is made in a C-shaped fashion. The incision is carried anteriorly, and the ear canal is transected slightly medially to the bone-cartilage junction of the ear canal. Cartilage is removed from the ear canal to permit

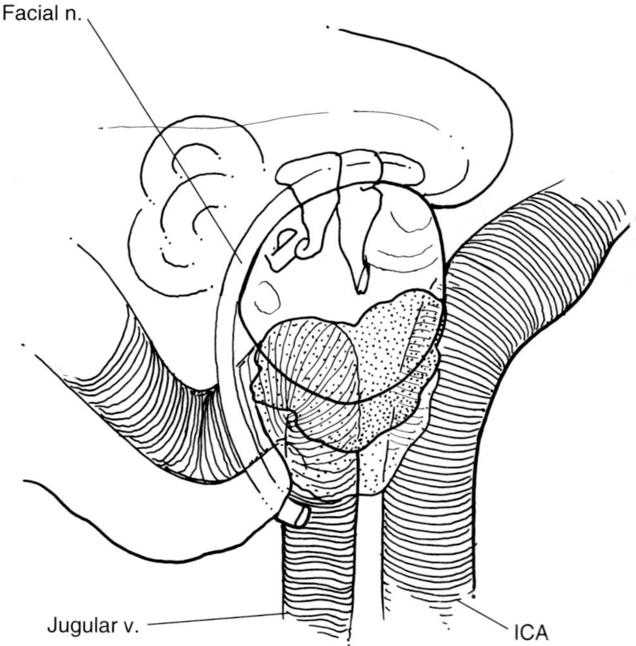

FIG. 14-6. Relationships of glomus jugulare to jugulare vein, carotid artery, facial nerve, and middle ear.

fashioning of the ear canal as a cuff that can be everted. The skin of the meatus is closed with 4-0 nylon sutures. The periosteum of the postauricular area is elevated as a flap and sutured behind the opening in the meatus to further reinforce the closure. Next, a mastoidectomy is completed, and the facial recess is opened to allow separation of the incudostapedial joint. The posterior wall of the ear canal can then be removed with rongeurs and cutting burrs. The remaining skin of the ear canal as well as the tympanic membrane, malleus, and incus are removed. Next, the facial nerve is decompressed from the geniculate to the stylomastoid foramen. An eggshell-thin layer of bone is left over the nerve itself. By use of cutting and diamond burrs, the bone of the tympanic ring is progressively removed, the level of the jugular bulb is identified, and the bone over the temporomandibular joint and vertical segment of the petrous carotid artery is removed anteriorly (Fig. 14-7).

Attention is then focused on the neck. The incision is continued vertically along the anterior border of the sternocleidomastoid muscle, the mastoid tip is removed as previously described, the jugular vein is identified, and ligatures are placed around the vein but are not yet tied at this point. The carotid artery is identified and marked with a ligature. The posterior belly of the digastric muscle is transected.

Next, the facial nerve is transposed. The transposition technique originally described by Fisch has been modified because of temporary and sometimes permanent residual facial weakness (27). Rather than exposing the facial nerve in the parotid, the surgeon transposes the nerve with periosteum of the stylomastoid foramen and elevates the entire tail of the parotid (28). After decompressing the nerve, the remaining egg shell–thin bone over the facial nerve is removed with a blunt instrument. The multiple fibrous connections along the descending portion of the nerve are transected sharply. The tympanic portion of the nerve does not have such adhesions, and this section elevates readily. The posterior belly of the digastric muscle is moved anteriorly because the fascia of this muscle contributes to the stylomastoid foramen periosteum. The nerve can then be transposed anteriorly along with the tail of the parotid. A large suture is placed through the periosteum of the stylomastoid foramen and attached to the soft tissues in the area of the root of the zygoma, thereby elevating the facial nerve and preventing it from being stretched when retractors are placed. The use of continuous facial nerve monitoring during this maneuver has significantly improved postoperative facial nerve function (Fig. 14-8) (29).

After the facial nerve is decompressed and elevated, a large Perkins retractor is placed beneath the angle of the mandible, and the entire mandible is retracted forward. This exposure usually avoids the need to resect the mandibular condyle, even in large tumors that extend into the infratemporal fossa extensively. The remaining bone over the distal sigmoid sinus, jugular bulb, and vertical portion of the petrous carotid artery can be removed with diamond burrs. Attention is once again focused in the neck, where the internal carotid artery is followed through the skull base into its intratemporal course. The lower cranial nerves (IX, X, and XI) are followed into the jugular foramen as well. The 12th cranial nerve is also identified and followed to its foramen.

The jugular vein is doubly ligated and transected between ligatures, and the external carotid artery is ligated. If the tumor extends intradurally, the proximal sigmoid sinus is doubly ligated with silk sutures. If the tumor is not intradural, then the sigmoid can be packed with Surgicel without violating the dura. The jugular vein is then elevated, and the tumor in the area of the jugular bulb is freed inferiorly to superiorly following the jugular vein into the jugular bulb. The tumor is freed from the carotid artery anteriorly, and bleeding from the caroticotympanic vessels is controlled with bipolar cautery. If the tumor is adherent to the internal carotid artery, it is best to leave a portion of it on the artery and remove

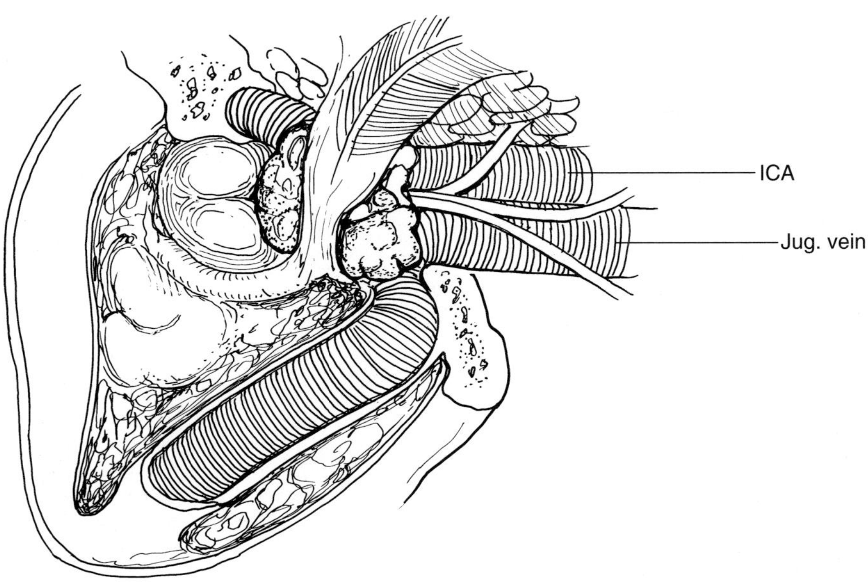

FIG. 14-7. Initial exposure in the infratemporal fossa approach. The mastoidectomy with resection of the tympanicum ring and dural sinus exposure has been completed.

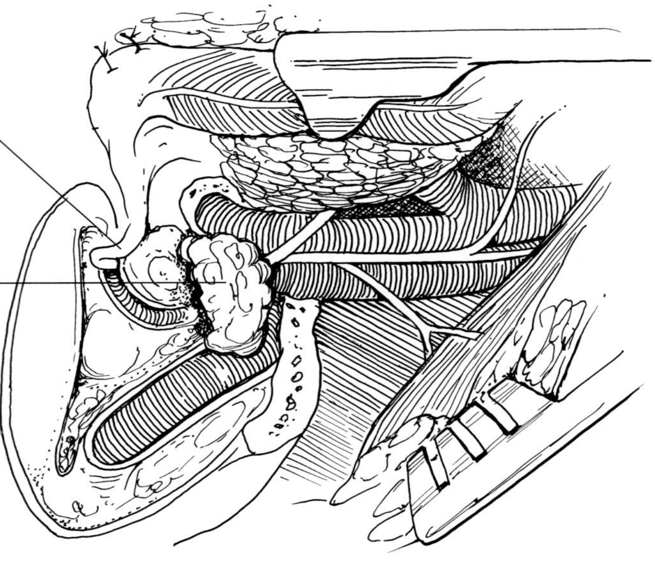

FIG. 14-8. Facial nerve transposition in the infratemporal fossa approach. The nerve is protected to prevent potentially damaging traction from excessive manipulation.

the bulk of the tumor. Tumor hemostasis is continued with bipolar cautery and oxidized cellulose packing of the inferior petrosal sinus; the tumor can be removed in continuity with the dome of the jugular bulb. If the last bit of the tumor from the carotid artery is not removed until the conclusion of the procedure, a small entry into the carotid artery that may occur at the location of the caroticotympanic artery can be repaired directly (Fig. 14-9).

Small intracranial tumor extensions are usually removed at the time of removal of the jugular bulb because this is the usual location of dural penetration. If there is extensive intracranial extension, however, a decision must be made about whether to attempt total removal of the tumor. The decision is largely based on the amount of blood lost up to this point in the operation. If blood loss has been limited to less than 3,000 mL, as is almost always the case, removal of the intracranial extension of the tumor may proceed. However, if the amount of blood loss has been greater, problems with bleeding may occur despite the replenishment of the known clotting factors with fresh frozen plasma and platelet packs. In such cases, a two-stage procedure with removal of the intracranial portion of the tumor at a later date is planned.

The removal of the intracranial portion of the tumor is often easier than the removal of tumor within the temporal bone. By the time one is ready for the removal of the intracranial extension, the blood supply has been obliterated. The blood supply to the intracranial portion of the tumor is often discrete and can be controlled with bipolar cautery as with other cerebellopontine angle tumors. If tumor has been left

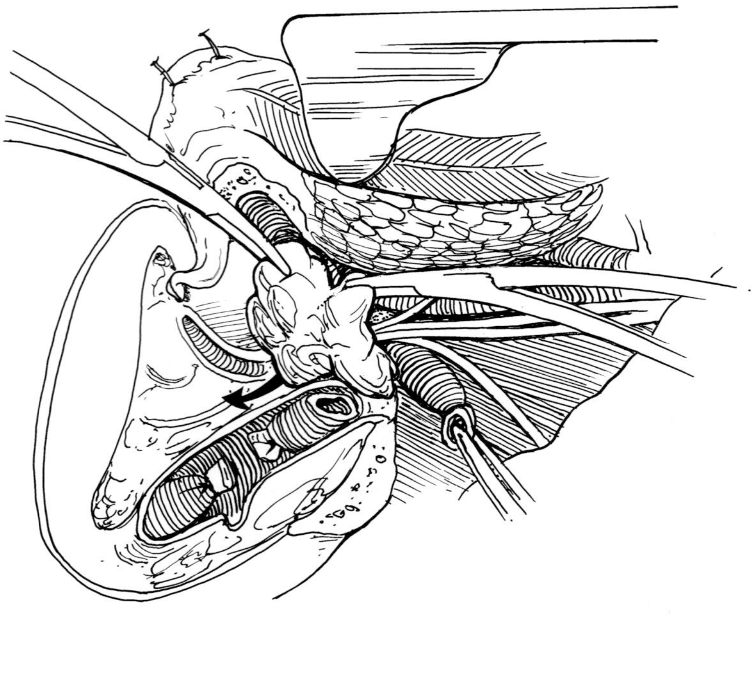

FIG. 14-9. Tumor resection proceeds systematically from inferior to superior. Tumor attachments to the carotid are removed last in the event of inadvertent carotid injury.

along the internal carotid artery, it is now removed. Closure is accomplished by closing the eustachian tube with oxidized cellulose and pieces of muscle. The mastoid is filled with strips of abdominal fat. A drain is left in the neck wound and removed on the first postoperative morning. A pressure dressing is placed for 4 postoperative days.

One technique with encouraging results in cases with large blood loss has been the use of the Cell Saver (Hemonics, Braintree, MA), which is commonly used in cardiovascular surgery. By use of this special irrigating suction device with a heparinized reservoir, intraoperative blood loss can be salvaged and prepared for replacement to the patient during the same procedure. Additionally, we routinely counsel patients on preoperative autologous donation of blood to minimize the need for banked blood replacement.

In jugular foramen tumors with a patent jugular bulb, preoperative occlusion of the inferior petrosal sinus and condylar vein may be performed to minimize the blood loss from these structures when the jugular bulb is opened (30). Care must be taken to perform this preoperative endovascular occlusion only when the surgeon is certain that the lesion requires resection of the jugular bulb.

A newer strategy for preservation of facial function in jugular foramen surgery is the fallopian bridge technique, in which the facial nerve is left in situ but the bone surrounding the nerve is almost completely removed (Fig. 14-10) (31). Although the technique is relatively new, it promises to decrease the number of cases requiring facial nerve translocations.

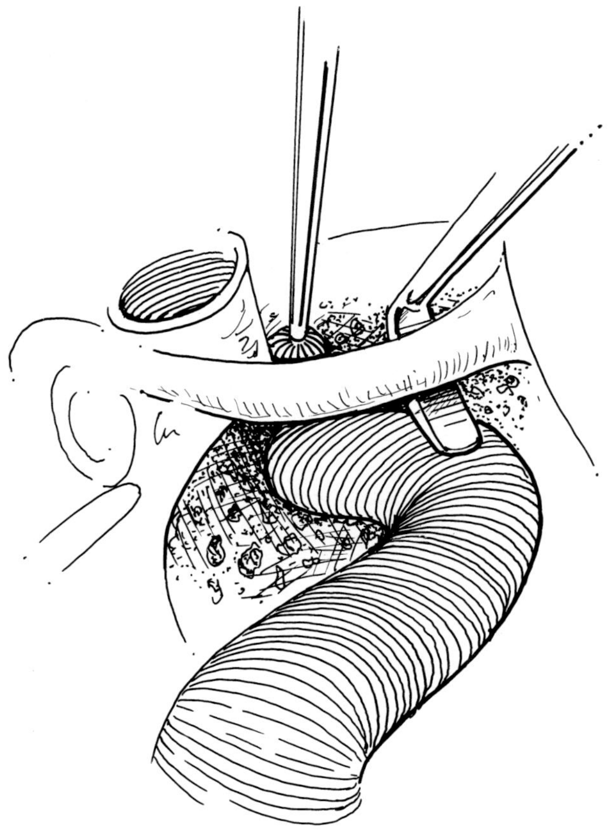

FIG. 14-10. Fallopian bridge technique. In this modification the facial nerve is dissected but left in situ without disturbing the tympanic membrane and middle ear.

Transcondylar Approach

In certain recurrent glomus jugulare tumors, the intracranial tumor may extend significantly toward the foramen magnum. In those situations, a wider exposure of the craniocervical junction is necessary. Although the transsigmoid translabyrinthine exposure offers a wide view, the craniocervical junction itself is not fully exposed with this procedure. In those cases, the transcondylar exposure is combined with the infratemporal fossa approach. The steps involved in the transcondylar approach (32) are initially extension of the muscular incisions of the posterior superior aspect of the upper neck to identify the vertebral artery posterior and inferior to the mastoid tip on the transverse process of C-1. Once this landmark is clearly identified, wide exposure of the occipital condyle and jugular tubercle permits full exposure of the hypoglossal nerve as well as wide infrajugular exposure and unlimited visualization of the craniocervical junction (Fig. 14-11). If more than half of the occipital condyle is resected, careful consideration should be given to a simultaneous cervical stabilization procedure. When transcondylar exposure is needed in addition to standard otologic exposure, we find the use of head-holding pins and a lateral position helpful for unimpeded access to the posterior superior skull base.

Complete Carotid Mobilization

In very rare cases of recurrent glomus jugulare tumors following previous surgery and radiation, the tumor may completely encase the petrous carotid artery with significant extension into the far anterior infratemporal fossa. In these cases, we have found the combination of the standard otologic (posterior) infratemporal fossa approach in combination with the preauricular infratemporal fossa approach quite useful. Specifically, an orbitozygotomy in continuity with the glenoid fossa is performed following a temporal craniotomy. In this fashion, the glenoid can be reconstructed at the conclusion of the procedure. The carotid canal can then be followed directly and fully from the base of the skull all the way to the cavernous sinus. In this way, the carotid artery can be mobilized anteriorly and inferiorly if necessary for complete tumor resection. Furthermore, this approach facilitates any carotid reconstruction if necessary.

Wound Management

Usually abdominal fat and temporalis muscle transposition provide adequate wound closure. If the surgery requires a large dural opening, or if the postoperative course is complicated by aspiration-related coughing, cerebrospinal (CSF) leakage can be troublesome. This problem is usually man-

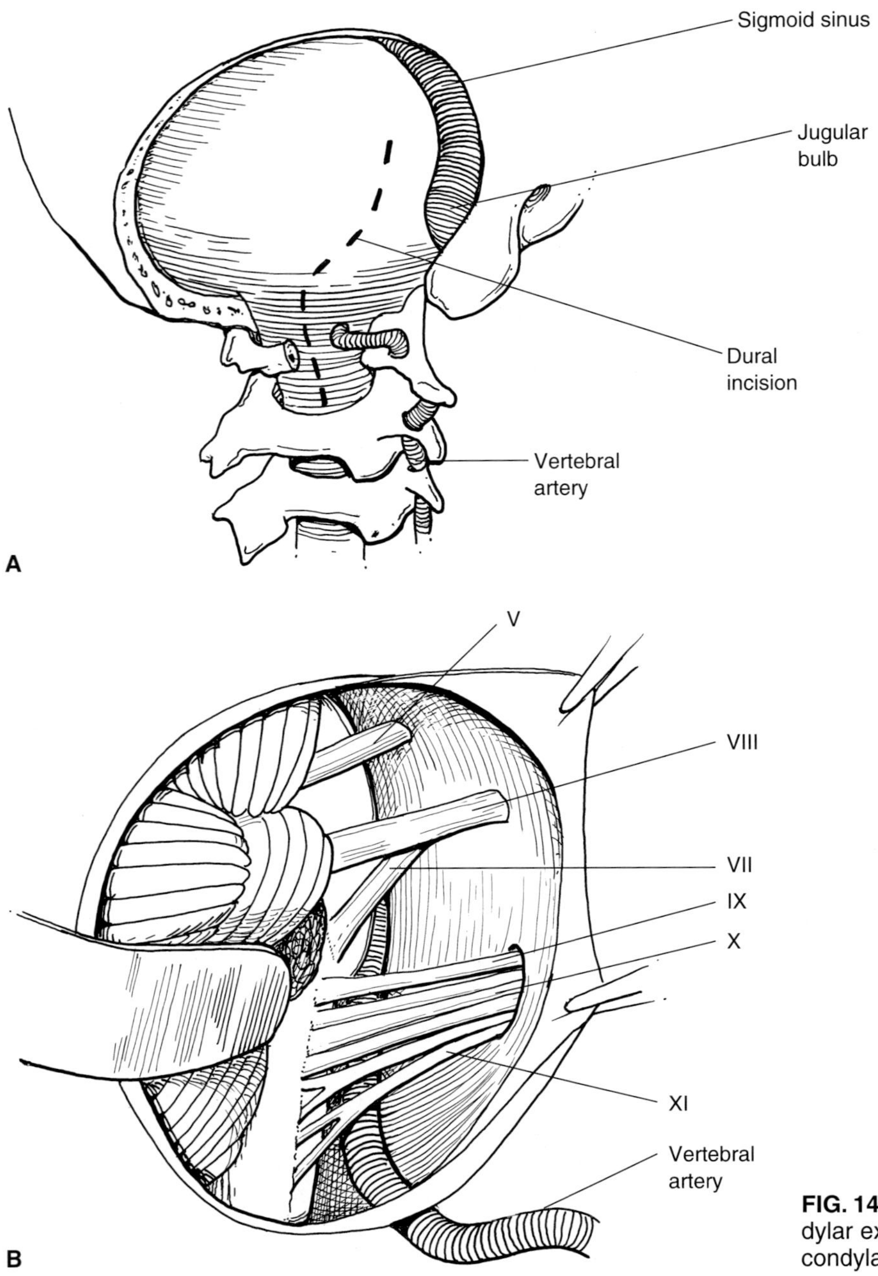

FIG. 14-11. A: Extradural relationships of transcondylar exposure. **B:** Intradural relationships of transcondylar exposure.

aged by a short course of lumbar CSF drainage. Wound revision is rarely required.

In reoperations, previously operated patients, or large deficits with limited local tissue available, free muscle grafts with microvascular anastomosis are the treatment of choice.

RESULTS

Glomus Jugulare Tumors

Green et al. (33) recently reviewed the treatment of patients with glomus jugulare tumors (jugular bulb, carotid artery involvement tumors, and intradural tumors); 52 patients who had undergone no prior radiotherapy or surgery were surgically treated for glomus jugulare tumors (33). The techniques involved were the infratemporal fossa approach in 83%, the mastoid-neck approach in 7%, and the mastoid-neck with limited facial nerve mobilization in 10%. Complete surgical removal was possible in 85% of the patients. Eight patients required transection of the facial nerve for complete tumor removal. These patients underwent segmental grafting or greater auricular nerve reconstruction. The mean intraoperative blood loss was 1,500 mL. Long-term facial function was good: over 94% of patients had grade I/VI or II/VI facial function at 1-year follow-up or greater. Nearly 20% of patients required a vocal cord augmentation procedure. However, no patient required a tracheotomy in the immediate postoperative period. Four patients required prolonged nasogastric tube feeding, and two ultimately requiring gastrostomy. Eighty-five percent of the patients were able to resume the same activity level as before surgery.

The morbidity in revision procedures is usually greater than in previously unoperated patients. Neural preservation is much more difficult in a scarred operative field with tumor infiltration of surgically created tissue planes.

Neurogenic Jugular Foramen Lesions

The results of neurogenic jugular foramen tumors are different than glomus jugulare tumors. Neurogenic tumors rarely affect the facial nerve, so facial function is less jeopardized. In contrast, since these tumors develop from the lower cranial nerve, ninth and tenth cranial nerve dysfunction is more common. In addition, these lesions generally have more intradural involvement than glomus jugulare tumors.

POSTOPERATIVE CARE

Just as the surgical care requires individualization, postoperative requirements are directly related to the operative findings and postoperative cranial nerve function. Patients with large extradural tumors or any intradural tumors are kept in the intensive care unit for at least one postoperative day before transfer to a regular nursing floor.

Patients with new-onset dysphagia from ninth and tenth cranial nerve dysfunction require early intervention. Speech pathologists with special expertise are consulted early to employ special swallowing strategies and formal swallowing studies. Early vocal cord medialization is also employed. Occasionally, tracheotomy and gastrostomy are still necessary although some centers find vocal cord medialization at the time of tumor removal helpful (34), we defer airway surgery until edema from tracheal intubation has resolved.

CONCLUSION

The management of jugular foramen tumors requires accurate preoperative evaluation with an individualized, multispecialty operative and postoperative management team. Glomus jugulare lesions are the most common neoplasms of this region; however, neurogenic lesions must also be considered. Modern diagnostic techniques with current skull base surgical approaches offer most patients an excellent outcome.

REFERENCES

1. Guild SR. A hitherto unrecognized structure in man. *Anat Rec* 1941; 79:(suppl 2):28.
2. Rosenwasser H. Carotid body tumor of the middle ear and mastoid. *Arch Otolaryngol* 1945;41:64–67.
3. Valvassori GE. Radiologic diagnosis neuro-otologic problems by tomography. *Arch Otolaryngol* 1969;89:57–60.
4. Alford BR, Guilford FR. A comprehensive study of tumors of the glomus jugulare. *Laryngoscope* 1962;72:765–787.
5. Fisch U. Infratemporal fossa approach to tumors of the temporal bone and base of skull. *J Laryngol Otol* 1978;92:949–967.
6. Glassock MC, Jackson CG, Harris PF. Glomus tumors: diagnosis, classification, and management of large lesions. *Arch Otolaryngol* 1982; 108:401–406.
7. Arriaga MA. Surgery for glomus tumors. In: Brackmann DE, Shelton C, Arriaga MA, eds. *Otologic Surgery*. Philadelphia: WB Saunders, 1994:580.
8. Gulya AJ. The glomus tumor and its biology. *Laryngoscope* 1993; 103(suppl 60):7–15.
9. Spector GJ, Ciralski R, Maisel RH, et al. Multiple glomus tumors in the head and neck. *Laryngoscope* 1975;85:1066–1075.
10. Borsaryi SJ. Glomus jugulare tumors. *Laryngoscope* 1962;72: 1336–1345.
11. Arriaga MA, Brackmann DE. Differential diagnosis of primary petrous apex lesions. *Am J Otol* 1991;12(6):470–474.
12. Arriaga MA, Lo WWM, Brackmann DE. Imaging case study of the month: magnetic resonance angiography of synchronized bilateral carotid body paragangliomas and bilateral vagal paragangliomas. *Ann Otol Rhinol Laryngol* 1992;101:955–957.
13. Rogers GP, Brackmann DE, Lo WWM. Magnetic resonance angiography, a technique for evaluation of skull base lesions. *J Otol* 1993;14(1): 56–62.
14. Janecka IP, Sekhar LN, Horton JA. General blood flow evaluation. In: Cummings CW, Fredrickson JM, Harker LH, et al., eds. *Otolaryngology head and neck surgery update II*. St. Louis: Mosby Year Book, 1990:54–63.
15. deVries EJ. A new method to predict safe resection of the internal carotid artery. *Laryngoscope* 1990;100:85–89.
16. Murphy TP, Brackmann DE. Effects of preoperative embolization on glomus jugulare tumors. *Laryngoscope* 1989;99:1244–1247.
17. Brackmann DE, House WF, Terry R, et al. Glomus jugulare tumors: effects of irradiation. *Trans Am Acad Ophthalmol Otolaryngol* 1972; 76:1423–1431.
18. Bickerstff ER, Howell JS. The neurological importance of tumors of the glomus jugulare. *Brain* 1953;76:576–693.
19. Steinberg N, Holz WG. Glomus jugulare tumors. *Arch Otolaryngol Head Neck Surg* 1965;82:387–394.
20. Brown JS. Glomus jugulare tumors revisited: a ten-year statistical follow-up of 231 cases. *Laryngoscope* 1985;95:284–285.
21. Spector GJ, Fierstein J, Ogura JH. A comparison of therapeutic modalities of glomus tumors in the temporal bone. *Laryngoscope* 1976;86: 690–969.
22. Horn KL, Honkinsan H. Tumors of the jugular foramen. In: Brackmann DE, Jackler RK, eds. *Neurotology*. Philadelphia: Mosby, 1994: 1059–1068.
23. Horn KL, House WF, Hitselberger WE. Schwannomas of the jugular foramen. *Laryngoscope* 1985;95:761–765.
24. Leonetti JP, Brackmann DE. Glomus vagale tumors: the significance of early vocal cord paralysis. *Otolaryngol Head Neck Surg* 1989;100: 533–537.
25. Kaye AH, Hahn JF, Kinney JE. Jugular foramen schwannomas. *J Neurosurg* 1984;60:1045–1053.
26. Fisch U. Infratemporal fossa approach for glomus tumors of the temporal bone. *Ann Otol Rhinol Laryngol* 1982;91:474–479.
27. Fisch U, Faga P, Valvanis A. The infratemporal fossa approach for the lateral skull base. *Otolaryngol Clin North Am* 1984;17(3):513–552.
28. Brackmann DE. The facial nerve in the infratemporal approach. *Otolaryngol Head Neck Surg* 1987;97:15–17.
29. Leonetti JP, Brackmann DE, Prass RC. Improved preservation of facial function in the infratemporal fossa approach to the skull base. *Otolaryngol Head Neck Surg* 1989;101:74–78.
30. Carrier D, Arriaga M, Dahlen R. Preoperative embolization of anastomosis of the jugular bulb: a new adjunct in jugular foramen surgery. *Am J Neuroradiol* 1997;18(7)1252–1256.
31. Pensak ML, Jackler RK. Removal of jugular foramen tumors. *Otolaryngol Head Neck Surg* 1997;117(6):586–591.
32. Fukushima T. *Manual of skull base dissection*. Pittsburgh: AF Neurovideo, 1996.
33. Green JD, Nguyen CD, Arriaga MA, et al. Technical modifications in the surgical management of glomus jugulare tumors. *Laryngoscope (in press)*.
34. Neterrville JD. *Primary thyroplasty in glomus jugulare surgery*. Oral presentation, American Neurotology Society Fall Meeting, Washington, DC, September 13, 1992.

Neurosurgical Issues in Otolaryngology: Principles and Practice of Collaboration,
edited by Moisés A. Arriaga and J. Diaz Day.
Lippincott Williams & Wilkins, Philadelphia © 1999.

CHAPTER 15

Contemporary Diagnosis and Management of Temporal Bone Encephalocele

Douglas A. Chen

OVERVIEW

Herniation of brain into the temporal bone, usually either temporal lobe or cerebellum, has been recognized since the early 1900s. Originally, the condition was associated with trauma and chronic suppurative otitis media, but with the decreasing incidence of otogenic intracranial complications, temporal bone encephaloceles have become an uncommon entity. In contrast, the contemporary otologic literature describes a myriad of presenting sign and symptoms, many of which are not associated with suppurative disease. Cerebrospinal fluid (CSF) leakage, ear mass, hearing loss, and seizures are a few of the presenting symptoms reported. Just as the presenting clinical picture has evolved over time, the nomenclature has also. Although *encephalocele* is currently the generally accepted term, brain fungus, meningoencephalocele of the mastoid, dural herniation, brain hernia, endaural encephalocele, brain prolapse, fungus cerebri, and mastoiditis cerebri have been used in the past. Fortunately, the incidence has decreased with fewer than 150 cases reported over the last 40 years.

PATHOGENESIS

Iurato et al. (1) reviewed 139 cases of temporal bone encephaloceles. They found that 21% were spontaneous, 59% occurred as a complication of mastoid surgery, 9% followed trauma, and 9% were a complication of chronic suppurative otitis media. Knowledge of the embryology of the temporal bone may aid in understanding the pathogenesis of spontaneous encephaloceles. The temporal bone embryologically consists of four ossification centers—the squamous, tympanic, petrous, and mastoid. The mastoid begins ossification at approximately the 30th week of gestation. Pneumatization of the mastoid follows and continues into adulthood. The formation of air cells consists of a process of marrow resorption, mucosal advancement, and bone remodeling. The occurrence of dehiscence in temporal bones can be explained as a disruption of normal ossification of the temporal bone, especially in the squamous and petrous portions. Persistent dehiscence of the petrosquamous suture line due to growth abnormalities, radiation, or chemotherapy may serve as a cause of encephalocele formation. Alternatively, an abnormality in the bone remodeling during pneumatization may cause dehiscence through which encephaloceles may develop. Ahren and Thuler (2) studied the incidence of such dehiscence and found that they occurred in 21% of 94 cadavers. In addition, 16% had very thin cortical bone in the tegmen area. Similarly, Ferguson et al. (3) observed a 22% incidence of tegmen defects. Multiple dehiscences within a temporal bone were observed and are consistent with the clinical reports of multiple and bilateral encephaloceles. Dura, however, is capable of supporting brain without herniation. Hence, the observation that a tegmen defect is necessary but not sufficient to cause encephalocele and some other factors must be involved. Increased intracranial pressure, aging, and low-grade inflammation have been proposed as associated factors.

Arachnoid granulations may also be involved in the formation of encephaloceles in the mastoid and sinuses. Arachnoid granulations are macroscopic enlargements of arachnoid villi that generally drain into venous sinuses and transport CSF. They increase in size and number with age and provide for resorption of CSF into the bloodstream. They can cause bone pits and depressions through bone resorption. Gacek (4) has reported on the clinical correlation of arachnoid granulations, temporal bone dehiscence, and CSF otorrhea.

D. A. Chen: Division of Otolaryngology, Section of Neurotology, Allegheny General Hospital, Pittsburgh, Pennsylvania 15212.

Encephaloceles related to chronic otitis media most frequently result as a surgical complication. In the early 20th century acute or chronic otitis media was a common cause of brain abscess. Without antibiotics the primary treatment was surgical drainage. Transmastoid trephination of peridural and brain abscesses was an accepted procedure. Fortunately, through a host of factors such as operating microscopes and antibiotics, surgically induced encephaloceles are less common today. Dural exposure is a necessary factor, but not sufficient as an isolated factor, to cause brain herniation. Violation of dural integrity, such as from a drill or cautery, most likely must occur, also. Primary repair should be performed to prevent brain herniation or CSF leakage, which can occur immediately or delayed. Head trauma resulting in brain herniation in similar fashion must involve skull base fracture with violation of dura.

Brain herniation may occur with chronic otitis media with or without cholesteatoma, although it is rare. Bone resorption and dural injury are most likely secondary to chronic inflammation and enzymatic degradation. Kamerer and Caparosa (5) reported on 15 cases of encephalocele, four of which did not have surgery. The diagnosis was unsuspected in several cases, and consequently the authors recommended histologic confirmation be obtained on all tissue adjacent to dura even when the gross appearance of the disease is consistent with granulation tissue.

Histologically herniated brain tissue is consistent with neural tissue, gliosis, and chronic inflammation. The tissue is considered devitalized and nonfunctional and can be excised without neurologic sequelae.

DIAGNOSIS

The diagnosis of temporal bone encephalocele is primarily clinical, with a host of tests that help confirm suspicions. Clinical findings include aural fullness, conductive hearing loss, middle ear effusion, persistent watery otorrhea, middle ear, or mastoid mass. More unusual findings include seizures (6), recurrent meningitis, and pneumocephalus. A previous history of ear surgery or head trauma is helpful.

A watery-appearing ear effusion or otorrhea is a typical presentation. In our unreported series of 11 cases between 1993 and 1996, seven presented with these findings. The discharge can be persistent or intermittent. When the leak is active, discharge may egress via the eustachian tube either down the pharynx or out the nose. An ear mass behind the tympanic membrane or in a mastoid cavity is suggestive of encephalocele and tends to be blue, pulsatile, and originating along the tegmen.

If present in sufficient quantity, CSF appears as a clear, thin, watery fluid and can be collected for laboratory evaluation. Glucose, protein, and chloride levels are time-honored methods for evaluating for CSF. A CSF glucose level 60% of serum levels, protein concentration less than 200 mg/dL, and chloride concentration greater than the serum concentration level are indicators of CSF. While these tests are helpful, many times there is insufficient quantity for collection or it is contaminated. β_2-transferrin is a protein produced by neuraminidase activity that is pathognomonic of CSF. It can be detected in small amounts even when the sample is contaminated with mucus and blood (7). Computed tomography (CT) with intrathecal injection of metrizamide can demonstrate extravasation of spinal fluid and its location. Generally the leak must be large for the test to become positive for an encephalocele.

Radiologic imaging with axial and coronal CT scans and magnetic resonance imaging (MRI) is frequently diagnostic. CT is especially sensitive in detecting bone defects in the tegmen. MRI, however, is more sensitive in distinguishing brain from other soft tissue such as granulation tissue or cholesteatoma. In many instances, both CT and MRI are complementary in the information they yield. Jackson et al. (8) recently reported on 35 patients with encephaloceles. Of the 32 patients with imaging, 22 patients had CT and 14 were positive. Ten patients had MRI, eight suggestive of brain herniation.

SURGICAL TECHNIQUE

The principles of encephalocele repair include amputation of the functionless brain hernia and watertight repair of the soft tissue and bone defects. Three surgical approaches have been described: transmastoid, middle fossa, or combined transmastoid–middle fossa (9). All of the approaches begin with the patient in the supine position with the head turned toward the opposite side. Head pins are not necessary. The transmastoid approach begins with a wide cortical mastoidectomy, with confirmation of the encephalocele as well as its location and size. Posterior and lateral hernias can be managed via the transmastoid approach alone. The encephalocele is amputated and the dura is elevated through the bone defect. Fascia can then be insinuated through the bone defect and secured between the exposed dura and bone defect. The pressure of the temporal lobe keeps the fascia in place. For rigid support, surgical Silastic sheeting, cartilage, or cortical bone has been advocated (10).

If the hernia is anterior, medially based, or large, the middle fossa can be exposed either as a separate procedure or in combination with the transmastoid approach (Figs. 15-1 and 15-2). The skin incision is extended to provide exposure of the middle fossa. A large piece of fascia is harvested from the temporal muscle for dural repair. The temporal lobe is elevated and the dura is repaired either intradurally or extradurally primarily or with soft tissue. A portion of the squamous temporal bone flap is then sized to repair the skull base defect, and more soft tissue is used to cover the bone flap.

Other soft tissue options other than fascia include pericranium, pedicled temporalis muscle flap, and abdominal fat. Synthetic materials for rigid support have been reported, such as silicone sheeting, Marlex mesh, and methyl methacrylate, but there is concern of higher incidence of infection

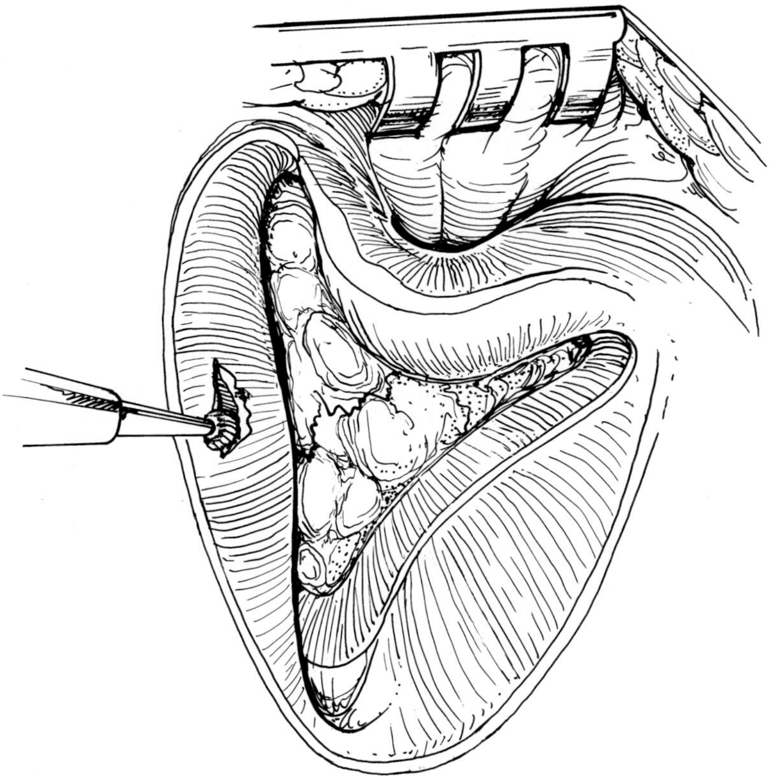

FIG. 15-1. Bony tegmen defect with dural defect approached via a mastoid approach.

or extrusion than there would be with bone. Hydroxyapatite cement has been recently approved by the Food and Drug Administration for repair of CSF leaks and appears well suited for the rigid reconstruction repair of brain hernias (11). We have limited but encouraging results with this material for encephalocele repair.

Our experience with temporal bone encephaloceles over the last 8 years is summarized in Table 15-1. The most common presenting symptom is a middle ear effusion with persistent clear watery otorrhea following placement of a tympanostomy tube. β_2-transferrin has been especially helpful in the diagnosis of spinal fluid leaks from encephaloceles. In

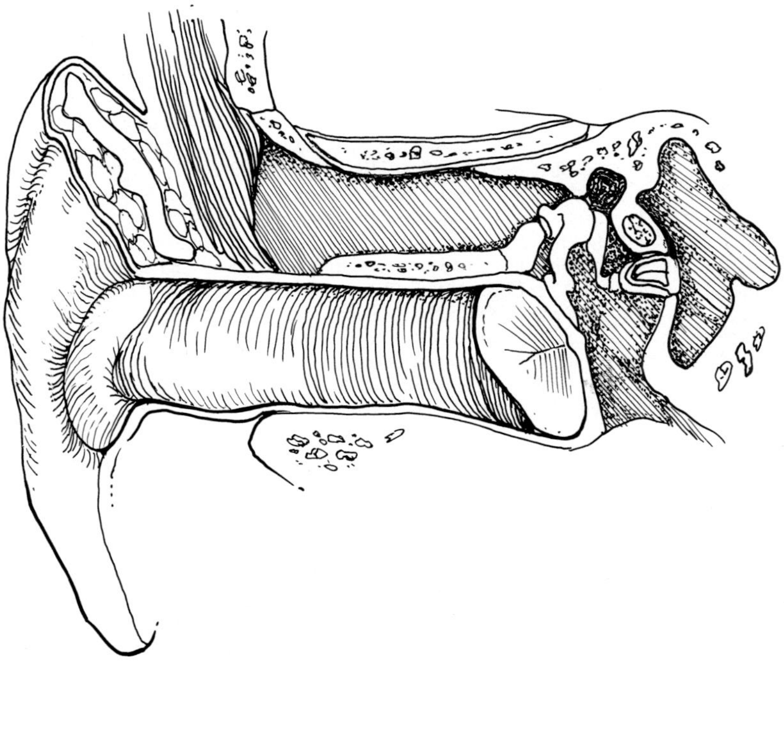

FIG. 15-2. Encephalocele repair through middle fossa craniotomy approach.

TABLE 15–1. *Temporal bone encephaloceles*

Patient number	Etiology	Presenting symptoms	Approach	Repair	Outcome
1	Head trauma	Meningitis	Middle fossa mastoid	Silastic/fascia	3 years NED
2	Spontaneous	Effusion	Middle fossa, mastoid	Methyl methacrylate/fascia	3 years NED
3	Spontaneous	Effusion	Middle fossa, mastoid	Cortical bone/fascia	2 years
4	Spontaneous	Effusion	Mastoid	Silastic/fascia	8 years
5	Spontaneous	Effusion	Middle fossa, mastoid	Silastic/fascia	1 year
6	Spontaneous	Effusion	Middle fossa, mastoid	Silastic/fascia	1 year
7	Spontaneous	Meningitis	Mastoid	Tragal cartilage	1 year
8	Spontaneous	Seizure Pneumocephalus	Mastoid	Hydroxyapatite cement/fascia	1 year NED
9	Previous surgery	Effusion	Mastoid	Silastic/fascia	5 years
10	Spontaneous	Effusion	Middle fossa, mastoid	Split calvarium bone/fascia	1 year
11	Previous surgery	Mass in mastoid cavity	Middle fossa, mastoid	Split calvarium bone/fascia	1 year

NED, No evidence of disease.

most cases the discharge can be collected on a small Gelfoam pledget placed in the ear canal adjacent to the tube. An intracranial complication was the presenting symptom in the remainder of the cases, in two patients meningitis and pneumocephalus, and seizure in a third. All patients underwent imaging preoperatively with either computed axial and coronal tomography of the temporal bone, MRI, or both (Fig. 15-3).

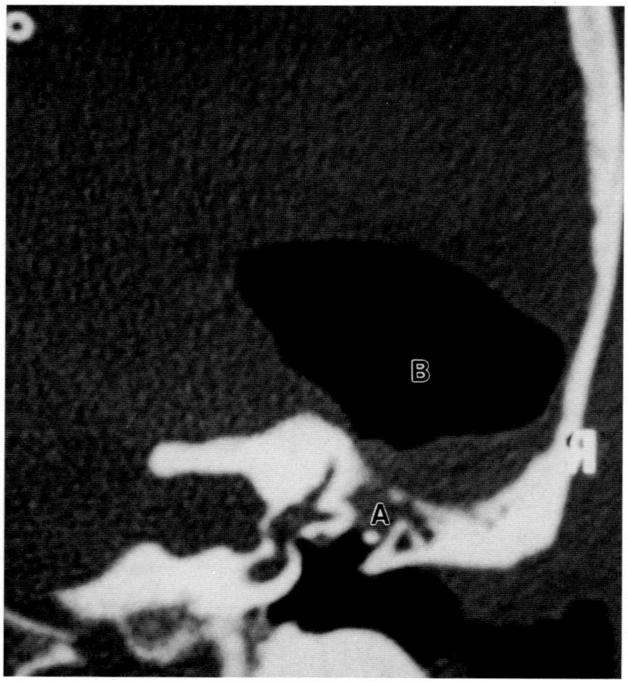

FIG. 15-3. A patient with an encephalocele **(A)** and resulting pneumocephalus **(B)**.

All patients underwent a soft tissue repair of the dural defect with fascia. The rigid repair of the bone defect was more diverse. Thick Silastic, methyl methacrylate, cortical bone, tragal cartilage, and hydroxyapatite cement were used for the rigid bone defect repair usually through a combined middle fossa and mastoid approach.

Fortunately, once repaired, recurrence or persistence appears uncommon, however, our longest follow-up is only 8 years.

REFERENCES

1. Iurato S, Ettore GC, Selvini C. Brain herniation into the middle ear: two idiopathic cases treated by a combined intracranial-mastoid approach. *Laryngoscope* 1989;99(9):950–954.
2. Ahren C, Thuler CA. Lethal intracranial complications following inflation in the external auditory canal in treatment of serous otitis media and due to defects in the petrous bone. *Acta Otolaryngol* 1965;60:407–421.
3. Ferguson B, Wilkins R, Hudson W, Farmer J. Spontaneous CSF otorrhea from tegmen and posterior fossa defects. *Laryngoscope* 1986:96.
4. Gacek RR. Arachnoid granulation cerebrospinal otorrhea. *Ann Otol Rhinol Laryngol* 1990;99:854–862.
5. Kamerer DB, Caparosa RJ. Temporal bone encephalocele—diagnosis and treatment. *Laryngoscope* 1982;92:878–882.
6. Hyson M, Andermann F, Oliver A, Melanson D. Occult encephaloceles and temporal lobe epilepsy: developmental and acquired lesions in the middle fossa. *Neurology* 1984;34(3):363–366.
7. Irjala K, Suombaa J, Laurent B. Identification of CSF leakage by immunofication. *Arch Otolaryngol Head Neck Surg* 1979;105:447.
8. Jackson CG, Pappas DG, Marolidis S, et al. Brain herniation into the middle ear and mastoid: concepts in diagnosis and surgical management. *Am J Otol* 1997;18:198–206.
9. Lalwani A. Temporal bone encephalocele. In: Jackler R, Brackmann D, eds. *Neurotology*. St. Louis: Mosby, 1994:1149–1155.
10. Graham MO, Lundy LB. Dural herniation and cerebrospinal fluid leaks. In: Brackmann D, Shelton C, Arriaga M, eds. *Otologic surgery*. Philadelphia: WB Saunders, 1994:278–288.
11. Kveton J, Friedman C, Constantino P. Indications for hydroxyapatite cement reconstructive in lateral skull base surgery. *Am J Otol* 1995;16(4):465–469.

Neurosurgical Issues in Otolaryngology: Principles and Practice of Collaboration,
edited by Moisés A. Arriaga and J. Diaz Day.
Lippincott Williams & Wilkins, Philadelphia © 1999.

CHAPTER 16

Intracranial Complications of Infections Related to the Paranasal and Mastoid Sinuses

Matthew R. Quigley

The paranasal and mastoid sinuses are air-filled cavities that penetrate the skull and in many places are separated from the dura by only thin bone. Thus they represent a potential nidus of epidural or intracranial infection. This chapter discusses primarily the sequelae of paranasal or mastoid infection, which has been community acquired, not iatrogenic secondary to surgical procedures. For purposes of definition, a chronic infection is one lasting longer than 3 months, and a suppurative otitis is associated with drainage and a perforated tympanic membrane (1). No specific recommendations are given as to the choice of antibiotics. In general, late-generation cephalosporins are utilized and often combined with metronidazole and/or vancomycin as guided by cultures and sensitivity results, but recommendations change frequently based on new antibiotic availability. These infections often represent potentially life-threatening situations and an infectious disease specialist should be consulted in all but the most straightforward cases.

The incidence of intracranial suppurative complications following nasal/sinus infection has significantly declined in the last 50 years since the widespread adoption of antibiotics. Prellner and Rydell (2) estimate the change to be from 2% to 0.02%, a 100-fold decline, although Kangsanarak et al. (3) document a 0.36% incidence of intracranial infectious complications from otitis media alone in a modern series over a 13-year period from their clinic in Thailand. Clearly, however, the major complication in all series is meningitis (4) followed in variable frequency by epidural abscess, brain abscess, and subdural empyema. We also discuss two frequent sequelae of suppurative otitis media—transverse sinus thrombophlebitis and ''otic'' hydrocephalus.

M. R. Quigley: Department of Neurosurgery, Allegheny University Hospitals, Pittsburgh, Pennsylvania 15212.

MENINGITIS

The middle ear and mastoid are the most likely source of meningitis as opposed to the paranasal sinuses. The common presentation is following an acute otitis, usually in the pediatric population. Gower and McGuirt (5) recorded meningitis as 76 of 100 cases of intracranial complications of otitis media. Of this meningitis group, 80% were pediatric and all but four were secondary to acute otitis. The etiology of bacterial spread to the meninges in acute cases is believed to be secondary to bacteremia as opposed to direct extension, which is more common in chronic suppurative otitis. Extension through the inner ear via a labyrinth fistula or cholesteatoma is usually seen in chronic cases (6).

Diagnosis

The appearance of meningitis is heralded by fever, nucal rigidity, headache, and lethargy in the setting of otitis media. Lumbar puncture (LP) is performed to confirm the diagnosis and identify pathologic organisms. A contrasted head computed tomography (CT) or magnetic resonance imaging (MRI) should probably be obtained prior to LP in all patients with chronic otitis to rule out parenchymal or epidural brain abscess.

Treatment

For acute otitis, other than myringotomy, antibiotics are the mainstay of treatment. In the pediatric population agents are chosen for their effectiveness against *Haemophilus influenzae,* which may be causative 70% of the time (5). Chronic otitis often necessitates mastoidectomy, which is done when the patient has been stabilized medically.

Outcome

The mortality following acute otitic meningitis is low, ranging from 3% in recent studies (7) to 8% in somewhat older studies (5). Patients with meningitis subsequent to chronic otitis do not fare so well, as Gower and McGuirt (5) report a 30.7% mortality and Proctor (8) reports a fourfold increase in mortality compared to acute cases.

BRAIN ABSCESS

A brain abscess represents an area of encephalitis that subsequently encapsulates around an accumulation of pus (9). The inciting event is believed to be a retrograde thrombophlebitis (4). Both paranasal and mastoid sinus areas may harbor the source, with the latter more common. Of all causes of brain abscess, an otologic process is present between 19% and 33% of the time (10–12), and the vast majority follow chronic as opposed to acute otitis infections (5,13). The paranasal sinuses are implicated in 0.5% to 16% of all brain abscess cases (14–16).

The most common organisms cultured are *Proteus mirabilis, Pseudomonas aeruginosa, Staphylococcus aureus,* and *Bacteroides fragilis* (3) with multiple organisms the rule. Negative cultures may be obtained, however, in 30% of the cases when antibiotics are used beforehand (10,12). The abscess forms adjacent to the involved sinus in a frontal lobe site following a paranasal infection and temporal or cerebellar abscess on the affected side when otitis is present. The predominance of the temporal lobe over the cerebellum following otitis is reported to vary from 1:1 to 5:1 (3,7,12). Virtually all abscesses secondary to a paranasal or otic sources are solitary (17).

Diagnosis

Signs and symptoms of abscess may be general with fever, headache, and lethargy, or focal with motor weakness, speech involvement, ataxia, nystagmus, or seizure. Sampson and Clark (18) document a rapid (<2-week) course in 75%, and seizure is present in about half (10,15). Diagnosis is best made with contrasted CT or MRI, which may demonstrate low signal only or the classic ring enhancement depending on the patient's age and the stage of the process (9). LP is rarely helpful and may be dangerous. Morgan et al. (15) documents LP results in 44 patients with abscesses undergoing a spinal puncture and found seven deteriorated clinically and all but one of them died.

Treatment

The fundamental neurosurgical principles for treatment of brain abscesses from any source are identification of the etiologic organism and management of the mass effect. Both paranasal and otologic sources usually afford an easy opportunity to identify the causative bacteriologic agent by direct culture. The method and even the requirement to drain or remove the brain abscess itself remain controversial. Many brain abscesses resolve with antibiotic treatment alone (19), which one review estimated may be successful 75% of the time (20). The main determinant of success appears to be size, with 3 cm being the cutoff. The patient's clinical status ultimately determines the necessity of drainage, which affords an immediate control of the mass effect. This is most easily accomplished with aspiration as guided by stereotaxis under local anesthetic (21). This may need to be repeated multiple times during the course of the disease (11), but even large abscesses (110–190 mL) have been managed with one or two aspirations (22). The role of excision of abscess by craniotomy appears to be quite limited, useful mainly in cases associated with intraabscess air due to some extracranial fistula (23). Series that have examined the outcome of patients handled by a variety of surgical techniques have failed to establish the superiority of one approach over another (10,20).

The use of high-dose corticosteroids as part of the treatment regimen remains controversial. Studies have shown diminished capsule formation (24) and reduced CT contrast enhancement (9). Most clinicians, however, do use the drugs acutely to control serious mass effect and then taper them rapidly as the patient improves. Antibiotic treatment is maintained for 6 to 8 weeks with acquisition CT scans every 2 weeks during treatment, and then monthly thereafter until resolution (20). Scan response may be slow, but some improvement should be seen within 2 months and resolution by 6 to 12 months (Fig. 16-1). Management of the paranasal or otic source is directed toward drainage and/or excision when the patient has stabilized medically. A cholesteatoma is often encountered when the mastoid exploration is undertaken in this setting (25).

Outcome

Mortality following brain abscess is generally below 5% in modern series (11,12,20). Outcome, however, is directly related to neurologic grade on presentation, and may reach 35% to 50% mortality in patients presenting in extremis (18).

EPIDURAL ABSCESS

Suppurative processes of the paranasal sinuses or more commonly the mastoid may by direct extension invade the epidural space. Otitic disease can manifest as either a middle or posterior fossa process. Neely and Doyle (4) indicate that this is the second most common intradural complication of otitis media, although infrequently seen following paranasal sinus disease (14). Further sequelae can be meningitis and transverse sinus thrombosis, the latter especially associated with advanced mastoid disease. The diagnosis is suspected with any paranasal infection or otitis associated with headache or intracranial signs as well as orbital or retroauricular swelling. Both CT and MRI can be used for diagnosis, with MRI having the added advantage of directly visualizing flow within the sinuses (Fig. 16-2). Treatment consists of

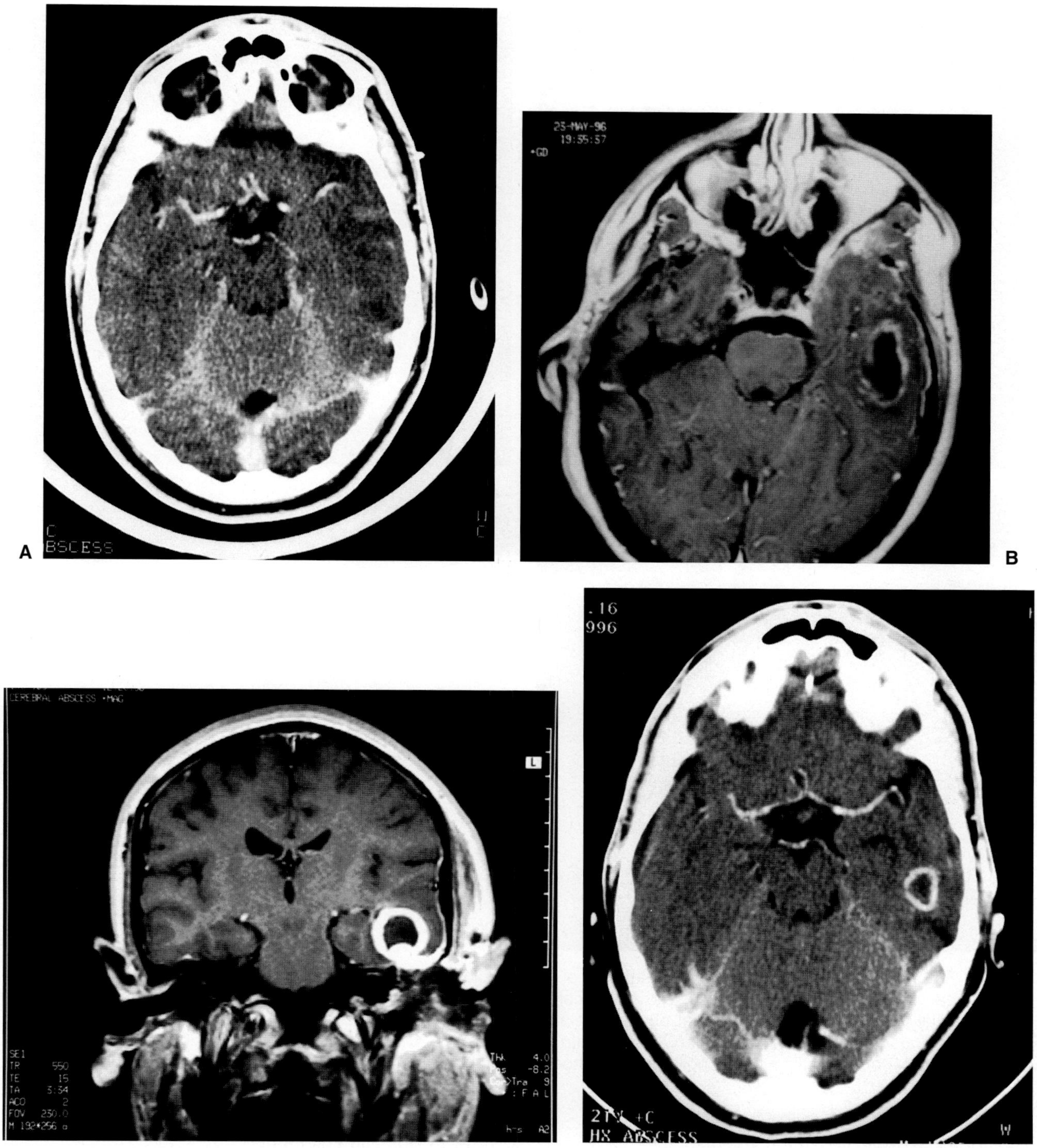

FIG. 16-1. **A:** Contrasted axial computed tomography (CT) in a 21-year-old man with a 1-month history of chronically draining ear treated with antibiotics. This scan was obtained when he presented with a grand mal seizure and lethargy. Note only low signal changes in left temporal lobe. **B:** Magnetic resonance imaging (MRI) scan performed 3 days later demonstrating ring-like enhancement pattern of an abscess. **C:** Contrasted coronal MRI following 2 months of appropriate antibiotic treatment. Note diminution of abscess size, thickening of the wall, and reactive dural changes along inferior aspect of middle fossa. A left mastoidectomy has been performed. **D:** Axial contrasted CT 5 months following presentation. Note small residual cavity present despite adequate antibiotic treatment. Radiographic evidence of cavity persisted for over 1 year (not shown).

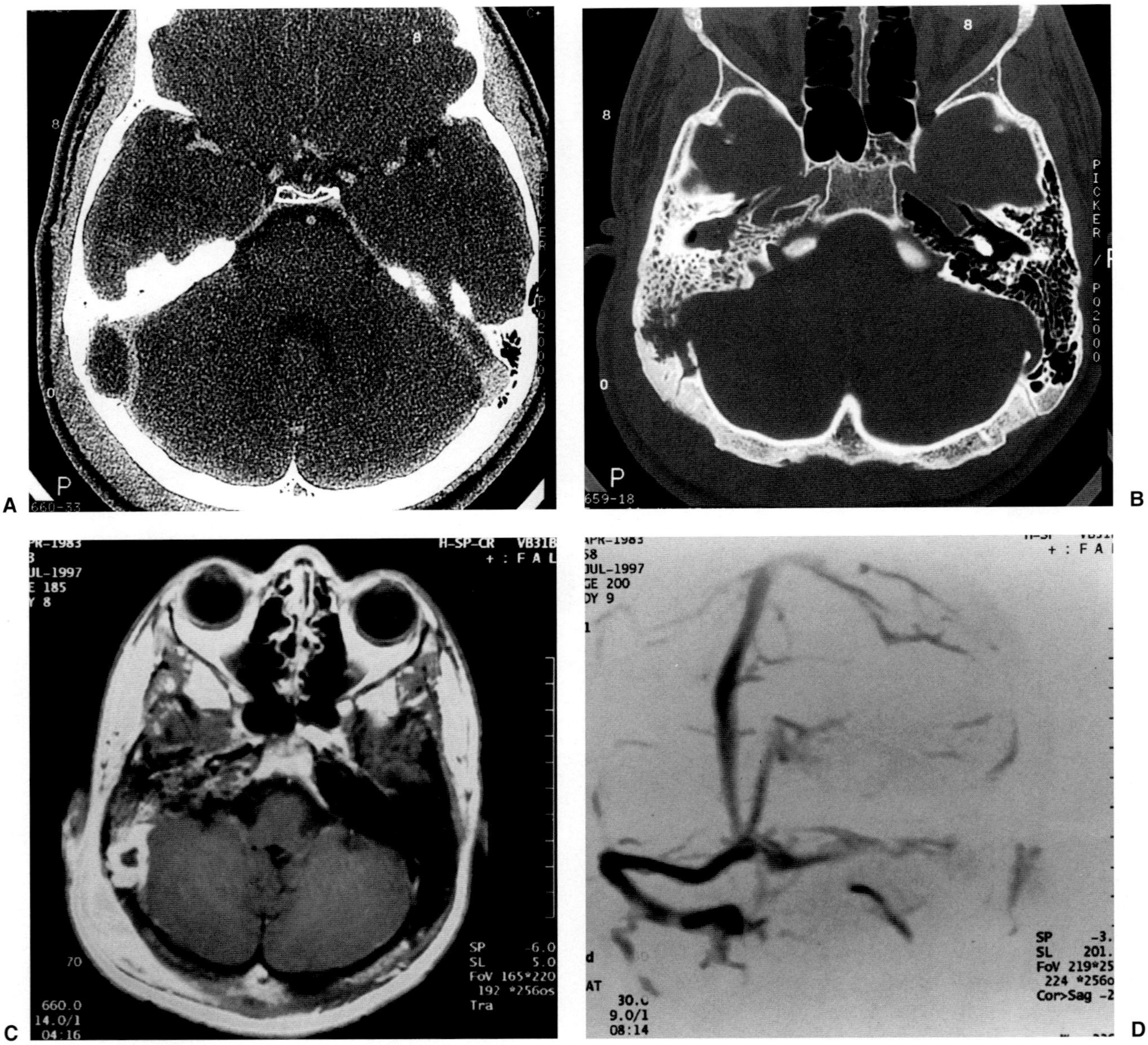

FIG. 16-2. Images taken on presentation of a 14-year-old boy with a 2-week history of a draining right ear, treated with oral antibiotics, and a new complaint of retroauricular swelling. **A:** Thin-cut contrasted axial CT demonstrating epidural abscess related to the right mastoid. **B:** Bone window CT showing obvious destruction of mastoid and erosion into posterior fossa. **C:** Contrasted axial MRI clearly showing epidural process. **D:** Slightly oblique MR venogram demonstrating occlusion of right transverse sinus.

excision of the associated epidural granulation tissue, which may be the only infectious manifestation as frank pus is not always found. Care is taken not to violate the dura or venous sinuses, and the excision is taken back to normal dura. A radical mastoidectomy or drainage of the affected paranasal sinus is usually performed at the same sitting. If frontal sinusitis is the cause of an abscess, a direct communication from the sinus through the dura is sought, and, if found, sinus removal is performed.

SUBDURAL ABSCESS (EMPYEMA)

This is a very uncommon suppurative complication of sinus disease usually seen as a sequela of a frontal infection (26). In Bok and Peter's (27) series, there was a 2.5:1 preponderance of paranasal sinus sources compared to mastoid disease in their review of 90 patients. The empyema is thought to arise either through direct extension of the sinus infection or retrograde thrombophlebitis (28). Signs and symptoms include headache, fever, orbital swelling, lethargy, and/or focal neurologic deficit in a patient with advanced sinus disease. Seizures are encountered in about one-third. The diagnosis is made by CT and/or MRI. LP is nonspecific and may be dangerous. Pus collections can be loculated, situated over the entire hemisphere or interhemispheric (27). Treatment is emergency evacuation under appropriate antibiotic coverage. Although the early literature, which predates CT, favors craniotomy for pus evacuation, recent series have demonstrated excellent outcomes with multiple burr holes instead. Bok and Peter (27) achieved an 86% good recovery and an overall 7.7% mortality among the 50 patients presenting with a good neurologic grade; with coma score of 12 to 15, there was only one death. Drainage of the sinus disease can be performed in the same sitting or deferred until the patient has defervesced.

INFECTIOUS SEQUELAE

Transverse Sinus Thrombophlebitis

The original description of this entity from the preantibiotic era of weight loss, anemia, tender sternocleidomastoid muscle, a chronic draining ear, and a picket fence fever due to periodic release of β-hemolytic strep is of historical interest only (29). Modern-day presentation is ordinarily that of a complication of chronic mastoid disease (5,30), often associated with the presence of cholesteatoma, in 40% to 86% (31,32). Headaches and otalgia are common as is retroauricular swelling (Griesinger's sign); palsies of the sixth and seventh nerves are infrequently noted. Mathews (31) estimates the incidence of transverse sinus pathology among patients with mastoiditis is 17%. The older literature stressed the requirement for angiography or retrograde venography for diagnostic purposes, but MRI with time-of-flight vascular imaging sequences is the method of choice for noninvasive testing (Fig. 16-2D) (33). MRI can also assess the extent of mastoid disease and possible epidural extension of the infection.

Recommendations for treatment appear clouded by reference to preantibiotic regimens. Certainly all agree with radical mastoidectomy under antibiotic coverage, but management of the venous system is controversial. Although the older literature advocated internal jugular ligation and heparin administration, since septic emboli were a common occurrence, in the antibiotic era these methods have been abandoned except in cases of intractable septic pulmonary emboli (30). Interestingly, this maneuver was necessary in 14% of Mathews's (31) series, 11% of the series of Samuel and Fernandes (32), and none of Teichgraeber et al.'s (30) patients; all were treated with antibiotics. These authors also advocate exploration and excision of the exposed transverse sinus during mastoidectomy, but the rationale for this in the face of adequate antibiotic coverage is lacking. At present, our practice is to leave the sinus untouched during mastoidectomy unless recurrent septic emboli have been documented.

Cultures from surgery often show mixed flora containing *Streptococcus, Bacteroides, Enterobacter,* and other gram-negative rods. Sterile cultures are also common if antibiotics were administered preoperatively. Mortality from transverse sinus thrombophlebitis varies between 0% and 36%, but as pointed out by Mathews (31), death from this disease is virtually always due to intracranial sepsis from concomitant meningitis or abscess formation.

Transverse and sigmoid thrombophlebitis may propagate proximally via the superior and/or inferior petrosal sinuses, causing the rare but dramatic presentation of proptosis, chemosis, and ophthalmoplegia due to cavernous sinus thrombosis. Both Dawes (34) as well as Seid and Sellars (35) record the incidence of this complication in less than 5% of transverse sinus thromboses, although Kangsanarak et al. (3) found a 25% occurrence in their series from Thailand. Diagnosis is made by the clinical signs as well as CT and/or MRI (36). Treatment requires addressing the primary infection source (mastoid, ethmoid) under antibiotic coverage. Prolonged anticoagulation with heparin and Coumadin should be strongly considered in these cases (as opposed to simple transverse sinus thrombosis) as they are the mainstays of treatment for cavernous sinus thrombosis due to other causes (37).

Otic Hydrocephalus

This is a very confusing term originally coined by Symonds (38) in 1931 to describe increased intracranial pressure (ICP) in association with infectious ear disease. Despite the term *hydrocephalus,* ventricular size is normal, but ICP is elevated and patients present with headache, falsely localizing signs (fourth or sixth nerve palsy), and visual symptoms from papilledema. Therefore, it is often considered under the general category of "pseudotumor" with other conditions causing elevated ICP with normal CSF and no obstructing lesions on scan (39). Some controversy regarding the etiology of otic hydrocephalus exists. Although Gower and McGuirt (5) state the "physiology of the elevated ICP is not known" and "lateral sinus thrombosis ... is not to be confused with otic hydrocephalus," other modern authors disagree. Lenz and McDonald (40) reviewed their own and others' (41,42) experiences and found a very high correlation between transverse sinus thrombosis and otic hydrocephalus, especially with involvement of the right side, which is frequently the dominant drain of the sagittal sinus. Gower and McGuirt's own clinical material documents three clear-cut cases of otic hydrocephalus among five patients with transverse sinus thrombosis, two of whom underwent subtemporal decompression for treatment of elevated ICP. Although often considered rare, the incidence of otic hydrocephalus following transverse sinus thrombophlebitis was 33% in Teichgreuber et al. (30) and 18% in Mathews's (31) series.

Treatment of the hydrocephalus per se is directed toward symptomatic relief of headache, palliation of cranial nerve palsies, and visual preservation. The first line of therapy is medical, with furosemide and acetazolamide diuretics and dexamethasone in resistant cases. Serial LPs to relieve pressure have been advocated. Careful ophthalmologic evaluation is mandatory as an enlarged blind spot, diminished acuity, and visual obscurations can progress to permanent visual loss. Surgery is reserved for resistant cases especially with frequent obscurations. Dandy (43) was the first to surgically treat pseudotumor via bitemporal craniectomies, but this approach has been virtually abandoned. Placement of a lumboperitoneal shunt is a low-morbidity procedure that has been associated with excellent control of ICP. Continued function of this device is hard to assess, however, requiring reexploration in questionable cases. Optic sheath fenestration through a lateral orbitotomy is another surgical alternative, although the mechanism by which it reduces papilledema is obscure, since little CSF can be absorbed via the orbit. Corbett et al. (44) successfully reversed papilledema of pseudotumor in 86% of their cases with visual improvement or stability. Results diminished if visual acuity was beyond 20/200. Bilateral symptoms can be ameliorated even with fenestration of only one eye (45). A frequent complication of this procedure is tonic pupil associated with variable accommodation paresis.

CONCLUSION

With the advent of antibiotics, intracranial complications of paranasal or otitic infections have become unusual. Clinical suspicion for such disease should remain high, however, in any patient with headache, orbital or retroauricular swelling, and/or focal neurologic signs, especially if associated with a chronic partially treated infectious process. CT or MRI should be obtained for diagnostic purposes in all but the most straightforward meningitis cases, which is also the only place for lumbar puncture. Associated complications such as transverse sinus thrombosis should be sought and can now be easily diagnosed with MR venography.

REFERENCES

1. Bluestone CD, Klein JO. Otitis media with effusion atelectasis and eustachian tube dysfunction. In: Blueston DC, Stool SE, eds. *Pediatric otolaryngology,* vol 1. Philadelphia: WB Saunders, 1990:320–322.
2. Prellner K, Rydell R. Acute mastoiditis: influence of antibiotic treatment on the bacterial spectrum. *Acta Otolaryngol* 1986;102:52–56.
3. Kangsanarak J, Navacharoen N, Fooanant S, Ruckphaopunt K. Intracranial complications of suppurative otitis media: 13 years' experience. *Am J Otol* 1995;16:104–109.
4. Neely JG, Doyle KJ. Facial nerve and intracranial complications of otitis media. In: Brackmann DE, Jackler RK, eds. *Neurotology*. St. Louis: Mosby, 1994:905–918.
5. Gower D, McGuirt WF. Intracranial complications of acute and chronic infectious ear disease: a problem still with us. *Laryngoscope* 1983;93: 1028–1033..
6. Nisson AJ, Bui H. Complications of chronic otitis media. *Ear Nose Throat J* 1996;75:224–292.
7. Friedman EM, McGill TJ, Healy GB. Central nervous system complications associated with acute otitis media in children. *Laryngoscope* 1990; 100:149–151.
8. Proctor CA. Intracranial complications of otic origin. *Laryngoscope* 1966;76:288–308.
9. Britt RH, Enzmann DR. Clinical stages of human brain abscesses on serial CT scans after contrast infusion. *J Neurosurg* 1983;59:972–989.
10. Mampalam TJ, Rosenblum ML. Trends in the management of bacterial brain abscesses: a review of 102 cases over 17 years. *Neurosurgery* 1988;23;451–458.
11. Ng PY, Seow WT, On PL. Brain abscess: review of 30 cases treated with surgery. *Aust NZ J Surg* 1995;65;664–666.
12. Yen P, Chan S, Huang T. Brain abscesses: with special reference to otolaryngologic sources of infection. *Otolaryngol Head Neck Surg* 1995;113:15–22.
13. Meyers EN, Ballantine HT. The management of otogenic brain abscess. *Laryngoscope* 1965;75:273–288.
14. Bradley PJ, Manning KP, Shaw MDM. Brain abscess secondary to paranasal sinusitis. *J Laryngol Otol* 1984;98:19–25.
15. Morgan H, Wood MW, Murphey F. Experience with 88 consecutive cases of brain abscess. *J Neurosurg* 1973;38:698–704.
16. Yang S. Brain abscess: a review of 400 cases. *J Neurosurg* 1981;55: 794–799.
17. Samuel J, Fernandes CM, Steinberg JL. Intracranial otogenic complications: a persisting problem. *Laryngoscope* 1986;96:272–277.
18. Sampson DS, Clark K. A current review of brain abscesses. *Am J Med* 1973;54:201–210.
19. Heineman HS, Braude AI, Osterholm JL. Intracranial suppurative disease. *JAMA* 1971;218:1542–1547.
20. Rosenblum ML, Mampalam TJ, Pons VS. Controversies in the management of brain abscesses. *Clin Neurosurg* 1986;33:603–632.
21. Dyste GN, Hitchon PW, Menezes AH, VanGilder JC, Greene GM. Stereotaxic surgery in the treatment of multiple brain abscesses. *J Neurosurg* 1988;69:188–194.
22. Stephanov S, Joubert MJ. Large brain abscesses treated by aspiration alone. *Surg Neurol* 1982;17:338–340.
23. Young RF, Frazee J. Gas within intracranial abscess cavities: an indication for surgical excision. *Ann Neurol* 1984;16:35–39.
24. Quartey GRC, Johnston JA, Rozdilsky B. Decadron in the treatment of cerebral abscess: an experimental study. *J Neurosurg* 1976;45: 301–310.
25. Mathews TJ, Marus G. Otogenic intradural complications (a review of 37 patients). *J Laryngol Otol* 1988;102:121–124.
26. Remmler D, Boles R. Intracranial complications of frontal sinusitis. *Laryngoscope* 1980;90:1814–1824.
27. Bok AP, Peter JC. Subdural empyema: burr holes or craniotomy? *J Neurosurg* 1993;78:574–578.
28. Courville CB. Intracranial complications of otitis media and mastoiditis in the antibiotic era. *Laryngoscope* 1955;65:31–64.
29. Shambaugh GE. *Surgery of the ear.* Philadelphia: WB Saunders, 1967: 318–328.
30. Teichgraeber JF, Per-Lee JH, Turner JS. Lateral sinus thrombosis: a modern perspective. *Laryngoscope* 1982;92:744–751.
31. Mathews TJ. Lateral sinus pathology. *J Laryngol Otol* 1988;102: 118–120.
32. Samuel J, Fernandes CMC. Lateral sinus thrombosis (a review of 45 cases). *J Laryngol Otol* 1987;101:1227–1229.
33. Sze G, Zimmerman RD. The magnetic resonance imaging of infectious and inflammatory diseases. *Radiol Clin North Am* 1988;26:839–859.
34. Dawes JDK. Discussion on intracranial complications of otogenic origin. *Proc R Soc Med* 1961;54:315–320.
35. Seid AB, Sellars SL. The management of otogenic lateral sinus disease at Groote Schuur Hospital. *Laryngoscope* 1973;83:397–403.
36. Doyle KJ, Jackler RK. Otogenic cavernous sinus thrombosis. *Otolaryngol Head Neck Surg* 1991;104:873–877.
37. Levine SR, Twyman RE, Gilman S. The role of anticoagulation in cavernous sinus thrombosis. *Neurology* 1988;38:517–522.
38. Symonds CP. Otitis hydrocephalus. *Brain* 1931;54:55–71.
39. Sklaw FH. Pseudotumor cerebri. In: Wilkins RH, Rengachary SS, eds. *Neurosurgery*. New York: McGraw-Hill, 1996:357–362.
40. Lenz RP, McDonald GA. Otic hydrocephalus. *Laryngoscope* 1984;94: 1451–1454.
41. Foley J. Benign forms of intracranial hypertension—toxic and otic hydrocephalus. *Brain* 1955;78:1–14.
42. Wright JLW, Grimaldi PMG. Otogenic intracranial complications. *J Laryngol Otol* 1973;87:1085–1096.
43. Dandy WE. Intracranial pressure without brain tumor: diagnosis and treatment. *Ann Surg* 1937;106:492–513.
44. Corbett JJ, Nerud JA, Tse DT, Anderson RL. Results of optic nerve sheath fenestration for pseudotumor cerebri. *Arch Ophthalmol* 1988; 106:1391–1397.
45. Horton JC, Seif SR, Pitts LH, Weinstein PR, Rosenblum ML, Hoyt WF. Decompression of optic nerve sheath for vision-threatening papilledema caused by dural sinus occlusion. *Neurosurgery* 1992;31: 203–212.

Neurosurgical Issues in Otolaryngology: Principles and Practice of Collaboration,
edited by Moisés A. Arriaga and J. Diaz Day.
Lippincott Williams & Wilkins, Philadelphia © 1999.

CHAPTER 17

Contemporary Diagnosis and Management of Anterior Skull Base Cephalocele and Cerebrospinal Fluid Leaks

Scott E. Celin

OVERVIEW

Cephaloceles and cerebrospinal fluid (CSF) leaks of the anterior skull base occur infrequently, but, when present, must be managed effectively to prevent long-term sequelae. The term *cephalocele* is used to describe any abnormal herniation of the leptomeninges outside of the cranium. When the herniation contains brain tissue, it is called an encephalocele. When brain tissue is not present, the term *meningocele* is used. Cephaloceles may be grouped by anatomic location into occipital, sincipital, and basal. Sincipital variants occur between the frontal and ethmoid bones, and basal variants can occur anywhere along the cribriform plate, fovea ethmoidalis, sphenoid bone, or temporal bone.

Most anterior skull base encephaloceles are congenital in etiology, although traumatic and iatrogenic encephaloceles also occur. Large congenital cephaloceles are usually easily diagnosed at birth due to associated craniofacial deformities, nasal obstruction, and associated airway compromise. Smaller cephaloceles may go undetected until later in life when they are noted incidentally on imaging studies or become symptomatic.

Cerebrospinal fluid leaks in the anterior skull base may occur spontaneously, after trauma (blunt or surgical), or may be related to small congenital cephaloceles that spontaneously develop leaks. Advanced skull base neoplasms can also result in spontaneous spinal fluid leaks. Leaks related to blunt trauma most often resolve with bed rest and reduction of facial fractures, sometimes utilizing a ventriculostomy catheter or lumbar drain to decrease intracranial pressure. When gross displacement of the skull base fragments occurs, repair using conventional neurosurgical techniques at the time of facial fracture repair is indicated. Iatrogenic CSF leaks most commonly follow endoscopic sinus procedures, transsphenoidal surgery, aneurysm surgery, or removal of skull base tumors. Although most of these leaks will be immediate, delayed leaks or delay in diagnosis is not uncommon. Spontaneous CSF fistulas may present only with unilateral rhinorrhea or may have associated meningitis, often on a recurrent basis.

S. E. Celin: Allegheny University of the Health Sciences, Pittsburgh, Pennsylvania 15212.

HISTORICAL MANAGEMENT

Large sincipital encephaloceles are usually diagnosed soon after birth and are treated with conventional neurosurgical techniques. These typically would include a bifrontal craniotomy with reduction of functional brain tissue into the intracranial compartment and repair of the defect using bone grafts, fascia grafts, and dural repair. Craniofacial reconstructive procedures are often necessary to repair the associated nasofrontal deformities. Small pedunculated basal encephaloceles typically present later in life when complications such as CSF leaks, meningitis, or headaches develop. The recommended treatment is resection as encephaloceles usually do not contain functional brain tissue. In the past, it was difficult to localize the site of smaller encephaloceles and CSF fistulas, and correction often required wide exploration to identify the site of the lesion. Although transnasal exposure using an external ethmoid approach as described by Montgomery was advocated by some otolaryngologists (1), most neurosurgeons preferred wider exposure provided by a craniotomy. Despite these techniques, failure rates for CSF rhinorrhea remained as high as 30%.

The development of nasal endoscopic techniques, skull

base imaging, and specialized diagnostic studies has allowed precise localization of smaller cephaloceles and CSF leaks. With precise localization, wide exposure is no longer necessary to diagnose the site of the lesion. As many of these patients have relatively few symptoms, endoscopic, endonasal techniques to resect cephaloceles and repair CSF fistulas have been developed. These techniques avoid the risks and expected sequelae of craniotomy, which include anosmia, frontal lobe retraction, visual changes, intracranial hemorrhage, and visible external scars. When appropriately selected, endonasal techniques have a high success rate (>90%) and extremely low recurrence rate (2,3). These techniques are described here.

ADVANTAGES OF TEAM SURGERY

Cooperation between neurosurgeons and otolaryngologists is important when managing these patients. These patients may present to either specialty, and the diagnosis often requires careful evaluation of neurologic and sinus symptoms and precise examination of the endonasal anatomy and baseline neurologic status of the patient. Depending on the clinical presentation (meningitis, active CSF leak, pneumocephalus, postoperative complication, asymptomatic clear rhinorrhea, etc.), the patient may or may not be hospitalized. Good initial communication will allow expedient diagnosis with focused diagnostic testing. Initial imaging studies typically include computed tomography (CT) scans or magnetic resonance imaging (MRI) of the anterior skull base. Often both studies are necessary to provide adequate information about the bony and soft tissue anatomy. Confirmation of active leaks may be done with radionucleotide studies or with β_2-transferrin evaluation of nasal drainage. Communication with qualified radiologists helps when deciding on the diagnostic imaging protocol. Nasal endoscopic exam is also important and may detect active leakage, the location of leak, or polypoid lesions to suggest cephalocele. Biopsy of polypoid tissue when a cephalocele is a possibility is not recommended until the appropriate diagnostic studies are complete and preparations have been made for definitive repair.

Definitive repair requires the availability of both the neurosurgeon and otolaryngologist. Endonasal surgery using endoscopes requires considerable knowledge of the endonasal anatomy (Fig. 17-1), skill using endonasal instruments, and the ability to work off of a videoscreen. Atraumatic technique is required to prevent bleeding, which obscures visibility and may prevent completion of the procedure. Most neu-

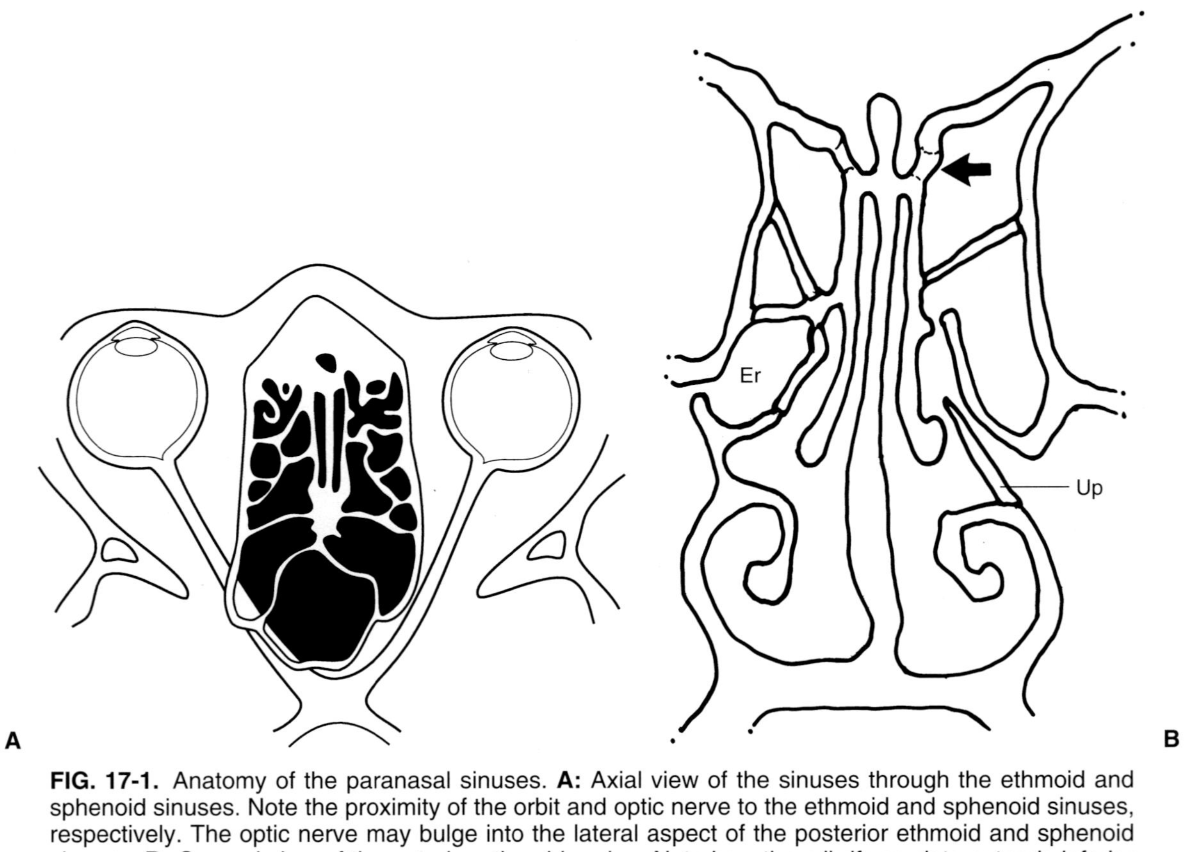

FIG. 17-1. Anatomy of the paranasal sinuses. **A:** Axial view of the sinuses through the ethmoid and sphenoid sinuses. Note the proximity of the orbit and optic nerve to the ethmoid and sphenoid sinuses, respectively. The optic nerve may bulge into the lateral aspect of the posterior ethmoid and sphenoid sinuses. **B:** Coronal view of the anterior ethmoid region. Note how the cribriform plate extends inferior to the roof of the ethmoid sinuses. The lateral aspect of the cribriform region (*arrow*) where the middle turbinates attach is the thinnest and is easily injured during endoscopic sinus surgery by otolaryngologists. UP, uncinate process; ER, ethmoid roof.

rosurgeons are not trained in endoscopic nasal surgery and so most of the procedure is performed by the otolaryngologist. The neurosurgeon must be available should a craniotomy become necessary to control bleeding or some other emergency problem. Lumbar drains are placed in most patients, and most otolaryngologists are not facile in placement or management of these postoperatively.

SURGICAL TECHNIQUE

Management of anterior skull base cephaloceles and CSF leaks is typically performed under general anesthesia. The nasal cavity is anesthetized and decongested both topically and using infiltration of lidocaine with epinephrine, as would be done for endoscopic sinus surgery. Care is taken to atraumatically pack topical anesthetic pledgets into the region of the leak, and the medications are allowed to work for at least 10 to 15 minutes. Sequential packs may be useful to achieve maximal vasoconstriction. If a lumbar drain is used, this is a good time for it to be placed. Intrathecal fluorescein may be used to localize an active CSF leak if the site is not identified on imaging studies, but all efforts should be made to identify the site preoperatively. The fluorescein must be acceptable for intravenous use (not the topical ophthalmic preparation) and is typically mixed as 0.1 mL of 10% fluorescein with 10 mL of the patient's CSF, which is withdrawn then reinjected sterilely through the lumbar drain. It takes approximately 30 minutes for the solution to circulate intracranially.

Endoscopic exposure of the site of the lesion is first performed. The frontal sinus, anterior ethmoid sinuses, and maxillary sinus drain into the space between the middle turbinate and lateral nasal wall called the middle meatus. Leaks in this area require removal of the uncinate process, bulla ethmoidalis, and the anterior ethmoid air cells. The middle turbinate may also need to be removed to provide adequate exposure. Leaks in the posterior ethmoid region require additional removal of the basal lamella (the partition that separates the anterior and posterior ethmoids), and removal of the vertical partitions in the posterior ethmoid air cells. Lesions in the cribriform plate (medial to the middle turbinate), as shown in Fig. 17-2, can be approached by removing a portion or all of the middle turbinate. This usually can be accomplished without ethmoidectomy. When the CSF leak is inside the sphenoid sinus, the sphenoid may be approached directly in the sphenoethmoidal recess. Often, the posterior half of the middle turbinate must be removed to provide adequate space for instrumentation. The sphenoid is entered medially to minimize risk of injuring the optic nerve and carotid artery. The anterior wall of the sphenoid can be safely taken down once the level of the roof and borders of the lateral wall are identified. If the site of lesion is not known, wide exposure of the skull base on the suspected side is necessary. This typically includes careful unilateral removal of all of the ethmoid partitions and the middle turbinate to have complete exposure of the skull base.

The green fluorescein is visible if an active leak is present. Otherwise, CSF can be detected by a ''washout'' sign (clear drainage that washes away the surrounding blood). The anesthesiologist can perform a Valsalva maneuver to increase intracranial pressure and increase the flow rate, which can aid in identification of the leak. Cephaloceles are removed in pieces. Bipolar cautery can be used for bleeding but typically small cephaloceles have narrow stalks and scant blood supply, which doesn't bleed significantly. If a leak was suspected but could not be identified, the area is left to heal as in an endoscopic sinus procedure. If the leak later reactivates, which occurred in one patient in our unpublished series, the site is then easily visible on office endoscopy.

After the cephalocele has been resected or the leak has been identified, the mucosa surrounding the perimeter of anterior skull base defects is removed to provide a 5 to 10 mm wide surface around the defect to allow adhesion and vascularization of a mucoperiosteal graft. When the leak is within the cribriform plate, removal of the surrounding mucosa has in the author's experience resulted in other small areas of leakage through olfactory nerve perforations. These additional sites are also covered with the graft. When large bony defects are present (greater than 1 cm^2), a layered repair is usually attempted (Fig. 17-3). Temporalis fascia or other fibrous tissue layer (preserved dura) can be placed through the defect above the skull base dura or between the dura and skull base to provide a watertight layer. This can be supported with a bone graft placed through the defect. Creation of this type of layered closure is very difficult and is not necessary or possible with small skull base defects or with defects within the sphenoid sinus.

Free mucoperiosteal grafts are then applied to the defect. These grafts are typically harvested from the nasal septum on the contralateral side of the nose. The graft should be slightly larger than the defect to allow for some contraction of the graft after it is harvested. The donor site can be cauterized lightly if necessary and will heal as long as a through-and-through defect is not created. The grafts are laid over the bone, which has been denuded of mucosa similar to the technique used in tympanoplasty. Surgicel or some other absorbable packing is then applied to the mucosal surface of the graft to hold it in the right position. Some CSF can be remove to help reduce the flow rate during this portion of the procedure, or the patient may be placed in the reverse Trendelenburg position if a lumbar drain has not been placed. The Surgicel is then supported with an expandable nasal sponge tampon (Mericel) that is the appropriate size to provide support to the area of repair. Multiple sponges may be necessary. They are infiltrated intraoperatively with antibiotic/saline solution (typically 450 mg clindamycin in 500 mL saline). This solution is also irrigated onto the sponges in the postoperative period three times daily to reduce bacterial colonization within the nasal packing.

Leaks within the lateral sphenoid sinus must be handled differently. These lateral leaks (skull base fracture, removal of clinoid process for aneurysm surgery) are dangerously

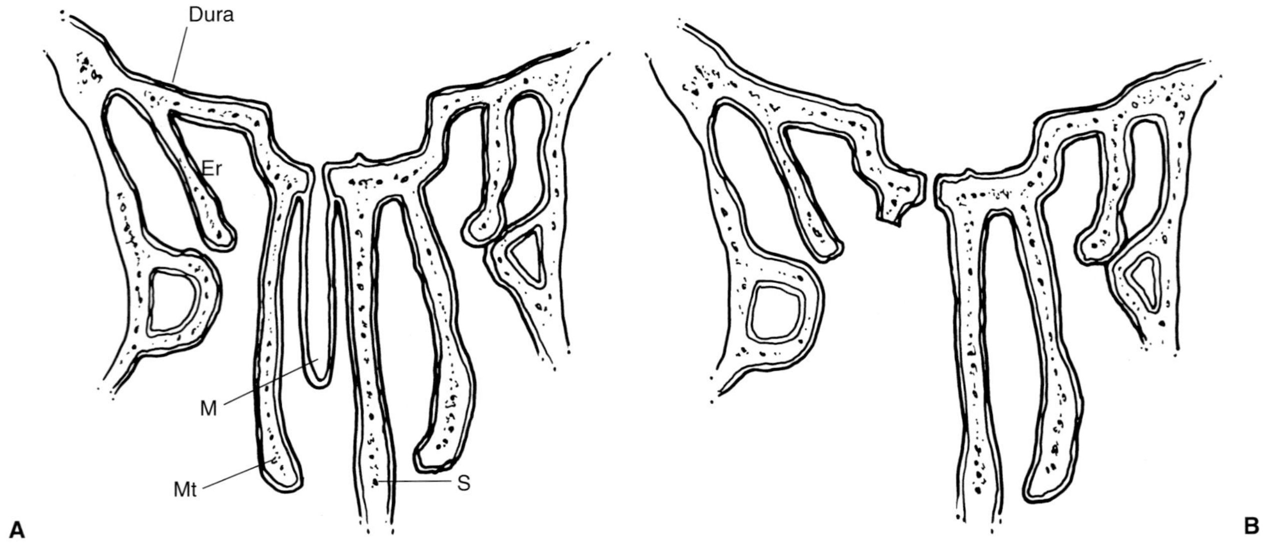

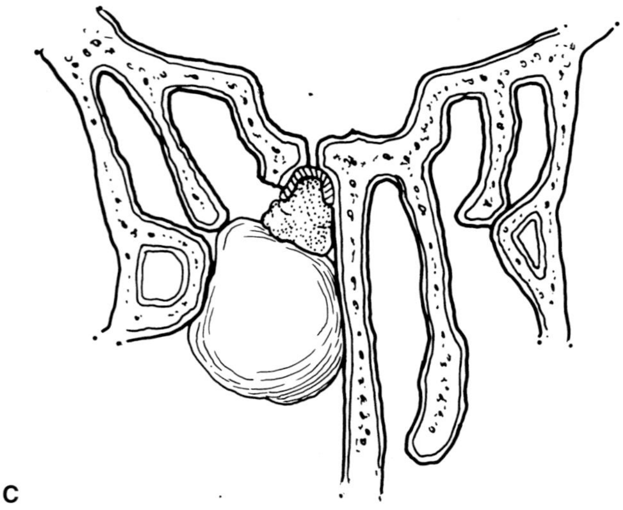

FIG. 17-2. Endoscopic closure of a cribriform meningocele. **A:** Coronal diagram of a cribriform meningocele as seen in two of our patients. Dural herniation through cribriform bony defects were present and actively leaking cerebrospinal fluid (CSF). MT, middle turbinate; M, meningocele; S, nasal septum; ER, ethmoid roof. **B:** To allow access to the cribriform region, the middle turbinate is resected up to a point close to its attachment at the skull base. The meningocele has been resected and the mucosa surrounding the defect has been removed. Active leakage of CSF is controlled with lumbar drainage or reverse Trendelenburg position. **C:** The mucoperiosteal graft is obtained from the nasal septum or the resected portion of the middle turbinate. It is positioned over the defect and packed into place with absorbable packing such as Surgicel (Su), which is reinforced with nonabsorbable nasal packing (P) such as Mericel nasal tampon.

close to the optic nerve and carotid artery. It is often too dangerous or not physically possible to remove the mucosa around the defect. The carotid artery is usually covered with a very thin layer of bone that, if fractured, will lacerate the internal carotid artery. Occasionally, the internal carotid may be covered only with mucosa. In these cases, a fat graft is used to ''plug'' the defect and temporarily obliterate the sphenoid while the defect is healing. It has been the author's experience that these grafts remain in place long enough to allow a fibrous layer to form at the dural defect, although the fat grafts eventually liquefy and resorb, usually with restoration of patency of the sphenoid ostium. The fat grafts are held in place either by preserving most of the mucosa over the rostrum of the sphenoid sinus by elevating through a posterior septal incision or by wedging a free bone graft over the sphenoidotomy site. An expandable sponge nasal tampon (Mericel) is then placed within the nasal cavity over the mucosal flap or bone graft to help hold them in place.

There are indications for traditional, open treatment of cephaloceles and CSF leaks. When the leak is into an otherwise intact frontal sinus, it is not possible to expose these lesions endoscopically. Lesions within the frontal sinus require open approaches through a frontal sinusotomy (osteoplastic, extended trephination) or frontal craniotomy. The latter is more likely to be necessary in traumatic lesions when multiple leaks or extensive dural tears are likely. When the anatomy of the sphenoid sinus has been extensively altered, such as in skull base resections for tumor, the normal anatomy of the carotid artery and brain may be extensively altered. These cases also may benefit from an open approach.

Close monitoring is required to prevent complications or recurrence. The patients are hospitalized postoperatively and remain at bed rest. The length of time necessary is left to clinical judgment due to the lack of controlled studies. The author currently keeps his patients at bed rest for 2 days at least. If a lumbar drain has been placed, it is left just above head level and drains continuously and usually remains in place for 48 hours. The author's preference is to leave the

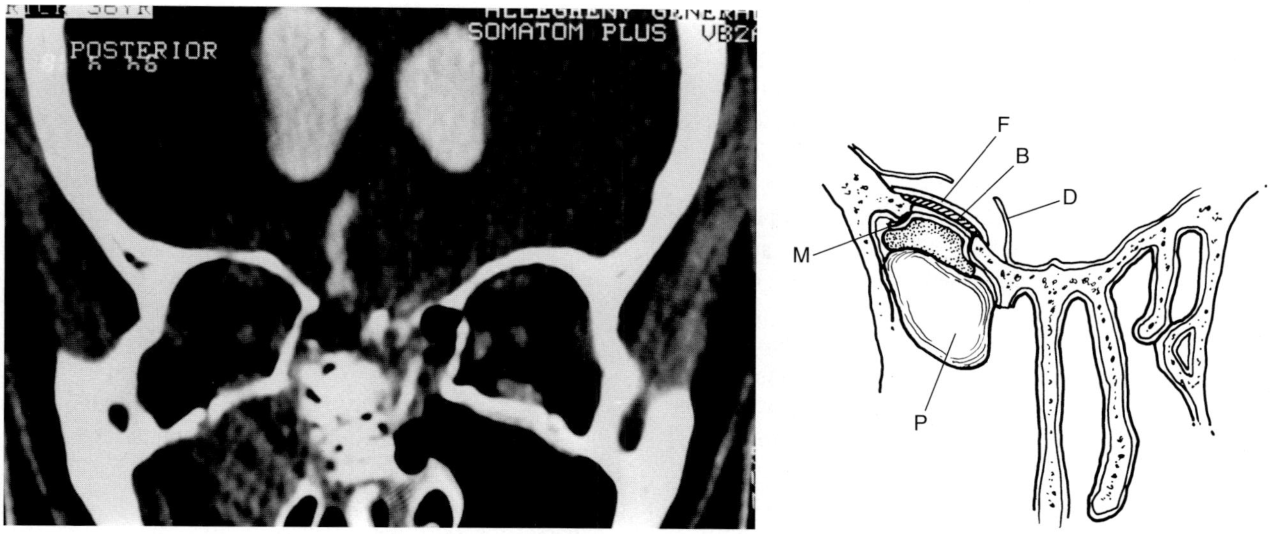

A B

FIG. 17-3. Repair of a large ethmoid roof defect. **A:** Coronal CT with intrathecal contrast showing a large iatrogenic defect in the ethmoid roof created during endoscopic sinus surgery. Nasal packing (NP) was in place at the time of transfer. Before the error was recognized, the surgeon ventured into the brain and a trail of CSF is visible in the defect (D). **B:** Diagram of the type of repair utilized. The dura was elevated through the bony defect from the bone surrounding the defect. A fascia graft (F) was then placed through the defect between the bone and dura. A septal bone graft (B) was then inserted to support the fascia. The area was then covered with a mucoperiosteal graft (M), Surgicel (S), and nonabsorbable packing (P).

nasal packing in place for 7 to 14 days and to irrigate it several times a day with antibiotic saline solution until it is removed. Several endoscopic nasal examinations are performed in the postoperative period to remove crusting, which may cause bacterial overgrowth. Perioperative intravenous antibiotics are given for 48 hours and are then continued orally until the nonabsorbable packing is removed.

CLINICAL RESULTS

A recent review of our results is currently under way. Thirty-two patients have been evaluated over the last 6 years for CSF rhinorrhea with or without cephaloceles. Twenty-three of them failed conservative therapy of bed rest and lumbar drain and required surgical intervention. Fourteen of the patients were successfully treated entirely through the endoscopic route. Five patients had leaks in the sphenoid sinus, eight in the ethmoid or cribriform region, and one from the frontal sinus; the last patient had undergone prior craniotomy for tumor with cranialization of the sinus and removal of the sinus mucosa. All of the leaks and cephaloceles treated endoscopically were closed after one endoscopic attempt, and there have been no recurrences. Two additional patients were successfully repaired using the operating microscope for exposure. One was a CSF leak after pituitary surgery and another had an iatrogenic defect created in the cribriform plate during exposure for revision pituitary surgery. Of the seven patients treated with open procedures, five had lesions in the frontal sinus and two had complex sphenoid defects after skull base resections. The success rate for these cases was also very high, with only one recurrence in a complex sphenoid leak.

POTENTIAL PITFALLS

Transnasal, endoscopic repair of basal encephaloceles and CSF leaks carries significant risks inherent with any skull base procedure. The entire surgical team, including anesthesia, operating room staff, and the surgeons, should be experienced in techniques required for craniotomy. The endoscopist should be very experienced in nasal endoscopic surgery and possess the skills necessary to dissect and repair the skull base. Experience with open skull base surgery allows the otolaryngologist to be familiar with intracranial anatomy and the anatomy of the carotid artery and optic nerve, and to have a good working relationship with neurosurgeons. Manipulation of the skull base requires familiarity with the instruments used within the frontal recess, and also often requires some of the neurosurgical dissectors, forceps, and elevators used in microscopic skull base procedures. Traditional nasal endoscopic instrumentation is often inadequate by itself to complete these procedures.

Preoperative imaging is critical to have an accurate "road map" of the skull base. Axial and coronal CT images obtained with fine, continuous cuts provide the anatomic detail required. When cephaloceles are present, MRI may enhance information regarding the size and location of the stalk of the lesion. If at all possible, CSF leaks should be localized with imaging studies and the presence of CSF should be confirmed with diagnostic studies (β_2-transferrin). Real-time CT imaging may be useful if the skull base anatomy is complicated or if revision procedures are performed.

Intracranial bleeding is possible both intraoperatively and postoperatively. The intracranial compartment should never be probed blindly, and bipolar cautery should be available to control hemorrhage from the skull base.

The patient should be closely monitored postoperatively for signs of infection, bleeding, altered mental status, or pneumocephalus. A specialized neurosurgical unit or intensive care setting is usually necessary to provide this level of care. If a lumbar drain is used, the staff should be familiar with its use to prevent inadvertent removal of too much CSF, which could result in pneumocephalus, brain herniation, or infection. The patient should be followed by both the otolaryngologist and neurosurgeon.

Nasal packing is usually left in place for 1 to 2 weeks postoperatively. Bacterial colonization of the packing may provide a source of intracranial infection and nasal antibiotic irrigations appear to minimize this. Systemic antibiotics are also provided, although the need for these is controversial.

Nasal endoscopic debridement is required after the packing is removed. The Surgicel that is placed over the mucoperiosteal graft remains in place for several weeks after the packing is removed and must be carefully debrided as it separates. The patient should be followed endoscopically until all of the crusting is resolved and the area of repair can be easily examined. The role for postoperative imaging is controversial but may be useful to rule out pneumocephalus or recurrent encephalocele.

MANAGEMENT OF COMPLICATIONS

Significant complications have not occurred in the author's unpublished series of patients, and this appears to be consistent with other published reports. Lanza et al. (2) report that 12 of 28 patients who were referred with active skull base defects had complications including meningitis, pneumocephalus, and severe headaches related to the defect itself, prior to surgical repair. These problems resolved after repair of the skull base defect.

Meningitis must be diagnosed quickly, necessitating close observation in the postoperative period. Fevers, mental status changes, and hemodynamic instability should be pursued aggressively with CSF and blood cultures, empiric broad-spectrum intravenous antibiotics, and possibly removal of the nasal packing. Failure to respond may require return to the operating room for exploration and revision of the repair.

Pneumocephalus may be related to aggressive removal of CSF, and may be indicated by mental status changes. Decreasing the amount of CSF removed will usually correct this. Tension pneumocephalus can occur if a ''ball valve'' exists at the skull base, which permits entry of air but not egress from the cranial vault. This must be treated rapidly to prevent brain injury. Removal of nasal packing and possible placement of a nasal airway may be beneficial as temporizing measures. Definitive neurosurgical intervention may be required.

Recurrent CSF leak occurs infrequently. Should this occur, a second attempt at repair is typically successful. The long-term success at closing CSF fistulas and removal of cephaloceles is extremely high, and there is no indication that long-term recurrence of these problems will occur.

REFERENCES

1. Donald PJ. Cerebrospinal fluid rhinorrhea. In: *Current therapy in otolaryngology—head and neck surgery*. B.C. Decker, 1990:304–307.
2. Lanza DC, O'Brien DA, Kennedy DW. Endoscopic repair of cerebrospinal fluid fistulae and encephaloceles. *Laryngoscope* 1996;106: 1119–1125.
3. Mattox DE, Kennedy DW. Endoscopic management of cerebrospinal fluid leaks and cephaloceles. *Laryngoscope* 1990;100:857–862.

Neurosurgical Issues in Otolaryngology: Principles and Practice of Collaboration,
edited by Moisés A. Arriaga and J. Diaz Day.
Lippincott Williams & Wilkins, Philadelphia © 1999.

CHAPTER 18

Pituitary Adenomas: Open Approaches

Raimund Rueger, J. Diaz Day, and Joseph C. Maroon

Technical and pharmacologic advances during the last 60 years have made it possible to perform pituitary surgery as an extracranial, transsphenoidal operation with minimal morbidity and mortality. Collaboration between neurosurgeons and otolaryngologists has lessened the functional and cosmetic consequences of earlier approaches to the sella turcica and has reduced hospitalization to 1 to 3 days.

INDICATIONS

The indications for pituitary surgery have changed in recent years. No longer are normal pituitary glands excised for pain control in metastatic breast or prostate cancer, nor for disseminated melanoma or diabetic retinopathy. Today, most pituitary surgery is for excision or debulking of pituitary adenomas, marsupialization of sellar cysts, removal of craniopharyngiomas, and closing of cerebrospinal fluid (CSF) leaks. Other lesions in the sphenoid sinus such as chordomas, mucoceles, and others may be removed transsphenoidally. Suprasellar extension of an adenoma is no longer a contraindication for this approach (at least for nonfibrous tumors), as the lesion can often be accessed from the sella by suctioning or curettage, or can be depressed into the vicinity of the sella by introduction of subarachnoid air (1).

With careful dissection, the extracranial approach can be repeated for tumor recurrence (Table 18-1). It can also be used in most patients after previous nasal surgery. Poor pneumatization of the sphenoid sinus (presellar and conchal types) does not preclude this operation, since it is possible to reach the pituitary fossa with a drill fitted with a diamond burr.

Absolute contraindications (2) are (a) acute sinusitis, (b) large suprasellar tumors in the presence of a normal-sized sella (because then too much normal gland would have to be sacrificed), and (c) very large extension of tumors above and within the sella.

HISTORICAL REVIEW

Surgery on the pituitary gland developed soon after the description of acromegaly by Marie (1886). The first approach was transcranial (lateral subtemporal) as described by Caton and Paul (1893) (3). Their patient died during surgery. Between 1904 and 1916, Horsely (4) operated on ten patients via a lateral middle fossa approach, with a mortality of 20%—an outstanding achievement at the time, when most other surgeons reported a mortality of 50% to 80%. Cushing (5) attempted this operation six times, and was able to visualize the optic chiasm only once. In 1909, Krause developed the frontal transcranial approach, on which most of today's transcranial operations are based (3,6). In Hardy's (7) words, "It will always remain a major operation because of the craniotomy, the exposure of the brain and optic chiasm, surrounded by main cerebral vessels of the circle of Willis, with the brainstem nearby."

Facing the prohibitive mortality for transcranial operations at that time, surgeons early on were attracted by the proximity of the sella turcica to the sphenoid sinus, and a multitude of extracranial transsphenoidal operations were developed. It is remarkable that all these different pathways had been described before World War I. The first operations used large incisions in the face, moved the nose aside on a pedicle flap, or split it down the middle vertically, and resulted in severe functional and cosmetic deficiencies (Fig. 18-1). Initially, all intranasal structures were removed. In 1897 Giordano was the first to propose an osteoplastic removal of the anterior wall of the frontal sinus, reflection of the nose, and resections of ethmoid sinuses, septum, and turbinates (3). Proust even introduced a forehead flap to cover the sella (6).

Schloffer (8) simplified the procedure by not resecting the

R. Rueger and J. C. Maroon: Allegheny General Hospital, Pittsburgh, Pennsylvania 15212.

J. D. Day: Department of Neurological Surgery, House Ear Clinic, Los Angeles, California 90057.

TABLE 18–1. *Extracranial open approaches to the pituitary gland*

Approach
Sublabial transseptal transsphenoidal
Transseptal transsphenoidal
Transnasal transsphenoidal (septal pushover)
Transethmoido-transsphenoidal or combined with transnasal or transseptal

frontal sinus or the floor of the anterior cranial fossa. Kocher and von Eiselsberg (9) modified it further by choosing a periorbital paranasal incision and by incorporating Killian's submucous resection, making it into a transseptal pathway (10). Kanavel (11) used a subnasal incision. MacBeth and Hall (12) utilized a bilateral external ethmoidectomy incision, connected across the nasal dorsum, to displace the nasal bones upward as a flap (Fig. 18-1). Netzer and McCoy (13) described a lateral rhinotomy approach to the septum. This was also used by Petruson and Elverson (14). All these operations required large facial incisions and are today obsolete.

Chiari (15) had developed a transethmosphenoidal operation, which was used in modern times by Kirchner and Van Gilder (16). Montgomery (17) added a posterior septal flap to cover the sella. Angell-James (18) and Briant (19) used a combined transethmosphenoidal and transnasosphenoidal pathway, observing with the microscope and suctioning through the ethmoidectomy opening, while passing instruments through the nose. The posterior septum was sometimes resected for better access.

Bateman (20) combined the transethmoidal and the transseptal pathway, again using the ethmoid portal for observation and suctioning, the transseptal passage for instrumentation. The advantage of this method was that it took advantage of a short distance to the sella. The disadvantages included an external scar, an oblique approach that reduced the safe distance between operative fields and vital structures, and possible damage to the optic nerve.

Preysing (21) in 1913, Tiefenthal in 1920, and Trible and Morse in 1965 approached the pituitary through the hard palate and septum (6). This approach had the advantages of utilizing the shortest, most direct pathway to the pituitary

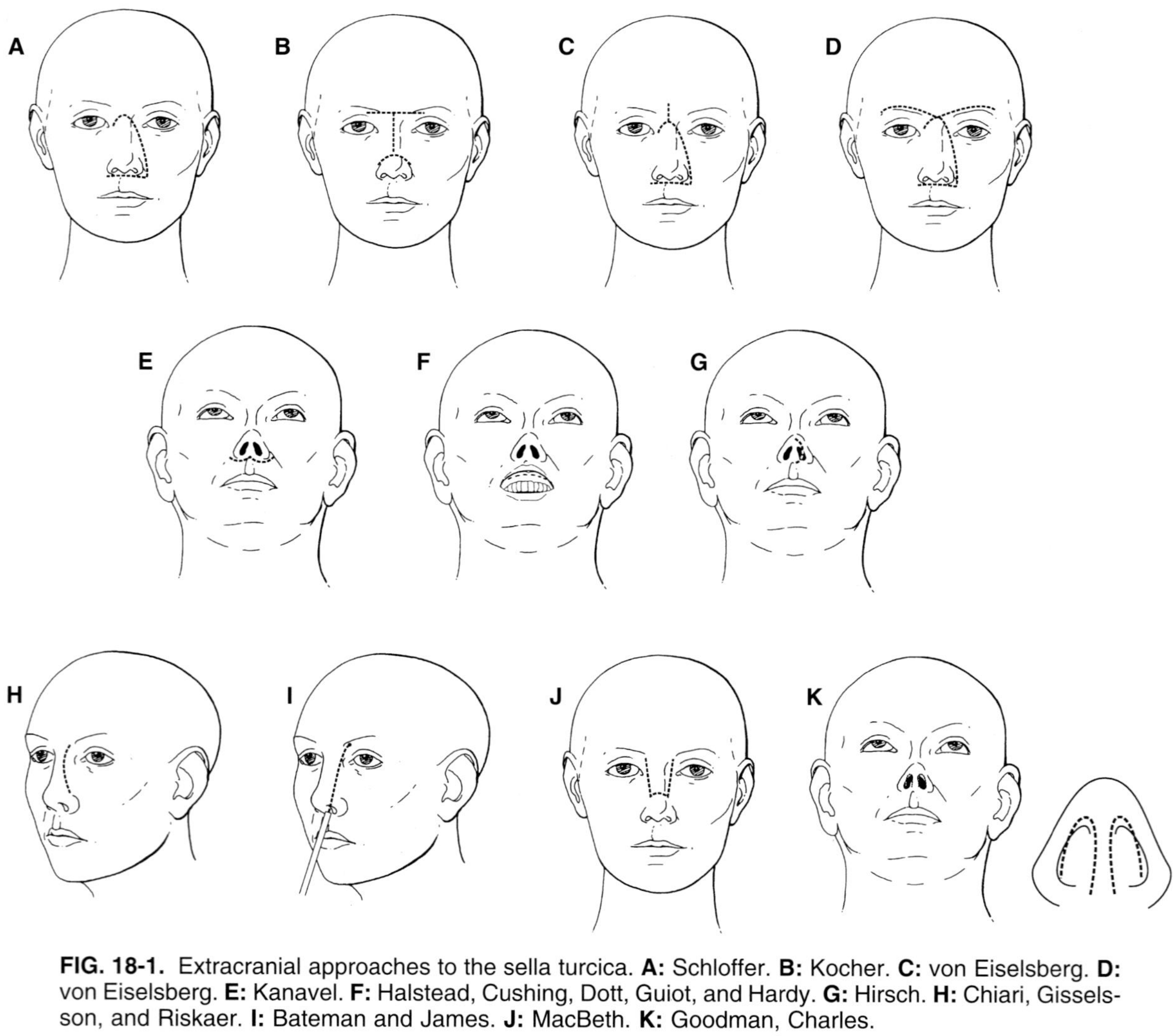

FIG. 18-1. Extracranial approaches to the sella turcica. **A:** Schloffer. **B:** Kocher. **C:** von Eiselsberg. **D:** von Eiselsberg. **E:** Kanavel. **F:** Halstead, Cushing, Dott, Guiot, and Hardy. **G:** Hirsch. **H:** Chiari, Gisselsson, and Riskaer. **I:** Bateman and James. **J:** MacBeth. **K:** Goodman, Charles.

fossa and a wide operative field. There was also no external scar. Unfortunately, these advantages were overshadowed by the difficulty of using the microscope, unsuitability if the patient had trismus or macroglossia (e.g., in acromegaly), and its increased postoperative morbidity in comparison to the other approaches. Furthermore, the approach required traversing the oral cavity and its attendant flora.

Fein and Denker in 1910 chose a transantro-ethmo-sphenoidal pathway (22), which was again popularized in 1955 by Hamberger et al. (23). Again, there was no external scar. However, this method required traversing the longest distance to the sella. The approach angle was also oblique, at an angle of about 25 degrees. Further, it was not suited for using the microscope and unsuitable if the sphenoid was poorly pneumatized. Patients suffered numbness of the upper incisors postoperatively.

Hirsch (24) split the columella vertically and continued with a transseptal transsphenoidal pathway to the sella. This operation has been modified by McCurdy and Van Sant (25), who used an open rhinoplasty approach, which is in current use (26,27). A different transnasal pushover technique was introduced by Griffith and Veerapen (28), which is also of current interest (29).

Cushing (5) developed the standard sublabial transseptal transsphenoidal approach by combining the techniques of his contemporaries, using Halstead's sublabial incision, Kocher's and von Eiselsberg's submucous resection, Kanavel's headlight, and he out-fractured rather than resected the turbinates. He was able to lower the mortality to 5.6% in 231 operations. Still, visualization was poor, and infection accounted for most of the mortality. By 1926 he switched to transcranial approaches, which by this time had become better developed, and which gave him better visualization and better ability to decompress the optic chiasm or to remove lateral extensions of tumors, which also seemed to delay recurrences. Mortality was reduced to 4.5% and was mainly due to postoperative hemorrhage and cerebral edema. Collins (3) reported that at his 70th birthday celebration Cushing was overheard to remark that the transsphenoidal approach, because of its many advantages, would possibly return.

Meanwhile, the transsphenoidal approach was used with excellent results in Europe by Hirsch (24), Hamlin, Dott, Guiot, and others (6). Jules Hardy (7), from Montreal, after working with Guiot, reintroduced the sublabial transseptal transsphenoidal operation on the North American continent in 1965. By now, the introduction of antibiotics, cortisone, image intensifier, and the operating microscope had lessened considerably the dangers and technical difficulties that had beset the transcranial approach in the past. Excellent reviews of the evolution of pituitary surgery, with extensive bibliographies, were published by Collins (3), Hardy (7), Kern et al. (30), Lee (6), and Welbourne (10). They should be consulted for more details. The advantages and complications of the transsphenoidal approaches are listed in Tables 18-2 and 18-3.

TABLE 18–2. *Advantages of the transsphenoidal approaches*

Direct pathways to the sella with minimal morbidity and mortality
Applicable to wide range of age
Tolerated by patients with serious other illnesses, who would not be candidates for craniotomy
Allows binocular vision through operative microscope
Allows surgeon to use both hands for surgery
Use of drill safer
Safer in presence of abnormal position of carotid arteries
Allows microdissection of small adenomas with preservation of pituitary function
Preservation of olfaction
Less chance of injury to optic chiasma or optic nerve
Ability to remove pituitary tumor, which has herniated into sphenoid sinus

Current Extracranial Open Approaches to the Pituitary Gland

Sublabial Transseptosphenoidal (Fig. 18-2)

The patient is orotracheally intubated in the recumbent position. We prefer a wire-reinforced endotracheal tube, which is then taped to the midline of the chin. The eyes are covered, and the head is placed in a horseshoe extension of the operating table and there positioned by the neurosurgeon. The face and an area over the right lower quadrant of the abdomen are prepared and draped. An adhesive drape is placed over the face to hold the towels in place, eliminating the need for towel clips. A window is cut into the drape

TABLE 18–3. *Potential complications of the transsphenoidal approaches*

Neurosurgical
Meningitis (6,30,32,35)
Diabetes insipidus (transient or permanent)
Cerebrospinal fluid leak
Intracranial hemorrhage
Injury to carotid artery (with transsection or formation of pseudoaneurysm)
Mycotic aneurysm of carotid artery (following sinus infection) (36)
Tension pneumoencephalos (37)
Hypo- or anosmia (6,30,32)
Worsening of vision or of visual fields (38)
Rhinologic
Septal hematoma
Septal abscess
Septal perforation
Saddle nose or retraction of nasal columella
Intranasal adhesions or crusting
Epistaxis
Numbness of upper lip, central incisors, tip of nose
Loss of upper buccal vault, leading to denture problems
Diplopia (from detachment of the trochlea)
Unsightly scar at columella or ala
Dehiscence of the sublabial suture line
Tendency for sinus infection

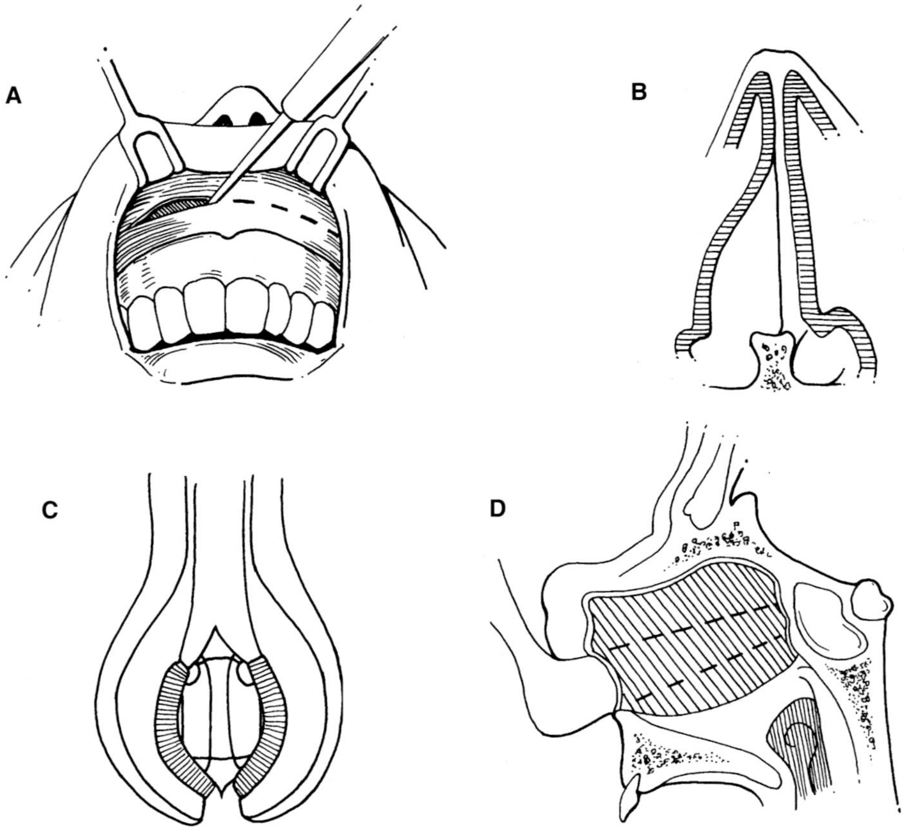

FIG. 18-2. Sublabial transsepto-sphenoidal approach.

over the site of operation. Xylocaine 2% with adrenaline 1:100,000, altogether six carpules of 1.8 cc each, is then injected in the upper buccal sulcus, the nasal columella, and into the mucoperichondrial and mucoperiosteal membranes of the nasal septum and nasal floor on both sides. No topical medication is used. The upper lip is then gently retracted, and with an electric knife in the cutting mode an incision is made through the mucosa of the upper lip, from the right to the left canine fossa, 5 to 8 mm distal to the gingivomucosal junction (a more peripheral incision leads to increased lip swelling). This assures preservation of the upper buccal vault and prevents problems with dentures (Fig. 18-2A). The incision is carried down to the bony premaxilla. Bleeders are electrocoagulated. The anterior nasal spine and the caudal end of the septal cartilage are palpated and dissected free, then an incision is made through the perichondrium of the septum on the right side.

With a Mackenty elevator, the periosteum of the premaxilla is swept up to the piriform apertures, the mucoperiosteum of the nasal floor is carefully detached from the bony lip of the piriform aperture, and is then elevated off the nasal floor bilaterally, up to the decussate fibers. With a Cottle dissector, the perichondrium is dissected off the cartilaginous septum on the right side, the decussate fibers are cut bilaterally (Fig. 18-2B), and the cartilaginous septum is then detached from the bony septum vertically (a Freer dissector is best suited for this). Dissection progresses posteriorly on both sides of the perpendicular lamina, until the rostrum of the sphenoid sinus is reached. The perpendicular lamina is then subtotally resected with Jensen forceps. The harvested bone is preserved for possible use in the reconstruction of the sellar floor. The mucoperiosteum is then elevated laterally off the anterior wall of the sphenoid sinus, until the natural ostia appear. The vomer, unless deformed, is left intact. It serves as a midline guide to the sella, and as such is especially valuable in reoperations. The cartilaginous septum is now displaced into the left nasal cavity, still covered by the intact left-sided perichondrium. A pituitary speculum is inserted (Fig. 18-2C,D) and the neurosurgical team is summoned. One should also realize that the maximal width that the pituitary speculum can be opened is the distance between the two median pterygoid plates [Lee (6)], and thus differs from patient to patient. Forceful attempts to gain greater width of exposure may lead to fracture of the median pterygoid plates or the medial walls of the maxillary sinuses, which has led to difficulty in treating malocclusion (31,32). The neurosurgeon then removes the rostrum, giving him an additional perception of the midline. In closing, the septal cartilage is repositioned on top of the maxillary crest and retained there with a suture of 4-0 catgut. The nasal cavity is inspected. Small unilateral tears are accepted as drainage openings, larger ones are sutured. The sublabial incision is closed with the interrupted 4-0 chronic catgut sutures. Nasal splints are inserted and secured by a transfixion suture of 4-0 silk. Folded Telfa is inserted lateral to each splint for packing.

We never lower the piriform aperture by bone removal, thus avoiding denervation of the central incisors (6,33). The anterior nasal spine is rarely an obstruction, since the biaxial light beams of the microscope bypass it. If removal is necessary, it is done with a chisel, and the spine is later wired back into place with no. 32 wire. This prevents retraction of the columella. In narrow noses, the newly introduced Fukushima speculum is of great help. It is more slender and it incorporates an upper lip retractor. Special care needs to be applied in patients with Cushing's disease, as their tissues are more fragile, with greater tendency to bleed and to bruise.

The mean operating time for this exposure in our hands is 35 minutes, the time for closure 10 minutes. Packing is removed on the following day, the splints after 5 to 7 days. Patient may resume wearing dentures after 2 weeks. Time in hospital is controlled by the endocrinologist, otherwise discharge would be possible on the day after surgery.

Transseptal Transsphenoidal

This operation was originally introduced by Hirsch (24) (Fig. 18-1G), who split the columella vertically and then proceeded with a septoplasty approach, saving a caudal strut of cartilage, but resecting most of the cartilaginous and all of the bony septum. The operation was changed to an open rhinoplasty approach by McCurdy and Van Sant (25) (Fig. 18-1K) as follows: Under general orotracheal anesthesia the patient is positioned in the recumbent position. The face is prepped and draped; 1% lidocaine with adrenaline 1:100,000 is infiltrated into the columellar skin, the intercrural area, the dome, and the mucoperichondrium and mucoperiosteum of the septum and floor bilaterally. Cotton pledgets moistened with 0.05% of oxymetazoline hydrochloride are placed into the nose for vasoconstriction. A standard open rhinoplasty incision with the inverted V of Goodman and Charles (Fig. 18-1K) is made, and the "elephant trunk" is elevated onto the dome. The intercrural ligaments between the medal crura are separated with iris scissors, exposing the caudal edge of the septal cartilage. Upper and lower tunnels are fashioned by raising the perichondrium of the septum on one side, the decussate fibers are cut, the mucoperiosteum of the nasal floor is elevated, the bony septum is subtotally resected, and the cartilaginous septum is dislocated in the opposite naris. The neurosurgical part then follows. In closing, the septum is repositioned, and the skin incision closed meticulously with 6-0 nylon or 5-0 chromic suture, followed by septal splints and packing.

This operation can also be performed through a regular hemitransfixion incision, with entry into the septum at the caudal end of the septal cartilage, or more posteriorly (34). In narrow noses, this approach may require an alotomy for adequate exposure. This approach is easy in acromegalics.

Transnasal Transsphenoidal (Fig. 18-3)

First described by Griffith and Veerapen in 1981 (28), it has gained acceptance in England. It is somewhat modified by Cooke and Jones (29). The technique is as follows: Under general orotracheal anesthesia in the recumbent position, the patient's head is positioned. The nasal mucosa is coated with cocaine paste to reduce vascularity, and an image intensifier is positioned to give a lateral image of the sphenoid sinus, pituitary fossa, and facial skeleton. The skin is prepped and draped and covered with a plastic foil. Under microscopic guidance, a short nasal speculum is then introduced into the right nostril, after its tips have been lubricated with povidone-iodine solution. The nasal speculum is passed between the middle turbinate laterally and the nasal septum medially. Opening the speculum fully compresses the right middle turbinate laterally and enables the slightly everted tips of the second (Hardy) speculum to pass without abrading the nasal mucosa (Fig. 18-3A). When the posterior nasal cavity is reached, the tips of the speculum are opened and the posterior part of the septal bone is fractured across to the left as closely as possible to the anterior surface of the sphenoid bone. This is achieved by forcefully turning the blade tips of the speculum to the left, and usually results in an associated tear in the septal mucosa close to the rostrum of the sphenoid bone (Fig. 18-3A). The Hardy speculum is then expanded and the "prow" of the sphenoid comes into view (Fig. 18-3B,C), giving a useful guide to the midline. Bleeding from the torn mucosa is controlled with bipolar cautery, the anterior wall of the sphenoid sinus is removed, and the pituitary surgery can begin.

In closing, the Hardy speculum is removed and briefly inserted into the left naris to reposition the septum in the midline. Packing is inserted bilaterally, more on the left side. It is removed after 48 hours. If the nasal passage did not admit a Hardy speculum, a Killian's nasal speculum was used, and occasionally an alotomy was done. Operating time was given as 5 to 6 minutes for exposure. The authors claim that in uncomplicated cases they have been able to enter the sphenoid sinus 10 minutes after starting the procedure.

Transethmoido-Transsphenoidal (Fig. 18-4)

A routine external ethmoidectomy is performed (Fig. 18-4A,B), preserving, if possible the middle turbinate. The most posterior ethmoid cell is entered directly below the posterior ethmoid foramen, and through its posterior wall the sphenoid sinus is entered. The anterior wall of the sphenoid sinus is removed, which sometimes requires resection of the most posterior part of the septum (Fig. 18-4C). Although the distance of the dissection from the optic foramen is only 2 to 3 mm, few difficulties have been encountered in expert hands. Some authors combine this approach with a transnasal or

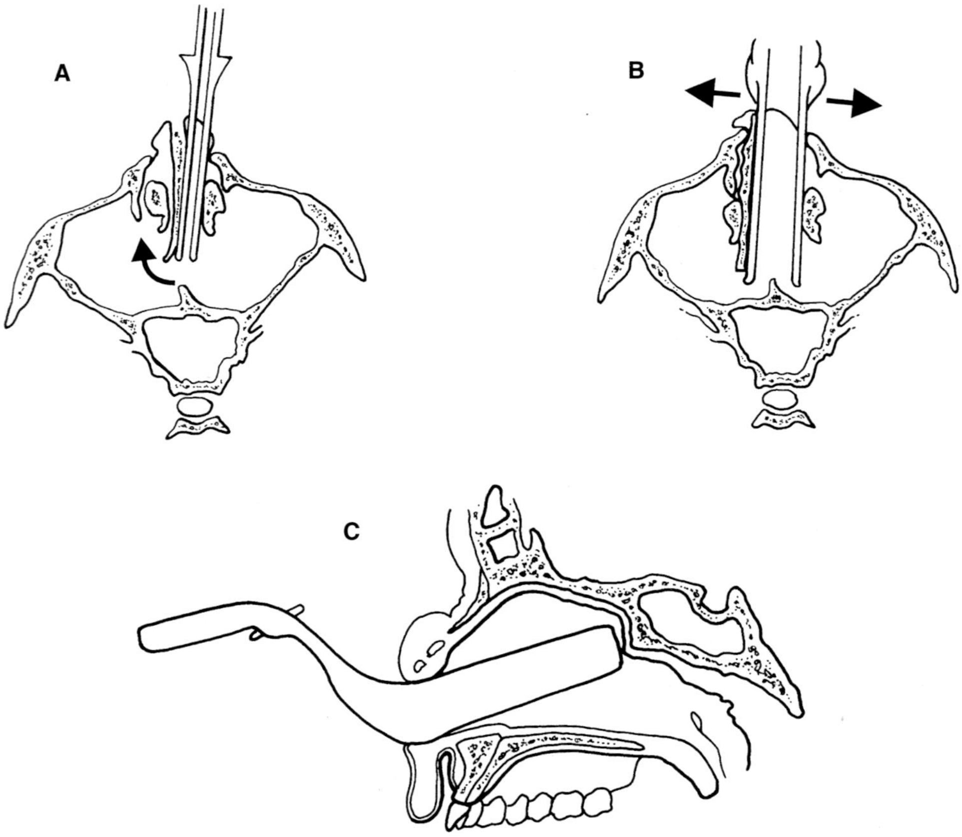

FIG. 18-3. Transnasal-transsphenoidal approach.

transseptal one and then utilize the above-described pathways.

Neurosurgical Resection

The technique of resection is similar for all the above-described approaches. Upon reaching the sella floor, a rectangular opening is made to expose the dura. The floor is thinned in the case of large tumors and is easily removed with fine rongeurs. When the floor is thick, the high-speed drill is used to expose the dura.

The dura is then opened in a cruciate fashion to expose gland and tumor. The tumor capsule is defined with a fine dissector, and an attempt is made to circumferentially free capsule from gland by sweeping around the tumor. Ring curettes are then utilized to remove tumor. This is usually performed in a stepwise, orderly fashion, working on each side. Once the lateral margins are freed, the superior and anterior aspect of the mass is addressed. As in the case of macroadenomas, arachnoid will fall into the sella when the suprasellar portion is decompressed. In some cases, cavernous sinus extension requires resection out of a direct line of view. This is done with a rounded-edge ring curette.

At the conclusion of tumor resection, a determination is made of the necessity of a dural patch graft and adipose graft placement in the sphenoid sinus. The primary determinant is the presence or absence of an intact arachnoid membrane. Any evidence of CSF leakage triggers the decision to place a fascial graft on the defect to separate the subarachnoid space from the sphenoid sinus and nasopharynx. The sphenoid sinus is then completely obliterated with adipose tissue.

Lumbar spinal drainage is necessary for 24 to 48 hours to allow the graft to begin sealing off the compartments. Lowered CSF pressure promotes an adequate seal forming early. The patient's head is kept elevated approximately 30 to 45 degrees at all times for 1 to 2 days. An alternative to a lumbar drain is to perform a lumbar puncture in the recovery room. This is done utilizing a large-bore (18-gauge) needle and draining 30 to 40 cc of CSF. Several punctures are made in the dura before withdrawal to promote temporary fistula formation. This method is quite successful and obviates the hindrance a lumber drain poses to the patient's immediate postoperative mobility.

Operative Results

Between 1984 and 1997, we performed 232 transsphenoidal operations (231 sublabial transseptal, 1 transseptal) at

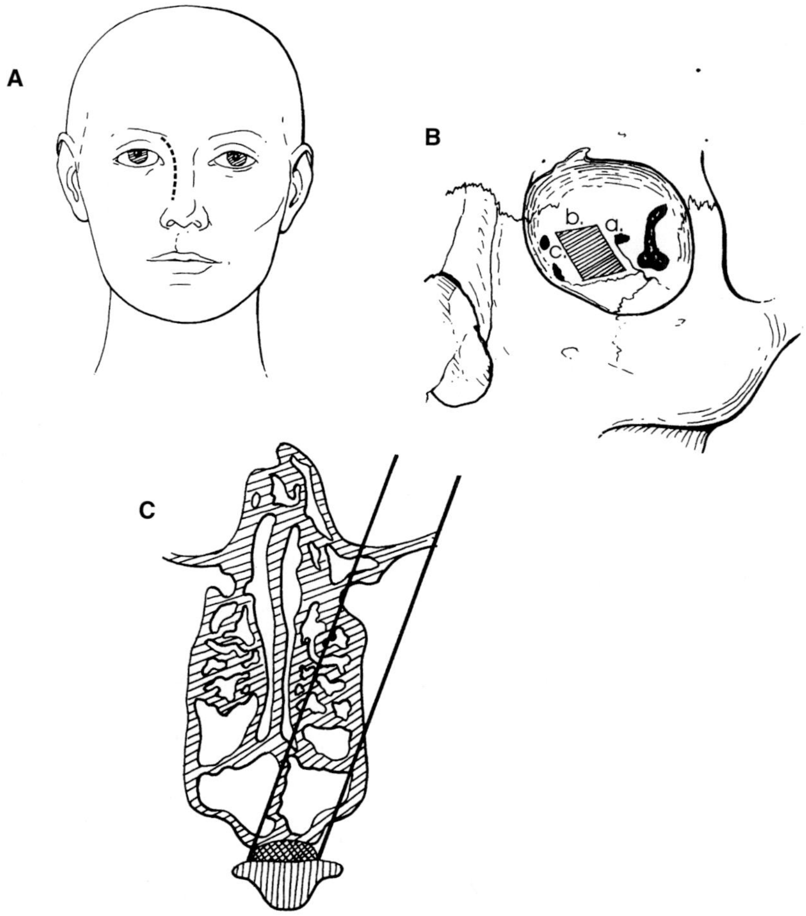

FIG. 18-4. Transethnoidal-transsphenoidal approach.

Allegheny General Hospital. The patients ranged in age from 12 to 82. Two-hundred seventeen operations were done for neurosurgical indications, 15 for lesions of the sphenoid sinuses. Adequate records could be evaluated for 216 patients (201 and 15), of which 192 had follow-up examinations with the ENT Service. These two subsets form the basis of this analysis.

The distribution of cases is illustrated in Tables 18-4 and 18-5. The majority of pituitary tumors were large, with suprasellar extension. Eleven patients had had septal surgery in the past, two of whom also had septal perforations preoperatively (one of which could be closed).

Four had severe septal deformities, which were corrected at the time of surgery. There were 22 repeat sublabial operations, one of them through the left side of the septum. The indications were tumor recurrence (16 cases), CSF leaks (three cases), reformation of sellar cyst (one case), and hematoma formation (two cases). Three of the repeat operations were second repeat procedures. Eight of the 22 patients have had their initial sublabial operations at other institutions.

TABLE 18–4. *Distribution of intrasellar lesions*

Lesion	Number
Nonfunctional adenomas	144
Prolactinomas	31
Acromegaly	17
Cushing's	8
Craniopharyngioma	4
Sellar cyst	3
Empty sella syndrome	2[a]
Rathke's pouch cyst	5
Metastasis to pituitary	3[b]
Total	217

[a] One case also contained a growth hormone secreting adenoma.
[b] One lung, one breast, one undifferent. Adenoca.

TABLE 18–5. *Distribution of sphenoid lesions*

Lesion	Number
Nonresolving acute sphenoiditis	1
Chronic fungal sphenoiditis	2
Chronic nonfungal sphenoiditis	2
Mucocele	3
Extracranial meningioma in sphenoid sinus	2
Meningioma at skull base (biopsy only)	2
Squamous cell carcinoma	1
Fibrous dysplasia	1
Exploration for suspected tumor	1
Total	15

TABLE 18-6. *Recorded complications—neurosurgical (in 217 cases)*

Complication	Number
Death	1
Meningitis (recovered)	2
Diabetes insipidus	
Transient	25
Permanent	10
Present preoperative	2
Cerebrospinal fluid leak	
Temporary	11
Requiring surgery	6

There was one intraoperative death (intracranial bleeding into a very large tumor with extensive suprasellar and lateral extensions). No other intra- or perioperative deaths occurred.

Visual Outcomes

Twenty-two patients had visual field defects preoperatively. Of these, 13 improved or normalized, three were unchanged, and one developed a field defect briefly postoperatively (presumably from a small hematoma). His fields returned to normal later. Five were lost to follow-up.

Twenty-eight patients had decreased vision, of which 22 improved or normalized postoperatively, four were unchanged, one was lost to follow-up, and one worsened. Six patients had diplopia secondary to cranial nerve palsies (one ptosis, two sixth nerve, one third nerve, and two unspecified). Of these, three improved or normalized postoperatively, and three were unchanged. An additional patient with acute ophthalmoplegia recovered.

Our complications are listed in Tables 18-6 and 18-7. We attribute the low rate of complications to meticulous dissection and to avoidance of bone resection at the piriform aperture or anterior nasal spine (33). It is possible that heating of the premaxilla during cautery for bone bleeders contributes to sensory loss in the upper incisors. Mostly the numbness is temporary. Disturbance at the sublabial incision was caused by premature use of upper dentures. We now caution our patients not to wear upper dentures for 2 to 3 weeks postoperatively. Patient satisfaction is high. We have encountered no objections when a reoperation became necessary.

TABLE 18-7. *Recorded complications—rhinologic (in 192 cases)*

Complication	Number
Epistaxis	
Slight	5
Severe, requiring packing	3
Otis media	1
Sinusitis	4
Persistent numbness	
Central incisors	2
Upper lip	2
Septal perforation	4[a]
Septal hematoma	1
Septal deformity	
Worse postoperative	1
Wound dehiscence, mild	4
Wound dehiscence, requiring resuturing	1

[a] All were small and located at the sphenoid rostrum, functionally neutral.

REFERENCES

1. Spaziante R, deVitis E. Forced subarachnoid air in transsphenoidal excision of pituitary tumors (pumping technique). *J Neurosurg* 1989; 71:864–867.
2. Kirchner JA. Discussion. *Laryngoscope* 1984;94:1074.
3. Collins WF. Hypophysectomy: historical and personal perspectives. *Clin Neurosurg* 1972;21:68–78.
4. Horsley V. On the technique of operations on the central nervous system. *Br Med J* 1906;2:411–423.
5. Cushing H. Surgical experiences with pituitary disorders. *JAMA* 1914; 63:1515–1525.
6. Lee KJ. The sublabial transsphenoidal approach to the hypophysis. *Laryngoscope* 1978;88(suppl 10, pt 2)L1–L65.
7. Hardy J. Transsphenoidal surgery on the normal and pathological pituitary. Clinical neurosurgery. In: *Proceedings of the Congress of Neurological Surgeons, Toronto 1968.* Baltimore, MD: Williams & Wilkins, 1969:185–217.
8. Schloffer J. Erfolgreiche Operation Eines Hypophysentumors auf Nasalem Wege. *Wien Klin Wochenschr* 1909;59:636–638.
9. von Eiselsberg F. My experience about operations upon the hypophysis. *Trans Am Surg Assoc* 1910;28:55–72.
10. Welbourn RB. The evolution of transsphenoidal pituitary microsurgery. *Surgery* 1986;100:1185–1189.
11. Kanavel AB. Removal of tumors of the pituitary body by the intranasal route. *JAMA* 1909;53:1704–1707.
12. MacBeth R, Hall M. Hypophysectomy as a rhinological procedure. *Arch Otolaryngol* 1962;75:440–450.
13. Netzer HR, McCoy, Gordon: Transseptal-transsphenoidal hypophysectomy. *Arch Otolaryngol* 1967;86:28–31.
14. Petruson B, Elversson J. A lateral rhinotomy approach to the transsphenoidal hypophysectomy. *Clin Otolaryngol* 1988;13:251–258.
15. Chiari O. Ueber eine Modifikation der Schlofferschen Operation von Tumoren der Hypophyse. *Wien Klin Wochenschr* 1912;25:5–6.
16. Kirchner JA, Van Gilder JC. Transethmoidal hypophysectomy: some surgical landmarks. *Trans Am Acad Ophthalmol Otolaryngol* 1975;80: 391–396.
17. Montgomery WW. *Surgery of the upper respiratory system,* vol 1. Philadelphia: Lea & Febiger, 1971:71–94.
18. Angell-James J. Transethmosphenoidal hypophysectomy. *Arch Otol* 1967;86:256–264.
19. Briant TDR. Transethmoidal sphenoidal hypophysectomy. *Laryngoscope* 1968;78:649–653.
20. Bateman GH. Transsphenoidal hypophysectomy. *Otol Clin North Am* 1971;4:205–215.
21. Preysing J. Beitraege zur Operation der Hypophyse. *Verh Dtsch Laryngol Gesellsch* 1913;20:51–73.
22. Hardy J. Transsphenoidal hypophysectomy. *J Neurosurg* 1971;34: 582–594.
23. Hamberger CA, et al. Transantrosphenoidal hypophysectomy. *Arch Otol* 1961;74:2–8.
24. Hirsch O. Endonasal method of removal of hypophyseal tumors. *JAMA* 1910;55:772–774.
25. McCurdy JA, Van Sant TE. Transseptal-transsphenoidal hypophysectomy via the external rhinoplasty approach. *J Otolaryngol* 1978;7: 29–31.
26. Koltai PJ, Goldstein JC, Parnes SM, Price JC. External rhinoplasty approach to transsphenoidal hypophysectomy. *Arch Otolaryngol* 1985; 111:456–458.
27. Quilligan JJ, Everton DM, Burgess LP, et al. External (combination) rhinoplasty approach for transsphenoidal adenectomy. *J Otolaryngol* 1985;14:192–196.

28. Griffith HB, Veerapen R. A direct transnasal approach to the sphenoid sinus: technical note. *J Neurosurg* 1987;66:140–142.
29. Cooke RS, Jones RAC. Experience with the transnasal transsphenoidal approach to the pituitary fossa. *Br J Neurosurg* 1994;8:193–196.
30. Kern EB, Pearson BW, McDonald TJ, et al. The transseptal approach to lesions of the pituitary and parasellar regions. *Laryngoscope* 1979; 89(suppl 15):1–34.
31. Grayson RJ Jr, Johnson PA. Transsphenoidal hypophysectomy: an unusual complication. *Virginia Med* 1986;113:294–295.
32. Kennedy DW, Cohn ES, Papel ID, Holliday MJ. Transsphenoidal approach to the sella: the Johns Hopkins experience. *Laryngoscope* 1984; 94:1066–1073.
33. Watson SW, Sinn PB, Neuwelt EA. Dental considerations in the sublabial transsphenoidal surgical approach to the pituitary gland. *Neurosurgery* 1982;10:236–241.
34. Escajadillo JR, de Gortari E. Transseptal approach for the treatment of pituitary lesions. *Arch Otol* 1983;109:326–328.
35. Chan KH, Chau PY, Wang RY. Meningitis caused by flavobacterium meningosepticum after transsphenoidal hypophysectomy with recovery. *Surg Neurol* 1983;20:294–296.
36. Onishi H, Haruhide I, et al. Intracranial mycotic aneurysm associated with transsphenoidal surgery to the pituitary adenoma. *Surg Neurol* 1989;31:149–154.
37. Altinoers N, Ada N, et al. Tension pneumocephalus after transsphenoidal surgery: case report. *Neurosurgery* 1988;2:516–518.

Neurosurgical Issues in Otolaryngology: Principles and Practice of Collaboration, edited by Moisés A. Arriaga and J. Diaz Day. Lippincott Williams & Wilkins, Philadelphia © 1999.

CHAPTER 19

Pituitary: Endoscopic Transnasal Approach

Ricardo L. Carrau and Hae-Dong Jho

OVERVIEW

Historical Perspective

The first successful removal of a pituitary tumor was performed by Schloffer in 1907, using an transethmoidal-transsphenoidal approach. In 1909, Oscar Hirsch, from Vienna, reported the successful use of endonasal-transsphenoidal approach to the pituitary. Although Hirsch's first operation was a staged endonasal approach to the pituitary, he subsequently changed his technique to a sublabial transseptal approach (1). Other surgical approaches were reported with mixed results until 1910, when Cushing reported a sublabial-transseptal-transsphenoidal approach to the pituitary (2). The transsphenoidal approach, using the sublabial or transseptal route, became the standard approach to pituitary tumors (1,3–5). The transseptal-transsphenoidal approach, as known to contemporary surgeons, has changed little since Cushing's original description. This approach, however, has been complemented with technologic advances, such as the intraoperative fluoroscopy, as described by Guiot, the operating microscope, as described by Hardy, and most recently the use of intraoperative navigation devices and intraoperative magnetic resonance imaging (MRI) (1,4,6).

Briefly, the transseptal-transsphenoidal approach involves the use of sublabial or septal incisions, wide dissection of the mucoperiosteum of the floor of the nose and septum, and resection of the osseous septum and rostrum of the sphenoid sinuses to expose the anterior face of the sella turcica. The exposure is maintained with a self-retainer speculum, and the resection of the pituitary tumor is performed under microscope magnification and intraoperative fluoroscopic imaging (or intraoperative navigational device).

The microscopic approach is limited by the optical properties of the lens and illumination. The microscope has a restricted focal length, illumination, diameter of the visual field, and angle of visualization. Thus, despite the magnification provided by the microscope, the field of vision is restricted; thus, neurovascular injuries, such as carotid artery perforation (i.e., exsanguination, cerebrovascular accident), and optic nerve injury continue to be potential catastrophic complications of the transsphenoidal approach to the pituitary (3,5).

The sublabial-transseptal-transsphenoidal and the transseptal-transsphenoidal approaches are associated with postoperative sequelae that include facial and endonasal swelling and the frequent requirement of nasal packing and/or septal splints. Sinonasal complications such as sinusitis, nasal synechiae, septal perforation, and numbness of the upper incisors are common. Other rare but significant complications include sagittal fracture of the maxilla and bilateral optic nerve injury caused by the overenthusiastic use of the self-retainer speculum.

Hirsch's endonasal approach, using a microscopic technique, has been advocated by others, who claim a lower morbidity in regard to sinonasal complications (7–9). Among other approaches, the endoscopic-transsphenoidal approach, via transnasal or transseptal routes, has been the subject of sporadic reports, including small series of patients (10–16). We have applied endoscopic skills, acquired during surgery for inflammatory disease of the sinonasal tract, to the endoscopic-transnasal-transsphenoidal technique to pituitary surgery (17–21). Our endoscopic approach differs from other techniques, as we utilize an endonasal-transsphenoidal route without the use of a retractor or speculum, and the endoscope is the sole visualizing tool used during the entire operation.

R. L. Carrau: Department of Otolaryngology, University of Pittsburgh Medical Center, Pittsburgh, Pennsylvania 15213.

H.-D. Jho: Department of Neurological Surgery, University of Pittsburgh Medical Center, Pittsburgh, Pennsylvania 15213.

Perioperative Considerations

The surgical indications for endoscopic pituitary surgery are identical to those for conventional microscopic surgery.

Surgery is recommended for patients presenting with hormone-nonsecreting pituitary adenomas when those tumors cause hypopituitarism, visual disorders, or pituitary apoplexy, or when they show progressive growth in serial follow-up. Surgery is also indicated for hormone-secreting adenomas that do not respond to medical therapy.

Preoperative testing includes MRI of the brain/sella, a formal endocrine evaluation, and an ophthalmic examination, including evaluation of the visual fields. A computed tomography (CT) scan of the paranasal sinuses is obtained preoperatively in patients with complex anatomy of the sinuses (e.g., multiple septations, previous surgery, poorly pneumatized sphenoid).

Postoperative evaluation includes a nasal examination and a formal endocrine evaluation 2 to 3 weeks postoperatively, and an MRI of the brain 6 weeks after surgery. A postoperative visual evaluation is performed in patients who presented with a preoperative visual disorder.

Perioperative stress doses of steroids are used selectively for patients with anterior hypopituitarism. Patients presenting with anterior hypopituitarism are started on hormonal replacement preoperatively. Thyroid hormone replacement is maintained at least for 2 weeks postoperatively.

Intravenous perioperative prophylactic antibiotics with broad spectrum coverage (e.g., ceftriaxone) are administered before the induction of anesthesia and are continued for 24 hours after surgery. In addition, 600 mg of clindamycin-phosphate are diluted in 150 mL of normal saline solution, which is then used as the irrigation solution during the procedure.

Following surgery, the patient is admitted to a regular hospital room and observed overnight for the potential occurrence of diabetes insipidus. About two-thirds of our first 100 patients undergoing endoscopic pituitary surgery were discharged from the hospital the day following their operation. Two of our patients with microadenomas were discharged the day of the surgery.

Upon discharge from the hospital, patients are advised not to blow their nose, lean forward, strain, or lift anything over 20 lb for 4 to 6 weeks after surgery. The patient is prescribed oxymetazoline 0.05% nasal spray to be used twice a day for 5 days after the surgery and normal saline solution spray to be used six to eight times daily. During the early postoperative period, all patients enjoy an unobstructed nasal airway. Postoperative pain is minimal and most patients do not require any analgesic medication.

ADVANTAGES OF TEAM SURGERY

The neurosurgical team is experienced in microscopic techniques for intracranial surgery, including the resection of pituitary tumors. Intraoperative management of pituitary tumors and their possible complications is identical whether an "open" or endoscopic approach is used. In other words, the approach is different but the extirpative part of the surgery involves the same techniques and instrumentation as the transseptal-transsphenoidal approach. The otolaryngology team utilizes endonasal-endoscopic approaches to the sinonasal tract, including the sphenoid sinus, on a routine basis for indications that include inflammatory diseases, trauma, and tumors. Ample endoscopic skills and knowledge of the anatomy of the sinonasal tract ease the transition to the endoscopic approach and add to the margin of safety. The experience of both teams is combined to provide an approach that offers wide visualization of the tumor and surgical landmarks, and, hence, a safe extirpation with minimal postoperative morbidity.

SURGICAL TECHNIQUE

Surgery

General anesthesia is induced and paralysis is continued throughout the surgery. The patency of the airway is maintained by an orotracheal tube that is secured in place with surgical tape. The operating table is positioned perpendicular to the anesthesia staff, exposing the right side of the patient to the surgeon (Fig. 19-1). The position of the patient is similar to the one used for the microscopic technique. The patient is positioned supine with 20 degrees of hip flexion to provide slight elevation of the torso. The patient's head is slightly flexed, tilted to the left 10 degrees and turned to the right side 10 degrees. The head is fixed in this position using a three-pin head fixation system such as a Mayfield head holder. A C-arm fluoroscope is utilized selectively in cases with complex sinus anatomy (e.g., lack of pneumatization of the sphenoid sinus, previous surgery). The C-arm fluoroscope is positioned at the head of the table, providing a lateral image that includes the nasal cavity, sphenoid sinus, and sella turcica. Alternatively, an intraoperative navigational device can be used in lieu of the fluoroscope. The face, nasal vestibules, and lower abdomen are prepared with 5% povidone-iodine solution, followed by a 70% alcohol solution. The patient, the fluoroscope, and the endoscopic equipment are draped within a sterile field.

The nose is decongested with oxymetazoline 0.05%. The middle turbinate, posterior septum, and rostrum of the sphenoid are infiltrated with Xylocaine 1% and epinephrine 1/100,000, under direct visualization with a 0-degree sinonasal endoscope. The 0-degree endoscope is used to complete most of the surgical approach and removal of the tumor. The endoscope is attached to a videocamera connected to a closed circuit system to provide a continuous monitored view and to allow videotaping of the surgery. The 0-degree endoscope provides the surgeon with a view that is less distorted than the view provided by angled lenses. The straight visual axis aids the surgeon in maintaining a better anatomic orientation during the procedure. In addition, the surgeon can rotate the light-carrier cable of the 0-degree endoscope to be positioned opposite the camera cable. This allows the surgeon to manipulate the surgical instruments with ease, beneath and parallel to the endoscope rod. An irrigation-suction system (Endoscrub, Xomed-Treace, Jacksonville, FL) is also attached to

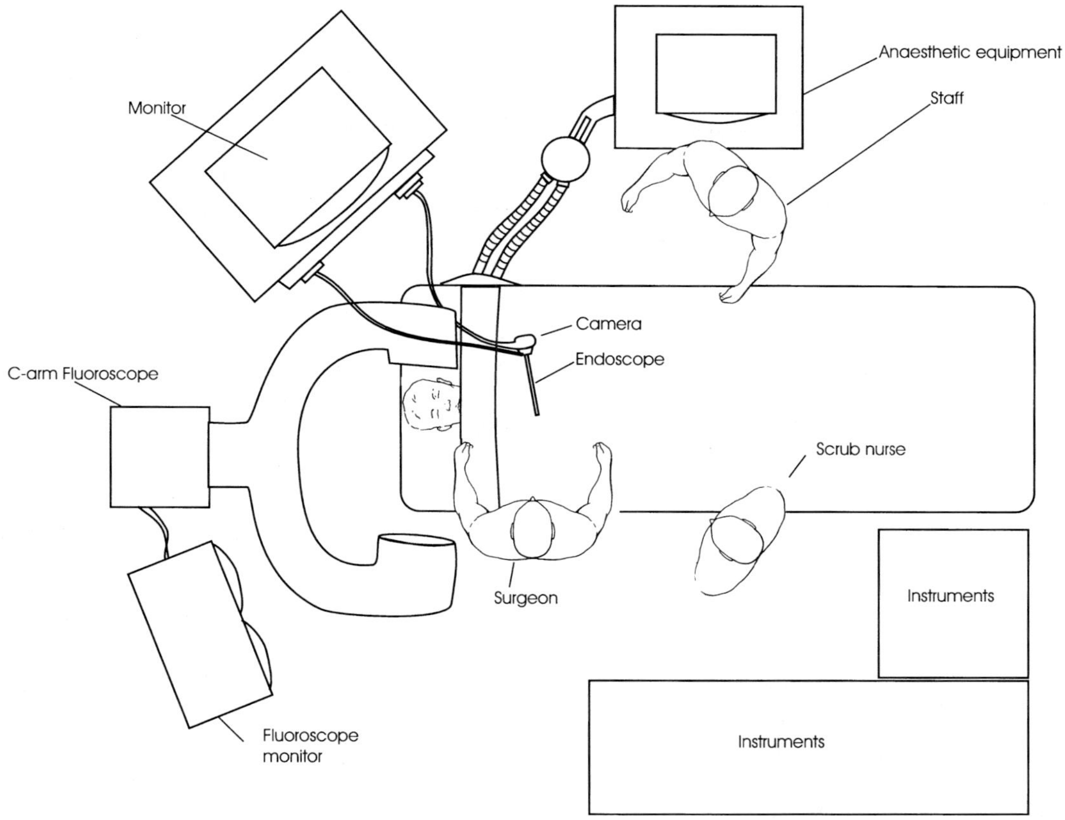

FIG. 19-1. Arrangement of personnel and equipment in the operating room. The surgeon should have an unobstructed view of the monitor.

the endoscope. This device uses an irrigation-suction system to clean the lens of the endoscope. The irrigation flow and suction can be adjusted according to the surgeon's preference. The surgeon controls the irrigation with a pedal, eliminating the need to remove the endoscope from the nose to clean the lens.

In the majority of cases, the surgery is performed through one nostril. The decision as to which nostril to use is made on the basis of the dimensions and anatomy of the nasal cavity. In our experience, only 2/100 patients required a bilateral approach due to a very narrow nasal cavity. Six to seven minutes after the injection of the Xylocaine 1% with epinephrine 1/100.000 (i.e., maximum vasoconstriction), the middle turbinate is out-fractured using the blunt end of the Cottle elevator (Fig. 19-2). It is prudent to avoid undue trauma to the middle turbinate that may lead to bleeding and thus affect the visualization of the sphenoethmoid recess. Thus, whenever possible, the middle turbinate should be protected with a 1/2″ × 3″ cotton pledget.

The natural ostium of the sphenoid sinus is then identified visually and its position is corroborated with the fluoroscope (Fig. 19-2). The mucosa surrounding the natural ostium is then coagulated using a bipolar cautery, and the ostium is fractured with the Cottle elevator in a medial and inferior direction, to allow the insertion of up-biting and down-biting

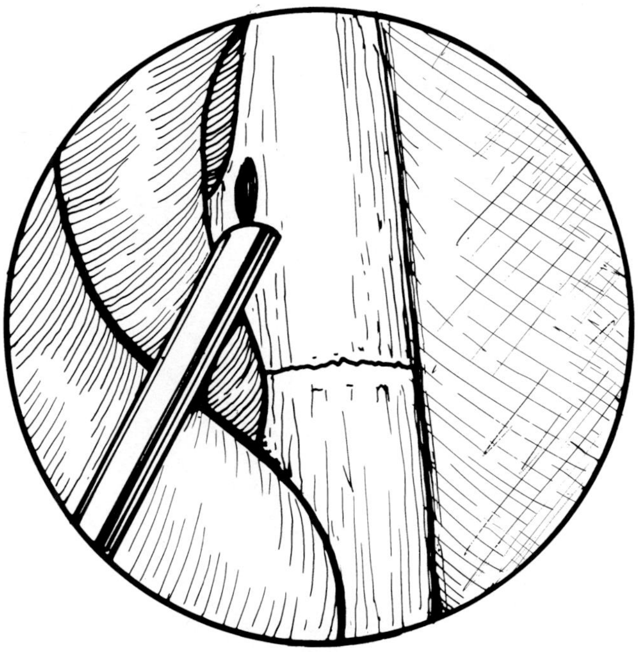

FIG. 19-2. The middle and superior turbinates are outfractured, providing an unobstructed view of the natural ostium of the sphenoid sinus. The natural ostium is usually identified posterior to the inferior edge of the superior turbinate.

Kerrison rongeurs. Kerrison rongeurs are used to enlarge the sphenoidotomy under direct visualization. The relationship of the rostrum of the sphenoid with the lateral wall is carefully assessed before enlarging the sphenoidotomy in this direction (Fig. 19-3). Once the ipsilateral rostrum of the sphenoid has been removed, allowing the concomitant passage of the endoscope and surgical instruments, the sphenoid sinus is inspected with 0-degree and 30-degree endoscopes to identify surgical landmarks, such as the carotid canal, optic nerve, opticocarotid recess, and clival indentation (this landmark identifies the midline) (22).

The posterior septum is then transfixed with an angled Cottle elevator. The vertical hemitransfixion incision is extended through the ipsilateral mucosa and the vomer bone/cartilage at its junction with the rostrum of the sphenoid. The mucosa over the rostrum of the contralateral sphenoid sinus is then elevated, following a submucosal plane, to identify the contralateral natural ostium (Fig. 19-3). A wide sphenoidotomy of the contralateral sinus is performed, as previously described, providing the surgeon with a view that includes both sphenoid sinuses and the sphenoid sinus septum (i.e., the same view obtained with a transseptal-transsphenoidal approach) (Fig. 19-4).

A free bone graft is then harvested from the septum of the sphenoid sinus, using parallel horizontal cuts with the turbinate scissors. This bone graft is utilized at the end of the extirpative surgery for the reconstruction of the floor of the anterior sella. The anterior wall of the sella is identified and its position corroborated with the fluoroscope before a small opening is performed with a microdrill or bone curette. The initial opening frequently can be created by biting off the sphenoid sinus septum that is in contact with the anterior sella. The sellotomy can then be enlarged using 1- or 2-mm Hardy punches or bone curettes. Occasionally, the bone of the anterior sella is thick enough to require using a chisel or a drill to open the fenestra. We have utilized the Xomed (Xomed-Treace) MPS 2000 electrical drill with a micro-long extender and a diamond burr or the Black Max drill system (Anspach Companies, Palm Beach Gardens, FL) with an extender and a diamond burr. Both of these drills offer a variety of bits, are relatively lightweight, and well balanced.

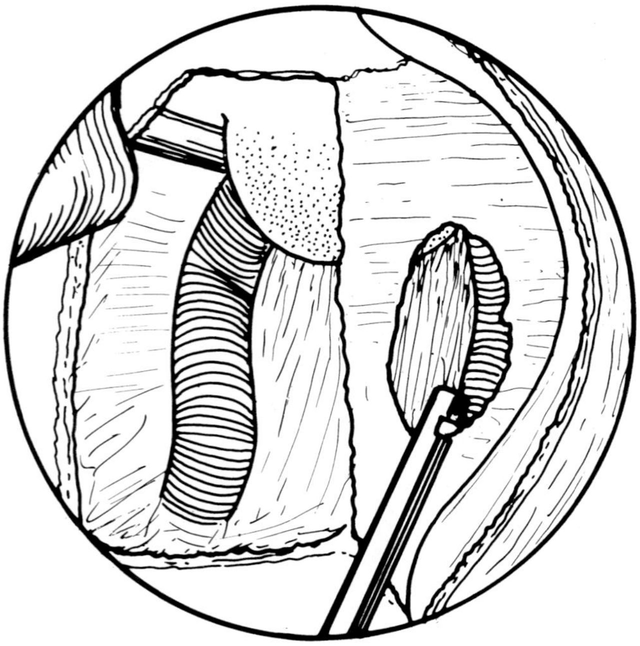

FIG. 19-3. A wide sphenoidotomy, including all the rostrum of the sphenoid sinus, facilitates the identification of the optic nerve, internal corotid artery, and sella. The nasal septum has been transfixed at its junction with the rostrum of the sphenoid and, after sub-mucosal dissection, the contralateral rostrum of the sphenoid sinus has been exposed and the natural ostium of the left sphenoid sinus is being enlarged with Kerrison rongeurs.

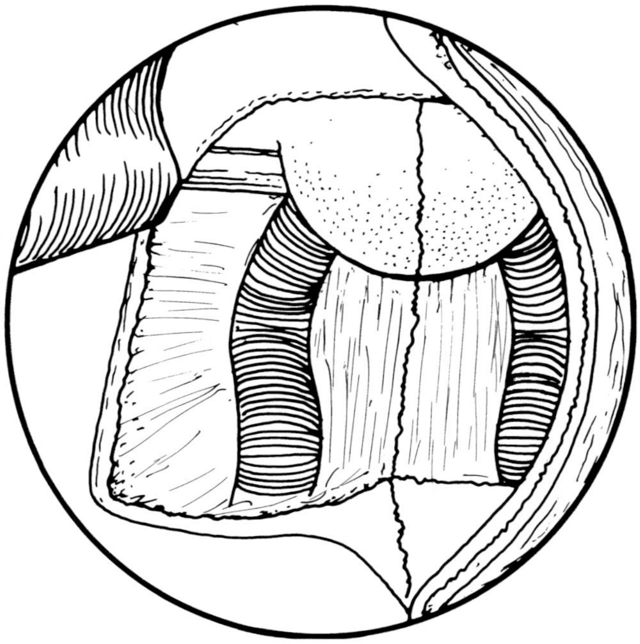

FIG. 19-4. Bilateral wide sphenoidotomies have been completed and the intersinus septum has been removed, allowing a bilateral visualization of the internal carotid arteries and the sella. This is a view that is similar to the one offered by the microscope when using a transeptal approach.

Once the intrasellar dura mater is exposed, the endoscope is placed in a Greenberg retractor modified to hold the endoscope with a C-clamp (Fig. 19-5). This system provides rigid stability for the endoscope at a position that allows full visualization of the surgical field and allows the neurosurgeon to use a bimanual technique. The endoscope can be advanced or retracted according to the surgeon's need for magnification or wide field view throughout the surgery. The focal length of the endoscope is from 2 mm to infinity; therefore, the focus of the surgical field is maintained during these movements. The dura mater is opened with a cruciate incision using a sickle knife or angled microscissors and the tumor is identified and removed using pituitary microrongeurs, microsuction, or pituitary curettes.

The resection of macroadenomas that extend out of the sella is facilitated by the insertion of a 30-degree endoscope

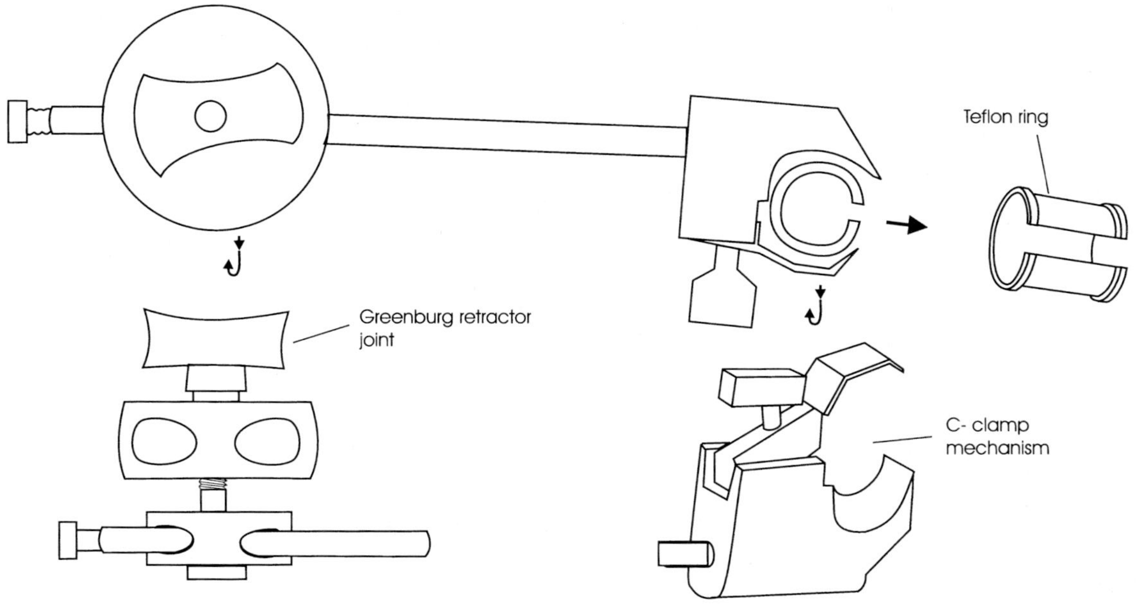

FIG. 19-5. Diagram illustrating the endoscope holder.

into the sella turcica (Fig. 19-6). The 30-degree endoscope enables the surgeon to visualize every corner of the sella to complete the tumor resection. This is in contrast to the operating microscope that does not allow direct visualization of the extrasellar tumor. The angle of view facilitates the tracing and removal of the extrasellar tumor, and the identification and preservation of the arachnoid membrane, surrounding neurovascular structures, and the normal pituitary gland. Large tumors encasing the carotid artery in the cavernous sinus may be completely excised under direct visualization of the carotid artery and of the lateral wall of the cavernous sinus. Similarly, tumors of the high clivus that invade the posterior fossa may also be excised using this technique (21).

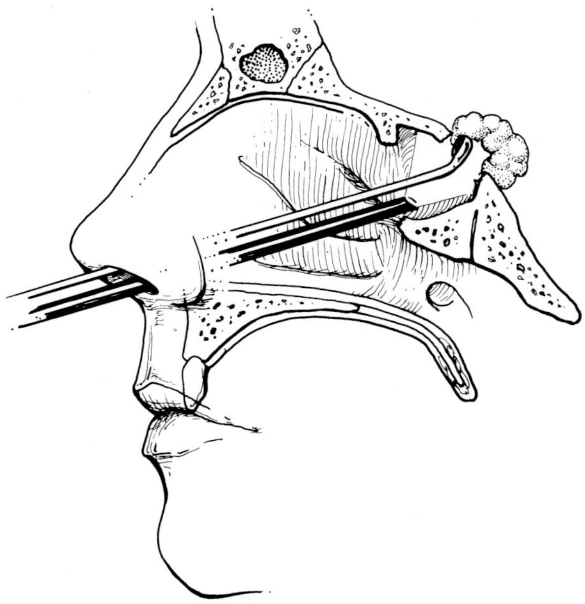

FIG. 19-6. Diagram illustrating a sagittal view of the removal of a supradiaphragmatic extrasella pituitary tumor under direct visualization with a 30° telescope. The telescope is positioned beneath the curette or forceps to allow direct visualization of the structure in question.

After the tumor is removed, the sella is reconstructed with free fat and bone grafts. The free fat graft is harvested through a 2-cm curvilinear incision made at the inferior margin of the umbilicus. The donor site is closed with subcuticular stitches and is dressed with a Band-Aid. The fat graft is then inserted into the sella and a watertight seal is confirmed by repeated Valsalva maneuvers. The floor of the sella is then reconstructed using a piece of the bone harvested from the sphenoid septum. Septal cartilage/bone, hydroxyapatite bone cement, or thin titanium mesh may be used to reconstruct the anterior wall of the sella when a bone-free graft is not available. A fat graft, however, is not necessary when the dural defect is small and a cerebrospinal fluid (CSF) leak is not encountered during the surgery or anticipated postoperatively. The sphenoid sinus can then be loosely packed with absorbable gelatin sponge (Gelfoam, Upjohn Company, Kalamazoo, MI) to control mucosal oozing. As we have gained experience with our endoscopic technique, this has become unnecessary in most cases.

We avoid the use of any type of nasal packing, although occasionally a piece of Telfa (Kendall Co., Mansfield, MA), or even Merocel is necessary to control the oozing at the sphenoidotomy site or turbinate. A Doyle septal splint (Xomed-Treece) is utilized only in rare occasions if the nasal septum and turbinates are significantly abraded during the surgery. The nasal packing is removed the evening of the day of surgery or the day after surgery. Doyle splints are usually left in place for 7 to 10 days.

Results

Although we have used this approach in over 100 patients, postoperative endocrinologic data are available for the first 76 patients. This group comprises 32 patients who presented with nonsecreting pituitary adenomas, nine patients with Cushing's disease, 23 patients with prolactinomas, two patients with acromegaly, and ten patients with various other lesions. Thirty-four were men and 42 were women, ranging in age from 14 to 88 years. The 66 patients presenting with pituitary adenomas included 19 patients with microadenomas, 21 patients with intrasellar macroadenomas, 15 patients with macroadenomas with suprasellar extension, and 11 patients with invasive macroadenomas involving the cavernous sinus and the suprasellar area.

Seven of nine patients with Cushing's disease had normal 24-hour urinary cortisol levels postoperatively. Two patients with residual hypercortisolism were treated with stereotactic gamma-knife surgery. One of these patients was one of two who required two endoscopic operations. The other patient, requiring two operations, needed cortisol and thyroid replacement treatment for anterior hypopituitarism.

Fourteen of 23 patients with prolactinomas improved clinically and their prolactin level returned to within normal limits. Twelve of them demonstrated postoperative prolactin levels below 10 ng/mL. Four patients improved clinically but persisted to show mildly elevated prolactin levels. The remaining five patients underwent a subtotal resection due to cavernous sinus invasion. Two of these patients were treated with stereotactic gamma-knife surgery and the remaining three patients were treated with bromocriptine. One of the patients who received postoperative gamma-knife surgery developed hypothyroidism. One patient with preoperative anterior hypopituitarism benefited from the return of a normal pituitary function postoperatively. Four patients with preoperative hypopituitarism continued to have hypopituitarism postoperatively.

Twenty-five of 32 patients with hormone-nonsecreting adenomas underwent a total resection and seven underwent subtotal resection. All seven patients who underwent a subtotal resection presented with tumors that invaded the cavernous sinus. One patient with residual tumor was treated with stereotactic gamma-knife surgery. Another patient with residual tumor was treated with fractionated external radiation therapy. The remaining five patients with residual tumors are being followed with interval MRI scans, due to their advanced age. Thirteen of 32 patients with hormone-nonsecreting adenomas presented with preoperative anterior hypopituitarism. Three of these 13 patients recovered normal pituitary function postoperatively. The remaining ten patients persisted with anterior hypopituitarism. Three patients with normal pituitary function preoperatively developed anterior hypopituitarism postoperatively.

POTENTIAL PITFALLS

Endoscopic Skills

Pituitary tumor surgery requires a solid fund of knowledge and expertise in neuro-oncology and neuroendocrinology in addition to the technical skills required to remove the tumor completely, while preserving the pituitary function. This is common to endoscopic and traditional techniques. The main disadvantage of endonasal-transsphenoidal-endoscopic pituitary surgery is that the endoscope occupies part of the surgical route, so that a surgeon has to learn to maneuver surgical instruments around the endoscope shaft. In addition, the endoscopic image is mono-ocular (i.e., two-dimensional) and when projected on the video monitor the resolution and sharpness is not as clear as that of direct microscopic visualization. However, the endoscope provides a continuous panoramic view of the complex anatomy of the posterior sphenoidal sinus, including anterior sella, optic protuberances, planum sphenoidale, cavernous sinuses, carotid artery protuberances and clival indentation. This makes it unlikely that a surgeon would accidentally injure the optic nerves or carotid arteries. As described earlier, direct visualization of the suprasellar structures under the 30-degree endoscope helps to avoid potential injury to the hypothalamus or to the optic nerves/chiasm (Fig. 19-6).

The learning curve for neurosurgeons who are not familiar with this endoscopic techniques is steep. Practice in the dissection laboratory is essential to master the basic skills of endoscopic surgery. Pituitary surgeons can also gain experience by using the endoscopes to complement traditional approaches. This provides a safe scenario where the surgeon can assess the advantages and disadvantages of the endoscopic techniques.

Sinonasal Complications

The perioperative nasal and facial edema and pain associated with "open" approaches is absent after endoscopic approaches. The endoscopic transnasal-transsphenoidal approach obviates the morbidity associated with the use of a self-retainer speculum and the wide dissection of the nasal and septal mucoperiosteum, such as septal perforation, necrosis of the mucoperiosteum, postoperative widening of the nasal base, maxillary diastasis, and compression injury of the optic nerves. Other potential perioperative morbidity of endoscopic transnasal transsphenoidal surgery that is similar to that of other approaches includes bleeding from sinonasal sources, sinusitis, and nasal synechiae.

Bleeding

Intraoperative nose bleeding is usually minor and of mucosal (i.e., capillary) origin. Capillary bleeding responds to vasoconstrictors, such as oxymetazoline 0.05% applied as a loose packing with 1/2″ × 3″ cottonoids that have been soaked in this solution. Alternatively, bipolar cautery can be used to achieve hemostasis. Indiscriminate use of cautery, however, will lead to necrosis of the mucosa with subsequent postoperative crustings and problems with nasal hygiene. Occasionally, the lateral septal artery is injured at the inferior margin of the sphenoidotomy, requiring bipolar cauterization and/or clipping of the artery or its origin, the posterior nasal artery.

Sinusitis

Sinus infections after sphenoid surgery using the endoscopic-transnasal approach are rare, as the integrity of the osteomeatal complex is preserved and the sphenoid drainage is assured by a wide sphenoidotomy. We have encountered two patients with delayed (4–8 months) postoperative sphenoiditis. Both of these patients had crusting formation that was acting as a foreign body. The infection resolved after removal of the crusting and a brief course (5–7 days) of broad-spectrum antibiotics.

Synechiae

Intraoperative abrasion or laceration of the turbinates and nasal septum should be avoided. Postoperative edema may place the surfaces of these two areas in contact, leading to the formation of synechiae as the surgical abrasions heal. In our experience, the synechiae are typically formed between the middle turbinate and the nasal septum, have been minor in nature, and do not compromise the nasal airway. We use Doyle septal splints, however, in those patients who are deemed to have significant nasal abrasions that include the septum and the inferior turbinate.

Neurosurgical

Potential neurosurgical complications are identical to those encountered during traditional techniques.

Cerebrospinal Fluid Leaks

Cerebrospinal fluid leaks noted during the extirpative surgery are managed by the meticulous reconstruction of the sella with fat and bone grafts. CSF leaks that persist after optimal reconstruction of the sella are managed by obliteration of the sphenoid sinuses using an abdominal fat graft, as follows. The mucosa of the sphenoid sinuses is meticulously removed under endoscopic visualization. A free fat graft, harvested from the abdomen, is then used to fill the volume of the sphenoid sinus. Alternatively, the sella or the sphenoid sinus may be obliterated with hydroxyapatite cement. However, this requires that the leak is of slow flow to allow the hydroxyapatite cement to set. The free fat graft is splinted with Surgicel and the sphenoidotomy is then protected with Gelfoam and/or Gelfilm. The nasal cavity is packed with 1/2″ nasal packing impregnated with antibiotic ointment. The packing is removed 5 days later (i.e., empirical timing). If the leak is of slow flow or the defect is small, the packing may be obviated. Postoperative lumbar drains or even ventriculoperitoneal shunts are recommended for those patients who are suspected to have a high intraventricular pressure, or in those in whom the described method has failed.

Three of 100 patients in our series developed a postoperative CSF leakage. All three were immediately repaired with sphenoid sinus obliteration using abdominal fat grafts. Spinal drainage was not required.

Bleeding

The common concern regarding uncontrollable bleeding through a "limited exposure" has not been a problem in our experience. Bleeding either from the tumor or a venous sinus has been managed under the endoscope as it would be managed under the operating microscope. The endoscope holder allows the surgeon to suction with one hand and use the bipolar cautery or any other instrument with the other (bimanual technique).

Endocrine

The most common endocrine complications include diabetes insipidus and panhypopituitarism, and may be transient or temporary. Hormone replacement is tailored to the deficit and its duration (i.e., vasopressin, cortisol, and thyroid hormone). Four patients developed transient diabetes insipidus requiring one or two doses of pitressin. One patient with craniopharyngioma developed permanent diabetes insipidus after total resection of the tumor as expected preoperatively. Other endocrine deficits were described above (see Surgical Technique: Results).

REFERENCES

1. Landolt AM. History of transsphenoidal pituitary surgery. In: Landolt AM, Vance ML, Reilly PL, eds. *Pituitary adenomas*. New York: Churchill Livingstone, 1996:307–314.
2. Rosegay H. Cushing's legacy to transsphenoidal surgery. *J Neurosurg* 1981;54:448–454.
3. Black PMcL, Zervas NT, Candia G. Incidence and management of complications of transsphenoidal operation for pituitary adenomas. *Neurosurgery* 1987;20:920–924.
4. Hardy J. Trans-sphenoidal approach to the pituitary gland. In: Wilkins RH, Rengachary SS, eds. *Neurosurgery*, 2nd ed. New York: McGraw-Hill, 1996:1375–1384.
5. Zervas NT. Surgical results in pituitary adenomas: results of international survey. In: Black PM, Zervas NT, Ridway EC Jr, et al., eds. *Secretory tumors of the pituitary gland*. New York: Raven Press, 1984: 377–385.
6. Guiot G, Rougerie J, Fourestler A, et al. Une nouvelle technique endoscopique. Exploration endoscopiques intracraniennes. *Presse Med* 1963; 71:1225–1228.
7. Cooke RS, Jones RAC. Experience with the direct transnasal transsphenoidal approach to the pituitary fossa. *Br J Neurosurg* 1994;8:193–196.
8. Griffith HB, Veerapen R. A direct transnasal approach to the sphenoid sinus: technical note. *J Neurosurg* 1987;66:140–142.
9. Stevens MH, Apfelbaum RI. Transnasal pituitary tumor surgery. *Laryngoscope* 1990;100:817–819.
10. Gamea A, Fathi M, el-Guindy A. The use of the rigid endoscope in trans-sphenoidal pituitary surgery. *J Laryngol Otol* 1994;108:19–22.
11. Helal MZ. Combined micro-endoscopic trans-sphenoid excisions of pituitary macroademomas. *Eur Arch Otorhinolaryngol* 1995;252: 186–189.
12. Janowski R, Auque J, Simon C, et al. Endoscopic pituitary tumor surgery. *Laryngoscope* 1992;102:198–202.

13. Liston SL, Siegel LG, Thienprasit P, et al. Nasal endoscopes in hypophysectomy [letter]. *J Neurosurg* 1987;66:155.
14. Sethi DS, Pillay PK. Endoscopic management of lesions of the sella turcica. *J Laryngol Otol* 1995;109:956–962.
15. Shikani AH, Kelly JH. Endoscopic debulking of a pituitary tumor. *Am J Otolaryngol* 1993;14:254–256.
16. Wurster CF, Smith DE. The endoscopic approach to the pituitary gland [letter]. *Arch Otolaryngol Head Neck Surg* 1994;120:674.
17. Carrau RL, Jho HD, Ko Y. Transnasal-transsphenoidal endoscopic surgery of the pituitary gland. *Laryngoscope* 1996;106:914–918.
18. Jho HD, Carrau RL, Ko Y. Endoscopic pituitary surgery. In: Wilkins RH, Rengchary SS, eds. *Neurosurgical operative atlas.* Park Ridge, IL: American Association of Neurological Surgeons, 1996;5:1–12.
19. Jho HD, Carrau RL. Endoscopy assisted transsphenoidal surgery for pituitary adenoma: a technical note. *Acta Neurochir (Wien)* 1996;138:1416–1425.
20. Jho HD, Carrau RL. Endoscopic endonasal transsphenoidal surgery: experience with 50 patients. *J Neurosurg* 1997;87:44–51.
21. Jho HD, Carrau RL, McLaughlin ML, Somaza SC. Endoscopic transsphenoidal resection of a large chordoma in the posterior fossa: a case report. *Acta Neurochir (Wien)* 1997;139:343–348.
22. Renn WH, Rhoton AL Jr. Microsurgical anatomy of the sellar region. *J Neurosurg* 1975;43:288–298.

Neurosurgical Issues in Otolaryngology: Principles and Practice of Collaboration,
edited by Moisés A. Arriaga and J. Diaz Day.
Lippincott Williams & Wilkins, Philadelphia © 1999.

CHAPTER 20

Cervical Spondylotic Myelopathy

Adnan A. Abla, Scott E. Celin, Joseph C. Maroon, and Max Medary

OVERVIEW

Surgical management of cervical spine degenerative disease has evolved through the years. The posterior surgical approach to the cervical spine was the major procedure for cervical spondylotic myelopathy. However, with the recent advances of radiographic imaging and microinstrumentation, surgeons are leaning more toward the anterior approach. This requires extensive knowledge, experience, and understanding of the anatomy of the anterior neck region. For the last 5 years neurosurgeons and ENT surgeons at our institution worked as a team in exposing the anterior cervical spine and excising osteophytic elements anterior to the spinal cord. This team approach minimized potential risks during the procedure and provided an excellent surgical exposure to the cervical spine.

HISTORICAL MANAGEMENT

Cervical spondylotic myelopathy (CSM) is a condition that affects the middle-aged and the elderly. Although degenerative changes in the cervical spine start to appear after the fifth decade, CSM is seen in only 5% to 10% of the population. Underlying pathophysiologic factors include the size of the spinal canal, vascular changes within the cord, repeated trauma, and biomechanical properties of the cervical spine. Although long recognized, it has only recently been described as a clinical entity (1).

Ferguson and Caplan (2) divided CSM into four distinct syndromes (2). The most common of these is the combined form of radicular and long tract sign involvement. The stooped, wide-base, somewhat spastic gait of the elderly along with numbness and weakness in upper extremity muscles are characteristics of this disease entity. The typical physical findings on examining these patients are weakness in upper extremity muscles and atrophy of hand muscles with hypo- or hyperreflexes at the level of compression. The Hoffmann reflex, inverted radial reflex, Lhermitte sign, clonus, Babinski, and alteration in position sense are indicative of myelopathy. Thus, patients with compression at one level will show lower motor neuron findings at the site of compression and upper motor neuron findings below the compression site. These findings are suggestive of demyelination and degeneration in the corticospinal tract and posterior columns as well.

Histologic studies on animal models and autopsy findings of patients with CSM showed a variety of alteration in the spinal cord: central cystic formation in the gray matter, demyelination in the lateral columns, and necrosis of the posterior columns (3,4). It is important to differentiate this disease from other conditions such as multiple sclerosis, amytrophic lateral sclerosis, low-pressure hydrocephalus, and spinal cord tumors (5). Magnetic resonance imaging of the cervical spine can be diagnostic of CSM and is an excellent diagnostic tool to rule out syrinx, congenital malformation, tumor, infarct, and lesions suggestive of multiple sclerosis. Although myopathies and neuropathies may affect gait, they are typically characterized by lower motor neuron findings and have distinctive electromyographic and nerve conductive studies.

The natural course of the disease is unpredictable, but once it's recognized, complete remission to normality never occurs, and spontaneous regression of neurologic deficit is highly uncommon. So is the treatment of the disease. Nonoperative management consists of immobilization of the cervical spine with rigid neck collars, Somi brace, and Minerva body jacket. Immobilization is used to prevent mobility of the cervical spine and reduce inflammation at the site of nerve compression (6,7). Their advantages are acceptable in patients with radiculopathy, but investigators doubted

A. A. Abla: Medical College of Pennsylvania–Hahnemann School of Medicine, Pittsburgh, Pennsylvania 15212.

S. E. Celin: Allegheny University of the Health Sciences, Pittsburgh, Pennsylvania 15212.

J. C. Maroon and M. Medary: Department of Neurosurgery, Allegheny General Hospital, Pittsburgh, Pennsylvania 15212.

their benefits in cases of myelopathy. Patient selection is very crucial in the nonoperative treatment of CSM because various investigators have found a tendency toward deterioration in symptomatic patients with conservative measures and have advocated earlier surgical intervention (8). Posterior approaches have been recommended for patients with multilevel compression of the spinal cord, congenital spinal stenosis, ossification of the posterior longitudinal ligament (OPLL), and in cases of hypertrophy of the ligamentum flavum. Laminectomy is usually performed along with 50% of the facet joint without compromising the integrity and stability of the cervical spine (9). The procedure is not advocated in patients with kyphosis because of further deterioration and angulation after the procedure.

Different techniques of laminectomy have developed, including open door laminoplasty, which preserves the lamina and expands the spinal canal (10). Advocates of the anterior approach felt that the results were better than with the posterior approach (11,12). With the recent advances in new radiologic technology and the use of microinstrumentation, the compression region in the cervical spine has become well identified. If the area of compression is anterior to the cervical spinal cord, then the anterior surgical approach would be one option. Similarly, if the compression is posterior, then a posterior approach would be more beneficial. In most cases, osteophyte formation anterior to the cord is the cause of CSM, rather than hypertrophy of the ligamentum flavum posteriorly. Despite the controversy surrounding the anterior or posterior approach, surgeons are leaning more toward the anterior approach, tailoring their surgery to sites of compression (13–16). Robinson and Smith (17) adopted excision of the disc, replacing it with tricortical iliac crest graft. They believed that the osteophyte would resorb once fusion takes place. Later, Claward (18) adopted removal of the disc and the compressive osteophyte. Since CSM is a degenerative condition that involves all discs, especially the mobile ones, spur formation will appear at all disc levels. Several large series have appeared in the literature that emphasize the value of radical disc excision and removal of all compressive structures to relieve pressure on the nerve roots and spinal cord (19–22).

Wide exposure of the anterior cervical spine requires a detailed understanding of the anatomy of the neck, particularly the region between the vascular and visceral spaces and the important vascular and nervous structures that pass through this region. To perform simultaneous, multilevel exposures and plating of the anterior spine, wide exposure is required (23–25). Because serious complications were encountered related to exposure of the spine (including vocal cord paralysis, pharyngoesophageal perforation with salivary contamination, and hematoma leading to airway compromise), a team approach was initiated with otolaryngologists–head/neck surgeons performing the anatomic exposure and closure for the neurosurgeons.

ADVANTAGES OF TEAM SURGERY

The advantages of the team approach are multiple. Otolaryngologists are familiar with the local neurovascular anatomy and commonly perform procedures on the larynx, pharynx, and deep structures within the neck. These procedures allow easy identification and preservation of the superior laryngeal nerve, recurrent laryngeal nerve, thoracic duct, and the pharyngoesophagus. The operative time required to provide this exposure is reduced because of the otolaryngologist's familiarity with the local anatomy. Additionally, the functional results appear to be improved, including better voice, reduced risk of aspiration, decrease incidence of serious dysphagia, and shorter hospitalization. Inadvertent entry into the pharyngoesophagus is avoided, which minimizes the risk of infection, loss of bone grafts, and osteomyelitis with the resulting need for additional surgical procedures.

The otolaryngologist, as part of the team, also assists in postoperative monitoring of speech and swallowing problems. Patients are closely observed for aspiration and significant dysphagia.

Operative Technique

After general endotracheal anesthesia and with the patient in the supine position, the neck is moderately extended and turned to the left 30 degrees. Evoked potentials are used prior and after extensions of the neck to make sure there are no changes from positioning. We have not used cervical traction in any procedure. Exposure of the anterior spine is always from the right side. Muscle relaxants and anesthetics that affect stimulation of the recurrent and superior laryngeal nerves are avoided. Lateral radiographs or scout films are reviewed to estimate the relationship between the larynx and the cervical spine. Because many of these patients have flexion deformities of the neck, the larynx may be low lying and not over the expected vertebral body levels. The shoulders are retracted inferiorly with surgical tape attached to the sides of the operating table to allow for C-arm images intraoperatively including the lower cervical spine levels. Perioperative antibiotics are administered based on the neurosurgeons preference.

A variety of skin incisions can be used: an extended transverse incision, a diagonal incision paralleling the anterior border of the sternocleidomastoid muscle, or a "hockey stick" (Fig. 20-1) incision beginning at the mastoid tip and coursing diagonally then transversely into the lower neck. The incisions are chosen based on the level of cervical exposures required, presence of prior surgical scars, aesthetic factors, and surgeon preference. Our neurosurgeons prefer to work from the right side of the neck. If the right side is used to expose C5-6 and C6-7, special attention must be paid to the recurrent laryngeal nerve, which courses obliquely on the right from the subclavian artery to the larynx. The nerve

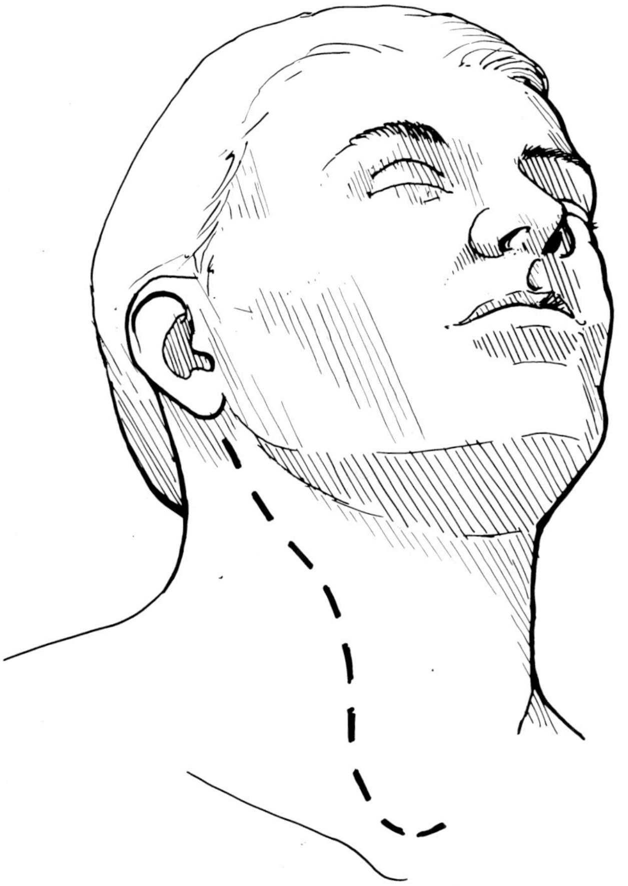

FIG. 20-1. Hockey stick skin insicion for exposure of anterior cervical spine.

must be identified and then atraumatically dissected free from the surrounding tissue. This allows the laryngotracheal complex to be retracted to the left without traction injury to the nerve. If the left side of the neck is used, there is a lower chance that the recurrent laryngeal nerve will be injured since it remains within the tracheoesophageal groove. However, the thoracic duct is in danger of injury due to its course from the thorax to the internal jugular vein. The risks of complications between the right and left sides of the neck appear equal, so this choice is left to the neurosurgeon. The horizontal component of the incision is centered around the midportion of the cervical spine levels to be exposed.

The incision is carried through the platysma muscle, and flaps are elevated superiorly and inferiorly. The ipsilateral strap muscles are then exposed by making a vertical incision through their overlying fascia. This plane is then followed posteriorly between the visceral and vascular spaces, leaving the fascia over the carotid artery and jugular vein intact. The omohyoid muscle is transected if the spine is to be exposed below the C4 level. The superior laryngeal nerve must be identified, dissected free of surrounding tissue, and preserved when exposing C2 or C3 (Fig. 20-2). The nerve is most easily identified just lateral to the thyrohyoid membrane. It can then be dissected posteriorly behind the carotid artery where it branches from the vagus nerve. The hypoglossal nerve also must be identified and dissected when exposing C2 and sometimes for C3. When exposing these levels, branches of the external carotid artery and venous communications with the internal jugular vein usually have to be sacrificed to allow the larynx to be adequately retracted for maximal exposure. This can be done safely because of the collateral circulation from the contralateral side. The hypoglossal and superior laryngeal nerves should be identified prior to ligation of these vessels to avoid accidental injury. In addition to the carotid branches, sensory and motor branches of the cervical plexus, which course medially in the neck, must be sacrificed to achieve maximal exposure. These include sensory branches of the vagus nerve, which are often seen entering the pharyngoesophagus at various levels between the superior and recurrent laryngeal nerve. Sacrifice of these nerves is well tolerated.

When exposing the C5, C6, and C7 levels, the superior thyroid artery and the superior and middle thyroid veins are usually ligated. The retropharyngeal space is then entered and blunt finger dissection is performed inferiorly. The fibrofatty soft tissue pedicle between the cricoid cartilage and the jugular vein contains the recurrent laryngeal nerve and the inferior thyroid artery and veins. This tissue is dissected to expose the recurrent laryngeal nerve. If neuromuscular paralysis is not used, a nerve stimulator can be used for positive identification. As the recurrent laryngeal nerve is

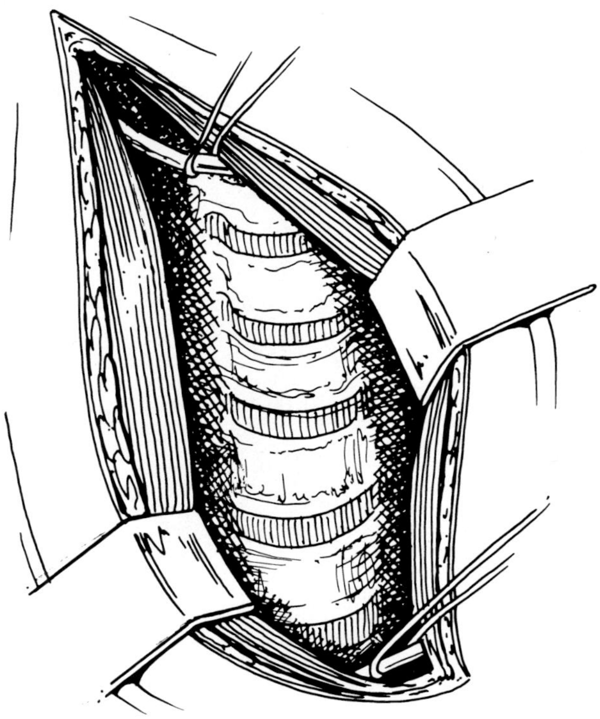

FIG. 20-2. Anterior cervical spine exposed with identification of superior laryngeal nerve (above) and recurrent laryngeal nerve (below).

stimulated, the movement of the ipsilateral arytenoid cartilage can be palpated at the cricoarytenoid joint. As previously mentioned, the nerve must be skeletonized and dissected inferiorly almost to the subclavian artery to allow for laryngotracheal retraction without excessive traction on the recurrent laryngeal nerve, which can result in neuropraxia and subsequent postoperative aspiration and hoarseness. A vessel loop is now passed around the dissected nerves and gently used to retract the nerves either superiorly or inferiorly out of the path of exposure to the spine.

A lateral neck x-ray is now taken with a spinal needle inserted into an intervertebral space to identify the cervical spine level. After taking the x-ray, the needle is removed and that level is marked with either electrocautery or a marking pen. The longis colli muscles are then divided in the midline and elevated from the anterior surface of the cervical spine while waiting for the x-ray to be developed. The Thompson Farley retractor is then applied with its blades under the longis colli muscles (Fig. 20-3). This retractor provides excellent exposure from C-2 to T-1 and protects the esophagus and trachea medially and the carotid sheath laterally. The superior laryngeal and recurrent laryngeal nerve are also protected by applying two additional blades superiorly and inferiorly.

Thorough examination of the radiographic studies determines the extent of surgery in terms of discectomy, osteophytectomy, partial or total corpectomy, and the number of discs or vertebral bodies needed to be excised. The operative microscope is brought into the field after excision of the disc material for magnification and better illumination in the region of the nerve roots and spinal cord. For simple disc degeneration and osteophytes that do not extend more than 3 mm above and below the disc level, we perform a simple discectomy and osteophytectomy using the Midas Rex (Fort Worth, TX) instrumentation and special drills. The end plates are always excised down to the cancellous portion of the vertebral body. When the spinal canal is compromised less than 50% of the spinal cord, a hemicorpectomy is performed. Corpectomy is reserved for situations in which the osteophyte compromises more than 50% of the spinal canal and extends beyond the middle vertebral body; the posterior longitudinal ligament is excised and removed. If the ligament is adherent to the dura, we leave the ligament in place. The width of bone removed is approximately 14 mm, and

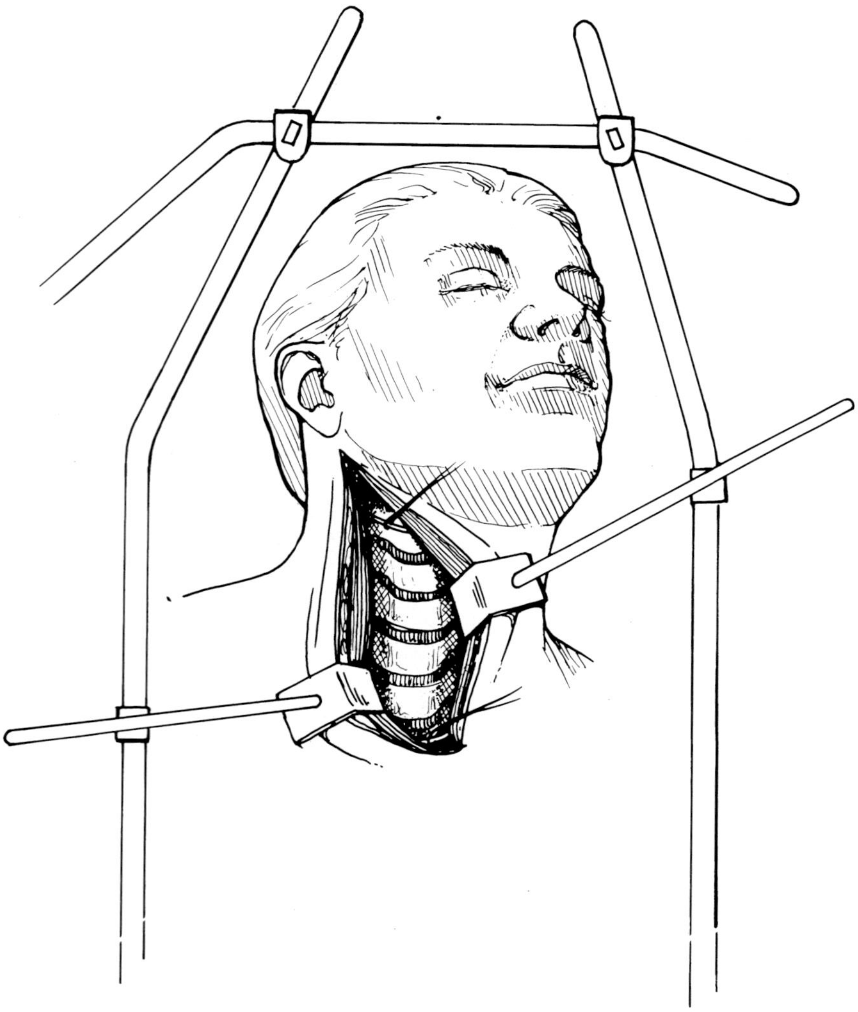

FIG. 20-3. Application of Thompson Farley retractor.

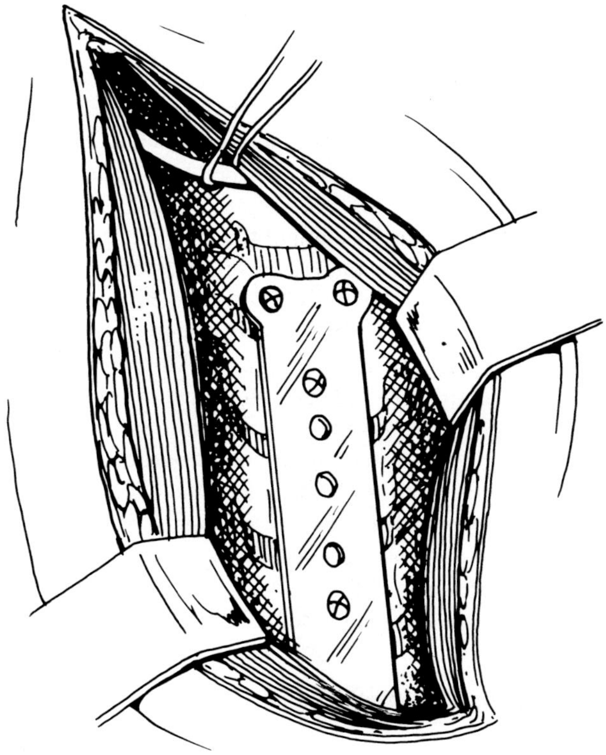

FIG. 20-4. Application of Synthes plate with screws after completion of procedure.

a generous foramenotomy is performed using Kerrison nos. 1 and 2 rongeurs. Fibular bone allograft is then cut and inserted in the bony defect. Manual traction on the neck or the application of the Casper bone spreader is routinely used for insertion of the bone graft. The size of the graft used ranges from 6 to 40 mm. Synthes plates (Synthes Spine System, Paoli, PA) are then contoured and applied to span the defect (Fig. 20-4). Different sizes of screws are used along with the locking screw system.

After the neurosurgical portion of the procedure is completed, the otolaryngologist reenters the operating room and surveys the pharyngoesophagus and the exposed neurovascular structures. The pharyngoesophagus is examined for evidence of perforation, excessive traction, or other injury. The superior and recurrent laryngeal nerves are released from their vessel loops and may be stimulated with a nerve stimulator if neuromuscular paralysis has not been induced. The nerves are otherwise examined for anatomic integrity. The wound is then copiously irrigated with saline and it is assured that all bleeding has been stopped. Suction drains are then inserted into the retropharyngeal space where venous oozing may sometimes persist from the vertebral bodies or prevertebral musculature. It is important to evacuate this fluid, as it can result in a retropharyngeal collection and airway compromise. Although these drains are not necessary for routine single-level anterior disc procedures, the extensive dissection performed for multilevel or rigid plate fixation creates a large potential space that can compromise the airway if a hematoma develops. The drains typically remain in place for 2 or 3 days until the output decreases to acceptable levels (typically less than 30 cc per 24 hours). There were initially concerns from our neurosurgeons regarding the possibility of introducing infection by leaving the drains in place with the presence of implanted hardware and bone grafts. The incidence of postoperative infection is reduced in head and neck surgery if potential fluid spaces are drained, and there have been no postoperative wound infections in our patients attributable to drains. The platysma muscle, subcutaneous layer, and skin are then closed in a layered fashion. A dressing and rigid cervical collar are then applied.

Patients remain intubated and are observed in the recovery room and sometimes overnight in the intensive care unit until they are fully awake and alert. Patients have some mild to moderate degree of laryngeal and hypopharyngeal edema, which, when combined with a depressed level of consciousness, may result in airway compromise. Because intubation is not easy under these circumstances, every effort should be made to assure that extubation occurs under ideal circumstances.

Potential Pitfalls

These procedures are associated with significant risks due to multiple factors. Many of these patients are elderly and have severe comorbid diseases such as coronary artery disease, pulmonary problems, limited cervical spine mobility (difficult intubation), and sleep apnea. Preoperative medical consultation is imperative to identify and optimize the medical conditions of these patients. The consultant should be available to assist with ventilator management if necessary and to help manage complicated medical problems.

Intraoperative pitfalls can be divided into those related to the exposure and those related to the cervical spine procedure itself. The most significant intraoperative event potentially would relate to injury to the carotid artery or jugular vein. Accidental entry into the carotid artery may disrupt plaque and result in intimal dissection or embolic stroke. By following a plane of dissection outside of the fascia overlying the major vessels, the risk of major vessel injury may be minimized.

It is important that the hypoglossal, superior laryngeal, and recurrent laryngeal nerves be identified and preserved when working at cervical levels adjacent to them. Transection or excessive traction of these nerves results in significant morbidity, which, when added to the minor dysfunction of sacrifice of the ansa cervicalis, results in significant swallowing dysfunction, aspiration, and possibly pneumonia or airway compromise. Enteral tube feedings, gastrostomy tube placement, extensive swallowing rehabilitation, or vocal cord medialization surgery may be necessary. Every effort should be made to identify and dissect these nerves gently to preserve their function. Good communication between the otolaryngologist and neurosurgeon will prevent inadvertent excessive retraction or transection during the spinal portion of the procedure.

Hemostasis is important, along with placement of adequate drainage to prevent hematoma formation. A small hematoma, combined with expected postoperative laryngohypopharyngeal edema, will result in airway compromise. Emergency intubation is very difficult in the presence of edema, retropharyngeal hematoma, and cervical spine immobilization. Anoxic complications may result if the airway cannot be secured quickly. One of our patients suffered disruption of cervical plates with displacement of fixation screws through the posterior wall of the hypopharynx during emergency intubation related to previously undiagnosed sleep apnea superimposed on a normal amount of postoperative edema. This necessitated return to the operating room, replacement of bone grafts and fixation plates, and extensive hospitalization.

Surgical procedures for the anterior cervical spine require understanding of the anatomy of the cervical spine in terms of vertebral body and disc dimension. Pathologic changes that distort the normal anatomy could lead to improper surgical procedures and inadequate removal of pressure on the spinal cord. The complexity of the cervical spine entails tremendous hazards and pitfalls for those who are not familiar with this surgical field. One of the potential pitfalls is operating on the wrong disc level. This can be avoided by taking a proper lateral cervical x-ray or, if needed, C-arm fluoroscopy. It is very important to obtain a lateral x-ray with delineation of the C-1–C-2 junction. Patients with thick or short necks present major difficulties in viewing the whole cervical spine. In these conditions obtain a preoperative x-ray, which should include C-1–C-2 and count down to the cervical body or disc seen on the x-ray. Insert a spinal needle on that disc and repeat the x-ray. Always remove soft tissue and osteophyte anterior to the disc to avoid insertion of the needle in bone. It is imperative to compare preoperative x-ray with the interoperative one to confirm the site of pathology. In cases where previous surgery was performed and two vertebral bodies were fused, avoid inserting a needle in the fused area. Always put the spinal needle at the disc above the fusion.

Osteophytes anterior to the disc must be shaved down to the disc level without excision of bone from the vertebral body. Where the disc has collapsed, try to shave as little as possible of the anterior vertebral body in order to see the end plates and then try to insert the needle between the end plates. All these maneuvers avoid the potential of excising the healthy bone that is needed for good fusion.

Another pitfall is inserting a screw in soft tissue, especially the disc. This would lead to poor screw incorporation and loosening with time, thus creating a major site of instability and poor fusion. To avoid this pitfall, always delineate the full height of the vertebral body and insert the screw in the middle. A third potential pitfall is excision of more bone than is needed. This pitfall can be avoided by carefully studying the radiographs to determine how much bone to drill. For good incorporation of screws, the height of the vertebral body should be greater than the screw diameter. A fourth potential pitfall is insertion of loose bone graft. This situation could lead to poor fusion, slippage of the graft either anteriorly or posteriorly, weakness in the construct, and potential breakage of the screws. This can be avoided by drilling the end plates of the disc down to the cancellous portion of the vertebral body, and application of traction. The graft should fit tightly in place after the traction is released.

Major potential pitfalls can be avoided in placement of screws and plates. These constructs help support the stability and avoid slippage of the bone grafts. The screws should always be incorporated in bone and should not compromise the spinal canal. Always measure the width of the vertebral body and choose screws that do not go beyond that width. Inserting a screw into the spinal canal could lead to hemorrhage, cerebrospinal fluid leak by tearing the dura, and injuries to the spinal cord. Try to put the screws as close as possible to the center of the vertebral body to avoid penetration of the nerve root and vertebral artery.

Management of Complications

Because of the complex nature of these spinal problems, complications may be minimized but they cannot be avoided entirely. Odynophagia and mild dysphagia are almost universal complaints with extensive dissection in the retropharyngeal space. These symptoms are usually easily overcome without consultation for speech or swallowing therapy. Prolonged or more significant dysphagia has occurred in approximately 15% of our patients. Causes include vocal cord paralysis, superior laryngeal nerve dysfunction (unilateral loss of supraglottic sensation), excessive edema, and preexisting swallowing dysfunction (presbyesophagus, abnormal peristalsis) with additional postoperative disability. Patients experiencing swallowing problems should undergo fiberoptic laryngoscopy and a modified barium swallow to attempt to identify the problem. Consultation with a speech and swallowing therapist is useful for swallowing therapy when problems are identified on modified swallow.

Vocal cord paralysis has occurred when the dissection included the C-5 to C-6 and C-6 to C-7 levels despite identification, dissection, and careful retraction. When significant dysphagia and aspiration are not present, observation for recovery is recommended. Recovery of function has occurred in all cases in our series where the nerve was identified and dissected. Recovery usually occurs over a period of a few weeks to 3 months. Patients are followed closely during this period for signs of aspiration and recovery. Vocal cord medialization can be considered if patients have significant aspiration, even if eventual recovery of vocal cord function is expected. If a thyroplasty is chosen, this should be delayed for 2 to 3 weeks to allow for reduction of the postoperative laryngeal edema. A Gelfoam injection can temporarily provide vocal cord medialization, but this must be performed transcutaneously or under fiberoptic laryngoscopy because cervical extension cannot be performed for rigid, direct laryngoscopy. Gelfoam injection will provide approximately 4 to 6 weeks of vocal cord medialization and, because it is temporary, it may have to be repeated if recovery does not occur in this period of time.

Although the majority of our patients have been successfully extubated in the recovery room, airway compromise has occurred infrequently. All or our patients are observed overnight in a special unit whose staff is trained to observe for stridor or depressed respiration. When intubation is necessary in the postoperative period, it should be performed by the most senior person immediately available because of the difficult nature of these airways. Intubation must be accomplished without accidental neck extension, which may dislodge plate fixation screws. This occurred in one of our patients, with the screws displaced through the posterior hypopharyngeal wall, creating salivary contamination of the surgical site and unstable spine, necessitating further surgery. Two patients were reintubated due to retropharyngeal fluid collections, causing airway obstruction. One of these events occurred early in our series before drains were used on every patient. The control occurred 1 week postoperatively in a patient who had been successfully discharged but had a delayed hematoma 3 days after drain removal. This was felt to be secondary to a severe, preexisting coagulopathy related to liver disease.

Wound infections have not occurred in any of our patients. We use meticulous dissection around the pharyngoesophagus, careful hemostasis, and suction drains to prevent fluid collection, and we practice good maintenance of intraoperative sterility. Should infection occur, incision and drainage should be performed along with administration of systemic antibiotics. One should maintain a high suspicion of salivary contamination and consider barium swallow or wound exploration depending on the clinical events.

Complications related to spinal surgery were minor and did not require further surgical intervention over a 5-year period. We operated on 85 patients with severe CSM. Multiple discectomy, osteophytectomy, hemicorpectomies, and corpectomies were performed. Bone allografts were used along with the Synthes plating systems. The length of allografts varied from 6 to 40 mm. Allografts were used in 296 discectomies, 24 partial corpectomies, and 18 corpectomies. Early fusion appeared after 3 months in two-level discectomies and in 6 months in corpectomies. All cases showed solid corpectomies. The graft shifted posteriorly 3 mm with no deterioration in clinical condition. Four of the grafts in multilevel discectomies slipped up to 2 mm anteriorly and did not require any surgical intervention. All of the patients with two-level corpectomies had an increase in kyphosis by 4 degrees. This leads to minimal shifting in the plates and pullout of the screws. Synthes plates were used as a means of internal fixation. These plates were 24 to 75 mm in length and were contoured to fit against the vertebral bodies. Eight plates were 2 to 3 mm away from the bone and five were more than 5 mm. This interface was mainly in the center of the kyphotic deformity, which was not corrected. Six plates were off-center by 2 to 3 mm, and eight plates were difficult to contour at the top of the fusion area, thus creating 2 to 3 mm of interface.

Twelve plates shifted secondary to microsettling. None of the plates broke or was removed. Three hundred and forty screws were applied; the length of the screws varied between 14 and 16 mm, and the diameter was 4.0 to 4.35 mm. Screws were applied to mid-vertebral bodies in 70% of cases, and in the rest were close to the top of the vertebral body, but never in the disc space. In cases of multilevel discectomies, we incorporated two screws in each vertebral body. In cases of corpectomies, we avoided incorporating any screws in the allograft. Fifteen of the screws pulled out 2 to 3 mm from the plate and ten pulled out 6 mm. None of the screws was removed and none caused any adverse effect. One screw broke 10 months after surgery but did not affect the fusion. One screw tore the esophagus and appeared in the stomach on a chest x-ray. This was the result of excessive extension of the neck for a patient with sleep apnea that required emergency reintubation.

ACKNOWLEDGMENTS

The authors would like to acknowledge Adib and Abir Abla for typing the manuscript. Also, thanks to Synthes Plates for use of their instrumentation.

REFERENCES

1. Brain WR, North Field DW, Wilkinson M. The neurologic manifestations of cervical spondylosis. *Brain* 1952;75:187–225.
2. Ferguson RJC, Caplan LR. Cervical spondylitic myelopathy. *Neurol Clin North Am* 1985;3:373–382.
3. Bohlman HH, Bahniuk E, Raskulinecz G, Field G. Mechanical factors affecting recovery from incomplete cervical spinal cord injury. *Johns Hopkins Med J* 1979;145:115–125.
4. Ono K, Ota H, Tada K, Yamamoto T. Cervical myelopathy secondary to multiple spondylotic protrusions. A clinicopathologic study. *Spine* 1977;2:109–125.
5. Epstein JA. Management of cervical spinal stenosis, spondylosis, and myeloradiculopathy. *Contemp Neurosurg* 1985;2:1–6.
6. Johnson EW. Conservative treatment of cervical disc disease. In: Dansker SB, ed. *Cervical spondylosis.* New York: Raven Press, 1981: 145–153.
7. Naylor JR, Mulley GP. Surgical collar: a survey of their prescription and use. *Br J Rheumatol* 1991;30:282–284.
8. Philips DG. Surgical treatment of myelopathy with cervical spondylosis. *J Neurol Neurosurg Psychiatry* 1973;36:879–884.
9. Raynor RB, Pugh A, Shapiro I. Cervical facetectomy and its effects on spine strength. *J Neurosurg* 1985;63:278–282.
10. Hirabayashik, Satomi K. Operative procedure and results of expansive open-door laminoplasty. *Spine* 1988;13:870–876.
11. Guidetti B, Fortuna A. Long-term results of surgical treatment of myelopathy due to cervical spondylosis. *J Neurosurg* 1969;30:714–721.
12. Bohlman HH. Cervical spondylosis with moderate to severe myelopathy. Spine 1977;2:151–162.
13. Saunders RL, Bernini PM, Shiffeffstg K, Reeves AG. Central corpectomy for cervical spondylotic myelopathy. *J Neurosurg* 1991;74: 163–170.
14. Hanai K, Kenji, Fujiyoshi F, Fuminori, Kamei K. Subtotal vertebrectomy and spinal fusion for cervical spondylotic myelopathy. *Spine* 1986;11:310–315.
15. Whitecloud TS. Anterior surgery for cervical spondylotic myelopathy. Smith, Robinson, Cloward, and vertebrectomy. *Spine* 1988;13:863.

16. Brown JA, Havel P, Ebraheim N, Greenblatt SH, Jackson WT. Cervical stabilization by plate and bone fusion. *Spine* 1988;13:235–240.
17. Robinson R, Smith G. Anterolateral cervical disc removal and interbody fusion for cervical disc syndrome. *Bull Johns Hopkins Hosp* 1955;96:223–224.
18. Claward R. The anterior approach for the removal of ruptured cervical disc. *J Neurosurg* 1958;15:602–617.
19. Bertalanffy H, Eggert HR. Clinical long term results of anterior discectomy without fusion for treatment of cervical radiolopathy and myelopathy: a follow up of 164 cases. *Acta Neurochir* 1988;90:127–135.
20. Hoff JT, Wilson CB. Microsurgical approach to the anterior cervical spine and spinal cord. *Clin Neurosurg* 1979;26:513–528.
21. Kojimat, Waga S, Kubo N, et al. Anterior cervical vertebrectomy and interbody fusion for multilevel spondylosis and ossification of the posterior longitudinal ligament. *Neurosurgery* 1989;24:864–872.
22. Mann KS, Khosla VK, Gulati DR. Cervical spondylotic myelopathy treated by single slope multilevel anterior decompression. *J Neurosurg* 1984;60:81–87.
23. Riley LH. Surgical approaches to the anterior structures of the cervical spine. *Clin Orthop* 1973;91:16–20.
24. McDonnell DE. Anterolateral cervical approach to the craniovertebral junction. *AANS Operative Atlas* 1991;1(3):147–164.
25. Robinson RA, Southwick WO. Surgical approaches to the cervical spine. In: American Academy of Orthopedic Surgeons, ed. *Instructional course lectures.* St. Louis: CV Mosby, 1960:299–330.

Neurosurgical Issues in Otolaryngology: Principles and Practice of Collaboration,
edited by Moisés A. Arriaga and J. Diaz Day.
Lippincott Williams & Wilkins, Philadelphia © 1999.

CHAPTER 21

Cervical Spine Trauma

Karl D. Schultz, Jr., Regis W. Haid, and David Masel

OVERVIEW

Instability of the bony and ligamentous components of the cervical spine can produce devastating lifelong physical and psychologic disability. A spinal cord injury, unless accompanied by a significant head injury, leaves its victim fully cognizant of the severity and implications of the event leading to this injury. The physiologic impairments produced by a severe spinal cord injury not only affect daily activities but also markedly influence the psychologic well-being of the individual. Furthermore, the expense to society, in 1987 dollars, for treatment of a spinal cord injury varies from $50,000 to $250,000 for paraplegics and high-level, respiratory-dependent quadriplegics, respectively (1). The personal tragedy and loss of productivity are immeasurable and underline the need for a systematic approach to the diagnosis and treatment of acute injuries of the cervical spine.

The incidence of cervical spine injury (CSI) in patients who have sustained major trauma is reported to be between 1.5% and 3.0% (2,3), with neurologic deficits occurring in up to 40%, mostly from fracture dislocations (4). Most spinal cord injuries occur secondary to motor vehicle accidents (42%–56%), falls from a height (19%–30%), gunshots (12%–21%), and sports-related activities, primarily diving (6%–7%) (5,6). Greater than two-thirds of the patients are males with an average age of 35 (7).

Despite recent advances in the understanding of neuronal injury, repair, and plasticity, our ability to effect and promote significant neuronal repair remains limited. Therefore, the efforts of physicians taking care of trauma patients with possible CSIs must be directed toward preventing not only initial injury to the spinal cord but also secondary insults by maintaining an optimum environment for neuronal healing in those individuals who have already sustained a spinal cord injury. This chapter provides an overview of the basic tenets in managing CSI, with particular emphasis on current standards for the initial immobilization, diagnosis, classification, and definitive management of traumatic CSI. A brief discussion of modern surgical therapy is also presented.

FUNDAMENTAL CONCEPTS

Emergency Room Assessment

In a landmark retrospective study in 1979, Bohlman (8) reported that 100 of 300 cervical fractures ultimately treated at a tertiary care center were missed during the initial emergency department evaluation. Unfortunately, some of the individuals admitted with minor neurologic deficits developed progressive neurologic symptoms including paraplegia and quadriplegia due to poor medical management. Since that time, widespread promulgation of basic management tenets has greatly diminished unnecessary morbidity.

As with any trauma victim, the initial management of the individual with possible spinal column or cord injury should follow the basic ABCs (airway, breathing, circulation) set forth by the American College of Surgeons Committee on Trauma (9). The physician should remember the very important concept that all trauma victims have a spinal column injury until proven otherwise. Strict immobilization of the entire spinal axis must be instituted and maintained from the time of initial field evaluation by emergency medical personnel through the emergency room trauma assessment. In addition, no spinal segment should be mobilized until that particular region has been cleared through clinical and radiographic evaluation. By establishing and maintaining strict immobilization of all segments of the spine throughout the primary and secondary surveys, injuries to the axial skeleton can be ''neutralized'' while the initial resuscitation is performed.

When faced with a patient with an obvious neurologic injury, it is important to avoid focusing exclusively on this

K. D. Schultz, Jr., and R. W. Haid: Department of Neurosurgery, Emory University School of Medicine, Atlanta, Georgia 30322.
D. Masel: Neurosurgical Center, El Paso, Texas 79902.

injury. Instead, addressing the adequacy of the airway and gas exchange while maintaining hemodynamic stability through the control of major hemorrhage is imperative. The nervous system is particularly susceptible to hypoxic injury, and it is critical to monitor the patient's vital signs and avoid even mild periods of hypotension and hypoxia in the acute setting. Whereas such periods of hypoperfusion may be inconsequential to other organ systems, there is growing evidence that even brief periods of hypotension can significantly increase mortality and decrease chances for optimal recovery in individuals suffering from spinal cord injury (10).

Spinal Immobilization

Anatomic studies of normal individuals have shown that application of a soft collar alone allows 92% of the normal lateral range of motion and 75% of full flexion and extension. Rigid cervical collars limit the full range of flexion and extension motion to 29% of normal (11). The persistent mobility offered by these orthoses make them suboptimal for immobilizing the cervical spines of trauma patients.

Spinal immobilization instituted in the field involves placing the victim on a rigid backboard and gently positioning the head in a neutral position. Sandbags are placed alongside the head and then taped with the forehead to the backboard. The modern designed two-piece hard cervical collar can then be applied with little additional neck movement. This combination provides the most effective immobilization of the entire spine and, if necessary, allows for safe and rapid exposure to the airway (12). When a conscious victim holds his head in a position other than neutral due to pain, no attempt should be made to straighten it. Instead, the head should be immobilized in the position of comfort. Such a head position, due to either cervical muscle spasms or a conscious effort, often represents an attempt on behalf of the individual to stabilize a spinal column injury and prevent secondary insult. The marked reduction in the ratio of quadriparesis to paraparesis among multiple trauma victims has been attributed to the addition of these rigid practices to the initial trauma assessment (2).

Emergent Treatment

Due to the potentially severe derangements of the autonomic nervous system, sensorimotor systems, and respiratory function in individuals with cervical spinal column injury, the management of the airway and circulatory systems can be quite challenging. The fact that aspiration and shock are the primary causes of death during the early postinjury period in spinal cord injury patients attests well to the importance of properly managing the ABCs (13). Guidelines exist that need to be followed when dealing with a victim who has known or uncertain spinal instability.

Individuals who are alert and able to maintain an adequate airway need no more than oxygen supplementation via a nasal cannula or face mask. In managing an obstructed airway, neck extension or a jaw thrust maneuver should be avoided in an individual whose cervical spine status is unknown. Instead, the chin lift maneuver should be performed. If this maneuver fails or if ventilatory effort is compromised due to diaphragmatic paralysis or depressed level of consciousness, the patient should be intubated. Intubation in this setting is most safely performed with the aid of an assistant providing in-line stabilization of the cervical spine. Regardless of the technique used for intubation, the head should be kept in neutral position and axial traction should be avoided. Modest axial traction can cause significant vertebral body distraction in an unstable cervical spine (see Fig. 21-6) (14).

Under current advanced trauma life support (ATLS) guidelines (9), if the integrity of the cervical spine is unknown, blind nasotracheal intubation is preferred over the orotracheal route and surgical airway. A significant growing body of literature now suggests that orotracheal intubation can be safely performed in these individuals by adequately trained individuals (15,16). Orotracheal intubation is often most easily performed using a rapid sequence induction (i.e., neuromuscular blockade and potent sedation) and can be performed either with a laryngoscope or, preferably, with the use of a flexible bronchoscope. Proponents of this technique emphasize that individuals performing the procedure must be competent in performing rapid sequence inductions and proficient with the laryngoscope or flexible bronchoscope. Finally, if the airway cannot be secured with either one of the above methods, a surgical cricothyroidotomy is recommended.

The maintenance of adequate circulation and cardiac function is essential and minimizes secondary spinal cord injury due to hypoperfusion. Multitrauma victims with evidence of neurologic injury may suffer from shock, which can be neurogenic, hypovolemic, or both.

Neurogenic shock associated with a cervical spinal cord injury is due to disruption of the descending sympathetic outflow from the hypothalamus. The loss of peripheral sympathetic tone diminishes normal vasoconstrictor tone, resulting in hypotension, venous pooling, and a decrease in cardiac preload. Vagal predominance causes bradycardia (heart rate usually below 60), which aids in distinguishing neurogenic shock from the tachycardia and hypotension due to sepsis or hypovolemia.

Resuscitation from neurogenic shock begins with placing the victim in the Trendelenburg position, which reduces venous pooling and increases the central venous pressure. A military antishock trouser (MAST) pneumatic counterpressure suit can aid in this effort if precautions are taken to avoid lower spine manipulation. Finally, atropine sulfate (0.5–1.0 mg) can be prescribed to overcome the vagal output. Fluid resuscitation should proceed with caution, as these patients have a normal blood volume and simply suffer from distribution difficulties. Congestive heart failure could complicate the initial resuscitation if the patient's fluid status is not appropriately monitored.

Neurologic Assessment

Once the ABCs have been addressed and the victim is stabilized, the secondary assessment can begin. The entire spine from occiput to sacrum should be palpated, as the patient is log rolled from the backboard, noting any obvious deformities in spinal alignment, interspinous space widening, bruising, crepitance, or areas of tenderness and spasm. Because of the large paraspinous muscles in the cervical region, the spinous processes above C-7 are difficult to appreciate. However, any tenderness in this area may represent soft tissue injury and could preclude clearing the cervical spine. Removing the patient from the backboard as soon as possible prevents further skin breakdown that can occur on the occiput and sacrum with relatively short periods of backboard immobilization.

A thorough neurologic assessment should be undertaken as soon as possible so as to document a baseline of the patient's degree and level of deficit. The neurologic exam must assess both spinothalamic (pain, temperature) and dorsal column (vibration, proprioception, light touch) sensory functions as well as motor power and reflex activity. As CSI can present with varying degrees of spinal cord injury as well as with a radiculopathy (nerve root compression), the symmetry of findings is very important.

Fine touch can be examined using a cotton tip applicator, and all dermatomes should be tested bilaterally. When a sensory change is discovered, that level should not only be recorded on the medical chart but also, ideally, marked directly on the patient for comparison with future exams. Dermatomes are useful in determining spinal cord levels (Fig. 21-1). One particular subtlety to the dermatomal chart is the

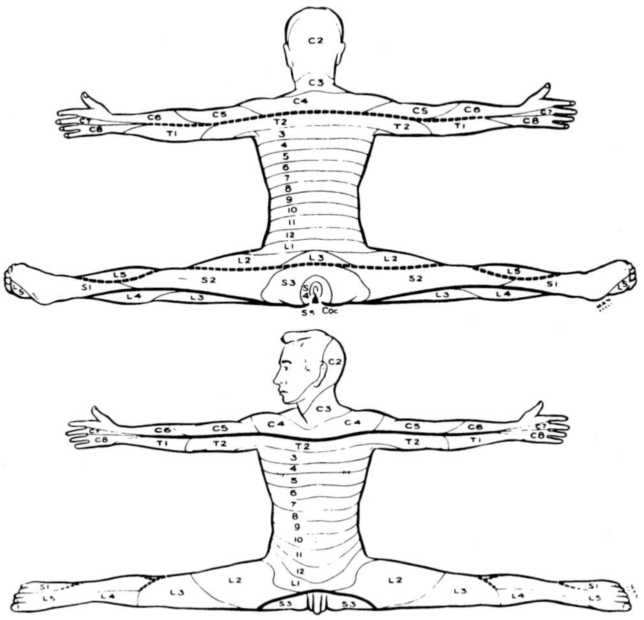

FIG. 21-1. Cutaneous innervation dermatomes representing individual spinal segments. Note the "C-4 cape" on the anterior and posterior chest. (From ref. 60, with permission.)

TABLE 21–1. *The Medical Research Council of Great Britain grading scale, the most commonly used scale for grading motor function in individual muscle groups*

Grade 0	No motor activity
Grade 1	Palpable muscle contraction; No joint motion
Grade 2	Complete range of motion with gravity eliminated
Grade 3	Complete range of motion against gravity
Grade 4	Complete range of motion against gravity with some resistance
Grade 5	Complete range of motion against gravity with full resistance

Grade 4 is sometimes subdivided into 4−, 4, and 4+ to reflect varying degrees of weakness against resistance.

C-4 "cape," where the C-4 dermatome covers the upper shoulders and abuts the T-2 dermatome of the upper chest. If a sensory change is found at this level it is important to continue the examination onto the upper extremities where the C-5–T-1 dermatomes lie to avoid falsely identifying a C-4 level.

Vibratory/joint position sense can be tested with a 128-Hz tuning fork. Again, side-to-side differences should be noted. It is this portion of the exam that is most likely to be affected by underlying medical conditions such as diabetes or alcohol-related peripheral neuropathy.

Motor examination is critically important as it is the most objective portion of the exam. The motor power of all major muscle groups should be tested in all four extremities and graded according to a reproducible scale such as that offered by the Medical Research Council of Great Britain Scale (Table 21-1). The status of voluntary contraction of the anal sphincter should be included in this portion of the exam.

Deep tendon reflexes (DTRs) should be examined in all extremities, noting not only their briskness but also their symmetry. DTRs are graded from 0 (absent) to 4 + (hyperactive with generalization or clonus). A single absent DTR suggests root impingement (peripheral nerve lesion), whereas symmetrical loss of DTRs of the lower extremities or, rarely, all four extremities suggests spinal shock. DTR hyperactivity simply represents an upper motor neuron lesion but does not confirm a particular spinal level.

Reflexes such as the anal wink and bulbocavernosus, as well as tonic, subconscious, muscle activity, such as anal sphincter tone, should always be tested. The presence of these reflexes in the setting of a spinal cord injury represents "sacral sparing" and is a good prognostic indicator of further recovery. Reflex penile erection, or priapism, may be present in males suffering from complete spinal cord injury. As it represents loss of descending inhibitory influence, its presence carries a much poorer prognosis for recovery.

The neurologic sequelae that can result from CSI include spinal shock, cervical root injury, and incomplete spinal cord injuries, including the Brown-Séquard, central cord, and the anterior cord syndromes. Spinal shock presents as complete loss of neurologic function below the cord lesion, including both segmental and polysynaptic reflex activity as well as autonomic function. It appears to be the result of a sudden loss of supraspinal facilitory input to the spinal circuitry. Although prognostically ominous, a thorough assessment of neurologic function distal to the site of spinal cord injury is not possible until it clears. Spinal shock generally resolves in 1 to 2 weeks, although it can last longer and can be permanent in as many as 15% of patients (33).

The Brown-Séquard syndrome results from an anatomic or functional unilateral cord hemisection (Fig. 21-2). Owing to the disruption of the descending corticospinal and ascending dorsal column tracts, both of which decussate in the medulla, paralysis and loss of vibratory and position sense ipsilateral to the lesion occur. Pain and temperature fibers in the spinothalamic tracts cross within several segments of their entry into the spinal cord, and thus unilateral injury causes the contralateral loss of these sensations below the level of injury. This type of injury is usually caused by penetrating injury such as gunshots and stab wounds, but hemicord dysfunction can also occur with a unilateral facet dislocation. One retrospective review of the literature demonstrated significant functional strength recovery in the lower extremities and functional walking capacity in 93% of victims at 6 months (17).

When the central or paracentral regions of the spinal cord are injured, the central cord syndrome can result. This syndrome usually occurs without evidence of spinal fracture or dislocation. Instead injury usually occurs in the presence of cervical spinal stenosis, either congenital or acquired from degenerative changes. Although the mechanism is unclear, an ischemic insult to the central portions of the cord from either restricted arterial inflow or reduced outflow from venous congestion seems plausible. The patient often presents in spinal shock and occasionally, after this clears, the syndrome presents itself. Classically, motor strength is more involved than sensory, with weakness of the upper extremities exceeding that of the lower extremities, and proximal function affected more than distal. This particular pattern is due to the laminated structure of the spinal cord, with motor neurons controlling the upper and lower extremities located centrally and laterally, respectively. Sensory involvement is variable, with the dorsal columns minimally involved and spinothalamic tracts showing dysfunction contralaterally below the injured segment. The prognosis for recovery is fair, with one study showing 59% of patients achieving functional recovery (18).

The anterior cord syndrome is rare after trauma unless cardiac arrest, aortic disruption, or a period of profound hypotension or hypoxia occurs as a result of the trauma. Occasionally, a flexion injury or vertebral burst fracture will cause this syndrome. Decreased perfusion of the spinal cord in the anterior spinal artery distribution is characterized by dysfunction of the spinothalamic sensory and corticospinal motor systems, while dorsal column function (proprioception and vibration sense) is spared. The prognosis for significant recovery is poor (19).

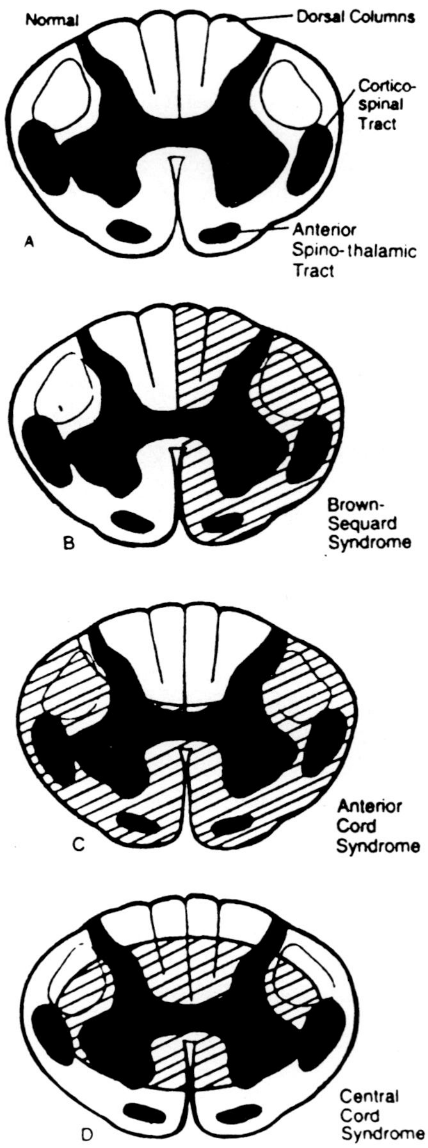

FIG. 21-2. Incomplete spinal cord injury syndromes. **A:** Normal anatomy with the ascending dorsal columns (proprioception and light touch), descending corticospinal tract (motor), and ascending anterior spinothalamic tract (pain, temperature) identified. **B:** The Brown-Séquard syndrome. Injury to half the cervical spinal cord can lead to ipsilateral loss of motor and dorsal column function, and loss of contralateral pain and temperature sensation. **C:** Anterior cord syndrome. Neural function of the anterior two-thirds of the spinal cord is disrupted. Proprioception and the sense of vibration and light touch are maintained while all motor function, pain, and temperature sensation below the level of the lesion are lost completely. **D:** Central cord syndrome. Injury to the central portion of the spinal cord results in greater loss of neurologic function in the arms than in the legs with distal function worse than proximal. The lumbar and sacral tracts are spared because of the lamination of fibers within the anterior spinothalamic and lateral corticospinal tracts where the cervical fibers lie medial to the lumbosacral fibers.

The cervical root syndrome is an isolated deficit in a specific nerve root. All motor and sensory modalities subserved by the root are compromised. It commonly occurs with an acute disk herniation or a facet fracture/dislocation.

Pharmacologic Treatment of Spinal Cord Injury

If spinal cord injury is confirmed or strongly suspected, the current standard of care for a nonpenetrating injury is the intravenous administration of methylprednisolone as an initial bolus of 30 mg/kg of body weight over 15 minutes, followed by an infusion of 5.4 mg/kg per hour for the next 23 hours. In the Second National Acute Spinal Cord Injury Study (NASCIS II) trial, the use of this steroid provided improved neurologic outcome compared with the administration of naloxone and placebo at 6-month and 1-year follow-up (20,21). Interestingly, patients who were started on methylprednisolone more than 8 hours postinjury actually did statistically worse than those administered placebo. Therefore, steroids are recommended for use only when begun within the first 8 hours postinjury. Most recently, results from the NASCIS III trial have been reported. The study continues to support the use of methylprednisolone for 24 hours postinjury when patients are started on the protocol within 3 hours postinjury. However, the study found improved neurologic outcome at 6 months when methylprednisolone was continued for 48 hours in those patients instituted on therapy between 3 and 8 hours postinjury (22). Although the authors have no experience with these newer guidelines at the time of publication, the guidelines will likely become the standard of care in the use of methylprednisolone for spinal cord injury.

Associated Injuries

Due to common mechanisms, the detection of a CSI should alert the physician to the possibility of additional spine-related injuries. For example, multiple, noncontiguous spinal fractures have been said to occur in 4% to 5% of cases and are frequently missed during the initial assessment (23,24). Therefore, when one spinal column injury is found, a thorough radiographic evaluation of the remaining spinal column must be performed. Particular attention must be paid to both ends of the spinal column as almost half of these secondary fractures occur at C-1, C-2, L-4, and L-5 (23).

Additionally, mechanisms causing CSI also predispose individuals to both vertebral and carotid artery injuries. The vertebral artery may be directly injured from fractures that extend through the foramen transversarium from C-1 to C-6. The carotid, being relatively fixed at its origin from the great vessels and at the carotid canal in the skull base, is most likely to be injured at its proximal and distal ends. Moreover, hyperflexion, rotation, and distractive injuries to the cervical spine can stretch and kink these vessels, leading to dissection and/or thrombosis. Arterial insufficiency or ischemic strokes involving the brainstem and all three cerebral arterial territories can result. Therefore, symptoms of ischemia (blurred vision, dizziness, weakness) or overt stroke (hemiparesis, limb ataxia, cranial nerve deficits) should prompt an evaluation of the cervical vasculature.

A recent study reported a vertebral artery injury rate of 19% when all CSIs were prospectively evaluated (25). Higher rates of injury (46%–75%) have been found in the subset of patients with cervical spine dislocations (26,27). In light of the potentially devastating neurologic injury that can occur if these injuries go undiagnosed, the authors recommend that magnetic resonance angiography (MRA) or digital subtraction angiography of the cervical vessels be performed for patients with unexplained neurologic deficit, cervical spine subluxations and dislocations, and fractures extending through the foramen transversarium and in patients with unexplained neck pain after seemingly mild neck injury.

RADIOGRAPHIC ASSESSMENT AND CLEARANCE OF THE CERVICAL SPINE

Radiography is readily available in the emergency room setting, making plain radiographs the most practical and subsequently most widely used adjunct to the history and physical examination of the trauma patient. The overall incidence of positive cervical spine radiographs in trauma victims is relatively low, ranging from 1% to 10% by some reports (28,29). Nevertheless, early reports of "occult" or "asymptomatic" CSI spawned an aggressive use of cervical spine radiography in *all* blunt trauma patients. As the existence of asymptomatic cervical spine injury has subsequently been effectively argued against (30), the indiscriminate use of cervical spine films is no longer necessary. Nevertheless, some trauma centers continue this practice, resulting in a large number of negative radiographs and an expensive use of resources. Current standards of care allow the physician to determine clinically those patients needing further radiographic assessment, thereby providing safe and efficient evaluation of the trauma patient's cervical spine status.

Plain Radiography

Most authorities will concede that a single cross-table lateral (CTL) view will effectively diagnose between 57% and 85% of cervical injuries. As such, it is obviously inadequate as a sensitive screening tool (7). This study's limitations have been attributed to poor visualization of the C1-2 and C6-7 regions due to tissue overlap from bony structures such as the shoulder and occipital condyles. Today, a complete three-view cervical spine series consisting of the CTL, anteroposterior (AP), and open-mouth view is considered the most accurate method to screen for traumatic cervical spine injuries. A technically adequate study involves visualization of all cervical spine elements from the occipital condyles through and including the T-1 vertebrae in two views. Some centers will routinely add oblique views. Several studies have shown, however, that these additional views provide little additional information other than more clearly delineating injuries already detected on the three-view series (7).

It is important to note that the absence of radiographic abnormalities does not necessarily eliminate risk of CSI. Soft tissue structures vital to maintaining the integrity of the osseous components of the cervical spine (ligaments, facet joints, disks) are not visualized with plain radiography. Injury to these elements sometimes may be inferred by indirect evidence such as prevertebral soft tissue swelling, avulsion fractures, or neurologic deficit. Therefore, any radiographic or clinical evidence of CSI should be treated as an unstable lesion until proven otherwise. In these cases, the cervical spine must be immobilized in a neutral position despite a normal three-view radiographic analysis until further diagnostic workup can be performed.

Ancillary Radiographic Studies

The performance of additional radiographic studies including flexion and extension (F/E) views, supine oblique views, computed tomography (CT), and magnetic resonance imaging (MRI) are indicated when the standard three-view analysis (a) does not adequately visualize the entire cervical spine from the occiput to T-1 vertebral body due to anatomic difficulties, or (b) fails to explain symptoms of cervical pain or existing neurologic deficits. In addition, these studies may be employed for purposes of preoperative planning.

F/E views can be particularly helpful in evaluating the alert, neurologically intact, blunt trauma victim with cervical spine pain or tenderness whose initial three-view x-ray series is normal. If the patient can provide full excursion with minimal or no pain, these views can effectively rule out instability related to ligamentous injury. Supine oblique views can supplement the traditional three-view series by providing better detail of the posterolateral elements of the vertebral bodies, particularly the pedicles, laminae, and intervertebral foramina.

Thin-section (3–5 mm) axial CT imaging of the cervical spine can aid in visualizing and diagnosing bony injuries particularly to the occiput–C-1–C-2 and cervicothoracic regions, which, due to tissue overlap, are often difficult to evaluate on plain radiography. Furthermore, spinal canal contents and associated anatomic structures are easily appreciated allowing visualization of extradural compression by retropulsed bone, disk fragments, and hematomas. Axial CT imaging is limited in evaluating fractures and dislocations in the axial plane. As such, coronal and sagittal reconstructions provide invaluable anatomic details regarding fracture patterns and bony alignment in this plane. Myelography may be added to this study if MRI is either unavailable or contraindicated. A CT myelogram is best at indirectly identifying cord compression from extradural lesions such as a hematoma or disk or bone fragments.

MRI allows for direct visualization of the spinal cord, disks, and ligaments. In addition to compressive lesions, MRI can delineate cord injuries such as transection, contusion, and edema, thereby providing useful prognostic information for the clinician in regard to expected outcome. MRI is also able to define the integrity of the ligamentous structures such as the anterior and posterior longitudinal, transverse, and interspinous ligaments. The status of the ligaments, which until now could only be inferred from plain films and CT, is often very important in decision making regarding treatment.

Clearing the Cervical Spine

Unfortunately, there are no completely specific or sensitive indicators of CSI in regard to history, physical examination, and mechanism of injury. Jacobs and Schwartz (31) have retrospectively studied variables that statistically correlated with the presence of a CSI. Among others, a history of motor vehicle accident, fall of less than 10 feet, and physical findings of neck tenderness, neck spasm, or any neurologic deficit positively correlated with the presence of CSI. Contrastingly, a history of a fall more than 10 feet, loss of consciousness, low-energy accident, and physical findings of head trauma or facial injuries did not. These data are not to be interpreted to mean that CSI can be ruled out when no "statistically significant" variable is present. Instead, the data underscore the fact that the presence of a CSI cannot be predicted based solely on mechanism, history, or physical examination.

Our apparent inability to predict who needs further radiographic assessment of the cervical spine has led some authors to ask instead, "Who does not?" (32). Current prospective reports cumulatively numbering several thousand patients have shown that no alert patient who has no complaints of neck pain on questioning or palpation, is devoid of neurologic deficit, and has no potentially distracting injuries has been found to have sustained a CSI. Such patients should be considered at low risk for CSI and need not be studied radiographically (33). Instead, their cervical spine collars should be removed and the patients observed while they flex and extend; if they have no pain with these maneuvers, the cervical spine can be cleared clinically.

Contrastingly, current evidence indicates that trauma patients with an alteration in mental status of any etiology (e.g., drugs, hypoxia, head injury, etc.) or with any neurologic deficit require further cervical spine radiography. Cervical spine fractures have been found in 4% to 6% of these individuals, two-thirds of which are unstable (34–36). Similarly, alert patients with no alteration in level of consciousness or neurologic deficit but with complaints of cervical region discomfort on questioning or palpation, as well as those with distracting injuries should receive full radiographic evaluation (33). The latter patients should undergo traditional three-view cervical spine imaging and, if negative, F/E films. If this proves asymptomatic, the cervical spine can be cleared. If the patient cannot fully flex and extend his neck with normal range of motion, the cervical spine cannot be considered stable. The inability to fully flex and extend may be due to severe muscle spasm and splinting, masking underlying ligamentous instability. It is thus imperative that the patient be maintained in a rigid cervical collar until full and unencumbered F/E films are revealed to be normal. Patients who can provide full excursion on F/E films without abnormality can be cleared of gross instability. However, it is the practice of the senior authors to utilize cervical spine collars for those alert patients with unexplained cervical pain and normal F/E films until the cervical pain resolves. On occasion, follow-up F/E films will demonstrate ligamentous instability initially masked by cervical splinting.

Patients who demonstrate altered levels of consciousness should likewise undergo three-view radiographs of the cervical spine. If normal, these patients must still be kept rigidly immobilized as they may not be able to reliably relate existing cervical pain suggestive of ligamentous instability. In these patients, who often demonstrate concomitant head injuries, it is the practice of the authors to perform flexion and extension views under fluoroscopy. If these studies are normal, the cervical collar is removed. It is important to clear the cervical spine as safely and soon as possible. In the pediatric population, significant skin breakdown can occur due to pressure and excoriation from the rigid orthosis if left in place for even short periods of time (≥24 hours).

Those individuals with an abnormality on plain films or F/E views as well as those with neurologic deficit have unstable cervical spines until proven otherwise. These patients should be kept in a rigid cervical orthosis while further radiography or treatment is performed. Typically, patients will need further CT evaluation of the fracture or subluxed area seen on plain films and/or MRI evaluation for assessment of a neurologic deficit not explained by plain films or CT.

Assessing Spinal Stability

The major concern after trauma to the cervical spine is to determine its stability. Clinical instability, as defined by White and Panjabi (37), is the loss of the ability of the spine to maintain its orientation so that there is no initial or subsequent neurologic injury, no deformity, and no incapacitating pain during normal activity. In the majority of cases, instability can be diagnosed acutely by clinical history, neurologic examination, static and dynamic radiographs, and thorough consideration of the biomechanics of the injury. On occasion, however, an initial injury may produce new spinal mechanics that fail only after repeated loads, and instability may be diagnosed in a delayed manner through follow-up.

Most of the radiographic criteria utilized to diagnose cervical spine instability are based on biomechanical laboratory testing of load to failure studies. These studies support the view that although ligaments cannot be directly visualized on plain radiographs, their integrity can be indirectly assessed.

In the upper cervical spine, the transverse atlantal ligament (TAL) is the primary determinant of stability. It is generally accepted that if the atlantodental interval (ADI) is greater than 3 to 4 mm in adults on a lateral radiograph, the TAL is probably ruptured. The normal ADI is slightly larger in children, with greater than 95% having ADIs less than 5 mm, due to the increased ligamentous laxity found in children. Likewise, on the open-mouth odontoid view, if the combined overhang of the lateral masses of C-1 on C-2 is greater than 7 mm, then the TAL is likely to be ruptured. This rule, known as "Spence's rule," has recently been debated through MRI and CT evidence of TAL rupture without C-1 lateral mass displacement of greater than 7 mm. The authors of this study evaluated 39 patients with C-1 fractures and demonstrated a false-negative rate of 61% on plain radiographs using this rule. They concluded that the "7 mm rule" is unreliable and should be abandoned as a screening tool. Instead, their report suggested that both static and dynamic plain radiographs as well as CT and MRI provide more accurate assessment of the integrity of the TAL (38).

In the subaxial spine, several criteria have been experimentally derived and have proven sensitive predictors of instability and hence need for surgical intervention: radiographic abnormalities of greater than 11 degrees of sagittal plane angulation and greater than 3.5 mm of sagittal plane translation at a motion segment, interspinous process widening, loss of facet parallelism, greater than 50% compression of vertebral body height, loss of the normal cervical lordosis, and dynamic cervical spine films showing excessive translation or angulation (39).

In addition to radiographic abnormalities, the presence of neurologic deficit implies that the spinal cord was subjected to either a vascular or mechanical insult. Although clinical instability is not guaranteed in the traumatic case with neurologic involvement, the clinician should be attuned to the radiologic clues that might confirm such instability. Some investigators have suggested that if the trauma is significant enough to injure neural elements, then the integrity of the supporting structures has been altered, possibly permitting reinjury, and an unstable spine exists (37).

EMERGENT TREATMENT OF CERVICAL SPINE INJURY

If a fracture or dislocation is seen on plain films, the goals include (a) arriving at a definitive diagnosis and (b) producing and/or maintaining safe anatomic realignment of the spinal column, thus protecting the spinal cord. If there is no need for reduction, a CT scan including one level above and below the abnormality should be obtained with the patient immobilized. MRI may then be performed if necessary to further define ligamentous or spinal cord injury.

Emergent Reduction

If reduction is necessary, a prereduction CT myelogram or MRI is recommended for purposes of (a) evaluating associated fractures and fracture planes and (b) ruling out an associated retropulsed disk fragment that, if unrecognized, can present a significant risk to the cervical cord during reduction. The presence of such an abnormality may indicate that an anterior approach for decompression might be needed as an initial therapeutic maneuver.

If no contraindications to closed reduction exist, the patient should be placed into Gardner Wells (GW) tongues (Zimmer, Warsaw, IN) and traction for purposes of reducing and maintaining anatomic alignment of fractures and dislocations before further diagnostic tests are done. If a halo is likely to be used after definitive treatment, a MRI-compatible halo ring can be placed for initial traction/reduction and later converted to the vest.

The general principle of acute reduction is to re-create the force vector that produced the injury, i.e., distraction /flexion, extension. The pins of the GW tongues are placed 3 to 4 cm above the pinna, just above the temporalis muscle. If in-line reduction is indicated, the pins are placed in the same coronal plane as the external auditory meatus (EAM). If flexion or extension is needed for reduction, the pins can be adjusted 2 to 3 cm posterior or anterior, respectively, to the EAM. Traditionally, the weight used is approximated by multiplying the number of cervical vertebrae above the level of the abnormality by three. For example, a fracture dislocation at C4-5 can be reduced by starting at 4 × 3, or 12 pounds. Thereafter, 5-pound weights can be added every 10 to 15 minutes until reduction is obtained, not to exceed 10 pounds per vertebral level.

A lateral cervical spine film must be immediately taken after instituting or changing the traction weight. This avoids overdistraction of the vertebral bodies due to incompetent ligamentous structures and a subsequent stretch injury to the spinal cord. Often, sedatives such as midazolam or lorazepam can be used along with narcotic analgesics to allow the cervical musculature to relax and aid reduction. Once reduction is obtained, all weight except for 10 to 15 pounds can be removed. At this point, the patient should be kept in traction until definitive treatment is performed. One injury that needs special attention is that of atlanto-occipital dislocation. This highly unstable and usually fatal injury can be overdistracted with minimal traction, sometimes as little as 3 to 5 pounds, causing iatrogenic injury to the cervicomedullary junction. Occasionally, a spinal fracture cannot be reduced with this method, usually because of facet fracture fragments or other soft tissues interposed between the facets. Open surgical reduction and fusion are then required.

Managing Life-Threatening Injuries with an Uncertain Cervical Spine Status

The need to perform emergency procedures (e.g., tracheostomy, craniotomy for acute epidural hematoma, etc.) before full clearance of the cervical spine is not uncommon. In this situation, patients should be treated as if their cervical spine is unstable until complete radiographic evaluation can be obtained.

Once again, the ABCs are of primary importance and should guide the initial treatment of these victims. In the event that an emergent tracheostomy is needed, the cervical spine should be immobilized in the neutral position either by an assistant providing in-line stabilization, or by placing foam blocks or sandbags next to the head and taping these along with the forehead to the backboard. Although slight extension of the neck may be necessary for a proper surgical approach, and in most instances is safe to perform, overt hyperextension of the cervical spine should be avoided. In this position, an emergency tracheostomy can be performed in almost any environment.

For individuals requiring lifesaving procedures that need to be performed in the operating room, patient transport and positioning are important. The patient's entire spinal axis should be maintained in neutral alignment by keeping the patient on a rigid backboard with the cervical spine immobilized by a rigid hard collar, sandbags, and tape. The patient can then be moved to the operating room table and the backboard removed in one easy motion. The cervical spine should be kept in neutral position, again with either a rigid collar, or, should the neck need to be exposed, with sandbags and tape while the procedures are being performed. Once completed and the patient's condition is stabilized, full cervical spine films can then be obtained and treatment decision making can be initiated as directed above. By following these procedures, the cervical spine can be stabilized and further neurologic injury avoided in the event an unstable injury exists.

SPECIFIC INJURY PATTERNS AND THEIR TREATMENT

Trauma to the cervical spine involves a complex set of variables whose interaction ultimately determines whether the external force applied will adversely affect the integrity of the spinal column. In addition to the direction and magnitude of the traumatic force, other factors such as the length of time over which the force is applied, the instantaneous posture of the head and neck, and the anatomic location of load impact will determine the eventual injury pattern. Furthermore, the anatomic characteristics of the upper cervical spine [occiput (Occ)–C-1–C-2] are quite different from the subaxial cervical spine (C-3–C-7). These anatomic differences account for not only the distinct difference in motions between these two segments but also the consequences of trauma.

Atlanto-Occipital Dislocations

Injuries to the craniocervical junction are usually produced as a result of high-energy impact and are usually fatal due to injury of the respiratory centers within the brainstem. An increasing number of survivors are now being reported (41), most likely due to improved resuscitation by emergency medical services (EMS). The shallowness of the occipital condyles and superior C-1 facets, the inherent ligamentous laxity, and the poorly developed cervical musculature found in the pediatric population predispose children to this injury.

The injury mechanism is complex, but hyperextension, rotation, and distraction are usually implicated. Rapid deceleration with impact of the head invariably occurs. The injury involves variable ligamentous disruptions at the Occ–C-1–C-2 junction including the atlanto-occipital articular capsular ligaments. The resultant craniovertebral dislocation is highly unstable and can lead to brainstem compression and vertebral artery injury.

Findings on plain film radiography may include Occ–C-1 longitudinal distraction as well as anterior and posterior translation of the occiput on the atlas. Whereas the normal Occ–C-1 articulation is not well visualized due to overlying soft tissue and the mastoids in adults, the longitudinally distractive forces can cause a ''bare'' or ''naked'' appearance of the occipital condyles and superior facets of the atlas. Prevertebral soft tissue swelling is invariably present and should raise suspicion of an injury at this level particularly with individuals who demonstrate high cervical spinal cord injury or altered mental status. Several measurement techniques have been developed for assessing normal and abnormal relationships of the skull base and cervical spine on lateral radiographs. Despite the use of such techniques, the diagnosis of Occ–C-1 dislocation by plain film radiographs has been shown to be only 50% to 75% accurate (41). For this reason the additional use of CT with sagittal and coronal reconstructions to image the Occ–C-1 joint directly is useful. MRI can also be used to document ligamentous injury but is most useful in assessing the neural axis to explain neurologic deficits.

Although halo immobilization can be used to provide acute stability for the craniovertebral junction while other life-threatening injuries are treated, these injuries are purely ligamentous and do not heal well with immobilization alone. Consequently, these patients remain at risk for further neurologic deterioration due to recurrent subluxations. Long-term stability requires fusion of the occiput to the upper cervical spine.

Among survivors, the long-term prognosis of these patients depends on the initial severity of the injury. Neurologic recovery has been reported in over 60% in a most recent study, including several patients who presented with severe spinal cord injuries. Patients suffering from complete spinal cord injuries and patients suffering concomitant head injuries often have a poor outcome (41).

Fractures of the Atlas

Acute atlas fractures account for 3% to 13% of all cervical spine fractures. Of these fractures, 56% are isolated to the atlas, 44% are combined C-1/C-2 fractures, and 9% are combined C-1/subaxial fractures (42). The Jefferson fracture is the best known of the atlantal fractures (43), although isolated lateral mass fractures can occur. Jefferson originally described an injury pattern of bilateral fractures of both the anterior and posterior arch (i.e., four fracture lines). However, the advent of CT imaging has shown that the ring of C-1 may only be fractured in two or three sites.

The major injury vector in atlas fractures is axial compression from a direct blow to the vertex of the head, classically from a diving injury. The oblique orientation of the lateral masses of C-1 between the occipital condyles and the superior facets of C-2 directs axial forces laterally, pushing the facets of the atlas apart until the ring fractures. If hyperextension occurs, the posterior arch of the atlas may be fractured as it is compressed between the occiput and the posterior arch of the axis, or an avulsion injury of the anterior tubercle of C-1 can occur. The spinal canal is not compromised by any of these fracture patterns, and subsequently fractures of C-1 are associated with a low incidence of spinal cord injury. However, commonly associated head trauma can cause significant morbidity and mortality.

Radiographically, atlas fractures are classically diagnosed by noting lateral displacement of the C-1 articular masses on the frontal view although isolated posterior arch fractures are best visualized on lateral projections. As the TAL spans the distance between the lateral masses, widening of the lateral masses indicates disruption of this ligament and hence C-1–C-2 instability. Through an in vitro laboratory analysis, Spence et al. (44) demonstrated rupture of the TAL when the combined overhang of the lateral masses of C-1 on C-2 was on average 6.3 mm. The results of this study have been used clinically to indirectly determine the integrity of the TAL on open-mouth odontoid views and has become known as ''Spence's rule.''

Most isolated atlas fractures can be treated successfully with an external orthosis. Traditional treatment protocols regarding the type of orthosis have relied on indirect evidence of TAL integrity, and hence stability. A stable injury, defined as combined lateral mass displacement less than 7 mm, can be treated with a simple rigid collar, whereas unstable injuries, with lateral mass displacement greater than 7 mm, are best treated with halo immobilization. Using external orthosis in this manner has resulted in bony union of the atlas fracture in 95% of cases (42). Surgical treatment, involving either C-1–C-2 fusion or occipitocervical fusion has classically been reserved for cases of continued C-1–C-2 instability despite external bracing.

This treatment algorithm has recently been debated. For reasons discussed above (see Assessing Spinal Stability), Dickman and colleagues (38) recommend that both static and dynamic plain radiographs as well as CT and MRI be used to accurately assess the integrity of the TAL. The TAL's integrity, in turn, should guide therapy. Under Dickman et al.'s new proposal, patients in whom the TAL was torn within its substance should undergo early surgery, as the likelihood of ligamentous healing is poor. However, if the C-1 lateral mass is comminuted and the tubercle for ligament insertion is simply disconnected, leaving the ligament structurally intact, a rigid orthosis alone could achieve long-term stability over 74% of the time. As a result of studies such as these, our understanding and rationale for treatment continues to evolve.

Atlantoaxial Subluxation and Dislocation

In the absence of an odontoid fracture, subluxation or overt dislocation of C-1 in relation to C-2 may either be rotatory or translational (most commonly anterior). Translational subluxation requires bilateral displacement of the lateral masses of the atlas in the same direction, whereas rotatory subluxation requires the lateral masses to be in different points within the sagittal plane, one anterior or posterior to the other. Translational dislocation of both lateral masses can occur only with TAL instability as seen with traumatic rupture of the TAL and inherent laxity without rupture. Rotatory subluxation can occur spontaneously, with minor or major trauma, or as a result of ligamentous laxity due to inflammatory diseases, e.g., rheumatoid arthritis and upper respiratory infections. Although atlantoaxial subluxation and dislocation may occur as isolated injuries, they are most commonly associated with C-1 and C-2 fractures.

The mechanism of anterior dislocation is flexion and anterior translation by an impact to the occiput, similar to the mechanism of an odontoid fracture. If there is no associated dens fracture, then the spinal canal diameter will narrow significantly between the posterior arch of C-1 and dorsal aspect of the dens, resulting in various degrees of neurologic injury or even death. If an associated fracture of C-2 exists, neurologic injury is less likely.

As its name implies, traumatic rotatory subluxation is caused by a rotatory force and most likely indicates failure of one or both alar ligaments (45). Patients with rotatory subluxation will usually present with a ''cock robin'' appearance in which the patient's head is flexed, rotated approximately 20 degrees to one side and laterally flexed toward the other side. These patient's cervical spine should not be manipulated until full radiographic evaluation has been performed.

Radiographically, translational displacement has been classically diagnosed using the ADI. With an ADI of greater than 3 mm (in adults), the TAL is considered incompetent and hence unstable. Using thin-slice MRI to directly visualize the TAL, however, some authors report that an ADI of greater than 3 mm predicted only 74% of TAL ruptures (38). Additionally, if the patient is positioned supine on a backboard with even slight extension of the cervical spine, the increased ADI may not be evident. Hence, other radiographic clues should be sought such as retropharyngeal soft tissue swelling or a small fleck of bone that may be visible on open-mouth views where the TAL was avulsed from its insertion site on the lateral mass of C-1. Unless the above studies suggest gross instability, most patients will require additional studies. In patients who complain of neck pain but are neurologically intact, flexion and extension views under physician-directed supervision are necessary, but internal splinting may hide the injury. In this case, and in cases where neurologic impairment exists, CT can be used to identify evidence of TAL avulsion, and MRI can evaluate the ligament directly along with the neural axis.

Similarly, traumatic rotatory subluxations and dislocations can be difficult to diagnose radiographically. If plain films are studied closely, the open-mouth view may show asymmetry of the lateral masses, with the more anterior lateral mass appearing wider and closer to the dens compared with the contralateral lateral mass. In general, however, plain film x-rays often are difficult to interpret and multiplanar CT reconstructions through this area are an invaluable tool.

Rotatory subluxation has been classified into four subtypes (Fig. 21-3). Type I injuries are the most common and demonstrate rotation of the atlas about the dens with a normal ADI. Range of motion is limited but within normal range. Some authors have questioned the pathologic significance of this lesion. Type II injuries involve rotatory subluxation with one lateral mass subluxed anteriorly, while the contralateral lateral mass acts as a pivot. The TAL is usually deficient and the ADI often measures 3 to 5 mm. The rotation allowed by this injury is supraphysiologic. Type III injuries occur when the TAL and secondary atlantoaxial ligaments are deficient. In this type both lateral masses are subluxed anteriorly, one more than the other, and the ADI is greater than 5 mm. Type IV injuries are unique in that they occur

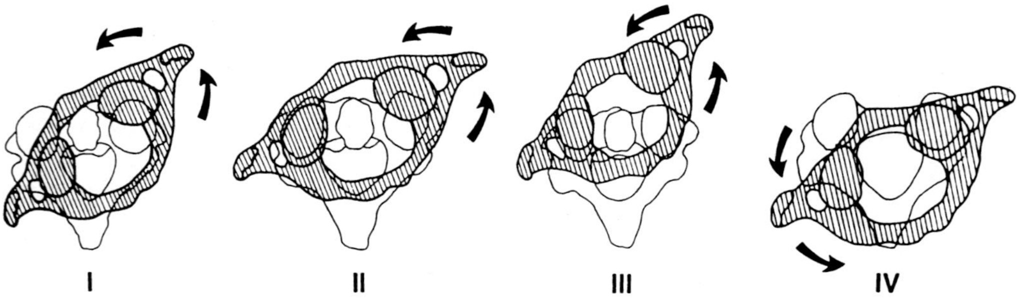

FIG. 21-3. Atlantoaxial rotatory subluxation. **A:** Type I—anterior displacement of atlas <3 mm. **B:** Type II—anterior displacement 3 to 5 mm. **C:** Type III—anterior displacement >5 mm. **D:** Type IV—posterior displacement of the atlas. (Adapted from ref. 45, with permission.)

when the dens is deficient due to either trauma or inflammatory diseases. In this case the lateral masses are displaced posteriorly and rotated (40).

Treatment of type I rotatory injuries involves traction to reduce the lesion followed by external immobilization with a sterno-occipital mandibular immobilizer (SOMI) or rigid collar. Type II lesions warrant further investigation with MRI, CT, and even lateral flexion and extension plain films. If the TAL is intact, then reduction with traction followed by more rigid immobilization with a halo is recommended. If the TAL is ruptured, most authorities recommend atlantoaxial fusion. Similarly, type III and IV lesions are highly unstable and should be treated with reduction followed by fusion. Should rotatory subluxation be diagnosed more than 3 months after injury, fusion should be obtained in situ as reduction can be dangerous.

Surgical treatment options for obtaining atlantoaxial fusion include a variety of posterior C-1–C-2 wiring constructs (see Fig. 21-9), clamps, or transarticular screws placed across the C-1–C-2 articulations bilaterally. The purpose of these constructs is to provide immediate stability of the C-1–C-2 region while fusion occurs. Unfortunately, eliminating the movement at C-1–C-2 eliminates 40% to 50% of axial rotation. Therefore, more conservative options such as external bracing should be utilized if indicated.

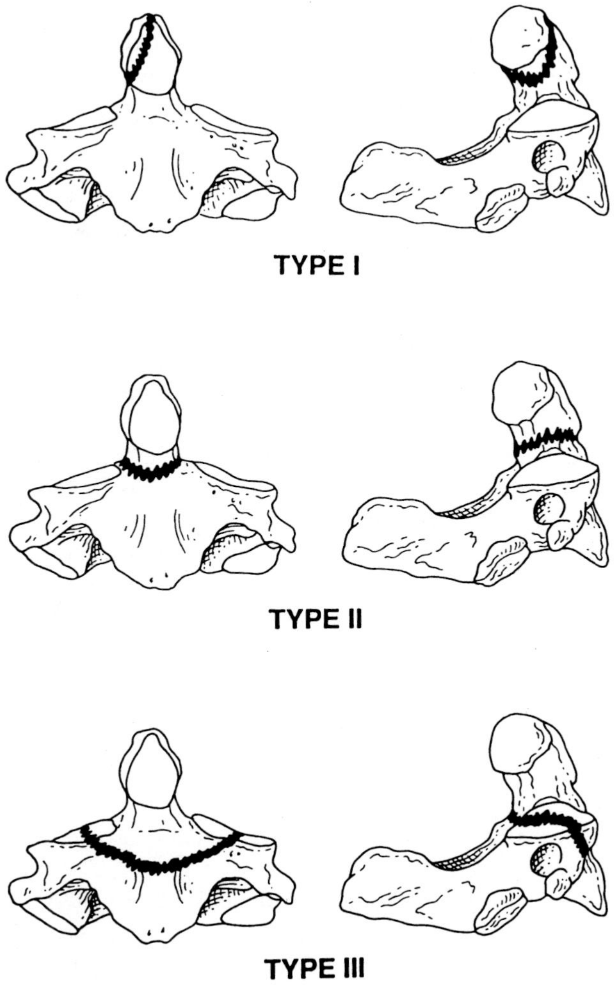

FIG. 21-4. Odontoid fractures. (Adapted from ref. 46, with permission.)

Odontoid Fractures

Odontoid fractures constitute 10% to 15% of all cervical spine fractures. Hyperflexion and hyperextension produce anteriorly and posteriorly displaced lesions, respectively. Symptoms include neck pain, spasm, and sometimes pain in the distribution of the greater occipital nerve (C-2). Unlike the previously discussed fractures, the diagnosis is usually readily made on plain films. CT with sagittal and coronal reconstructions can help delineate precise fracture planes.

Anderson and D'Alonzo (46) classified odontoid fractures into three categories (Fig. 21-4). Type I fractures involve only the tip of the odontoid, superior to the TAL. This injury simply represents an avulsion fracture caused by the alar ligament and are usually stable injuries. Type II fractures are the most common odontoid fracture and occur at the junction of the dens and body, inferior to the TAL. These lesions are considered unstable. Type III fractures are actually horizontally oriented superior C-2 body fractures that render the dens incompetent. They are the second most common odontoid fracture and are usually stable.

Because of the rarity of type I fractures, few series exist comparing treatment options. Flexion and extension films as well as MRI may be indicated as there have been reports of this fracture associated with atlanto-occipital instability (47). In the absence of such instability, rigid collars have proven adequate for proper healing. Recommendations for definitive treatment of type II injuries are controversial. In general, the older the individual and greater the displacement between the two fragments, the lower the rate of fusion obtained with external orthosis. The authors tend to use operative treatment for patients greater than 65 years old who are in otherwise good medical condition, for fractures displaced more than 4 to 6 mm in any direction, and for fractures unable to be maintained in alignment with a halo. In addition, we offer surgery to patients with other type II fractures as an alternative to halo immobilizaton. Treatment of type III lesions are generally nonoperative. Presumably, the relatively large bony surface area involved at the fracture site permits spontaneous fusion to occur with the use of external immobilization. Although halo immobilization has achieved 90% to 100% fusion rates in some series, others have had equivalent results with simple rigid collar immobilization (48).

Surgical treatment for type II and III have classically involved C-1–C-2 posterior fusion as mentioned above for atlantoaxial dislocation. A newer technique involving placement of a screw across the odontoid fracture from an anterior approach to C-2 has been developed (see Fig. 21-10). Early results from the senior author's own unpublished series suggest that for certain fracture patterns and individuals this method provides high rates of fusion with minimal morbidity. The advantage of the odontoid screw over traditional posterior procedures is that it preserves rotation at the C1-2 joint.

Traumatic Spondylolisthesis

C-2 fractures involving the pars interarticularis have been labeled in many colorful ways, including a ''hangman's fracture'' coined by Schneider et al. (49) in 1965, who elucidated the mechanisms involved in producing this fracture pattern. These lesions represent 20% of all axis fractures, and are rarely associated with direct neurologic injury. However, about one-third of all patients have a concurrent cervical spinal injury at another level. Like odontoid fractures, the diagnosis can usually be made on plain films. If there is angulation, displacement, or neurologic deficit, then CT to define the bony anatomy and MRI to rule out a ruptured C-2–C-3 disk are warranted. While the mechanisms of hyperextension and distraction combine to produce the classic hangman's fracture, hyperextension and axial loading, usually as a result of a motor vehicle accident, is more common.

A classification system of these fractures has been developed by Effendi et al. (50) and later modified by Levine and Edwards (51). This system addresses the displacement between the bony fragments as well as the degree of disruption of the C2-3 disk space and facets and is used to guide treatment (Fig. 21-5).

Type I fractures, the most commonly seen pattern, are fractures of the pars interarticularis with displacement less than 2 mm, leaving the C2-3 disk space intact. Type II traumatic spondylolisthesis represents fractures of the pars interarticularis with greater than 2 mm displacement. The mechanism involves axial loading with hyperextension followed by flexion. These injuries have been subtyped according to the predominant force and resulting position of the fractured fragments: flexion, extension, and listhesis (i.e., displacement). With these fractures, the stability of the C-2–C-3 disk may be compromised. Commonly, the disk disruption becomes evident as C2-3 disk space widening once the patient is placed into traction (Fig. 21-6). Type III fractures are the most uncommon type but carry the highest risk of neurologic injury and mortality when they do occur. The body of the axis is dislocated in flexion with locked facets at C-2–C-3 and severe disruption of the C-2–C-3 disk. The mechanism is flexion with axial loading.

Treatment of these injuries is based on the findings described by the above classification schema. For type I injuries, most authors recommend a SOMI brace or hard collar, reserving a halo for noncompliant patients. Type II lesions are treated according to the degree of disruption of the soft tissues and disk space, fragment displacement, and dynamic film stability. If only moderate displacement exists (less than 5 mm) with minimal angulation (less than 15 degrees) and the C2-3 disk space appears stable with flexion and extension views, patients will usually heal with a halo orthosis. Operative stabilization can be reserved for those who fail such treatment and for patients with greater than 5 mm of displacement, angulation greater than 15 degrees, or traumatic C-2–C-3 disk herniation. Type III lesions are treated according to disk space disruption and the ability to externally reduce the lesion through traction. If the facets can be reduced, treatment with a halo is the rule. If reduction cannot be obtained or the patient fails to fuse with a halo brace, then operative intervention including reduction and fusion is indicated. When surgical intervention is indicated for any type II or III fracture, anterior diskectomy and fusion with plating from C-2 to C-3 is preferred over posterior C-1–C-2 fusion procedures as the anterior approach allows continued axial rotation at C-1–C-2.

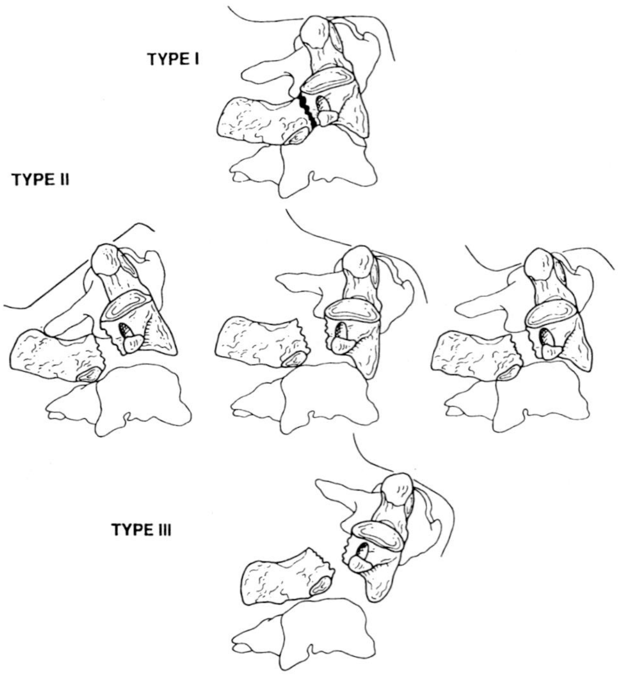

FIG. 21-5. Classification of traumatic spondylolisthesis. Type I—minimally displaced fracture fragments <2 mm. Type II—displaced fracture fragments >2 mm. Note subtypes of flexion, extension, and listhesis (translation) of C-2 body on C-3. The C-2–C-3 disk is variably disrupted. Type III—dislocated fragments. Note the anterior displacement of the C-2 body with invariable disruption of the C-2–C-3 disk space and the jumped C-2 facets on C3. (Adapted from ref. 50, with permission.)

Subaxial Spine Fractures and Dislocations

Injuries of the subaxial spine are best categorized by considering the mechanisms involved. Investigators have found that although many different forces may be involved in a single injury, it is the resultant force vector that will dictate the injury type. Thus, most spinal specialists consider subaxial spine injuries on a continuum (Fig. 21-7). Patients may suffer variations in the injury pattern given identical external forces depending on the inherent bone quality, posture of

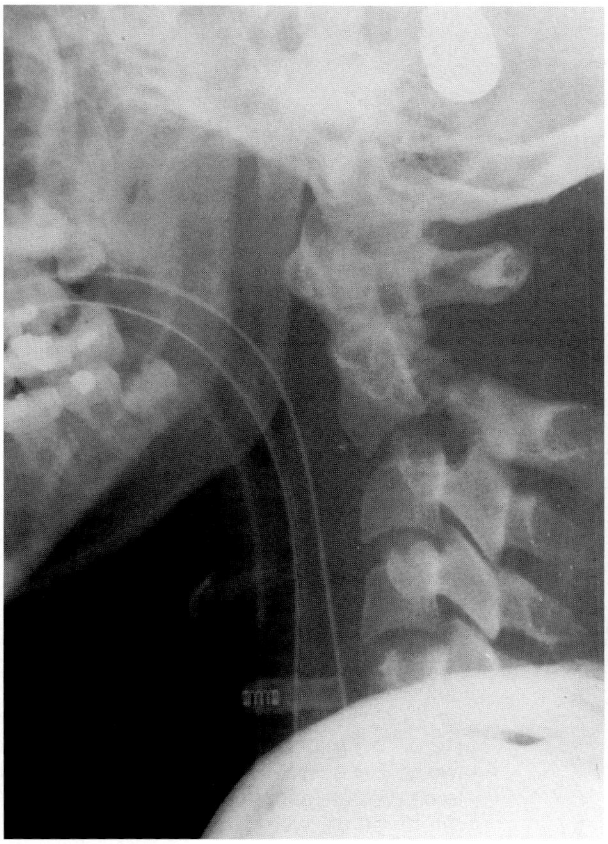

A

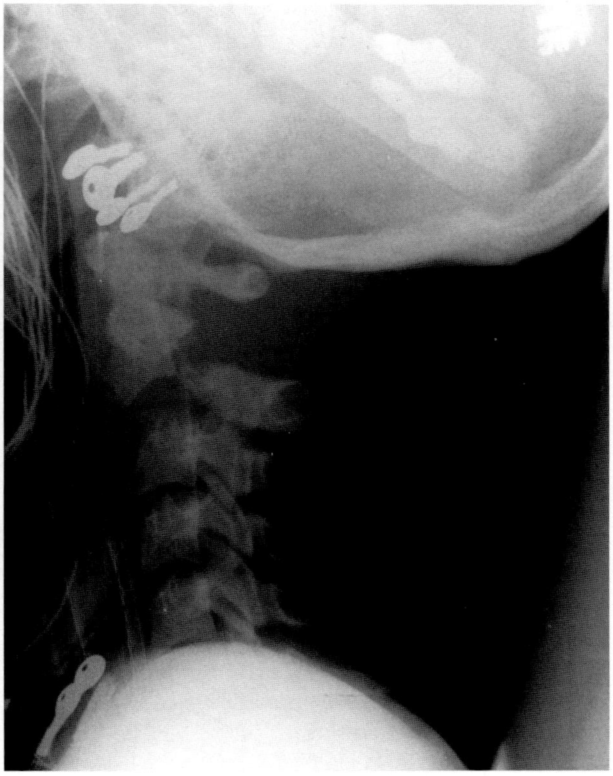

B

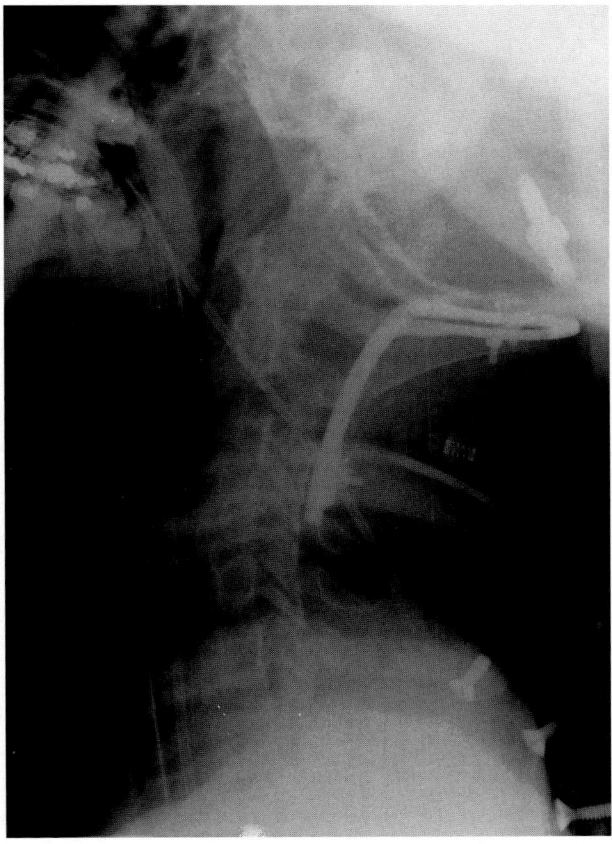

C

FIG. 21-6. Type II hangman's fracture. **A:** The initial lateral cervical spine film demonstrates a fracture through the pars interarticularis of C-2 with >2 mm of fragment displacement and anterior angulation. The C-2–C-3 facet joint is still relatively intact. **B:** After instituting 5 pounds of traction with Gardner-Wells tongues, the C-2–C-3 disk disruption becomes apparent. The traction weight was immediately reduced. **C:** Postoperative radiograph after an occipital to C3 posterior fusion demonstrating restoration of the normal occipital cervical alignment. An occipital cervical loop was chosen over an anterior C-2–C-3 diskectomy and fusion because of associated atlanto-occipital instability. However, this patient ultimately required an anterior C-2–C-3 diskectomy, fusion, and instrumentation due to continued instability at C-2–C-3.

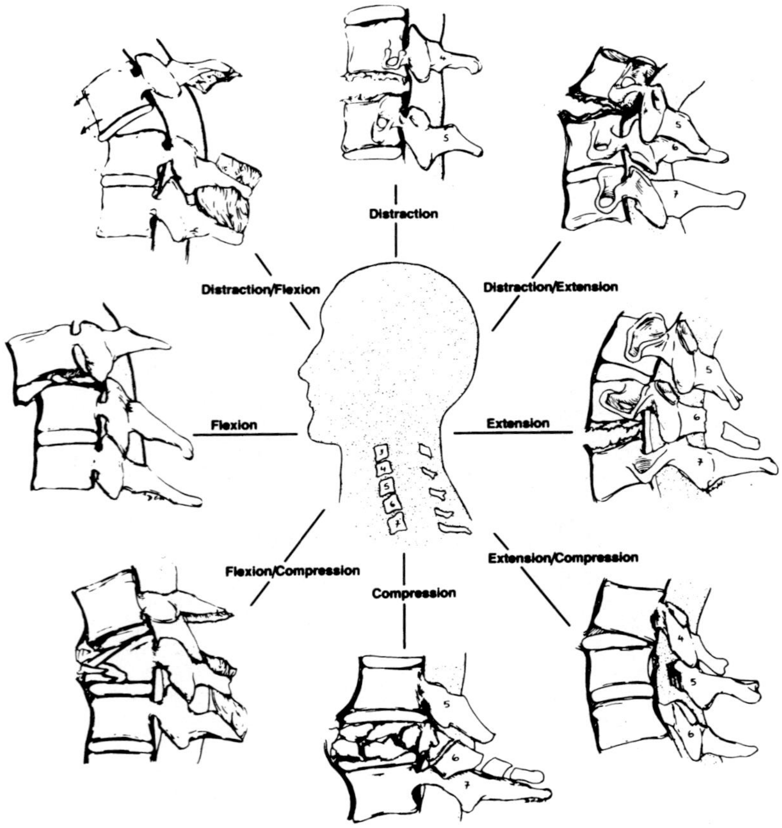

FIG. 21-7. Subaxial spinal fractures exist along a spectrum of injury patterns. This clock diagram outlines the four major mechanisms of injury: flexion (9 o'clock), extension (3 o'clock), distraction (12 o'clock), and compression (6 o'clock). When two of these forces occur together, the resultant force vector determines the fracture pattern. (From ref. 61, with permission.)

the neck on impact, preexisting degenerative diseases, and slight variations in the force vector. Allen et al. (52) have proposed such a classification based on the major injury vector and includes vertical compression, compression flexion, distractive flexion, compressive extension, distractive extension, and lateral flexion injuries.

Vertical compression injuries result from pure axial loading. This force vector results in compression or ''burst'' fractures as the vertebral body ''explodes'' under the force. Consequently, bony fragments may be retropulsed into the spinal canal. Less commonly, a simple wedge compression fracture may occur, reducing the anterior body height with possible fractures through the superior or inferior end plates. As these injuries usually cause only bony disruption and leave the ligaments intact, they are generally considered stable.

Compression/flexion injuries are common in clinical practice. The spectrum of radiographic findings ranges from mild anterior vertebral body fractures to the ''teardrop'' fracture. The latter is commonly seen in the typical diving injury in which the spine is hyperflexed while a compressive force is delivered to the head. In this injury, a small teardrop-shaped fracture of the anterior inferior segment of the more cephalad vertebral body occurs. Unfortunately, a retropulsed fragment of the posterior vertebral body not uncommonly impinges on the spinal cord, producing various neurologic injuries including complete and incomplete deficits and possibly an anterior spinal artery syndrome. Posterior arch fractures occur in up to 50% of compression flexion injuries (45). Although a small amount of distractive forces are applied to the posterior structures, ligamentous instability does not ensue. Therefore, these are generally considered stable injuries.

Distractive flexion injuries range from the hyperflexion sprain to bilateral jumped facets. As distractive forces are applied to the cervical spine, the posterior ligaments are injured first, with resultant interspinous process widening noted radiographically. As the forces increase, the facet capsules and anterior ligaments may fail. If axial rotation or a lateral bending force is superimposed, then unilateral locked facets may occur. While vertebral body fractures are uncommon, the ligamentous injury can be severe. As such these injuries are highly unstable. The much milder hyperflexion sprain implies a stable ligamentous injury and often heals with conservative management.

Compressive extension injuries occur when the head receives an axial load with the neck in an extended posture. Isolated vertebral arch fractures are one of the more common injury patterns. As the force increases in magnitude, however, the anterior ligaments fail and a fracture dislocation may occur. In this situation, the compressive forces cause fractures of the lateral masses, pedicles, and lamina while the extension component causes a vertebral body avulsion fracture of the superior aspect of the inferior vertebral body. If the anterior ligaments are intact, isolated vertebral arch fractures are stable. If the anterior ligaments are injured, the lesion is considered unstable.

Distractive extension injuries constitute hyperextension without a compressive force. The whiplash injury is a common result of this mechanism in which the anterior longitudinal ligament (ALL) and the anterior cervical musculature have been torn in some cases (53). Another common scenario for this injury pattern is the elderly individual who falls from bed striking the forehead and suffers a spinal cord injury, despite normal radiographs. The proposed mechanism is a pinching of the spinal cord between the vertebral bodies and the ''buckled'' ligamentum flavum. The ALL is often ruptured from the distractive force applied and may be manifest only as widening of the disk space anteriorly. Distraction injuries are stable in flexion, but, with disruption of the ALL, are unstable in extension.

Lateral flexion injuries result from an asymmetrically applied compressive force causing the spine to be bent laterally. This injury is most commonly seen in motor vehicle accidents and football injuries. The lateral mass, facet, lamina, and portion of the vertebral body opposite the side of impact receive compressive forces, while the ipsilateral elements are distracted. Common sequelae include lateral mass fractures, asymmetric vertebral body fractures, laminar fractures, and possibly unilateral facet subluxation or dislocation on the side receiving the distractive forces. Neurologic injury and spinal instability are common (45).

Treatment of Subaxial Spine Injuries

There is no ''cookbook'' approach to managing these cervical spine injuries. In general, evidence of severe ligamentous instability (e.g., bilateral/unilateral jumped facets), irreducible fracture dislocations, and compressive lesions (bone, blood) are indications for surgical intervention. However, in the patient with evidence of minor ligamentous injury and/or fractures without dislocation or neural compromise, the decision for treating operatively versus nonoperatively can be less straightforward. In these cases, the mechanism and findings on static and dynamic radiographs should receive equal consideration.

Surgical approaches to subaxial cervical spine trauma are limited to anterior, posterior, or combined. The choice of approach should be based upon the integrity of the bony elements, the location of neural compression, and the mechanism of injury. Anterior cervical stabilization is indicated for significant ventral cord compression from vertebrae or disk material as well as ligamentous instability. Compression fractures with significant kyphosis or traumatic disk herniation are two more common examples of indications for anterior approaches. A posterior approach is indicated for significant disruption of the posterior bony or ligamentous structures with little or no involvement of the vertebral body or disk. It is the preferred approach for spinal instability associated with flexion injuries, anterior dislocation, bilateral jumped facets, and unilateral jumped facets should closed reduction be unsuccessful. Occasionally, a combined approach is needed when both anterior and posterior structures are injured. Cases of severe flexion/compression injuries, vertical compression injuries with posterior ligamentous disruption, and bilateral facet dislocation associated with a disk herniation and cord compression are examples of where a combined approach is indicated.

The orthosis utilized both postoperatively and for stable injuries managed nonoperatively include the halo, SOMI brace, and rigid collar. Which particular othosis is used depends on the severity of the injury, perceived adequacy of internal stabilization, and patient issues such as compliance and bone quality. In the younger, healthy, compliant patient with a rigid internal fixation construct, a rigid collar will usually suffice. As compliance, bone quality, and the rigidity of the internal fixation construct decrease, the SOMI and halo braces are often used to supplement immobilization.

OPERATIVE MANAGEMENT OF CERVICAL SPINE INJURIES

Timing of Surgical Intervention After Cervical Spine Injury

In determining the exact timing of surgical intervention, three distinct factors should be considered. First, as mentioned above, the overall medical condition and need for lifesaving procedures should take precedence as most cervical spine injuries can be treated with immobilization or traction. Second, institutional factors such as the availability of the various spinal instrumentation systems can influence the technical aspects of performing such a surgical procedure. Furthermore, the familiarity of the operating room personnel with the surgical approaches and instrumentation techniques is critical in reducing operative time and surgical morbidity. Third, the neurologic condition of the patient, i.e., intact, partial, or complete spinal cord injury, at the time of assessment and on serial exams influences the expediency with which most surgeons will operate on the injury.

The single, most widely accepted indication for emergent surgical intervention is documented neurologic deterioration in association with ongoing spinal cord compression from bone or disk fragments, spinal hematomas, or nonreducible subluxation. Otherwise, the traditional neurosurgical approach to cervical spine injury has been to postpone surgery until the patient's medical condition has been optimized. Proponents of this policy cited lower rates of postsurgical morbidity including pulmonary embolism, gastrointestinal hemorrhage, and infection (54) as well as a reduced incidence of postsurgical neurologic decline (55) when surgery was delayed. This ideology led to prolonged immobilization, sometimes weeks, before intervention was attempted.

More recently, there have been renewed concerns over the systemic complications of prolonged immobilization, particularly in spinal cord-injured patients (21). As a result, investigators have reevaluated the efficacy of early surgery and have reported not only lower incidences of postoperative morbidity due to earlier mobilization and reduced hospitalization, but also improved neurologic outcome with earlier intervention (56). Of note, all studies to date investigating the effect of early or late surgical intervention on neurologic outcome are retrospective in nature and are not randomized with respect to many important variables that can affect neurologic recovery .

In summary, contemporary studies have shown that early surgery for cervical spine injury with neurologic injury does not increase the rates of postoperative complications. It is reasonable, therefore, to consider prompt spinal reduction and decompression with internal spinal stabilization so as to allow patients both with and without spinal cord injury the advantages of early mobilization. Ultimately, the decision to intervene surgically will depend on a number of patient- and institution-related variables, thus precluding a rigid protocol.

Surgical Considerations

When the neurologic condition of the patient is stable, operative intervention for the management of cervical spine trauma is indicated for unstable fractures, fractures that cannot be held in alignment satisfactorily with orthoses, fractures that have failed to heal with external orthoses (e.g., nonunion), and patients wishing to avoid rigid external immobilization. Internal fixation has several advantages. First, surgical stabilization produces immediate stability, obviating the need for prolonged bed rest and, in most cases, halo immobilization. Second, stabilization can be achieved with little associated surgical morbidity and mortality. Finally, the above two factors allow rehabilitation to be started sooner, which can ultimately reduce the overall cost of treatment.

The goals of spinal internal fixation procedures are to achieve anatomic alignment, to protect the neural elements, and to stabilize the spine yet preserve the motion of normal spinal segments. These goals may be attained only by achieving a satisfactory arthrodesis. It is important to recognize that instrumentation provides rigid yet temporary spinal fixation. Metallic wires, screws, plates, clamps, and rods are all susceptible to loosening, fatigue, and breakage. Therefore, it is imperative that the foundation for a solid osseous union (bone graft) be laid at the time of the operation to ensure long-term spinal stability.

Techniques of stabilizing the cervical spine have advanced significantly over the past decades. Although intended for treatment of traumatic unstable injuries, many of these techniques have since been applied to cases of neoplastic, degenerative, and postsurgical cervical instability as well. There are many instrumentation systems for surgery, and each has advantages and disadvantages. In general, titanium-based systems are replacing stainless steel systems as the metal of choice because titanium is MRI compatible, which allows for follow-up imaging. Ultimately, it is the role of the surgeon to choose the most appropriate technique(s) to assure that the goals of spinal instrumentation are met.

Just as the fracture patterns and biomechanics of the craniocervical region are different from those of the subaxial spine, procedures aimed at stabilizing these two regions are quite different. Although it is beyond the scope of this chapter to detail the operative technique for all methods described, a brief description of the options available will be presented for each of the two cervical spine regions.

Stabilization of the Craniocervical Region

Occipital-Cervical Fusion

Indications for occipital-cervical fusion include instability of the occipitoatlantal joint or atlantoaxial instability with a structurally deficient or fractured posterior atlantal arch. The posterior approach is most commonly used. The patient is positioned prone with the head held in a three-point skull fixator or a preoperatively placed halo device. Intraoperative x-rays of the cervical spine are obtained to assure proper alignment before proceeding. Next, through a midline incision, a subperiosteal exposure of the squamous portion of the occipital bone, rim of the foramen magnum, and the upper cervical vertebrae to be fused is performed.

Many techniques have been described. Historically, bone autograft either placed in an onlay fashion or wired between the occiput and C-2 regions provided successful fusions in approximately 80% of cases. These ''nonrigid'' methods, however, require prolonged postoperative halo immobilization. More recent trends have utilized ''rigid'' fixation devices in the form of plates and loops to immediately fixate the occiput to the upper cervical spine. Their advantage lies in the immediate rigid stability provided to the craniocervical junction, often obviating the need for halo immobilization. As a result of the rigid stabilization, higher fusion rates have been achieved.

Although various screw/plate methods have been described, the senior authors have recently preferred the use of titanium craniocervical loops (Fig. 21-8). Once the occiput and upper cervical spinal elements have been exposed and decompression performed, burr holes are placed bilaterally in the suboccipital region approximately 1 cm above the foramen magnum and lateral to the midline. Sublaminar braided titanium cables are then placed bilaterally at the cervical levels to be included in the fusion, usually down to C-2 or C-3. Once the loop has been properly molded to the craniocervical region, it is fastened by tightening the cables around the rod. Autograft bone is placed around the occiput and cervical levels to be fused and the wound is closed. The patient can then be placed into a rigid collar for 3 months until a solid arthrodesis can be demonstrated by plain films.

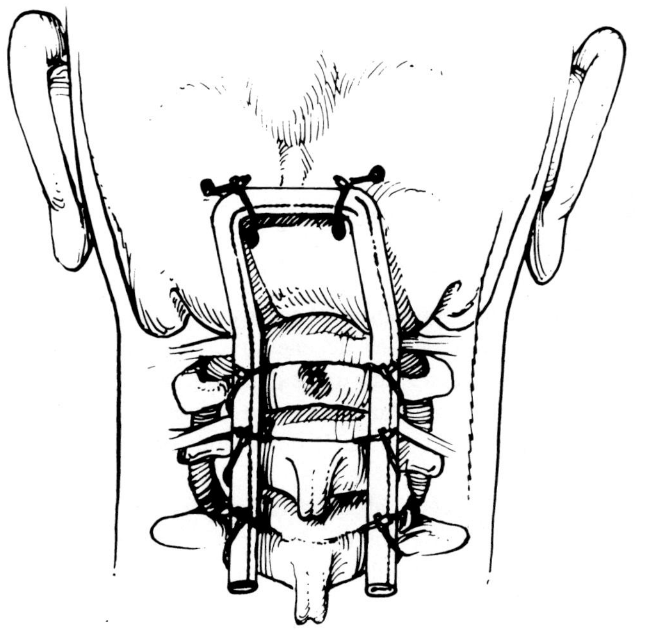

FIG. 21-8. Occipitocervical fusion from the occiput to C-3 with a titanium craniocervical loop. This technique allows for decompression, realignment, and immediate stabilization of the craniocervical junction. Application of bone autograft (typically iliac crest or rib) to this area allows for long-term stability.

Atlantoaxial Fusion

Atlantoaxial Wiring

Traditionally, posterior atlantoaxial fusion using wire and bone graft has been the most popular method to obtain internal fixation and arthrodesis. Although several configurations of wire and bone graft have been reported, the senior authors have the most experience and recommend the interspinous method described by Dickman et al. (57) (Fig. 21-9).

The arches of C-1 and C-2 are exposed through a standard midline posterior incision, being careful to avoid the vertebral artery that runs along the lateral margin of C-1. The ligamentum flavum, occipitoatlantal membrane, and the interspinous ligament are removed. The lamina of C-1 and C-2 are abraded with a drill to prepare the surface for the bone graft, which is ideally harvested as a bicortical piece of posterior iliac crest. This graft is then wedged between the inferior aspect of the C-1 arch and the superior aspect of the C-2 spinous process. Next, a looped titanium cable is passed superiorly under the arch of C-1, behind the graft, and secured beneath the base of the C-2 spinous process. The free ends of the wire, which are now anterior to the graft, are passed under the C-2 spinous process and tightened. This compresses the bone graft between C-1 and C-2 superiorly and inferiorly, and the wire strands anteriorly and posteriorly.

The resultant construct provides excellent rotational and translational stability while avoiding sublaminar wire passage at C-2, a feature of other wiring techniques. Patients are usually maintained in a halo until a solid arthrodesis forms.

Posterior Atlantoaxial Facet Screw Fixation

Posterior screw fixation rigidly couples the facets of the atlas and axis and is a biomechanically advantageous method to obtain immediate internal fixation of this joint. However, this technique is much more technically demanding than the interspinous wiring technique previously described and should only be performed by a surgeon experienced with the procedure.

The procedure essentially involves passing screws under both direct vision and fluoroscopic guidance through the C-2 pedicle and across the C1-2 facet joint, preferably bilaterally. As comminuted fractures of C-1 and C-2 as well as an anomalous medial course of a vertebral artery are absolute contraindications to the use of this technique, a complete

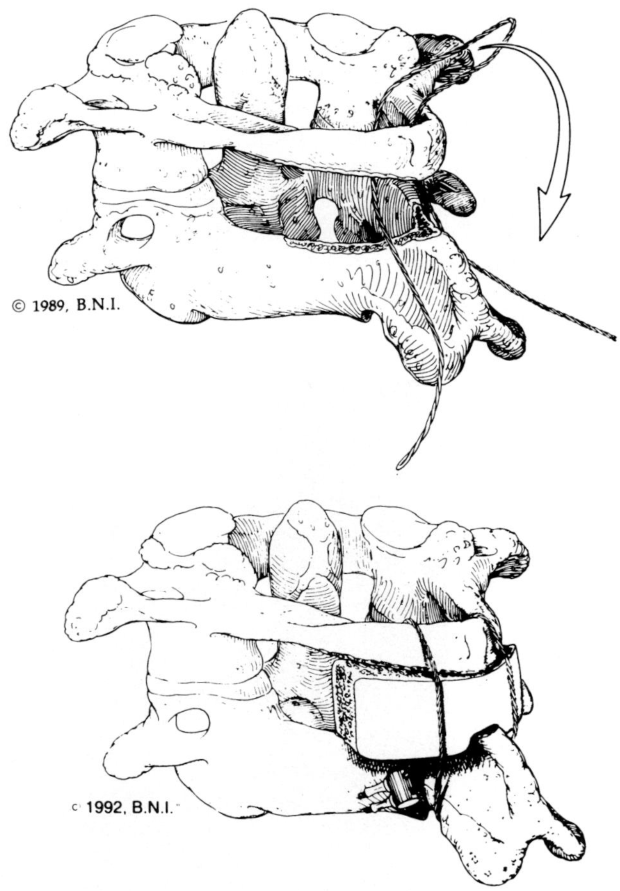

FIG. 21-9. Procedure of posterior C-1–C-2 fusion. **A:** Wire is looped in half and passed sublaminarly at C-1. **B:** A bicortical iliac crest autograft is appropriately fashioned and wedged between the inferior aspect of the C-1 arch and the spinous process of C-2. Finally, both free ends of the wire as well as the loop of wire are tightened around the spinous process of C-2. (Courtesy of the Barrow Neurological Institute.)

CT scan through the craniocervical junction should be performed and studied well before proceeding. This technique provides better rotational and translational stability than posterior spinous process wiring alone. The authors prefer to utilize both methods concomitantly, obviating the need for halo immobilization, and instead a rigid orthosis may be used postoperatively.

Anterior Odontoid Screw Fixation

When C-1–C-2 instability is due to an odontoid fracture, direct screw fixation of the odontoid can be performed with an anterior transcervical operative approach. This recently described technique is indicated for treatment of type II and some type III odontoid fractures. The odontoid fracture fragments must be able to be placed into alignment prior to the procedure or else the fragments will be malaligned. Additionally, the transverse ligament must be intact. If the transverse ligament is disrupted, fixating the odontoid process will not stabilize the atlas. If these conditions are met, this procedure is favored over posterior C-1–C-2 fixation as it spares C-1–C-2 rotation.

A standard anterior approach to the cervical spine is performed but obtaining access to the inferior aspect of the C-2 vertebral body can make this procedure difficult. Once the C2-3 disk space is exposed, a drill is passed into the anterior inferior aspect of C-2 and into the odontoid process under biplanar fluoroscopic guidance (Fig. 21-10). The goal is to pass a lag screw into the odontoid across the fracture line such that the threads are only in the distal fragment. This arrangement will allow for compression of the fragments into normal anatomic alignment as the screw is tightened. These patients can be managed postoperatively with a rigid orthosis.

Stabilization of the Subaxial Spine

Anterior Stabilization of the Subaxial Spine

The anterior approach has been used for decompression and stabilization due to degenerative diseases since the 1950s. More recently, this same approach has been used in combination with internal plates and screws for more complex decompression and stabilization after significant cervical spine trauma.

Most anterior cervical spine decompression procedures are coupled with insertion of a bone graft (autograft or bone bank iliac crest, rib, fibula) into the vertebral body defect or disk space to ultimately provide long-term stability through a solid fusion. However, when autograft is used alone in managing cervical spine trauma, graft extrusion rates of 10% to 29% and persistent postoperative deformity in 38% to 64% have been reported (58). This high rate of fusion failure resulted in the development of rigid anterior plating devices for use in the cervical spine. The concept was adapted from studies in the orthopedic literature demonstrating optimal results in plate osteosynthesis when absolute immobilization and compression of fracture fragments is achieved. Since the first attempt of applying a metal plate to the anterior cervical spine by Hermann (59) in 1975, several systems

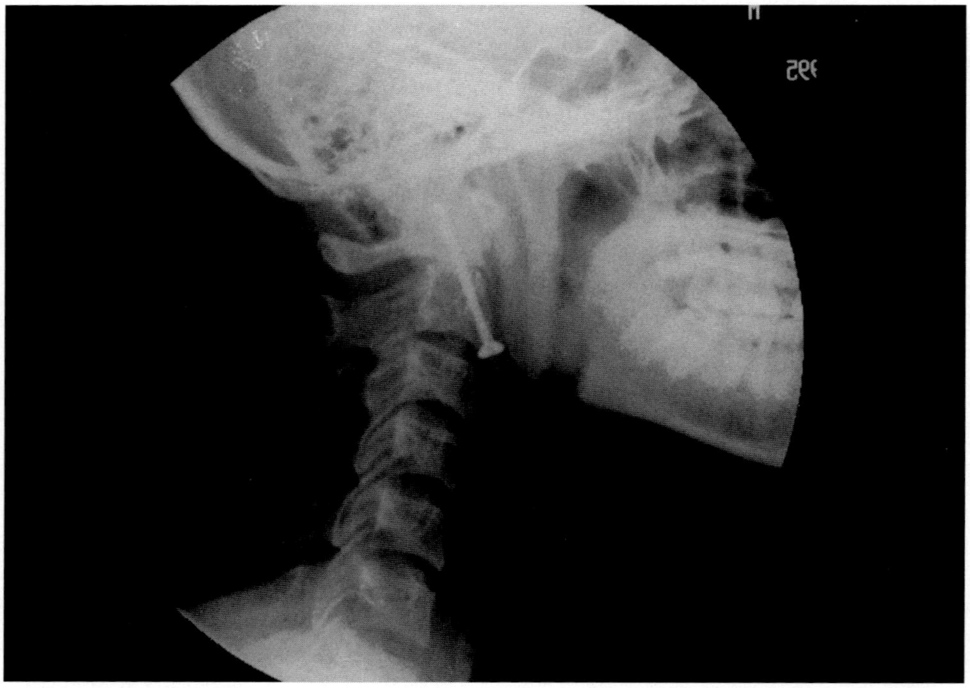

FIG. 21-10. Odontoid screw. A lag screw has been directed across a type II odontoid fracture and into the tip of the dens, realigning the fracture fragments.

have been developed each with variations of a common design.

The more common plate fixation systems of today are made of MRI-compatible titanium and are held in place with screws that enter only the anterior cortex of the vertebral body, reducing the risk of neural injury from screw penetration of the posterior cortex. The resultant construct resists flexion, extension, rotational, and lateral forces.

The procedure of applying this instrumentation involves exposure of the anterior vertebral bodies as described in Chapter 20. Decompression through diskectomy and/or corpectomy (vertebral body resection) is performed. A bone graft, either autograft iliac crest or allograft fibula, is positioned into the operative site. After graft insertion, an osteosynthetic plate of appropriate length is chosen and bent to match the cervical contour, being sure not to overlap adjacent disk spaces. Two holes are then drilled into the adjacent vertebral bodies at their midpoint, the holes are tapped, and the anchor screws are inserted through the ends of the plate and into vertebral bodies. Finally, various mechanisms can be used to lock the screw heads to the plate to prevent screw backout. Postoperatively, a hard cervical collar is typically worn for 8 to 12 weeks.

Posterior Stabilization of the Subaxial Spine

Posterior stabilization techniques vary significantly in design and materials compared with anterior techniques. Each method has certain advantages, disadvantages, and limitations. In general the presence or absence of the posterior elements (spinous process, lamina, facets) as well as fractures through these elements dictate the method that can be utilized.

Lateral Mass Plates and Screws

The use of plates and screws for internal fixation of the posterior cervical spine represents an important advancement in the management of spinal instability. The application of screws and plates is technically simple, produces immediate stability of the cervical spine without the need for rigid external orthosis, and is not dependent on the integrity of the laminae or spinous processes. In addition, this technique provides greater rotational stability than traditional wiring techniques. Osteoporosis, metabolic bone disease, and other conditions in which the bone is soft are the only relative contraindications to the use of screws and plates as screw pullout and loss of reduction is likely.

With the patient in a prone position and head fixated to the operating room table with either a three-pin head holder or a preoperatively placed halo, an x-ray is taken to confirm that appropriate spinal alignment has been maintained through the positioning process. The posterior spinal elements are approached through a midline incision and a decompression or open reduction is then performed as indicated. For C-3 to C-7, the entry point for the screws are 1 to 2 mm medial to the midportion of each vertebral body's lateral mass (Fig. 21-11). Various trajectories have been advocated to avoid the foramen transversarium and nerve roots, but the senior authors advocate the screw trajectory to be 30 degrees lateral and 15 to 20 degrees rostrally for C-3 to C-7. When C-2 is to be included, the screws are placed into the pars under direct visualization. Like anterior plates, they may be bent to match the cervical spine curvature. Once the plates have been fixated to the spine and autograft placed adjacent to the available decorticated elements, the wound can be closed. Finally, a rigid collar is applied.

Interspinous Wiring

Interspinous process wiring is the oldest method of stabilizing the subaxial spine from a posterior approach. It involves using stainless steel or titanium cables to fixate adjacent spinous processes at the levels of instability once a reduction has been performed. A 1.0- or 1.2-mm stainless steel wire or braided titanium or stainless steel cable is passed through the base of the spinous process of the more cephalad vertebrae by creating a hole with a towel clip or drill. The wire is then brought around the lower spinous process and tightened. Autograft is then placed over the laminae, which have been abraded using a drill. Postoperatively, the patient is placed in a rigid collar until an arthrodesis can be demonstrated by plain x-rays. Interspinous process wiring cannot be used when fractures of the lamina or spinous process are present. In addition, this method provides less rotational stability than lateral mass plates, as only the midline is fixated. The authors have used this technique infrequently since the advent of lateral mass plates, but it may be favored when bone quality is suboptimal for screws and plates.

Interlaminar Clamps and Sublaminar Wiring

Both of these techniques fixate the adjacent lamina at the level of instability. Halifax clamps have been more successfully utilized to fixate C-1–C-2, but have also been employed in the subaxial spine. Essentially two clamps are placed bilaterally around the laminae with autograft sandwiched between the clamp posteriorly and the lamina anteriorly. A screw mechanism is then used to tighten the clamps. With sublaminar wires, steel wire or braided titanium cable is passed bilaterally under the lamina of the vertebrae to be fused with an autograft placed in the interlaminar space. The ends of the wires are then twisted together.

Indications for these techniques include posterior ligamentous injury with minimal or no posterior bony element fractures. In addition, these techniques cannot be utilized when significant vertebral body fractures exist unless an anterior procedure is concomitantly performed. Although both the hooks of the clamps and the sublaminar wire hug the anterior aspect of the lamina, the narrow size of the subaxial spinal canal makes placement of any foreign body into the canal dangerous and risks spinal cord injury. Subsequently,

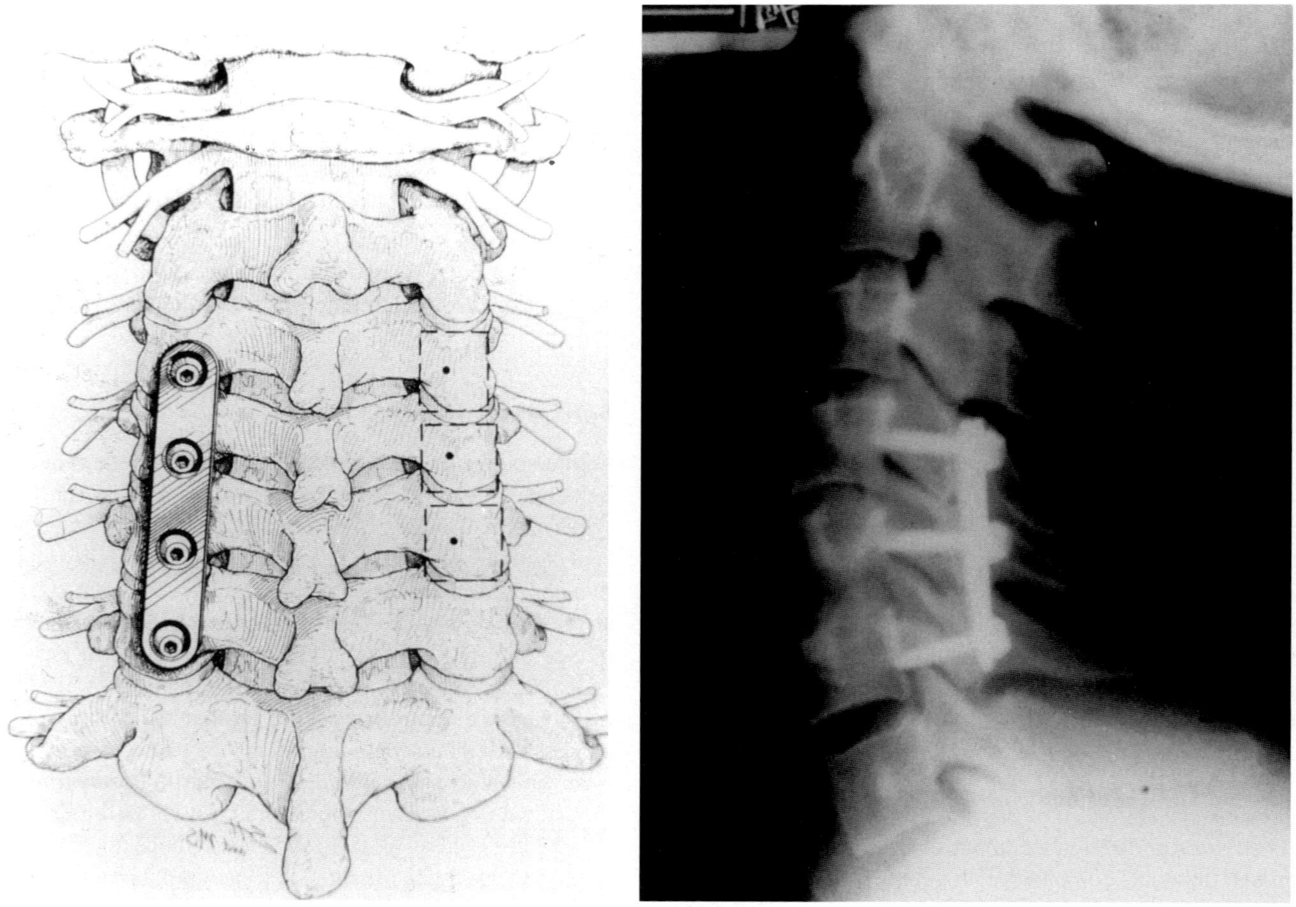

A B

FIG. 21-11. Lateral mass plating. **A:** The entrance point for the screws is 1 to 2 mm medial to the center of the lateral mass (*dotted outline*). The recommended trajectory of 30 degrees lateral and 20 degrees rostral from this point avoids direct injury to both the cervical nerve roots and vertebral body. **B:** Lateral radiograph of lateral mass plating from C-4 to C-6.

these techniques have been abandoned by most surgeons in dealing with subaxial spine injuries.

CONCLUSION

Considering the potential for substantial physical and emotional disability that can occur from injuries to the cervical spine neural elements, physicians must maintain a high index of suspicion for cervical spine injuries while managing trauma victims. The history and a meticulous clinical and radiographic evaluation of the patient are essential and, more often than not, will reveal the mechanism of injury. During the initial trauma assessment and emergency treatment, maintaining hemodynamic stability is crucial to prevent irreversible neurologic ischemic injury. Furthermore, controlled stabilization of the cervical spine will not only ''neutralize'' any existing spinal injury but also serve to prevent direct secondary injury. Finally, a thorough knowledge of spinal anatomy, biomechanics, and classification of cervical spine injuries is fundamental to successful management of victims of cervical spine injury.

REFERENCES

1. Whiteneck G, Menter R, Charlifue S, et al. Initial and long-term costs of spinal cord injury. *Paraplegia* 1988;26:135.
2. Roberge R, Wears R, Kelly M, et al. Selective application of cervical spine radiography in alert victims of blunt trauma. *J Trauma* 1988;28:784–787.
3. Kreipke D, Gillespie K, McCarthy M, Mail J, Lappas J, Broadie T. Reliability of indications for cervical spine films in trauma patients. *J Trauma* 1989;29:1438–1439.
4. Riggins R, Kraus J. The risk of neurologic damage with fractures of the vertebrae. *J Trauma* 1977;17:126–133.
5. Fife D, Kraus J. Anatomic location of spinal cord injury. *Spine* 1986;11:2–5.
6. Fine P, Kuhlemeier K, DeVivo M, et al. Spinal cord injury: an epidemiological perspective. *Paraplegia* 1979;17:237–250.
7. Sweeney T, Marx J. Blunt neck injury. *Emerg Med Clin North Am* 1993;11:71–79.
8. Bohlman H. Acute fractures and dislocations of the cervical spine: an analysis of three hundred hospitalized patients and review of the literature. *J Bone Joint Surg* 1979;61A:1119.
9. American College of Surgeons Committee on Trauma. *Advanced trauma life support course for physicians*. Chicago: 1990.
10. Meguro K, Tator C. Effect of multiple trauma on mortality and neurological recovery after spinal cord or cauda equina injury. *Neurol Med Chir* 1988;28:34–41.
11. Johnson R, Hart D, Simmons E, et al. Cervical orthoses: a study comparing their effectiveness in restricting cervical motion in normal subjects. *J Bone Joint Surg* 1977;59A:332–339.

12. Podolsky S, Baraff L, Simon R, Hoffman J, Larmon B, Ablon W. Efficacy of cervical spine immobilization methods. *J Trauma* 1983; 23:687–690.
13. Chesnut R. Emergency management of spinal cord injury. In: Narayan R, Wilberger J Jr, Povlishock T, eds. *Neurotrauma.* New York: McGraw-Hill, 1996:1121–1138.
14. Bivins H, Ford S, Bezmalinovic Z, et al. The effect of axial traction during orotracheal intubation of the trauma victim with an unstable cervical spine. *Ann Emerg Med* 1988;17:25–29.
15. Wood P, Lawler P. Managing the airway in cervical spine injury. *Anaesthesia* 1992;47:792–797.
16. Walls R. Airway management. *Emerg Med Clin North Am* 1993;11:(1):53–60.
17. Bosch A, Stauffer E, Nickel V. Incomplete traumatic quadriplegia: a ten year review. *JAMA* 1971;216:473–478.
18. Stauffer E. Neurological recovery following injuries to the cervical spinal cord and roots. *Spine* 1984;9:532–534.
19. Kuhn R. Functional capacity of the isolated human spinal cord. *Brain* 1950;73:1–51.
20. Young W, Bracken M. The Second National Acute Spinal Cord Injury Study. *J Neurotrauma* 1992;9(suppl 1):S397–S405.
21. Bracken M, Shephard M, Collins WJ, et al. Methylprednisolone or naloxone treatment after acute spinal cord injury: one year follow-up data. Results of the Second National Acute Spinal Cord Injury Study. *J Neurosurg* 1992;76:23–31.
22. Bracken M, Shepard M, Holford T, et al. Administration of methylprednisolone for 24 or 48 hours or tirilizad mesylate for 48 hours in the treatment of acute spinal cord injury. *JAMA* 1997;277:1597–1604.
23. Calenoff L, Chessare J, Rogers L, et al. Multiple level spinal injuries: importance of early recognition. *Am J Roentgenol* 1978;130:665–669.
24. Kewalramani L, Taylor R. Multiple noncontiguous injuries to the spine. *Acta Orthop Scand* 1976;47:52–58.
25. Giacobetti F, Vaccaro A, Bos-Giacobetti M, et al. Vertebral artery occlusion associated with cervical spine trauma: a prospective analysis. *Spine* 1997;22:188–192.
26. Louw J, Mafoyane N, Small B, Nesser C. Occlusion of the vertebral artery in cervical spine dislocations. *J Bone Joint Surg* 1990;72B: 679–681.
27. Willis B, Greiner F, Orrison W, Benzel E. The incidence of vertebral artery injury after midcervical spine fracture or subluxation. *Neurosurgery* 1994;34:435–442.
28. Sussman B. Fracture dislocation of the cervical spine: a critique of current management in the United States. *Paraplegia* 1978;16:15.
29. Fischer R. Cervical radiographic evaluation of alert patients following blunt trauma. *Ann Emerg Med* 1984;234:905–907.
30. Roberge R. Facilitating cervical spine radiography in blunt trauma. *Emerg Med Clin North Am* 1991;9:733–742.
31. Jacobs L, Schwartz R. Prospective analysis of acute cervical spine injury. *Ann Emerg Med* 1986;15:44–49.
32. Bachulis B, Long W, Hynes G, Johnson M. Clinical indications for cervical spine radiographs in the traumatized patient. *Am J Surg* 1987; 153:473–477.
33. Diliberti T, Lindsey R. Evaluation of the cervical spine in the emergency setting: who does not need an x-ray? *Orthopaedics* 1992;15: 179–183.
34. Michael D, Guyot D, Darmody W. Coincidence of head and cervical spine injury. *J Neurotrauma* 1989;6:177–189.
35. Hills M, Deane S. Head injury and facial injury: is there an increased risk of cervical spine injury? *J Trauma* 1993;34:549–553.
36. Williams J, Jehle D, Cottington E, Schufflebarger C. Head, facial, and clavicular trauma as a predictor of cervical-spine injury. *Ann Emerg Med* 1992;21:719–722.
37. White A III, Panjabi M. *Clinical biomechanics of the spine*, 2nd ed. Philadelphia: JB Lippincott, 1990.
38. Dickman C, Green K, Sonntag V. Injuries involving the transverse atlantal ligament: classification and treatment guidelines based upon experience with 39 injuries. *Neurosurgery* 1996;38:44–50.
39. White A III, Johnson R, Panjabi M, Southwick W. Biomechanical analysis of clinical instability in the cervical spine. *Clin Orthop* 1975; 109:85–96.
40. Fielding J, Hawkins R. Atlanto-axial rotatory fixation. *J Bone Joint Surg* 1977;59A:313–318.
41. Dickman C, Papadopoulos S, Sonntag V, Spetzler R, Rekate H, Drabier J. Traumatic occipitoatlantal dislocations. *J Spinal Disord* 1993;6: 300–313.
42. Martin G, Haid R Jr, Rodts G. Injuries of the atlanto-axial complex. *Contemp Neurosurg* 1997;19:(12):1–9.
43. Jefferson G. Fracture of the atlas vertebrae. *Br J Surg* 1920;7:407.
44. Spence K Jr, Decker S, Sell K. Bursting atlantal fracture associated with rupture of the transverse ligament. *J Bone Joint Surg* 1970;52A: 543–549.
45. Glasser R, Fessler R. Biomechanics of cervical spine trauma. In: Narayan R, Wilberger J Jr, Povlishock T, eds. *Neurotrauma.* New York: McGraw-Hill, 1996:1095–1112.
46. Anderson L, D'Alonzo R. Fractures of the odontoid process of the axis. *J Bone Joint Surg* 1974;56A:1663–1674.
47. Scott E, Haid R Jr, Peace D. Type I fractures of the odontoid process: implications for atlanto-occipital instability: case report. *J Neurosurg* 1990;72:488–492.
48. Polin R, Szabo T, Bogaev C, et al. Nonoperative management of types II and III odontoid fractures: the Philadelphia collar versus the halo vest. *Neurosurgery* 1996;38:450–457.
49. Schneider R, Livingston K, Cave A, Hamilton G. Hangman's fracture of the cervical spine. *J Neurosurg* 1965;22:141–154.
50. Effendi B, Roy D, Cornish B, et al. Fractures of the ring of the atlas. *J Bone Joint Surg* 1981;63B:319–327.
51. Levine A, Edwards C. Traumatic spondylolisthesis of the axis. *J Bone Joint Surg* 1991;67A:217–226.
52. Allen B, Ferguson R, Lehmann T, O'Brien R. A mechanistic classification of closed, indirect fractures and dislocations of the lower cervical spine. *Spine* 1982;7:1–27.
53. McNab I. Acceleration injuries of the cervical spine. *J Bone Joint Surg* 1964;46A:1797–1799.
54. Heiden J, Weiss M, Rosenberg A, et al. Management of cervical spinal cord trauma in southern California. *J Neurosurg* 1975;43:732–736.
55. Marshall L, Knowlton S, Garfin S, et al. Deterioration following spinal cord injury: a multicenter trial. *J Neurosurg* 1987;66:400–404.
56. Wolf A, Wilberger J. Timing of surgical intervention after spinal cord injury. In: Narayan R, Wilberger J Jr, Povlishock T, eds. *Neurotrauma.* New York: McGraw-Hill, 1996:1193–1199.
57. Dickman C, Papadopoulos S, Sonntag V, et al. The interspinous method of posterior atlantoaxial arthrodesis. *J Neurosurg* 1991;74:190–198.
58. Kalfas I. Cervical spine stabilization: surgical techniques. In: Narayan R, Wilberger J Jr, Povlishock T, eds. *Neurotrauma.* New York: McGraw-Hill, 1986:1179–1192.
59. Hermann H. Metal plate fixation after anterior fusion of unstable fracture dislocation of the cervical spine. *Acta Neurochir (Wien)* 1975;32: 101–111.
60. Haymaker W, Woodhall B, eds. *Peripheral nerve injuries,* 2nd ed. Philadelphia: WB Saunders, 1962.
61. Frymoyer JW, ed. *The adult spine,* 2nd ed. Philadelphia: Lippincott-Raven, 1991.

Neurosurgical Issues in Otolaryngology: Principles and Practice of Collaboration, edited by Moisés A. Arriaga and J. Diaz Day. Lippincott Williams & Wilkins, Philadelphia © 1999.

CHAPTER 22

Maxillofacial Trauma

William D. Clark and Joe B. Wiseman

The maxillofacial area is vulnerable to trauma from assaults, motor vehicle accidents, and sports injuries. Trauma that produces fractures of the maxillofacial skeleton may also produce brain trauma, cerebrospinal fluid (CSF) leaks, and intracranial hemorrhage.

A number of health care specialists treat maxillofacial trauma including otolaryngologists, oral surgeons, plastic surgeons, ophthalmologists, and neurosurgeons. Neurosurgeons are more often involved with the care of patients suffering frontal sinus fractures than other maxillofacial injuries.

NOSE

The nose is the most frequently fractured of the facial bones. Fractures may be limited to the external bony skeleton (nasal bones and frontal processes of maxilla), producing a cosmetic deformity with or without functional impairment. Such an injury may also include the nasal septum, usually causing nasal obstruction. The nasal bones are adjacent to the frontal bone superiorly. The perpendicular plate of the ethmoid, which is a part of the nasal septum, attaches to the cribriform plate. The cribriform plate is adjacent to the frontal bone anteriorly and the sphenoid bone posteriorly. Fractures of the nose or nasal septum may extend in the frontal bone/sinus, sphenoid sinus, roof of the ethmoid sinuses, fovea ethmoidalis, and the cribriform plate. These fractures are considered anterior skull base fractures rather than nasal fractures. These areas are densely adherent to dura. The bone of the anterior skull base is very thin especially in the region of the cribriform plate and fovea ethmoidalis. Thin bone in these areas fractures easily, penetrating dura, and disrupting the arachnoid resulting in a CSF leak. Moreover, the force from a traumatic blow is not easily absorbed by these thin bones and may cause direct dural disruption resulting in a CSF fistula. Therefore, a patient with a nasal fracture may present with CSF rhinorrhea.

Most cases of CSF rhinorrhea from trauma present early in the time course, usually within 1 week of injury (1). Initially, the CSF rhinorrhea is blood tinged but becomes clear after bleeding discontinues. Flow of CSF rhinorrhea can be a constant dripping or intermittent depending on the patient's position.

There are several ways to identify if the fluid from the nose is CSF. The target or double-ring sign is an initial clue to identify CSF. Bloody CSF is collected on filter paper or a pillowcase at the patient's bedside. A target or double-ring sign develops on the collected medium because CSF is less dense and migrates farther from the center than blood. The fluid can be tested for glucose with a urine dipstick but it is a nonspecific test. Levels greater than 30 mg per 100 mL are suggestive of CSF (1). Biochemical analysis of the fluid for glucose, protein, and potassium level and comparing it to serum levels is another method that is nonspecific. The most sensitive and specific indicator of CSF is the presence of β_2-transferrin in the collected fluid detected by electrophoresis.

Identification of the origin of a CSF fistula in the anterior cranial fossa can be difficult in those cases with intermittent low-output flows. Nasal endoscopy should be the first method employed since it is minimally invasive and the location of an active, high-output leak may be visualized. Conventional computed tomography (CT) scans at 1.5-mm intervals with coronal views may identify an isolated fracture site. CT cisternography using an intrathecal injection of contrast will identify a leak in 90% of patients with an active fistula. However, it is accurate in only 40% of patients with an inactive fistula (2). Radionuclide cisternography using intrathecal indium or technetium along with pledgets placed in the nose is another method employed. Radionuclide cis-

W. D. Clark: Department of Otolaryngology, Wilford Hall Air Force Medical Center, Lackland AFB, Texas 78236.

J. B. Wiseman: Department of Otolaryngology/Head and Neck Surgery, Wilford Hall Medical Center/Brooke Army Medical Center, Lackland AFB, Texas 78236-5300.

ternography is accurate in 70% with an active leak and 28% accurate in inactive fistulas (2). Fluorescein injected intrathecally can be visualized by corresponding fluorescence using nasal endoscopy or by nasal pledgets to localize the region of a fistula. Again, this method is inaccurate in patients with an inactive fistula. Currently the technique of choice to identify the origin of a CSF fistula is magnetic resonance (MR) cisternography. An intrathecal injection of contrast material is unnecessary for MR cisternography. Therefore, MR cisternography is noninvasive, and exposure to ionizing radiation is avoided. MR cisternography is a heavily T2-weighted fast spin echo technique with high spatial resolution using fat suppression and video reversal of images. A small number of individual sections are compressed into a composite image by a maximum-intensity projection algorithm providing better depiction of anatomy in three dimensions. MR cisternography enhances the signal intensity of CSF with suppression and subtraction of the background. MR cisternography identified the site of a CSF leak in 100% of patients with an inactive leak (3).

As in any other injury attention should first be directed toward the ABCs (airway, breathing, circulation) of trauma management. Once the patient is stabilized, then early management of anterior skull base fractures with CSF rhinorrhea can begin. Early nonoperative management includes avoidance of activities that increase intracranial pressure. Straining, coughing, and nose blowing are minimized. Bed rest and head of bed elevation to 30 degrees is required. Stool softeners are prescribed. If these measures fail to slow the leak after 24 to 72 hours, a lumbar drain can be employed to further reduce intracranial pressure (1). The patient can be observed for 7 to 14 days following trauma (1); 85% of anterior skull base CSF fistulas will close spontaneously within the first week (1,4). The use of prophylactic antibiotics to prevent meningitis is controversial. Opponents of prophylactic antibiotics cite several articles that demonstrate no significant difference in the prevention of meningitis and concerns on the emergence of resistant organisms. However, a recent meta-analysis by Brodie (5) did demonstrate a significant decrease in the incidence of meningitis when prophylactic antibiotics were employed.

If the anterior skull base fractures continues to leak CSF after 7 to 14 days, then surgical management is needed. One approach that should be attempted first with nasal fractures that result in CSF fistulas is a closed reduction of nasal fracture. Displaced bone fragments brought into proper anatomic alignment and kept immobile may terminate a CSF fistula. Surgery to repair fractures and dural lacerations of the anterior cranial fossa can be divided into extracranial and intracranial techniques. Intracranial approaches include a transfrontal craniotomy or facial translocation. These intracranial approaches provide maximum exposure and direct suturing of dural defects. Disadvantages include anosmia and frontal lobe retraction. Extracranial approaches include an osteoplastic flap and frontal sinusotomy, external ethmoidectomy, lateral rhinotomy, and nasal endoscopy. Advantages of the extracranial approach are a decreased incidence of anosmia and absence of brain retraction. The main disadvantage is decreased exposure.

Displaced nasal fractures are treated by closed or open reductions with external and/or internal splinting. An ideal timing for reduction is before edema sets in. Usually, this is impractical. The second choice for timing reduction is after some resolution of swelling but before the bony fragments have had time to heal in a malposition. The younger the patient, the shorter the interval between injury and healing. In adults, bony fragments are usually mobile for about 10 to 14 days, with many authors recommending that reduction take place in less than 7 to 10 days (6,7). In young children, the shorter mobile period has prompted the recommendation for reduction of the fractures within 2 to 4 days (7). The pitfall to avoid is unnecessary delay in treating a nasal fracture.

The only potentially life-threatening complication of a simple nasal fracture is hemorrhage. The brisk bleeding associated with most nasal fractures is almost always self-limiting. However, severe hemorrhage may occur, even days to weeks after the injury. This is thought to be due to a laceration of the anterior ethmoid artery and may result in exsanguination. The precaution here is to take seriously the patient's report of persistent bleeding from a fractured nose. If an endoscopic examination of the nasal cavities detects specific bleeding points, endoscopic cautery may control the hemorrhage. Otherwise, the treatment is transorbital ligation of the anterior and, possibly, posterior ethmoid arteries of the involved side and/or nasal packing. Rarely, transantral ligation of the terminal branches of the internal maxillary artery will be required to control primary or delayed hemorrhage from a nasal fracture (7).

Another serious, although uncommon, complication of nasal trauma is septal hematoma. It is important to diagnose and treat this complication early because it will lead to septal abscess with cartilage loss and saddle nose deformity in the majority of cases. Usually, there will be bilateral nasal obstruction with the septum bulging to the lateral walls of the nasal cavities bilaterally. Treatment consists of clot evacuation and space drainage with provisions to discourage reaccumulation such as bilateral splinting of the septum. An anitibiotic effect against resistant *Staphylococcus aureus* is prescribed for 7 to 10 days to reduce the chances of abscess formation.

MANDIBLE

The mandible is the second most common facial bone to be fractured. The typical patient is a young adult male injured in a fistfight. Patients with mandibular fractures needing neurosurgical attention are more likely to be victims of motor vehicular accidents or penetrating trauma and can be of any age or gender.

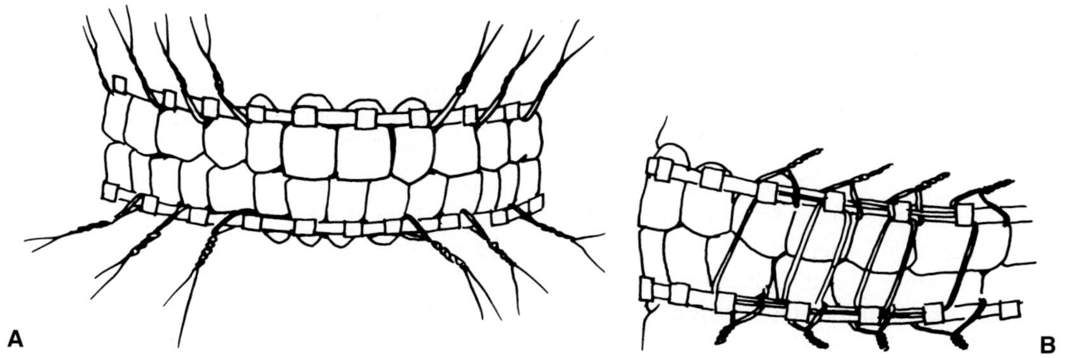

FIG. 22-1. Mandible fractures—maxillomandibular fixation (MMF). **A:** Arch bars are applied with dental wire ligatures. **B:** The dental arches are held together by either elastic bands (illustrated) or wire ligatures.

A rare complication of mandibular fracture of interest to the neurosurgeon is the displacement of a mandibular condyle into the middle cranial fossa. The magnitude of energy required to produce this injury will likely result in multiple head, neck, and facial injuries. The precautions here are to involve the maxillofacial surgeon early and be sure to preserve the mandibular condyle for possible use in the reconstruction of the mandible.

Treatment of mandibular fractures varies with the site and extent of injury as well as the age and dental status of the patient. The desires of the patient may influence the decision making in certain instances, especially in choosing between treatment involving maxillomandibular fixation (MMF) and open reduction with rigid internal fixation (ORRIF). MMF involves placing the teeth in occlusion and holding them there with hardware, most commonly arch bars and elastics (Fig. 22-1). ORRIF involves placing the teeth in occlusion, opening the fracture site(s), reducing the fracture lines, and rigidly holding the fractures in reduction with metallic hardware (Fig. 22-2). Therapeutic choices for mandibular fractures include various combinations of MMF, ORRIF, and open reduction with nonrigid fixation (8,9).

Multiple fractures of the mandible may produce airway compromise via several mechanisms. Pain and swelling often interfere with clearance of oral and pharyngeal secretions while posterior displacement of the anterior mandible permits posterior movement of the tongue base. Penetrating injuries to the mandible often include the tongue and/or floor of mouth with associated soft tissue swelling. Altered states of consciousness from central nervous system (CNS) trauma compound these problems.

Airway management may include frequent suctioning, early reduction of the fractures, and tracheotomy. The prudent neurosurgeon will involve an otolaryngologist early in the management of these patients.

Nasal airway devices have limited appeal in maxillofacial trauma cases. One must be alert to the possibility that part of the injury may include disruption of the skull base and/or pharyngeal mucosa. Nasal airways may find their way into the anterior cranial fossa or a submucosal location in such cases. The use of nasotracheal tubes carries a similar risk.

Plastic oral airways are also of limited value in the face of a mandibular fracture since they may produce pain and depend somewhat upon an intact mandibular arch for their stability and function.

When multiple fractures of the mandible are complicated

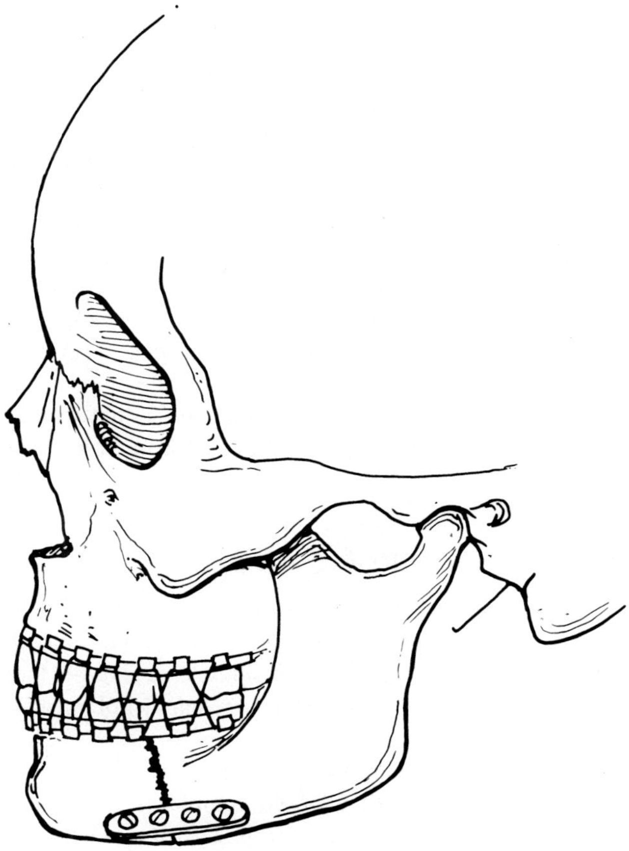

FIG. 22-2. Rigid internal fixation MMF was applied before placing a dynamic compression plate. The mandibular arch bar is left as a tension band device but other hardware can be removed.

by concomitant injury to the nose/midface producing both oral and nasal airway obstruction, tracheotomy is usually indicated.

ORBITAL FLOOR

Isolated orbital floor fractures have no neurosurgical implications. They are repaired, when indicated, via orbital exploration through the lower eyelid. Indications for repair include enophthalmus and inferior rectus muscle entrapment producing diplopia. Physical signs alerting one to suspect this injury include orbital swelling, orbital ecchymosis, and enophthalmus. Symptoms include diplopia and eye pain.

MALAR AREA

Malar area fractures are know by a number of names including zygomatic complex, zygomaticomaxillary complex, and tri-pod fractures. They have no direct neurosurgical ramifications. They should be suspected when there is malar area swelling and tenderness, especially with a lateral subconjunctival hemorrhage and a reduction of the malar eminence by palpation of the involved side. When displaced, they are treated by open reduction with internal fixation to reduce the chance of noticeable cosmetic deformity.

Indications for exploring/repairing the orbital floor in these injuries include persistent diplopia with evidence of orbital muscle entrapment, cosmetically significant enophthalmos, major comminution and/or displacement of the orbital rim, radiologic evidence of significant loss of orbital floor support (anticipation of eventual enophthalmos), combined orbital floor and medial orbital wall defects, radiographic evidence of soft tissue displacement (anticipation of eventual enophthalmos), comminution of the body of the zygoma, and physical or radiographic evidence of exophthalmos or orbital content impingement from displaced periorbital fractures (10).

The important point with these fractures is not to miss them or delay their treatment, as they are difficult to repair later.

LE FORT FRACTURES

Le Fort described three classes of bilateral midface fractures (11). The Le Fort I is a transverse fracture of the maxilla across the floor of both maxillary sinuses, freeing the hard palate and alveolar processes from the remainder of the maxilla (Fig. 22-3A).

The Le Fort II fracture involves the inferior and medial aspects of the orbits, the ethmoid complexes, and lateral aspects of the maxillary sinuses (Fig. 22-3B).

The Le Fort III (sometimes called craniofacial disjunction) has fracture lines through the medial and lateral orbital walls, the zygomatic arches, and posterior maxilla (Fig. 22-3C).

Some bilateral fractures of the maxilla are asymmetrical. For example, some produce the fracture lines of a Le Fort II on one side and a Le Fort III on the other. Bilateral malar area fractures combined with a Le Fort II produce the fracture lines for both the Le Fort II and III.

Le Fort fractures are usually high-energy injuries with an increased likelihood of associated injuries including CSF leaks, brain injury, and airway obstruction. They are treated by open reduction with rigid internal fixation, with strong consideration of restoring the integrity of the various facial buttresses (Fig. 22-3D) and utilizing plates and screws.

CSF leaks associated with these injuries are usually of the anterior skull base and often respond to reduction and fixation of the fractures.

FRONTAL SINUS

Fractures of the frontal bone often involve the frontal sinuses. Failure to recognize or adequately treat these injuries can result in a poor outcome and serious complications.

Treatment of these injuries is controversial and ever evolving. In general, it varies with the extent and location of the fracture lines and their degree of displacement. Each category of fracture will be discussed separately.

Anterior wall, nondisplaced to minimally displaced (Fig. 22-4A: Observation is the only treatment required of these injuries.

Anterior wall, displaced (Fig. 22-4B): Reduction is indicated for cosmetic and, sometimes, functional considerations.

Posterior wall, nondisplaced (Fig. 22-5A): Isolated posterior wall fractures are uncommon. Most feel that these injuries may be followed without treatment in the reliable patient. Some recommend exploration of these injuries via osteoplastic frontal sinusotomy.

Posterior wall, minimally displaced: These fractures are a source of controversy. Some experts feel that all should be explored and obliterated. Others write that they may be safely treated by observation. Repair of a concomitant anterior wall fracture may present the opportunity to view the posterior wall and nasofrontal duct areas directly.

Posterior wall and/or inferior wall with more than minimal displacement and/or involvement of the nasofrontal duct (Fig. 22-5B): Most feel that these injuries should be explored and the sinus obliterated with a fat graft.

Posterior wall, severely comminuted (Fig. 22-5C): The usual treatment for these injuries is cranialization (Fig. 22-6). Dural repair is often required in these injuries. This is the ideal setting for collaborative neurosurgical/otolaryngologic surgery.

Posterior wall with dural injury: Collaborative surgery is a must for these injuries. The neurosurgeon directs the repair of the dural injury, and the otolaryngologist directs the repair of the frontal sinus.

OBLITERATION OF THE FRONTAL SINUS

The mucous membranes of the frontal sinuses function differently from those of the other paranasal sinuses. They

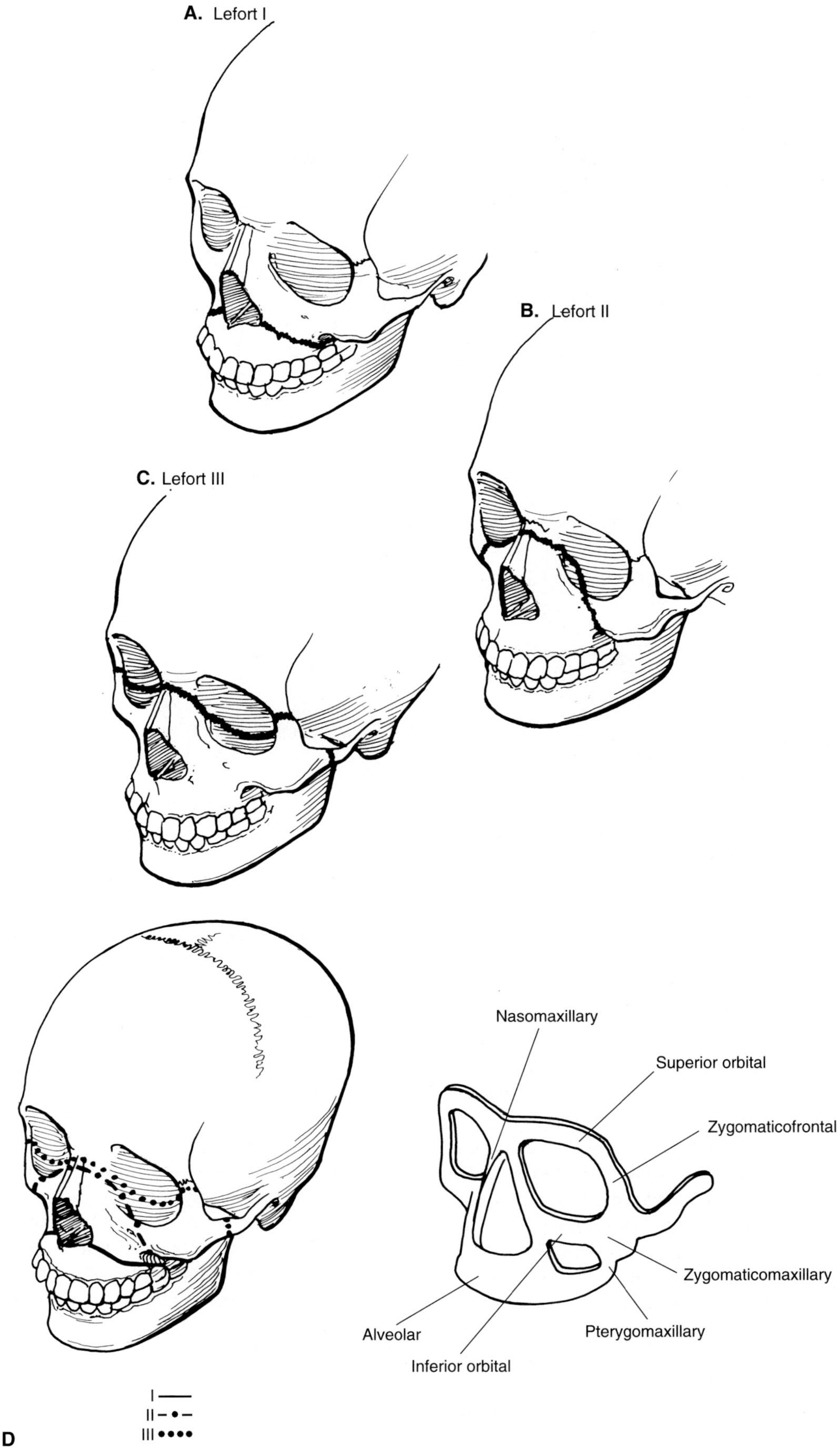

FIG. 22-3. Le Fort fractures. **A:** Le Fort I. **B:** Le Fort II. **C:** Le Fort III. **D:** Le Fort fracture lines and facial buttresses.

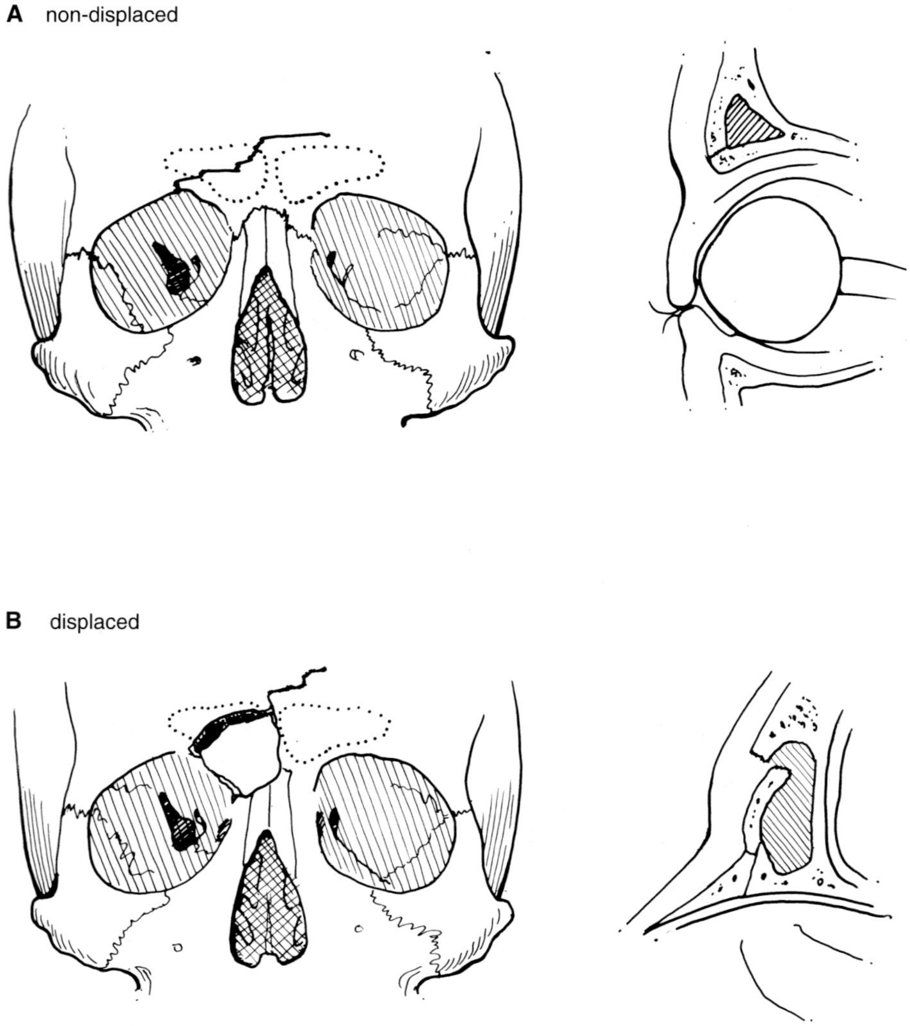

FIG. 22-4. Frontal sinus fractures—anterior wall. **A:** Nondisplaced. **B:** Displaced.

have a propensity to invade the intracranial cavity, given the opportunity (12). They also form cysts in association with fracture lines. Also, the natural drainage system of the frontal sinus follows a longer course and is more prone to troublesome obstruction than with the other sinuses.

Exploration and/or obliteration of the frontal sinus is performed via an osteoplastic frontal sinusotomy (Fig. 22-7). Lacerations over the frontal area may provide access to the frontal bone. Lacking such, a coronal incision provides excellent exposure to the area. In patients with prominent horizontal brow creases, a mid-forehead incision may be a viable alternative (13). The "butterfly" incision (bilateral eyebrow with extension across the bridge of the nose) is a less cosmetically desirable alternative. Access to the sinus cavity is gained via anterior wall fractures or by developing an osteoplastic flap including the anterior wall. Templates cut from a 6-foot Caldwell radiograph of the sinuses are helpful as guidance for the bone flap cuts. Transillumination of the sinus confirms the outline and may be used in place of the template.

Simple elevation of mucous membranes from the frontal sinus prior to obliteration is not adequate to remove all of the epithelium. Bony irregularities, including those associated with blood vessels, hide epithelial remnants and must be burred away to ensure complete removal (12). The operating microscope and diamond burrs are used to advantage to accomplish the task. It is thought that burring also provides for a better blood supply for tissue grafts.

The mucous membrane lining of the nasofrontal ducts is elevated and inverted upon itself prior to plugging the ducts with muscle and/or fascia grafts. The sinus cavity is usually filled with subcutaneous fat, freshly removed from the left lower quadrant of the abdomen. Recently, the use of hydroxyapatite paste has been reported as an alternative to fat grafts (14,15). The anterior wall of the sinus is replaced and held in position with miniplates or wire ligatures.

CRANIALIZATION OF THE FRONTAL SINUS

If the posterior wall is injured to the extent that requires this procedure, then the anterior wall usually has sustained

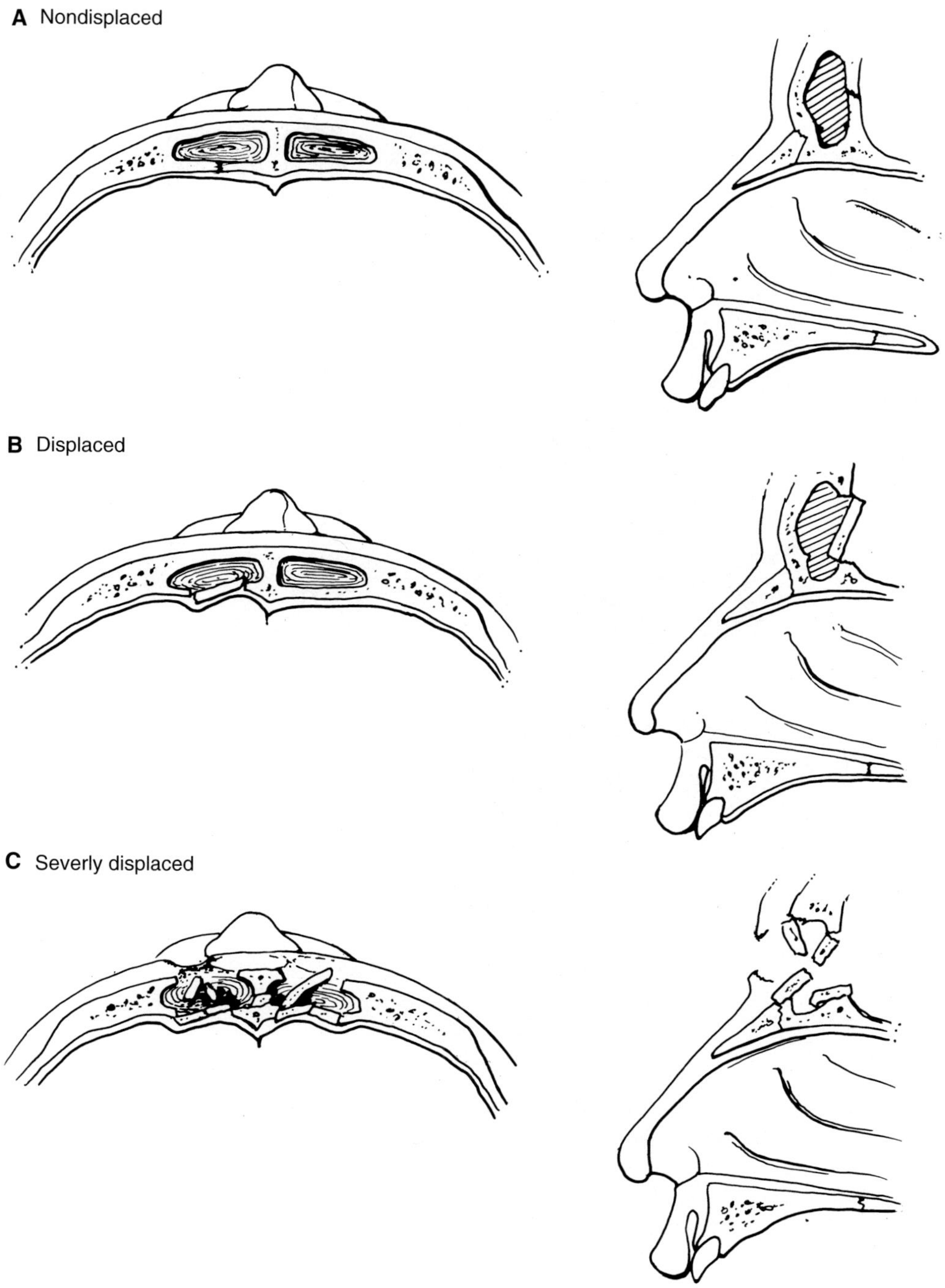

FIG. 22-5. Frontal sinus fractures—posterior wall. **A:** Nondisplaced. **B:** Displaced. **C:** Severely displaced.

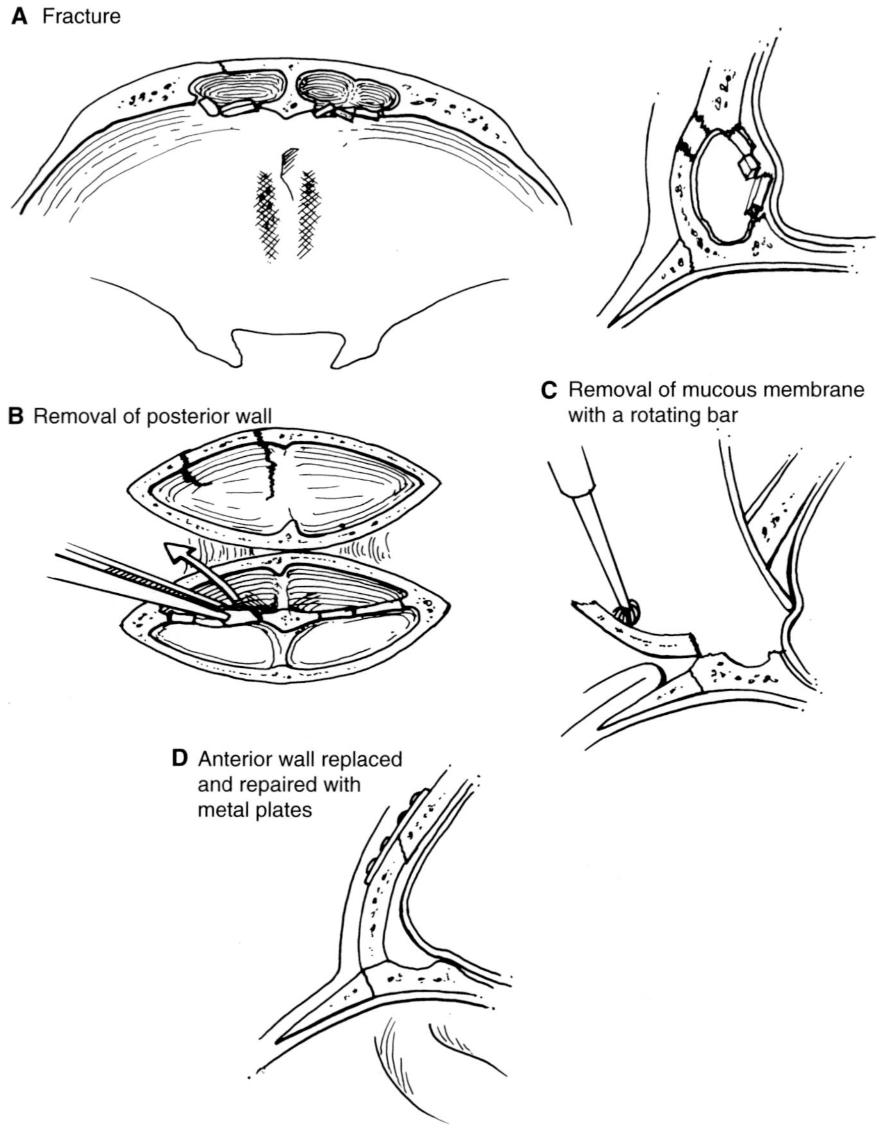

FIG. 22-6. Cranialization of frontal sinus. **A:** Fracture. **B:** Removal of posterior wall. **C:** Removal of mucous membrane with rotating burr. **D:** Anterior wall replaced and repaired with metal plates.

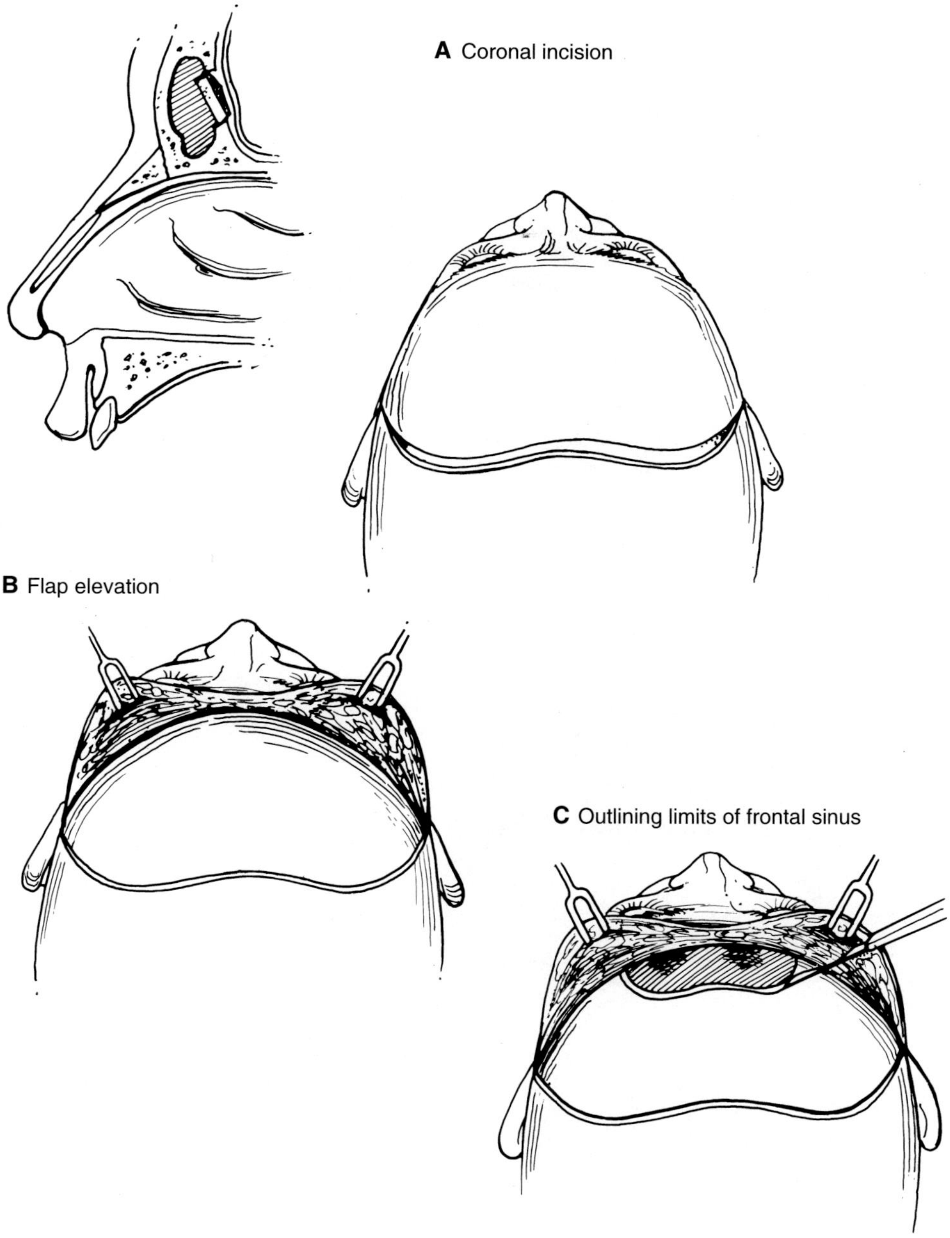

FIG. 22-7. Osteoplastic frontal sinusotomy with fat obliteration. **A:** The coronal incision. **B:** Flap elevation. **C:** Outlining limits of frontal sinus. *(Continued.)*

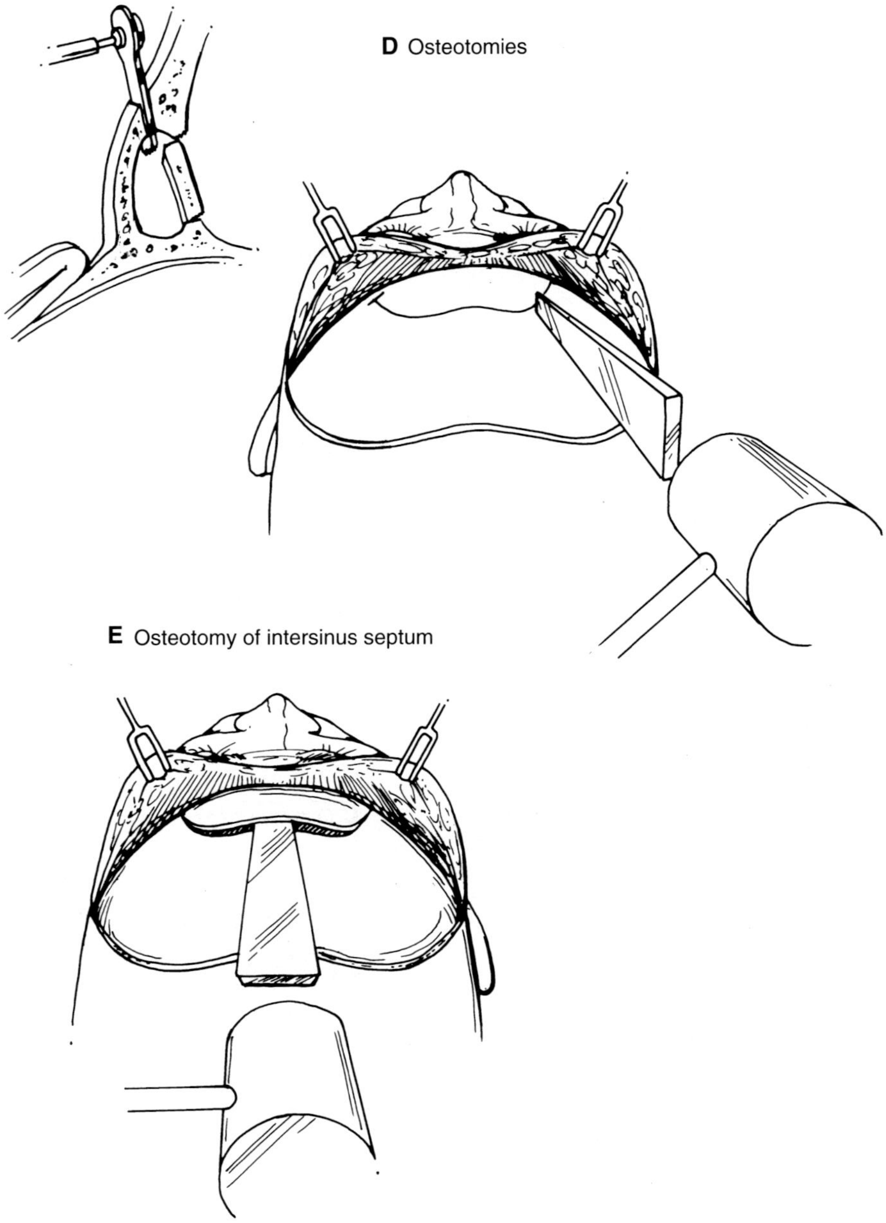

FIG. 22-7. *Continued.* **D:** Osteotomies. **E:** Osteotomy of intersinus septum. *(Continued.)*

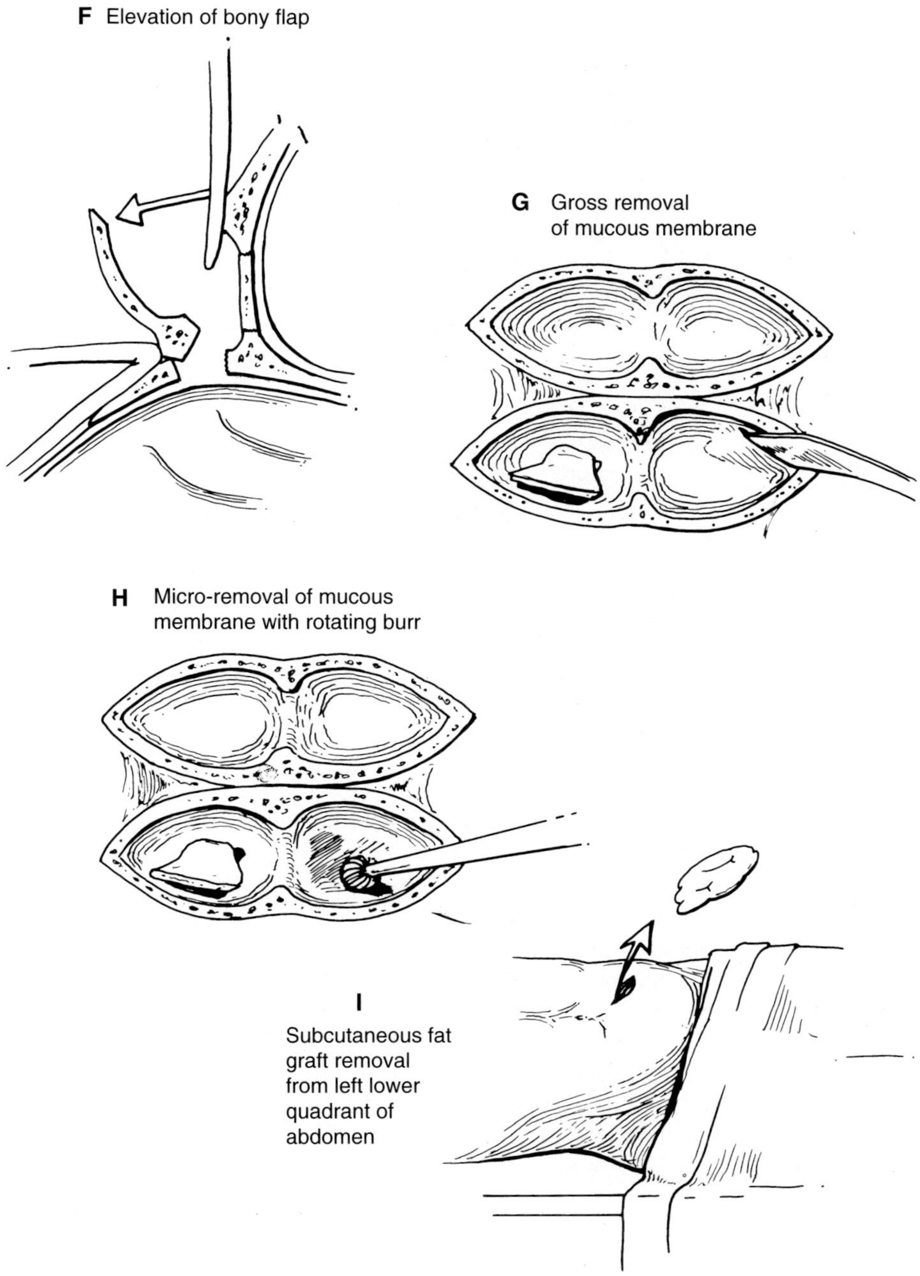

FIG. 22-7. *Continued.* **F:** Elevation of bony flap. **G:** Gross removal of mucous membrane. **H:** Microremoval of mucous membrane with rotating burr. **I:** Removal of subcutaneous fat graft from left lower quadrant of abdomen. *(Continued.)*

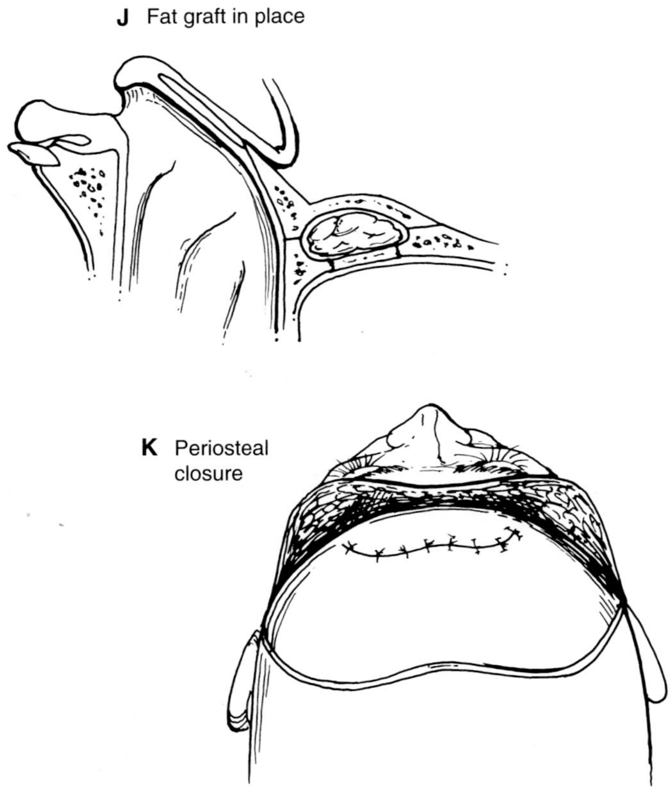

FIG. 22-7. *Continued.* **J:** Fat graft in place. **K:** Periosteal closure.

severe injury, too. Thus, access to repair these injuries is usually easily accomplished via the anterior wall fracture lines. The entire posterior wall of the frontal sinus is removed. The neurosurgeon may then inspect the dura and, perhaps, the brain parenchyma for injuries. While needed neurosurgical repair is taking place, the otolaryngologist may remove the sinus mucous membrane from the anterior fragments. This work is often facilitated by lifting out loose fragments and treating them under the operating microscope.

REFERENCES

1. Marentette LJ, Valentino J. Traumatic anterior fossa cerebrospinal fluid fistulae and craniofacial considerations. *Otolaryngol Clin North Am* 1991;24:151–163.
2. Wax MK, Ramadan HH, Ortiz O, Wetmore SJ. Contemporary management of cerebrospinal fluid rhinorrhea. *Otolaryngol Head Neck Surg* 1997;116:442–449.
3. Eljamel M, Pidgeon C, Toland J, Phillips J, O'Dwyer A. MRI cisternography and the localization of CSF fistula. *Br J Neurosurg* 1994;8:433–437.
4. Mincy JE. Post-traumatic cerebrospinal fluid fistula of the frontal fossa. *J Trauma* 1966;6:618–622.
5. Brodie HA. Prophylactic antibiotics for posttraumatic cerebrospinal fluid fistulae: a meta-analysis. *Arch Otolaryngol Head Neck Surg* 1997;123:749–752.
6. Bailey BJ. Nasal fractures. In: Bailey BJ, Johnson JT, Kohut RI, Pillsbury HC III, Tardy ME, eds. *Head and neck surgery—otolaryngology.* Philadelphia: JB Lippincott, 1993:991–1007.
7. Krause C. Nasal fractures: evaluation and repair. In: Mathog RH, ed. *Maxillofacial trauma.* Baltimore: Williams & Wilkins, 1983:257–265.
8. Clark WD. Management of mandibular fractures. *Am J Otolaryngol* 1992;13:125–132.
9. Clark WD, Bailey BJ. Management of fractures of the mandible. In: Mathog RH, ed. *Maxillofacial trauma.* Baltimore: Williams & Wilkins, 1983:148–161.
10. Shumrick KA, Kersten RC, Kulwin DR, Smith CP. Criteria for selective management of the orbital rim and floor in zygomatic complex and midface fractures. *Arch Otolaryngol Head Neck Surg* 1997;123:378–384.
11. Le Fort R. Étude experimentale sur les fractures de la machoire supérieure. *Rev Chir Paris* 1901;23:208–227,360–379,479–507.
12. Donald PJ. The tenacity of the frontal sinus mucosa. *Otolaryngol Head Neck Surg* 1979;87:557–566.
13. Cheney ML, Gliklich R, Topf P, Montgomery W. Midforehead incision: an approach to the frontal sinus and upper face. *J Craniofac Surg* 1995;6:408–411.
14. Friedman CD, Costintino PD, Jones K, Chow LC, Pelzer HJ, Sisson GA Sr. Hydroxyapatite cement. II. Obliteration and reconstruction of the cat frontal sinus. *Arch Otolaryngol Head Neck Surg* 1991;117:385–389.
15. Costintino PD, Friedman CD. Synthetic bone graft substitutes. *Otolaryngol Clin North Am* 1994;27:1037–1074.

Neurosurgical Issues in Otolaryngology: Principles and Practice of Collaboration,
edited by Moisés A. Arriaga and J. Diaz Day.
Lippincott Williams & Wilkins, Philadelphia © 1999.

CHAPTER 23

Management of Temporal Bone Trauma

Hilary A. Brodie

OVERVIEW

Epidemiology

Motor vehicle accidents account for 75% of severe head traumas evaluated in major trauma centers. The increased utilization of seat belts and the advent of air bags, however, may alter these statistics in the future. In the trauma patients with skull fractures, 14% to 22% sustain a temporal bone fracture (1,2). In a series of 820 temporal bone fractures, 31% of the temporal bone fractures resulted from motor vehicle accidents (3). Assault was the second most common cause, followed by falls and motorcycle accidents. Pedestrian injuries, bicycle accidents, gunshot wounds, all terrain vehicle accidents, sports injuries, and miscellaneous injuries accounted for 23% of the cases (Fig. 23-1). Temporal bone fractures occur disproportionately in males (male-to-female ratio 3 : 1) (3). The peak incidence of temporal bone fractures occurs in the third decade and 22% occur before 17 years of age.

Pathophysiology

A tremendous force is required to fracture the temporal bone. The force of lateral impact required to fracture the temporal bone of fresh cadavers is estimated at 1,875 pounds (4). Temporal bone fractures secondary to blunt trauma typically occur along structurally weakened points, such as the various foramina perforating the skull base. Fracture of the temporal bone often injures the structures contained within or coursing through the bone, resulting in cerebrospinal fluid (CSF) fistula, facial paralysis, sensorineural hearing loss, conductive hearing loss, vertigo, or meningitis. In addition to the peripheral injuries, some of the neuro-otologic symptoms result from shearing strain within the brain tissue with disruption of vessels, axons, synapses, and dendrites (5). Elevated intracranial pressure due to intracranial hemorrhage, cerebral edema, or hydrocephalus may also cause neuro-otologic manifestations (5).

The rate of mortality associated with temporal bone fractures is difficult to ascertain from the literature. Accurate data are often unavailable from patients dying of polytrauma in the field or in the emergency room. However, of patients with temporal bone fractures surviving beyond the emergency room, the mortality rate during the remainder of the hospitalization is 10% (3).

Classification

Temporal bone fractures have traditionally been divided into transverse and longitudinal, based on the relationship of the fracture line to the axis of the petrous ridge and otic capsule (6,7). Longitudinal temporal bone fractures, which spare the otic capsule, typically involve the squamosal portion of the temporal bone and the posterosuperior wall of the external auditory canal (EAC). The fracture passes through the mastoid air cells and middle ear and fractures the tegmen mastoideum and tegmen tympani. The fracture proceeds anterolateral to the otic capsule, typically fracturing the tegmen in the region of the facial hiatus. Longitudinal fractures typically result from a blow to the temporoparietal region.

Transverse temporal bone fractures passing through the otic capsule generally proceed from the foramen magnum across the petrous pyramid and otic capsule. The fractures often proceed through the skull base foramina including the jugular foramen, internal auditory canal (IAC), and the foramen lacerum. These fractures do not typically affect the ossicular chain or the EAC (8). Transverse fractures primarily result from a blow to the occipital region.

Transverse fractures constitute 10% to 30% of temporal bone fractures in the literature, and 70% to 90% are classified as longitudinal (7–13). Some authors argue that the majority

H. A. Brodie: Department of Otolaryngology, Head and Neck Surgery, University of California–Davis Medical Center, Davis, California 95616.

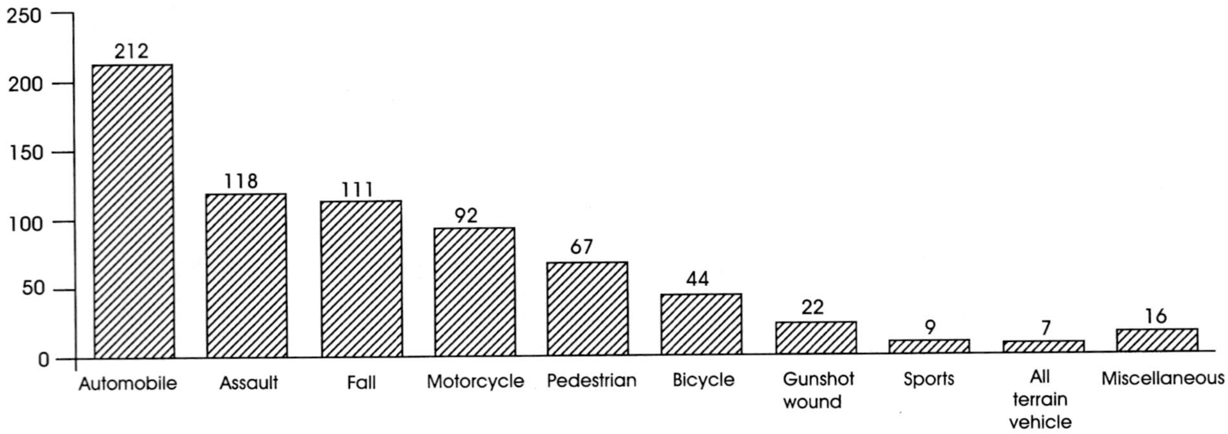

FIG. 23-1. Etiologies of temporal bone fractures.

of fractures are actually oblique as opposed to longitudinal and quite frequently mixed (14).

An important factor in the classification of temporal bone fractures that significantly influences the management of the various complications is whether the fracture passes through the otic capsule with consequent severe or total sensorineural hearing loss (6,15). Indications for surgical intervention for a CSF fistula and facial paralysis and the surgical approach to be utilized is significantly influenced by whether or not the otic capsule has been fractured. Consequently, it is more advantageous to classify the fractures into otic capsule disrupting and sparing fractures. In a recent large series only 2.5% of the fractures disrupted the otic capsule (3). Transversely oriented fractures that did not disrupt the otic capsule were categorized as otic sparing fractures.

Although otic capsule fractures (transverse fractures) constitute only a small proportion of temporal bone fractures, they manifest a much higher risk of complication. Facial nerve injuries are reported to occur in 30% to 50% of transverse fractures and 6% to 25% of longitudinal fractures (3,8,10). The outcome from facial nerve injury, however, does not differ significantly between the two groups aside from the difference in nerve transection. Fisch (16) reported a much higher incidence of nerve disruption in fractures involving the otic capsule. There is a twofold increased risk of CSF fistulas in otic capsule disrupting fractures (3). In addition to the increased risk of CSF fistulas, some authors have suggested that transverse fractures through the otic capsule carry a higher risk of delayed meningitis (17,18). Pollak et al. (18) reported on a 51-year-old man who died of meningitis, having suffered a transverse temporal bone fracture in childhood. The histopathology of his temporal bone revealed pus in the middle ear extending through an unhealed fracture line across the otic capsule. The fracture line contained loose fibrous tissue. The membranous bone along the tegmen has the capability to heal, whereas the enchondral bone of the otic capsule does not. Fractures through the otic capsule will generally partially fill with fibrous tissue and potentially seal with periosteal bone reaction on the surface of the otic capsule (18). Patients sustaining fractures to the otic capsule are at increased risk of developing delayed meningitis or brain abscess due to the presence of a persistent potential pathway between the middle ear and CSF space. Despite the theoretical increased risk, our review of our experience with over 800 temporal bone fractures revealed only four patients who developed delayed meningitis, all of whom had sustained otic capsule sparing fractures (3).

Sixty-two percent of temporal bone fractures are categorized as "open" fractures presenting with bloody otorrhea, brain herniation, or CSF draining from the EAC or penetrating wound site (3); 17% to 29% of temporal bone fractures are bilateral (3,19).

INITIAL EVALUATION

It is uncommon for temporal bone fractures to occur in isolation, and consequently the initial evaluation and management is focused on the emergent life-threatening issues of securing an airway, controlling hemorrhage, evaluating the neurologic status, and stabilizing and evaluating the cervical spine. Following or concurrent with this evaluation the neuro-otologic exam is performed. It is extremely important to assess facial nerve function in the emergency room as early as possible, prior to the administration of muscle relaxants, as will be discussed below. The ear exam focuses on the condition of the auricle, ear canal, tympanic membrane, and middle ear.

The auricles are inspected for lacerations and hematomas. Lacerations are closed after thorough cleaning and debridement of exposed cartilage. Hematomas are drained and pressure bolsters are sutured in place to close the dead space and prevent a recollection of blood. Untreated, the auricular hematomas will result in an auricular chondropathy or "cauliflower ear."

The ear canal is inspected for fractures along the roof, CSF otorrhea, degree of hemorrhage, and the presence of brain herniation. The ear is examined as aseptically as possible. Blood and cerumen in the ear canal should never be debrided with irrigation. Following stabilization in the emergency room and transfer to the ward or intensive care unit, the ear can be more carefully examined with the aid of an operating microscope. The ear canal is not packed initially unless packing is required for control of significant hemorrhage. If profuse hemorrhage cannot be controlled with packing, the patient is taken to either the operating room for carotid ligation or the angiography suite for balloon occlusion.

When severely traumatized ear canals are identified, particularly in the presence of a penetrating injury, the patient is at high risk of stenosis or cholesteatoma formation. Although the ear canal is not stented acutely, it is imperative that the problem be identified and the patient followed closely for the development of these complications. Early intervention with stenting at the onset of the stenosis can effectively prevent a problem that is much more difficult to address once the stenosis is mature.

The integrity of the tympanic membrane is assessed as is the presence of hemotympanum. Traumatic tympanic membrane perforations generally heal spontaneously and consequently no acute intervention is entertained.

The neuro-otologic exam should also note the presence or absence of nystagmus and the type of nystagmus. Peripheral vertigo generally manifests with horizontal or rotatory nystagmus and is suppressible with visual fixation. Central vertigo may present with vertical or direction-changing nystagmus that fails to suppress and may even enhance with fixation. The most common type of vertigo following head trauma is benign paroxysmal position vertigo, which manifests with transient rotatory nystagmus with the Halpike maneuvers (20). The nystagmus occurs with the affected ear down. There is a 2- to 10-second latency followed by 10 to 20 seconds of rotatory nystagmus. The nystagmus is fixed in direction and is fatigable. Central positional vertigo induces direction changing nystagmus, which has no latency and is nonfatigable. Interestingly, the incidence of vertigo does not closely correlate with the severity of the trauma (19,21).

Electronystagmography (ENG) is helpful in categorizing and localizing the vestibular injury; however, it is not obtained in the acute setting. The vast majority of posttraumatic vertigo resolves spontaneously. If the symptoms persist following discharge, the ENG can be obtained on an outpatient basis. A fistula test, which consists of applying positive and negative pressure in the ear canal and into the middle ear, is also not performed in the acute setting. The risk of additional iatrogenic injury and the potential for introducing infection or air into the inner ear outweighs the potential diagnostic benefits. If the patient continues to experience vertigo 1 week postinjury or is experiencing fluctuating or progressive hearing loss, the fistula test is performed at that time. The fistula test is not performed if there is evidence of a CSF fistula or infection in the middle ear.

Hearing is assessed clinically at the bedside with a progressively louder whispered voice and with the use of tuning forks, but audiograms are not typically obtained until the patient is stabilized. However, in the presence of complications of facial paralysis or a CSF fistula, an audiogram is required prior to the surgical intervention because the outcome of the audiogram significantly influences the treatment algorithm as discussed below.

Patients with severe head trauma of the magnitude required for a temporal bone fracture will generally already have had a computed tomography (CT) scan of the head to assess intracranial hemorrhage. Additional imaging of the temporal bone with axial and coronal fine-cut CT scanning is only indicated in the presence of facial paralysis or CSF leakage. Hearing loss, conductive or sensorineural, in the absence of other complications does not warrant additional temporal bone imaging. Demonstrating a transverse fracture through the otic capsule in a profound sensorineural hearing loss will not alter the treatment plan. Preoperative assessment with CT scanning in patients with a conductive hearing loss of sufficient magnitude to warrant exploration and ossicular reconstruction also will not alter the treatment plan. Conventional radiographs including Schuller, Towne-Chamberlain, Stenvers, and basal views as well as tomograms have been supplanted by fine-cut CT scanning and no longer plays a role in the evaluation of patients suspected of having a temporal bone fracture.

MANAGEMENT OF COMPLICATIONS

Facial Nerve Injury

Facial paralysis is a severely disfiguring complication of temporal bone fractures; 7% of temporal bone fractures result in facial paralysis of which one-fourth are complete (3). The reported incidence in the literature of up to 30% is exaggerated by sampling error in omitting simple uncomplicated temporal bone fractures that are not referred for otolaryngologic consult. The incidence of facial paralysis is also overestimated by including patients in retrospective reviews who have been referred to the tertiary care center for management of complications of temporal bone fractures such as facial paresis. Since the entire pool of temporal bone fracture patients is not included in the statistics, the incidence of complications becomes quite biased.

The type of fracture significantly affects the incidence of facial paralysis. Transverse temporal bone fractures have a fivefold increased risk of facial nerve injury compared with longitudinal fractures (3,8,10).

If head trauma patients are carefully evaluated in the emergency room upon admission, prior to the administration of muscle relaxants, 27% of the facial nerve injuries will present with immediate-onset facial paralysis. Seventy-three percent will have facial motion in the initial examination and then subsequently deteriorate (3). The latency of delay in onset of facial palsy ranges from 1 to 16 days.

Many aspects in the management of facial nerve injuries remain controversial. One of the main issues to be resolved is which patients should be surgically explored. Since the vast majority of traumatic facial palsies resolve spontaneously, the decision of who to explore is based on prognostic factors for poor outcome. The factors that are assessed in predicting recovery of facial function include timing of onset (delayed versus immediate onset), severity of injury (complete versus partial paralysis), degree of degeneration, type of injury (penetrating versus nonpenetrating), and the presence of associated infection.

The delay of onset of paralysis following temporal bone fracture is the most important of the predictive factors. In our series of 820 temporal bone fractures, there were 37 patients with delayed onset facial paralysis managed nonsurgically. Five patients were lost to follow-up. The rest recovered function to a House-Brackmann grade I or II (3). McKennan and Chole (22) described their experience with 17 patients with immediate-onset facial paralysis and 19 patients with delayed paralysis. Complete spontaneous recovery of facial function occurred in 94% of the patients with delayed-onset paralysis. The one remaining patient had a House-Brackmann grade II recovery. In contrast, 8 out of the 17 immediate-onset paralysis patients had facial nerve transections.

Turner (23) reviewed a large series of traumatic facial paralysis treated conservatively. His paper included 36 immediate-onset and 34 delayed-onset facial palsies. Complete recovery occurred in 94% of the delayed-onset cases and 75% of immediate-onset palsies. The one patient with delayed-onset paralysis who had no recovery of facial function developed the facial palsy coincident with acute otitis media. Maiman et al. (24), in contrast, found no correlation between immediate- or delayed-onset facial paralysis, treated nonsurgically, and outcome. Although 44 out of 45 of their patients (including both immediate or delayed onset) had satisfactory recovery. Review of the above literature argues strongly against surgical exploration and decompression of delayed posttraumatic facial paralysis. The natural course of delayed facial paralysis is almost always recovery of facial function to a House-Brackmann grade I or II. There are no data in the literature that demonstrates that surgical intervention in delayed-onset paralysis will increase the incidence of complete recovery of function.

May (25) describes the difficulty in differentiating immediate from delayed onset. He explored delayed-onset palsies and found on occasion a severed nerve. This observation highlights the necessity of a careful examination in the emergency room. Even in comatose patients, painful stimuli will generally induce a grimace. Admittedly, information regarding the immediate facial nerve function is not always available. Sometimes the exam is omitted due to attention to other life-threatening complications or because the patient has already received muscle relaxants with intubation. Some patients are not responsive to pain and a grimace cannot be induced. The critical issue is whether or not any facial function has been identified. If facial function is present in the emergency room and subsequently deteriorates, our experience is that the patient will recover without surgical treatment. When reliable information from the emergency room is unavailable, the patient is never documented to have facial function, and the diagnosis of facial palsy is delayed by a few days, these cases must be categorized as "unknown onset" and considered with the immediate-onset group.

The degree of facial nerve injury is also a critical factor in guiding the management algorithm. Incomplete paresis rarely fails to resolve spontaneously unless an additional insult to the nerve, such as infection, occurs (3). Consequently, only patients with complete paralysis of immediate or unknown onset are considered for surgical exploration.

The degree of injury can be assessed, not only clinically with facial motion but also with electrodiagnostic testing using the Hilger facial nerve stimulator, evoked electromyography (EEMG), and standard EMG. The role of electrodiagnostic testing is to assist the clinician in differentiating a neuropraxic injury from a neural degenerative injury and to assess the proportion of degenerated axons. Nerves sustaining a neuropraxic injury proximal to the stimulated portion of the nerve maintain electrical stimulability. Partial or complete disruption of the nerve results in wallerian degeneration and consequent decrease or loss of stimulability. However, the distal segment of the nerves maintains stimulability for 48 to 72 hours. Consequently, electrodiagnostic testing cannot reliably differentiate a neuropraxic injury from a laceration of the nerve for up to 3 days.

Sunderland (26) classified nerve fiber injuries in five categories: The first-degree injury is anatomically intact with a conduction blockade (neuropraxia). These lesions tend to recover completely. The second-degree injury transects the axons but maintains an intact endoneurium (axonotemesis). These lesions also tend to resolve without subsequent deficits. The third-degree injury transects the axon and endoneurium but maintains an intact perineurium (neurotemesis). Aberrant regeneration can occur with third-degree injuries, leaving patients with some weakness and synkinesis. Fourth-degree injuries transect the entire nerve trunk but maintain an intact epineural sheath (neurotemesis). Loss of the conduit of the epineural sheath allows regenerating axons to cross into adjacent fascicles, resulting in a loss of the topographic organization. A proportion of the regenerating fibers are also lost due to the healing process and scarring. These lesions result in a high incidence of residual weakness, synkinesis, and hyperkinesis. Complete transection of the entire nerve trunk and epineurium is classified as a fifth-degree injury (neurotemesis) and is associated with poor spontaneous recovery, if any, depending on the degree of diastasis of the nerve ends.

The Hilger facial nerve stimulator is used to perform both the minimal nerve excitability test (NET) as well as the maximal stimulation test (MST). The facial nerve is stimulated percutaneously adjacent to the stylomastoid foramen and the various distal branches. In minimal nerve excitability testing, the current is increased until threshold is reached, manifesting with facial twitching. A threshold difference of 3.5 mA or greater between the affected and nonaffected sides of the face suggests significant neural degeneration. The test is most useful between 2 and 14 days postinjury in patients with dense facial paralysis to differentiate between neuropraxic and degenerative injuries. The testing is unnecessary in incomplete paralysis in which there is almost always 100% recovery.

May et al. (27) argue that the MST provides a more reliable estimation of the degree of degeneration. In the MST, stimulation is performed similar to in the NET, but the intensity of the stimulus is increased until the amount of facial contraction plateaus or is limited by patient intolerance. The degree of contraction is subjectively assessed by the physician and compared with electrical stimulation of the unaffected side of the face. The difference in contraction is expressed as equal, mildly decreased, markedly decreased, or no response. The latter two categories are associated with poor prognosis. Similar to NET, MST is most useful between 2 and 14 days postinjury in patients with dense facial paralysis.

Evoked electromyography (EEMG) has been popularized by Fisch (28) and termed electroneuronography (ENoG). ENoG differs from EEMG only in the use of bipolar stimulating and recording electrodes. Both techniques measure the evoked compound muscle action potential (CAP) and provide similar information to the MST but in an objective fashion. The stimulating electrode is placed adjacent to the stylomastoid foramen and the recording electrode in the nasolabial crease. The diminution in the amplitude of the CAP is indicative of the percentage of degenerated nerve fibers. EEMG has been demonstrated to be the most accurate electrodiagnostic test for prognostic information (29). Fisch (30) reported that patients in whom the degeneration on EEMG reaches 90% within 6 days of onset of a traumatic facial paralysis have a poorer outcome and consequently should be decompressed. Sillman et al. (31) demonstrated a significant association between a CAP decline of greater than 90% and poor recovery of function for idiopathic paralysis, but demonstrated no significant association between CAP decline of greater than 90% and clinical outcome in traumatic paralysis.

The value of EMG in the acute management of traumatic facial paralysis remains controversial. Standard monopolar EMG is performed by insertion of an EMG electrode into the muscle and the spontaneous electrical activity recorded. Two types of information are obtainable: voluntary activity and fibrillation potentials. If voluntary activity is present in the acute postinjury period, the patient has a very high probability of good recovery (31). However, May et al. (32) reported only a 75% accuracy in predicting a poor recovery and 62% accuracy in predicting a favorable result. Fibrillation potentials result from denervation of the muscle but are delayed 2 to 3 weeks following the injury and consequently offer little additional information in the acute setting.

Following defining the at-risk population for poor recovery of function, the next question to answer is, Does surgical intervention alter the outcome? Turner (23) reported on 30 patients with complete facial paralysis treated nonoperatively. Good recovery occurred in 63% of the patients, incomplete recovery with synkinesis in 23%, and poor recovery in 13% (Table 23-1). Maiman et al. (24) reported on the outcome of 21 patients with posttraumatic complete facial paralysis. Full recovery occurred in 52% of the patients and incomplete recovery in 43%. One patient had a poor outcome. The overall rate of good recovery for patients treated conservatively was 63%. The outcomes for patients who underwent facial nerve decompression in various series as well as those receiving conservative management are summarized in Table 23-1 (3,23,24,31,33–35). The combined rate of good recovery of facial function following decompression was 55%. This figure excludes severed facial nerves. When comparing these results with those of nonoperative management, there appears to be little benefit from decompression. However, the criteria to be included in the surgical groups were that the nerves were no longer stimulable or demonstrated 90% degeneration. The patients included in the observation studies did not necessarily meet these same criteria.

TABLE 23–1. *Facial nerve outcome following surgical and nonsurgical management*

Treatment	*n*	Degree of recovery: Good	Incomplete	Poor	Transsected nerves
Conservative					
Turner	30	19	7	4	
Maiman	21	11	9	1	
Brodie	8	7	0	1	
Operative					
Kamerer	62	18	15	9	20
Lambert	17	11	0	0	6
Coker	12	5	4	1	2
Sillman	0	0	0	0	
Brodie	6	4	0	2	0

Since wallerian degeneration is not documented on electrodiagnostic testing for 2 to 3 days following the neurotemesis, it is not surprising that there is no good evidence in the literature demonstrating that decompression of a nonsevered nerve is efficacious. The key factor in the decision to surgically explore a facial nerve is whether the nerve is suspected of being severed or impaled with bone fragments. The incidence of transected nerves in the large series ranges from 7% to 47%. The high frequency of severed nerves in some of these reports is biased by patient selection. Patients are referred to the tertiary centers performing nerve explorations when they fail to spontaneously recover. However, the vast majority of patients do recover spontaneously and are not referred to tertiary centers.

The probability of severing the facial nerve is actually quite low but the outcome following observation alone of a transected nerve is poor. Since one cannot differentiate a Sunderland fifth-degree injury (severed nerve) from a third- or fourth-degree injury on the basis of electrodiagnostic testing, we advocate exploration only in patients with complete immediate-onset paralysis in whom electrical stimulability is lost.

The site of injury to the facial nerve in temporal bone fractures is in the perigeniculate region in 80% to 93% of patients (16,34,35). Lambert and Brackmann (34) found a second lesion in 4 out of 21 patients in the mastoid segment. Accordingly, the approach utilized for the nerve exploration must expose these regions. Fisch (30) advocates a translabyrinthine approach for transverse fractures and a combined transmastoid/middle cranial fossa approach for longitudinal fractures. May (36) described a transmastoid/supralabyrinthine approach to the region of the geniculate ganglion for facial nerve decompression. Goin (37) studied this approach in cadaveric temporal bones and found that he could consistently expose the distal labyrinthine segment and geniculate ganglion. However, the fundus of the IAC could be exposed in only 60% of the temporal bones. Yanagihara (38) applied the transmastoid/supralabyrinthine approach in 36 patients. Only five temporal bone fractures in his series of 41 patients required a middle cranial fossa approach to expose the geniculate region.

We utilize the translabyrinthine approach for facial nerve exploration in patients with profound hearing loss. The approach provides excellent exposure for decompression, nerve rerouting with direct reanastomosis, and cable grafting. In otic capsule sparing fractures with ossicular discontinuity, we would explore the nerve via a transmastoid/supralabyrinthine approach. This approach generally requires dislocation of the incus and ossicular reconstruction at the completion of the operation. If the patient has any contralateral hearing loss or the anatomy is not conducive for supralabyrinthine exposure, we would proceed with a middle cranial fossa approach.

Timing of facial nerve repair is also controversial. McCabe (39) advocated repairing the nerve within the first 3 days or delaying facial nerve reanastomosis for 20 days postinjury. This recommendation was based on the observation that regeneration and axoplasmic flow were greatest at 3 weeks postinjury. Barrs (40) studied the timing of facial nerve repair in micropigs and found no advantage of waiting the 3 weeks until the neuronal cell body metabolic activity was maximal.

Fisch (41) advocates exploration when the ENoG indicates 90% degeneration occurring within 6 days. He argues that decompression should be performed early to minimize further degeneration. May (25) also advocates early exploration. His series demonstrated a correlation of best results and shorter interval between injury and repair.

The range in latency to recovery of facial function varies from 1 day to 1 year. Fifty-nine percent of facial palsies that recover spontaneously do so within 1 month and 88% recover by 3 months postinjury (3).

Summary of Facial Nerve Treatment Algorithm

The patients with delayed-onset facial paralysis are placed on a 2-week course of systemic steroids (unless medically contraindicated) and observed (Fig. 23-2). Patients with complete paralysis of immediate onset are tested with the Hilger nerve stimulator on a daily basis. If no loss of stimulability occurs, the patients are observed. If the nerve loses stimulability within 1 week of the injury, facial nerve exploration is performed. Facial nerve injuries occurring in an otic capsule disrupting injury (transverse fracture) are explored via a translabyrinthine approach. In otic sparing fractures (longitudinal fracture), two surgical approaches are utilized. In patients with well-aerated mastoid air cell systems or with ossicular discontinuity, a transmastoid/supralabyrinthine approach is chosen. If the patient has a poorly aerated mastoid air cell system or total facial nerve decompression cannot be achieved by the transmastoid/supralabyrinthine approach, a combined transmastoid/middle cranial fossa approach is utilized. If a severed facial nerve is encountered using the transmastoid/supralabyrinthine approach and inadequate exposure for cable grafting occurs, a middle cranial fossa approach is performed.

The transmastoid facial nerve decompression begins with a complete mastoidectomy skeletonizing the tegmen mastoideum superiorly, the sigmoid sinus posteriorly, and the posterior EAC wall anteriorly. The antrum is opened, exposing the short process of the incus and the lateral semicircular canal. The semicircular canals are then skeletonized. The facial recess is opened and the facial nerve is skeletonized from the second genu to the stylomastoid foramen. If there is any evidence of bony trauma in this region, a complete decompression is performed; however, the nerve sheath is not incised. The buttress to the incus is subsequently removed and the tympanic portion of the nerve is decompressed. If there is adequate room to proceed, a supralabyrinthine decompression of the intralabyrinthine portion of the facial nerve is performed (Fig. 23-3). A laceration of the facial nerve in this region is cable grafted with a section of the greater auricular nerve. The cable graft is placed in the bony channel of the fallopian canal abutting the sharply incised edges of the facial nerve. To improve exposure, the eggshelled tegmen can be retracted superiorly. If the exposure remains inadequate, a middle fossa craniotomy is performed. If the fracture involves the proximal portion of the intralabyrinthine segment of the facial nerve, the middle fossa craniotomy is performed.

The squamosal portion of the temporal bone is exposed by extending the postauricular skin incision in a ''lazy S'' shape up to the vertex, first extending anteriorly, then posteriorly. The temporalis fascia is reflected inferiorly and the temporalis muscle is split vertically and elevated off of the squamosal portion of the temporal bone. Dissection should extend underneath the zygomatic arch, to allow adequate exposure for the craniotomy. The self-retaining retractors are adjusted to hold both muscle and skin. A bone window is created with a 5- or 6-mm cutting burr and suction irrigation. This bone window is 4 by 4 cm in size and is set at the level of the zygomatic root. Two-thirds of the window is anterior to the vertical plane of the EAC, and one-third

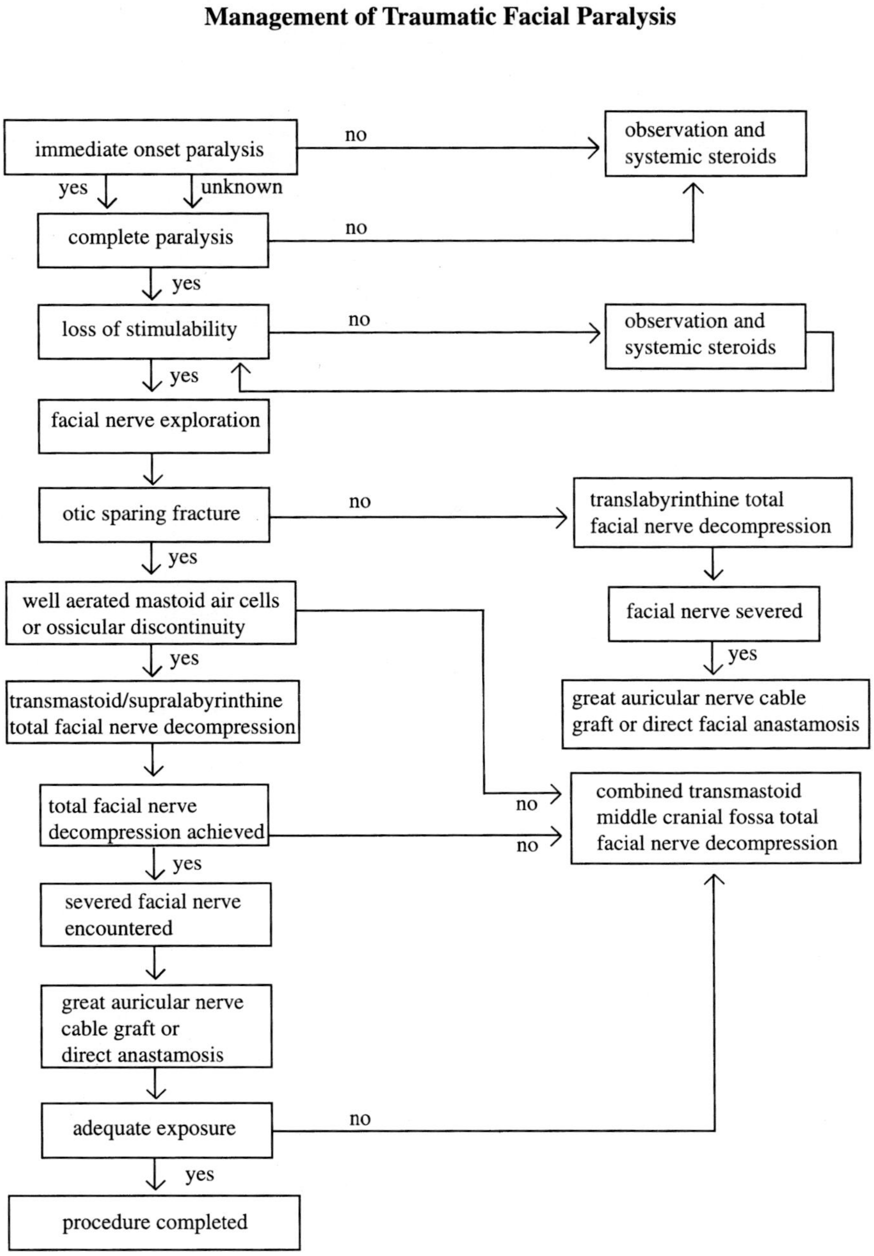

FIG. 23-2. Treatment algorithm for the management of facial nerve injuries.

of the window is posterior to the canal. A rongeur is used to remove the bone at the inferior edge of the craniotomy to the level of the middle fossa floor. This allows the optimal surgical line of site with minimal temporal lobe retraction. The House-Urban middle fossa retractor is engaged with the prongs in the edge of the craniotomy. The blade is gradually advanced, as the dura is elevated off the floor of the middle fossa. It is common to encounter dural venous bleeding at the anterior extent of the dissection. This can usually be controlled with a hemostatic agent such as Surgicel.

The landmarks in the middle fossa are the middle meningeal artery at foramen spinosum, the greater superficial petrosal nerve at the facial hiatus, and the arcuate eminence. The geniculate ganglion may be exposed without a bony covering on the floor of the middle fossa, so care should be exercised during dural elevation. The fracture line and hematoma is generally encountered in the region of the facial hiatus. The landmark for the superior semicircular canal is the arcuate eminence, but the precise location of the canal does not uniformly correspond with the arcuate eminence. A coronal CT scan may be helpful in ascertaining the relationship between the two. It will show the contours of the middle fossa floor, as they relate to the superior semicircular canal and the distance between the superior semicircular canal and the floor of the middle fossa. The canal may have very little bone coverage, and be seen as a blue line after simple dural elevation, or there may be a large number of air cells between the canal and the surface of the tegmen.

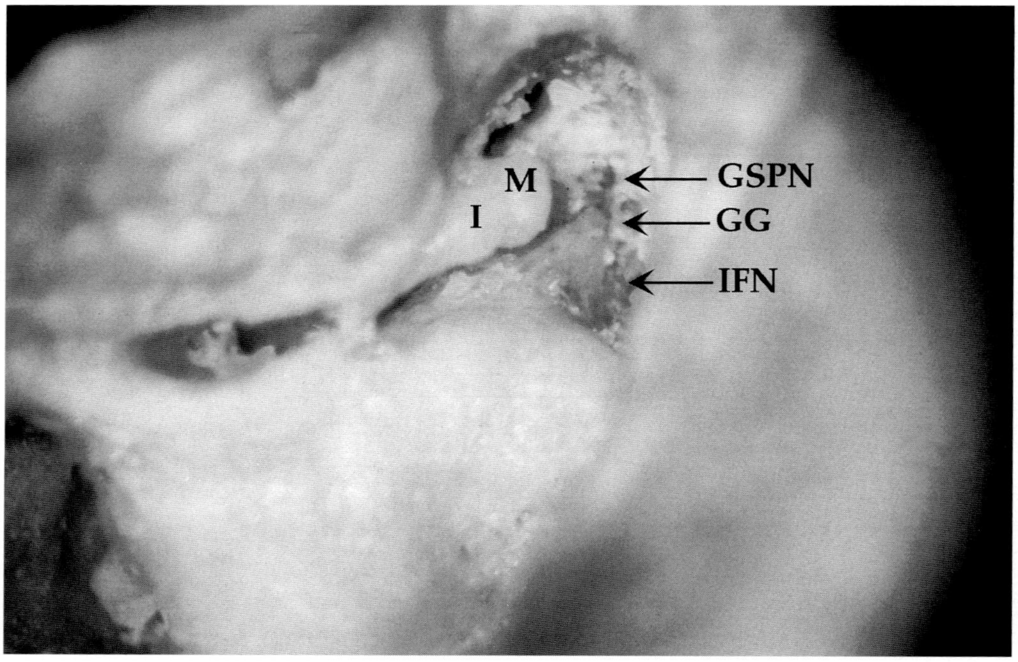

FIG. 23-3. Supralabyrinthine approach to the intralabyrinthine segment of the facial nerve, incus (I), malleus (M), greater superficial petrosal nerve (GSPN), geniculate ganglion (GG), intralabyrinthine portion of the facial nerve (IFN).

If the superior semicircular canal cannot be located by drilling over the arcuate eminence, two other methods may be considered. First, the tegmen tympani may be opened, exposing the ossicles. The location of the superior semicircular canal can be established by the spatial relationships. Second, the greater superficial petrosal nerve can be followed retrograde back through the facial hiatus to the geniculate ganglion. The intralabyrinthine portion of the facial nerve passes between the cochlea and the ampulla of the superior semicircular canal. The bone over the superior semicircular canal is removed using suction irrigation and diamond burrs. A light medial to lateral stroke is used until the blue line of the superior canal is identified. After the superior canal has been identified, dissection proceeds along the meatal plane, which is the bone within a 60-degree angle from the blue line of the superior canal (Fig. 23-4). Drilling within the confines of this plane will reduce the risk of inadvertent injury to the cochlea. Note that much wider drilling may be performed medially, whereas at the lateral extent of the IAC there is very little space between the cochlea and ampulla of the superior semicircular canal. The burr should hug the line of the superior canal as bone removal progresses. The

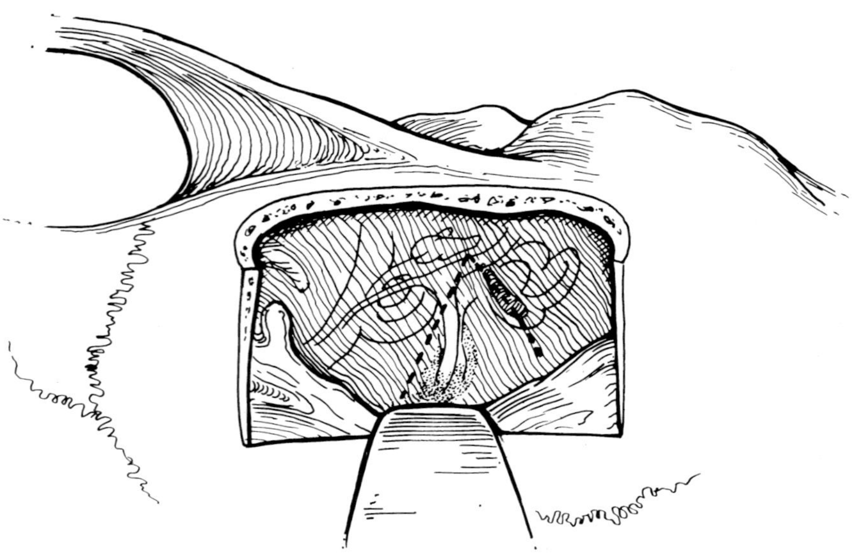

FIG. 23-4. Middle fossa approach to the internal auditory canal.

dissection will appear quite deep before the IAC is encountered. Bone should be removed 180 degrees around the IAC, from the lateral aspect of the meatus to the porus acousticus. An eggshell thickness of bone should be left on the dura. The last step in exposure of the canal is careful removal of this bone, and copious irrigation to remove bone dust.

At the most lateral extent of the IAC the vertical crest or "Bill's bar" is identified, with the facial nerve anteriorly and the superior vestibular nerve posteriorly. The dura of the IAC is incised in a longitudinal fashion, along the posterior edge, away from the facial nerve. If the facial nerve is lacerated, the proximal edge is freshened with microscissors. The nerve graft is secured proximally with a single 9-0 nylon suture and distally placed into the bony channel of the tympanic portion of the fallopian canal. A piece of temporalis fascia is placed over the graft. Bone wax is used to fill exposed air cells. A piece of temporalis muscle is placed in the bony defect, and the pedicled temporalis fascia flap is reflected over the floor of the middle cranial fossa. The temporal lobe is released, compressing the fascia over the bony defect. The bone flap is secured to the edges of the craniotomy with silk sutures. The temporalis muscle is closed superiorly, leaving a gap inferiorly where the temporalis fascia is passing and the skin is closed in two layers.

CSF Fistulae

CSF fistulae and the potential for meningitis are among the most serious of complications from temporal bone fractures. CSF fistulae occur in 17% of temporal bone fractures (3). CSF fistulae in longitudinal temporal bone fractures typically occur through the floor of the middle cranial fossa (tegmen tympani and tegmen mastoideum) into the epitympanum, antrum, and mastoid air cell tract. The CSF will flow out the ear canal if the tympanic membrane is disrupted or into the eustachian tube, resulting in CSF rhinorrhea. In transverse temporal bone fractures, CSF flows from the posterior cranial fossa through the disrupted otic capsule into the middle ear. In mixed fractures, the site of the fracture is often not clearly delineated until the time of surgical exploration of the mastoid and middle ear.

A unique characteristic of a fracture through the otic capsule is the absence of healing. The otic capsule is adult size at birth and undergoes minimal remodeling throughout life. Following a fracture, fibrous tissue will partially fill the crevice and the adjacent periosteal bone may seal off the fracture but the enchondral bone itself will not heal. The potential tract places the patient at continued risk of delayed meningitis.

The incidence of meningitis in patients with CSF leaks ranges from 2% to 88% (3,42–46). The wide range in incidence is a result of multiple factors, the most significant of which is the duration of leakage (42,44,46,47). Mincy (46) and Leech and Patterson (44) compared the incidence of meningitis in patients with CSF leaks continuing 7 days or less to those persisting for more than 7 days. Leech and Patterson found only a 5% incidence of meningitis in patients with CSF fistulae of less than 7 days' duration, and Mincy reported a similarly low incidence of meningitis in this group of 11%. The incidence of meningitis in patients with leakage for more than 7 days in Leech and Patterson's series was 55%, and 88% in Mincy's series. Spetzler and Wilson (47) demonstrated a 33% incidence of meningitis in persistent fistulae, and Grahne (42) found 54% of his patients with chronic CSF leakage developed meningitis.

Many studies over the past 25 years have demonstrated no benefit of prophylactic antibiotics in temporal bone fractures in the absence of CSF fistulas (44,45,48–55). The incidence of meningitis in this group is quite low. Rathore (56) pooled the data from many of these studies and found a 4% incidence of meningitis in patients with basilar skull fractures receiving prophylactic antibiotics and a 3% incidence in patients not receiving prophylactic antibiotics. Brodie and Thompson (3) demonstrated a 1% incidence of meningitis in the 578 patients with temporal bone fractures and no CSF fistulae (3). Hoff et al. (49) conducted a prospective randomized trial assigning patients with temporal bone fractures into a prophylactic antibiotic treatment group or to a no-antibiotic group. None of the patients in any group developed meningitis. All of these studies conclude that prophylactic antibiotics are not indicated, given the low incidence of meningitis in this group of untreated patients, and the lack of evidence demonstrating any benefit to prophylactic antibiotics in this situation. However, the risk of meningitis is significantly higher in patients with temporal bone fractures when CSF fistulae are present. Consequently, the role of prophylactic antibiotics must be examined in relation to this subset of trauma patients. Multiple studies over the past three decades have concluded that prophylactic antibiotics did not have a statistically significant effect on the incidence of meningitis in patients with CSF fistulae (45,47,48,50,51,55). However, the number of patients included in the various studies was inadequate for valid statistical analysis. Reevaluation of the literature over the past 25 years using a meta-analysis revealed a statistically significant reduction in meningitis using prophylactic antibiotics in patients with CSF fistula (57); 320 patients were included in the analysis. The incidence of meningitis in patients with posttraumatic CSF fistulae treated with prophylactic antibiotics was 2.1%. In patients who did not receive prophylactic antibiotics, the incidence of meningitis was significantly higher at 8.7% ($p < .02$). Individually, none of the studies included in the meta-analysis demonstrated a statistically significant effect of prophylactic antibiotics, which points out the pitfall of statistical analysis with inadequate numbers of patients.

In addition to the inadequate numbers of patients in these prior studies, there are significant problems inherent in this type of retrospective study. How do we define adequate prophylaxis? Do 3 days of perioperative antibiotics for repair of a concomitant open femur fracture constitute adequate prophylaxis of a CSF fistula that persists for 5 days? Do therapeutic antibiotics for a concurrent infection constitute adequate prophylaxis of a CSF fistula? One very important risk factor increasing the risk of meningitis in patients with CSF fistulae is the presence of a concurrent infection. Brodie and Thompson (3) found a 20% incidence of meningitis in patients with concurrent infection and a 3% incidence of meningitis in the absence of concurrent infection. In this study, in the absence of concurrent infection, no patients receiving prophylactic antibiotics developed meningitis within the first month postinjury. Clearly, these confounding variables must be controlled in a prospective multiinstitutional study to adequately address the question of the efficacy of prophylactic antibiotics.

The most common infecting organisms in meningitis occurring in the presence of a CSF fistula reported in the literature are *Pneumococcus* followed by *Streptococcus,* and *Haemophilus influenzae* (45,58,59).

Since acute posttraumatic CSF fistulae are associated with a high probability of early spontaneous closure and a low incidence of meningitis, they can be treated conservatively for 7 to 10 days. This treatment includes total bed rest with elevation of the head of the bed; stool softeners; instructions to avoid nose blowing, sneezing, and straining; and repeat lumbar punctures or lumbar drain if the leak persists. All of these measures are directed at maintaining the CSF pressure gradient below the healing tensile strength of the healing barrier. Due to the increased risk of meningitis following persistent CSF fistulae, closure of fistulae persisting greater than 7 to 10 days is recommended.

Closure of CSF Fistulae

The approach chosen to close a CSF fistula is influenced by many factors including the status of hearing in the affected and contralateral ear, the presence of brain herniation through the tegmen, and the location of the fistula. The treatment algorithm is presented in Fig. 23-5. In a patient with a fracture of the otic capsule resulting in profound sensorineural hearing loss, obliteration of the mastoid and middle ear is recommended (60,61). The ear canal, tympanic membrane, incus and malleus, and middle ear mucosa are all excised. The external auditory meatus is closed in a two-layer closure, and a complete mastoidectomy is performed. The mucosa of the eustachian tube is inverted and a muscle plug is inserted. The incus is then inserted as well, wedging the muscle into place. The eustachian tube and fracture line are covered by temporalis fascia, and the mastoid cavity and middle ear are obliterated with an abdominal fat graft.

The approach for closure of fistulae resulting from longitudinal fractures is dictated by the location of the fracture along the floor of the middle cranial fossa, the presence of brain herniation, and the status of the ossicular chain. Fistulae that occur laterally in the middle cranial fossa are accessible through a complete mastoidectomy and can be repaired by sealing the mastoid cavity off from the epitympanum and middle ear by placing a temporalis fascia graft over the antrum and facial recess and retrofacial air cell tracts. A second fascia graft is placed over the fistula and the mastoid cavity is obliterated with a fat graft. Fistulae that occur more medially along the tegmen tympani or are associated with brain herniation are addressed with a combined approach. When the temporal lobe herniates through the tegmen, the damaged brain is debrided via the transmastoid approach and the remaining brain and dura are elevated back up into the middle fossa by way of the middle fossa craniotomy. Temporalis fascia is placed over the floor of the middle cranial fossa. If a bony defect is present in the tegmen, the craniotomy bone window is split or thinned with a burr and placed along the floor of the middle cranial fossa superior to the fascia to prevent subsequent prolapse. A piece of Gelfilm is inserted through the mastoid cavity and antrum and placed over the top of the ossicles in the epitympanum in order to avoid adhesions and postoperative conductive hearing loss.

In the case of a fistula through the tegmen tympani in a patient with an ossicular discontinuity and the absence of brain herniation, the fistula can often be closed via a transmastoid approach alone. A tragal cartilage graft is inserted superior to the superior EAC wall extending to the tympanic portion of the facial nerve. The cartilage graft seals off the epitympanum and prevents herniation of tissue into the middle ear. The epitympanum is filled with a temporalis fascia graft.

Additional techniques have been advocated by other authors. Glasscock et al. (62) have advocated an intradural as opposed to an extradural approach for large defects, arguing that a better closure can be achieved intradurally. In our experience the combined mastoid and extradural middle fossa approach has provided uniformly good results.

There is a high risk of EAC stenosis and cholesteatoma formation when the ear canal is severely traumatized as seen with gunshot wounds to the temporal bone (63,64). In this situation, the CSF fistulae are generally closed with resection of the EAC and tympanic membrane and obliteration of the mastoid and middle ear as described above. Extreme care is taken to avoid leaving any fragments of epithelium that may subsequently lead to cholesteatoma formation. All mucosa is removed and the eustachian tube and external meatus are closed as described above.

Hearing Loss

Temporal bone trauma can cause a conductive hearing loss, sensorineural hearing loss, or mixed loss. Longitudinal fractures extend along the roof of the EAC, often tearing the tympanic membrane in the region of the notch of Ravinius. The fracture proceeds along the tegmen tympani and in 20% of patients disrupts the ossicular chain (7). The most common injuries to the ossicular chain is separation of the incudostapedial joint (82%) and dislocation of the incus (57%) followed by fracture of the stapes crura (30%) (65). The majority of stapedial fractures do not occur in isolation but are associated with incus dislocations (7). Fixation of the

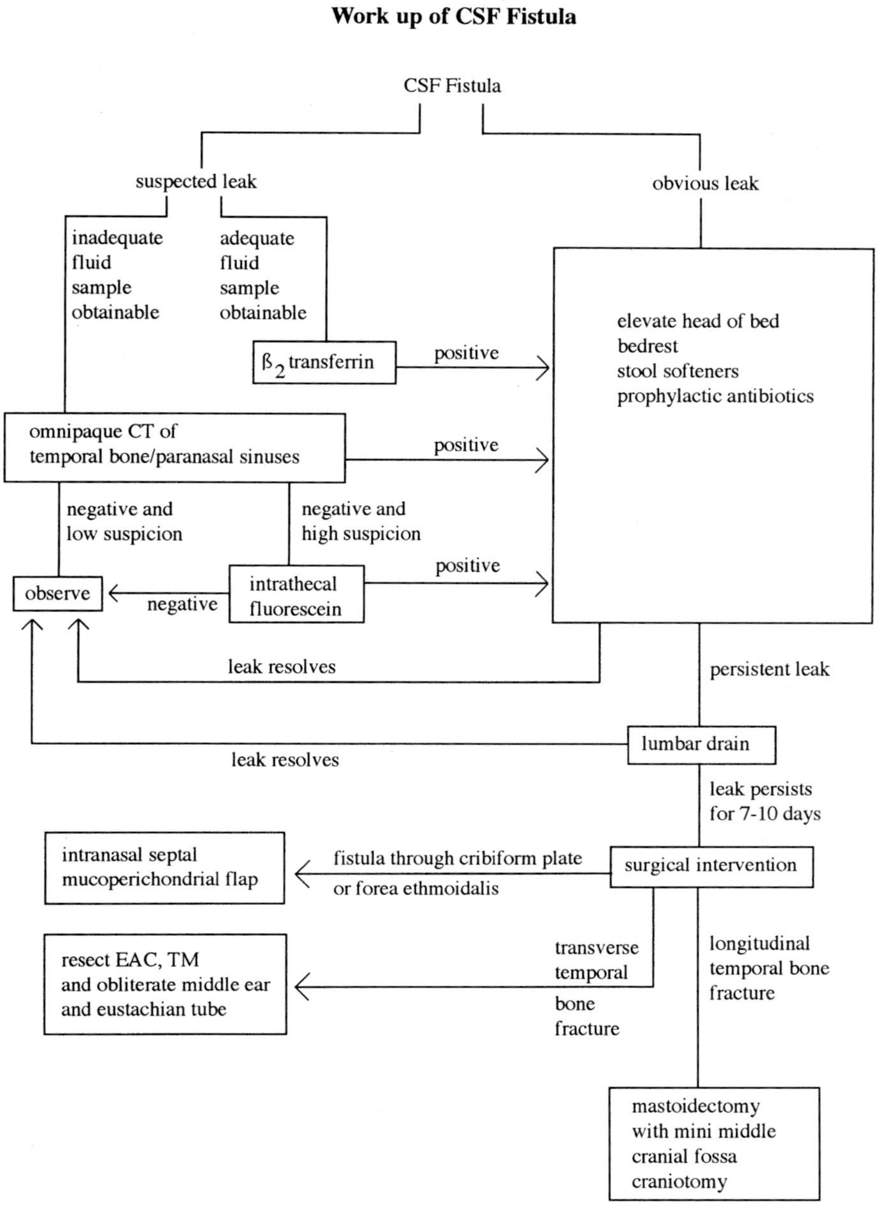

FIG. 23-5. Treatment algorithm for the management of posttraumatic CSF fistula.

ossicles in the epitympanum (25%) and fracture of the malleus (11%) occurs less frequently (65). One-third of the patients will have multiple concomitant middle ear pathology.

Almost universally, patients with temporal bone fractures will experience a hemotympanum with associated conductive hearing loss. Over a few days to few weeks postinjury, the middle ear will reaerate with resolution of the hearing loss attributable to the middle ear fluid. Factors that increase the duration of the middle ear fluid include endotracheal intubation, associated craniofacial fractures, and the presence of a CSF leak; 80% of cases of conductive hearing loss will resolve spontaneously without the need for surgical intervention (66). Residual conductive hearing loss following resolution of the hemotympanum and healing of the tympanic membrane suggests the possibilities of ossicular fracture or discontinuity. The indications for exploratory tympanotomy and ossicular reconstruction are conductive hearing loss greater than 30 dB that persists for more than 2 months postinjury. However, if the conductive hearing loss is in an only hearing ear, surgery is contraindicated. The audiogram in a mixed hearing loss must be critically assessed to establish the true potential benefit of ossicular reconstruction. If the bone conduction thresholds are more than 30 dB worse than in the contralateral ear, reconstruction, even with an excellent closure of the conductive component of the hearing loss, will provide minimal subjective improvement. In this scenario, the patient would still require a hearing aid to attain usable hearing in the surgical ear. Consequently, unless the mixed loss is profound and the patient cannot benefit preoperatively from a hearing aid, ossicular reconstruction is not recommended.

The most conducive injury for ossicular reconstruction is

a dislocation of the incudostapedial joint. In this situation an Applebaum hydroxyapatite prosthesis is inserted between the long process of the incus and capitulum of the stapes, generally resulting in near closure of the air-bone gap. Dislocation of the entire incus requires bridging the gap between the stapes suprastructure and the manubrium of the malleus. We prefer a sculpted incus interposition graft in this situation, although a variety of partial ossicular replacement prostheses are available and suitable for this type of reconstruction. The incus interposition is accomplished by drilling a cup in the end of the lateral process of the incus that will fit over the capitulum of the stapes. The long process of the incus is removed and the body sculptured. The articular surface is fashioned to fit under the manubrium. If, in addition to the incus dislocation, the stapes suprastructure is fractured, the long process of the incus is left intact and the body and short process sculptured. The superior surface of the body of the incus is fashioned to rest under the manubrium and the long process sits on the footplate. A variety of total ossicular replacement prostheses are also available for this purpose as well. A more unique problem occurs when the stapes suprastructure is fractured but the incus remains connected to the malleus. These patients are good candidates for a laser stapedectomy.

The hearing results following ossicular reconstruction for traumatic ossicular disruption are superior to those performed for chronic otitis media. Hough and Stuart (65) report closure of the air-bone gap to within 10 dB in 78% of patients and complete closure in 45%.

Transverse or otic capsule disrupting fractures typically result in severe to profound sensorineural hearing loss. Multiple pathogenic mechanisms can contribute to the deafness including disruption of the membranous labyrinth, avulsion or trauma to the cochlear nerve, interruption of the cochlear blood supply, hemorrhage into cochlea, and perilymphatic fistulae. Another proposed mechanism is endolymphatic hydrops resulting from obstruction of the endolymphatic duct by the temporal bone fracture (67). Acoustic-trauma associated with temporal bone fractures and incus dislocations frequently contributes to a sensorineural component to a mixed hearing loss; 50% of patients with traumatic incus dislocations will have at least 10 dB of sensorineural hearing loss and 18% will have more than 30 dB of loss (68). The loss occurs primarily in the 2,000- to 4,000-Hz range. The prognosis for recovery of function in patients with anacusis or profound deafness is extremely poor; however, patients with moderate to severe loss may have some recovery (66,69). Patients who are experiencing progressive or fluctuating sensorineural hearing loss, suggestive of a possible underlying perilymphatic fistula, may benefit from exploration and patching of the fistula (70).

Cholesteatoma and External Auditory Canal Stenosis

Cholesteatoma formation may occur many years after a temporal bone fracture (63,71). There are four pathogenic mechanisms responsible for posttraumatic cholesteatoma formation: (a) epithelial entrapment in the fracture line, (b) ingrowth of epithelium through the unhealed fracture line or rent in the tympanic membrane, (c) traumatic implantation of tympanic membrane skin into the middle ear, and (d) trapping of epithelium medial to a stenosis of the EAC. The typical location for cholesteatoma resulting from epithelium trapped within the fracture line is in the epitympanum and antrum. The fracture line along the posterior superior canal wall and scutum expands and then closes trapping the canal skin. As the trapped skin grows, it expands into the epitympanum and antrum forming a cholesteatoma. The ingrowth of epithelium through a displaced fracture line may also extend into the same region. Traumatic implantation of tympanic membrane skin will result in cholesteatoma formation within the mesotympanum. The fourth mechanism of cholesteatoma formation, trapping of epithelium medial to an EAC stenosis, results in a canal cholesteatoma. Posttraumatic canal cholesteatomas are the most preventable by careful follow-up, debridement, and stenting when narrowing progresses. The ear canal can be dilated with the insertion of increasing numbers of otowicks, saturated with Cortisporin, replaced every few days. Once the canal is adequately dilated, a larger Merocel sponge is inserted to maintain the lumen. A large vented custom ear mold is occasionally required to maintain the lumen following severe canal injuries. The mold is used throughout the day for 3 to 6 months. When the stenosis is complete, dilation is not possible and a canaloplasty and possible tympanoplasty are required. A lateral stenosis of the EAC must never be allowed to persist, even if completely benign in appearance, because of the very high probability of cholesteatoma formation.

Posttraumatic cholesteatoma involving the attic, antrum, or mastoid air cells will often grow for many years prior to detection. Until the cholesteatoma involves the ossicular chain with resultant conductive hearing loss, erodes into the labyrinth causing vertigo or sensorineural hearing loss, compresses the facial nerve resulting in facial paresis, or grows into the middle and can be visualized on physical examination, the growth will go undetected.

REFERENCES

1. Nageris B, Hansen MC, Lavelle WG, et al. Temporal bone fractures. *Am J Emerg Med* 1995;12:211–214.
2. Virapongse C, Bhimani S, Sarwar M. Radiography of the abnormal ear. In: Taveras JM, Ferrucci JT, eds. *Radiology: diagnosis—imaging—intervention,* vol 3. Philadelphia: JB Lippincott, 1987;9:1–19.
3. Brodie HA, Thompson TC. Management of complications from 820 temporal bone fractures. *Am J Otol* 1997;18:188–197.
4. Travis LW, Stalnaker RL, Melvin JW. Impact trauma of human temporal bone. *J Trauma* 1977;17:761–766.
5. Makashima K, Sobel SF, Snow JB Jr. Histopathologic correlates of otoneurologic manifestations following head trauma. *Laryngoscope* 1976;86:1303–1314.
6. Ulrich K. Verletzungen des Gehororgans bei Schadelbasis-frakturen. *Acta Otolaryngol Suppl (Stockh)* 1926;6:1–50.
7. Cannon CR, Jahrsdoerfer RA. Temporal bone fractures: review of 90 cases. *Arch Otolaryngol* 1983;109:285–288.

8. Wiet RJ, Valvassori GE, Kotsanis CA, et al. Temporal bone fractures. *Am J Otol* 1985;6:207–215.
9. Tos M. Course of and sequelae to 248 petrosal fractures. *Acta Otolaryngol (Stockh)* 1973;75:253–254.
10. Healy GB. Hearing loss and vertigo secondary to head injury. *N Engl J Med* 1982;306:1029–1031.
11. Fredrickson JM, Griffith AW, Lindsay JR. Transverse fractures of the temporal bone. *Arch Otolaryngol* 1963;78:770–784.
12. Ward PH. The histopathology of auditory and vestibular disorders in head trauma. *Ann Otol Rhinol Laryngol* 1969;78:227–238.
13. Hough JVD. Restoration of hearing after head trauma. *Ann Otol Rhinol Laryngol* 1969;78(2):210–226.
14. Ghorayeb BY, Yeakley JW. Temporal bone fractures: longitudinal or oblique? The cases for oblique temporal bone fractures. *Laryngoscope* 1992;102:129–134.
15. Kelly KE, Tami TA. Temporal bone and skull trauma. In: Jackler RK, Brackmann DE, eds. *Neurotology*. St. Louis: Mosby, 1994:340–360.
16. Fisch U. Facial paralysis in fractures of the petrous bone. *Laryngoscope* 1974;84:2141–2154.
17. Pearlman HB. Process of healing in injuries to the capsule of labyrinth. *Arch Otolaryngol* 1939;29:287–305.
18. Pollak AM, Pauw BKH, Marion MS. Temporal bone histopathology: resident's quiz. *Am J Otol* 1991;12:56–58.
19. Griffin JE, Altenau MM, Schaefer SD. Bilateral longitudinal temporal bone fractures: a retrospective review of seventeen cases. *Laryngoscope* 1979;89:1432–1435.
20. Schuknecht HF. Mechanism of inner ear injury from blows to the head. *Ann Otol Rhinol Laryngol* 1969;78:253–262.
21. Ylikoski J, Palva T, Sanna M. Dizziness after head trauma: clinical and morphologic findings. *Am J Otol* 1982;3:343–352.
22. McKennan KX, Chole RA. Facial paralysis in temporal bone trauma. *Am J Otol* 1992;13:167–172.
23. Turner JWA. Facial palsy in closed head injuries. *Lancet* 1944;246: 756–757.
24. Maiman DJ, Cusick JF, Anderson, AJ, et al. Nonoperative management of facial nerve palsy. *J Trauma* 1985;25:644–648.
25. May M. Trauma to the facial nerve. *Otolaryngol Clin North Am* 1983; 16:661–670.
26. Sunderland S. Some anatomical and pathophysiological data relevant to facial nerve injury and repair. In: *Facial nerve surgery*. Fisch U, ed. New York: Aesculapius, 1977, 47–61.
27. May M, Harvey JE, Marovitz WF, Stroud M. The prognostic accuracy of the maximal stimulation test compared with that of the nerve excitability test in Bell's palsy. *Laryngoscope* 1971;81:931–938.
28. Fisch U. Surgery for Bell's palsy. *Arch Otolaryngol* 1981;107:1–11.
29. May M, Klein SR, Taylor FH. Idiopathic (Bell's) facial palsy: natural history defies steroid or surgical treatment. *Laryngoscope* 1985;95: 406–409.
30. Fisch U. Management of intratemporal facial nerve injuries. *J Laryngol Otol* 1980;94:129–134.
31. Sillman JS, Niparko JK, Lee SS, Kileny PR. Prognostic value of evoked and standard electromyography in acute facial paralysis. *Otolaryngol Head Neck Surg* 1992;107:377–381.
32. May M, Blumenthal F, Klein SR. Acute Bell's palsy: prognostic value of evoked electromyography, maximal stimulation, and other electrical tests. *Am J Otol* 1983;5:1–7.
33. Kamerer DG. Intratemporal facial nerve injuries. *Otolaryngol Head Neck Surg* 1982;90:612–615.
34. Lambert PR, Brackmann DE. Facial paralysis in longitudinal temporal bone fractures: a review of 26 cases. *Laryngoscope* 1984;94: 1022–1026.
35. Coker NJ, Kendall KA, Jenkins HA, et al. Traumatic intratemporal facial nerve injury: management rationale for preservation of function. *Otolaryngol Head Neck Surg* 1987;97:262–269.
36. May M. Total facial nerve exploration: transmastoid, extralabyrinthine, and subtemporal indications and results. *Laryngoscope* 1979;89: 906–917.
37. Goin DW. Proximal intratemporal facial nerve in Bell's palsy surgery: a study correlating anatomical and surgical findings. *Laryngoscope* 1982;92(3):263–271.
38. Yanagihara N. Transmastoid decompression of the facial nerve in temporal bone fracture. *Otolaryngol Head Neck Surg* 1982;90:616–621.
39. McCabe BF. Facial nerve grafting. *Plast Reconstr Surg* 1970;45: 70–75.
40. Barrs DM. Facial nerve trauma: optimal timing for repair. *Laryngoscope* 1991;101:835–848.
41. Fisch U. Current surgical treatment of intratemporal facial palsy. *Clin Plast Surg* 1979;178:347–361.
42. Grahne B. Traumatic cranionasal fistulas persistent cerebrospinal fluid rhinorrhea and their repair with frontal sinus osteoplasty. *Acta Otolaryngol* 1970;70:392–400.
43. Hughes GB, Glasscock ME III, Hays JW, et al. Cerebrospinal fluid leaks and meningitis following acoustic tumor surgery. *Otolaryngol Head Neck Surg* 1982;90:117–125.
44. Leech PJ, Paterson A. Conservative and operative management of cerebrospinal fluid leakage after closed head injury. *Lancet* 1973;1: 1013–1015.
45. MacGee EE, Cauthen JC, Brackett CE. Meningitis following acute traumatic cerebrospinal fluid fistula. *J Neurosurg* 1970;33:312–316.
46. Mincy JE. Post-traumatic cerebrospinal fluid fistula of the frontal fossa. *J Trauma* 1966;6:618–622.
47. Spetzler RF, Wilson CB. Management of recurrent CSF rhinorrhea of the middle and posterior fossa. *J Neurosurg* 1978;49:393–397.
48. Klastersky J, Sadeghi M, Brihaye J. Antimicrobial prophylaxis in patients with rhinorrhea or otorrhea: a double blind study. *Surg Neurol* 1976;6:111–114.
49. Hoff JT, Brewin A, Sang H. Antibiotics for basilar skull fractures. *J Neurosurg* 1976;44:649.
50. Zrebeet HA, Huang PS. Prophylactic antibiotics in the treatment of fractures at the base of the skull. *Del Med J* 1986;58:741–748.
51. Frazee RC, Mucha P, Farnell MB, et al. Meningitis after basilar skull fracture. *Postgrad Med* 1988;83:267–274.
52. Einhorn A, Mizrahi EM. Basilar skull fractures in children. *Am J Dis Child* 1978;132:1121–1124.
53. Hellings TS, Evans LL, Fowler DL, et al. Infectious complications in patients with severe head injury. *J Trauma* 1988;28:1575–1577.
54. Ignelzi RJ, VanderArk GD. Analysis of the treatment of basilar skull fractures with and without antibiotics. *J Neurosurg* 1975;43:75–85.
55. Dagi TF, Meyer FB, Poletti CA. The incidence and prevention of meningitis after basilar skull fracture. *Am J Emerg Med* 1983;3:295–298.
56. Rathore MH. Do prophylactic antibiotics prevent meningitis after basilar skull fracture. *Pediatr Infect Dis J* 1991;10:87–88.
57. Brodie HA. Prophylactic antibiotics for posttraumatic cerebrospinal fluid fistulae. A meta-analysis. *Arch Otolaryngol Head Neck Surg* 1997;123:749–752.
58. Applebaum E. Meningitis following trauma to the head and face. *JAMA* 1960;173:1818–1822.
59. Kaufman BA, Tunkel AR, Pryor JC, et al. Meningitis in the neurosurgical patient. *Infect Dis Clin North Am* 1990;4:677–701.
60. Kveton JF. Obliteration of the mastoid and middle ear for severe trauma to the temporal bone. *Laryngoscope* 1987;97:1385–1387.
61. Coker NJ, Jenkins HA, Fisch U. Obliteration of the middle ear and mastoid cleft in subtotal petrosectomy. Indications, technique and results. *Ann Otol Rhinol Laryngol* 1986;95:5–11.
62. Glasscock ME III, Dickins JRE, Jackson CG, et al. Surgical management of brain tissue herniation into the middle ear and mastoid. *Laryngoscope* 1979;89:1743–1754.
63. McKennan KX, Chole RA. Post-traumatic cholesteatoma. *Laryngoscope* 1989;99:779–782.
64. Kronenberg J, Ben-Shoshan J, Modan M, et al. Blast injury and cholesteatoma. *Am J Otol* 1988;9:127–130.
65. Hough JVD, Stuart WD. Middle ear injuries in skull trauma. *Laryngoscope* 1968;78:899–937.
66. Tos M. Prognosis of hearing loss in temporal bone fractures. *Laryngol Otol* 1971;85:1147–1159.
67. Rizvi SS, Gibbin KP. Effect of transverse temporal bone fracture on the fluid compartment of the inner ear. *Ann Otol Rhinol Laryngol* 1979; 88:741–748.
68. Dommerby H, Tos M. Sensorineural hearing loss in posttraumatic incus dislocation. *Arch Otolaryngol* 1983;109:257–261.
69. Podoshin L, Fradis M. Hearing loss after head injury. *Arch Otolaryngol* 1975;101:15–18.
70. Lyos AT, Marsh MA, Jenkins HA, Coker NJ. Progressive hearing loss after transverse temporal bone fracture. *Arch Otolaryngol Head Neck Surg* 1995;121:795–799.
71. Freeman J. Temporal bone fractures and cholesteatoma. *Ann Otol Rhinol Laryngol* 1983;92:558–560.

Neurosurgical Issues in Otolaryngology: Principles and Practice of Collaboration,
edited by Moisés A. Arriaga and J. Diaz Day.
Lippincott Williams & Wilkins, Philadelphia © 1999.

CHAPTER 24

Acute Head Injury

Jack Wilberger

Head injury (HI) accounts for a disproportionate share of morbidity and mortality in traumatized patients. However, the past two decades have witnessed a significant decline in overall HI mortality from the mid-30% range in the 1970s to less than 20% in the 1990s. This improvement has paralleled an understanding of the secondary injury process—i.e., all neurologic damage does not occur at the moment of insult but evolves over the ensuing hours and days from various biochemical/molecular derangements. This understanding has led to the development of aggressive treatment strategies to prevent intracranial pressure (ICP) elevations and ischemia as well as to extensive clinical therapeutic trials to identify pharmacologic neuroprotective agents.

PATHOPHYSIOLOGY

The structural injury to the brain at the time of impact is rarely the sole determinant of outcome. A series of secondary clinical events—hypoxia, hypotension, mass lesions, increased ICP, ischemia—and biomechanical/molecular events—free radical production, excitotoxicity, loss of calcium homeostasis—ultimately determines eventual morbidity and mortality.

The frequent occurrence and deleterious effects of the secondary insults of hypoxia and hypotension have long been known (1,2). Mortality is doubled when these insults are superimposed on severe HI (Table 24-1). Similarly, the association between elevated ICP and outcome has been well established (3).

Recently, there has been considerable research into the biochemical/molecular mechanisms of secondary injury. While these events are multifactorial, interrelated, and time dependent, it becomes somewhat artificial, albeit necessary to separate out its component parts (Fig. 24-1).

There is widespread research on the contribution of oxygen free radicals to secondary injury (4,5). The specific free radicals generated—superoxide, hydroxyl, hydrogen peroxide, singlet oxygen, nitrous oxide—have the potential to do considerable damage to proteins and the phospholipid components of cell and organelle membranes. Additionally, extensive membrane depolarization, such as is seen with trauma, allows for a nonselective opening of the voltage-sensitive calcium (Ca) channels and an abnormal accumulation of Ca within neurons and glia. Such Ca shifts are associated with activation of lipolytic and proteolytic enzymes, protein kinases, protein phosphatases, dissolution of microtubules, and altered gene expression (6). Another method of abnormal Ca influx is via activation of excitatory amino acid receptors such as glutamate and aspartate—excitotoxicity—which occurs in a widespread fashion after trauma, resulting in cell swelling, vacuolization, and death (7).

EPIDEMIOLOGY/CLASSIFICATION

Closed HI leads to 500,000 hospitalizations per year, resulting in over 175,000 deaths and significant disabilities. While the statistics are somewhat variable, it is estimated that the incidence of HI currently approaches 222/100,000 population/year (8). The peak incidence occurs in men 15 to 24 years of age. For the most part, motor vehicular accidents still account for the majority of injuries; however, the increasing mandate for seat-belt use and availability of air bags appears to be having impact on this incidence. The incidence of penetrating HI from gunshot wounds (GSWs) is ever increasing and in some urban communities is now the most common type of injury seen.

A number of classification schemes have been developed for HI. The most reliable from a clinical and prognostic standpoint is based on the Glasgow Coma Scale (GCS) (Table 24-2):

GCS 3–7: severe
GCS 8–12: moderate
GCS 13–15: mild

J. Wilberger: Allegheny University of the Health Sciences, Pittsburgh, Pennsylvania 15212.

TABLE 24–1. *Effects of hypoxia and hypotension on head injury mortality*

Effect	Mortality (%)
Severe HI	20–30
Severe HI with hypoxia ($po_2 < 70$)	32–35
Severe HI with hypotension (SPB < 90)	50–55
Severe HI with hypoxia and hypotension	55–60

HI, head injury; SPB, systolic blood pressure.

TABLE 24–2. *Glasgow Coma Scale (GCS)*

Eye opening	
Spontaneous	4
To voice	3
To pain	2
None	1
Verbal response	
Oriented	5
Confused	4
Inappropriate	3
Incomprehensible	2
None	1
Motor response	
Obeys commands	6
Localizes pain	5
Withdraws	4
Flexion	3
Extension	2
Flaccid	1
Total	3–15

Mild HI has been generally considered a concussion, is infrequently associated with structural brain injury, and rarely leads to significant long-term sequelae. However, the postconcussion syndrome has been long recognized, and recent attention to neuropsychologic testing has shown the possibility of significant cognitive disability following a concussion (9).

Moderate HI may be associated with significant structural injury, such as hemorrhage or contusion, but death is uncommon.

Severe HI has an increasing mortality with a decreasing GCS and generally results in some form of cognitive and/or physical disability.

The accurate classification of HI is critical in both triage and management. It is important that severe HI be treated at facilities with appropriate neurotrauma resources. Similarly, moderate HI requires close clinical observation for neurologic deterioration. With mild HI the most important management issues relate to the need for computed tomographic

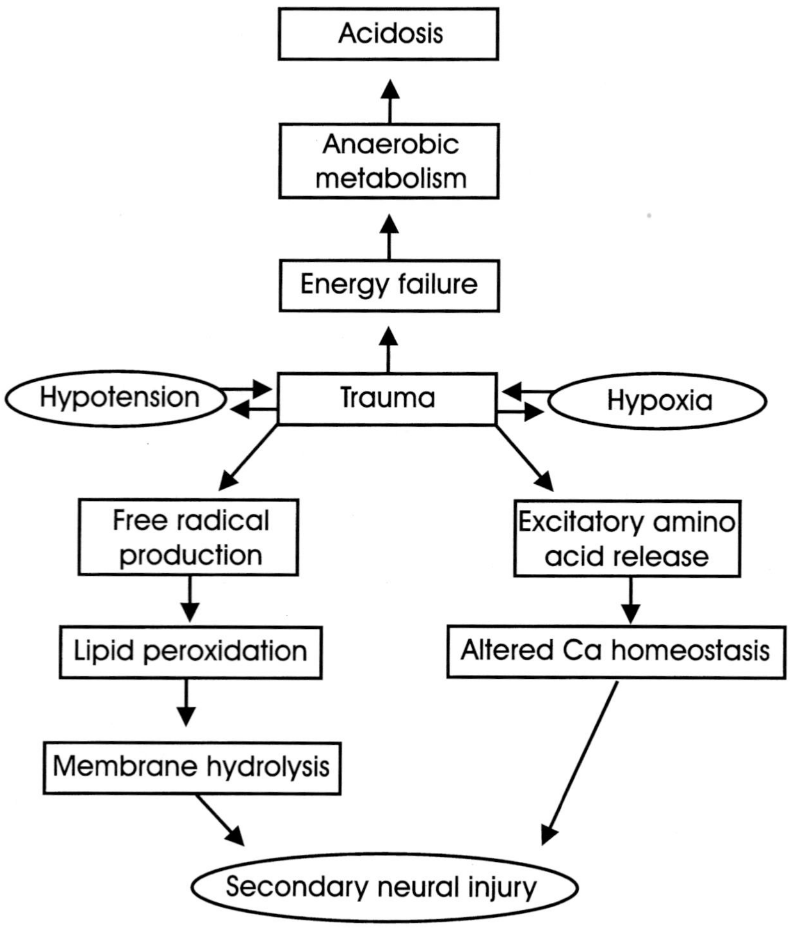

FIG. 24-1. Biochemical/molecular substrates of the secondary injury cascade.

(CT) scanning, possibly inpatient observation, and appropriate follow-up.

Clinical Considerations

Head injury is frequently associated with skull fracture. When associated with severe HI, linear fractures have little practical significance. However, with mild HI, the presence of a skull fracture increases the risk of an intracranial abnormality by as much as fourfold (10). Basilar skull fracture may be complicated by cerebrospinal fluid (CSF) leak, infection, and/or cranial nerve palsies, and generally warrants closer clinical monitoring than linear skull fracture. The exception to this is in infants and young children in whom linear fractures may be complicated by leptomeningeal cysts or "growing" skull fractures. When such occurs, a mass may develop over the fracture site as CSF collects from a disruption of the arachnoid underlying the injury. Such cysts always require surgical correction. Thus, it is important to follow young children for several months after linear fractures to be vigilant for this possible occurrence.

Epidural hematomas may complicate HI. The classically described lucid interval associated with this entity is currently rarely seen as most patients are unconscious from the time of injury. Most epidural hematomas require immediate surgical intervention; however, there are exceptions, particularly in alert pediatric patients (11).

Acute subdural hematomas occur in approximately 20% of severe HIs. Surgery within the first 4 hours after injury is generally associated with improved outcome; however, this basic tenet of HI management has been challenged (12,13).

Cerebral contusions are frequently associated with intracranial mass lesions, although they may occur as a result of the coup-contrecoup phenomenon, especially in the temporal and inferior frontal regions. Contusions per se rarely require surgical intervention; however, they necessitate careful clinical and CT follow-up as they may evolve into delayed posttraumatic intracerebral hematomas (14).

Diffuse axonal injury (DAI) is a frequent CT/pathologic correlate of severe HI and is usually associated with poor outcome (15). DAI is readily identifiable on CT as multiple punctate hemorrhages, typically in the deep white matter and corpus callosum and occasionally in the brainstem.

Approximately 10% to 15% of patients with clinically severe HI have a normal CT scan. In such situations, the possibility of extra- or intracranial vascular disruptions must be considered and angiography should be considered. Occasionally, magnetic resonance imaging (MRI) may demonstrate lesions not appreciated on CT in this setting.

ASSOCIATED DISORDERS

Approximately 5% to 10% of severe HI patients have an associated spine and/or spinal cord injury. Initial HI evaluation and management thus requires simultaneous evaluation and management of potential spinal injuries.

The majority of severe HI patients have multisystem injury. One must thus be continually alert for the possibility of other significant and potentially life-threatening injuries and establish treatment priorities accordingly.

Differential Diagnosis

Many nontraumatic disorders, such as drug or alcohol intoxication, metabolic disturbances, and subarachnoid or other types of intracranial hemorrhages, may mimic HI. Also, not infrequently a patient presents after an apparent traumatic event that itself was precipitated by primary underlying intracranial pathology, e.g., a stroke that causes loss of control while driving.

Evaluation

The primary evaluation of an HI patient necessitates a careful neurologic evaluation. However, since a significant number of these patients are multitraumatized, systemic evaluation and stabilization often takes precedence. The ABCs (airway, breathing, circulation) of trauma resuscitation must be followed [advanced trauma life support (ATLS)]. As noted previously, correction of hypoxia and hypotension has a significant impact on outcome from HI.

The neurologic evaluation of these patients is often complicated by many physical and iatrogenic factors. Severe ocular trauma may obviate examination of pupillary reflexes. Alcohol intoxication or the use of sedatives or muscle relaxants to facilitate patient transport adversely affects the neurologic findings. Extremity fractures limit the extent of the neurologic examination.

In spite of the above, the GCS has been the most reliable indicator of the severity of injury and deterioration or improvement. The initial GCS often influences early treatment decisions. Thus, an intimate familiarity with the examination essentials to establish the GCS is important (Table 24-2).

Once the GCS has been established, a more detailed neurologic exam can be pursued. Any laterality to the findings—e.g., a dilated pupil, hemiparesis—suggests a focal mass lesion. The higher the GCS, the more important a detailed mental status examination becomes in determining management.

For penetrating HI (GSW), there must also be a full and careful documentation of entry and exit wounds, evidence of powder burns, or the presence of any obvious foreign bodies.

In pediatric patients, the possibility of child abuse must be borne in mind, especially when the primary structural brain injury is subdural hematoma. When such concerns arise, there must be a careful systemic survey for evidence of other injuries—retinal hemorrhages, skin bruising, new and old long bone fractures.

The more severe the HI, the greater the urgency for CT

scanning as an integral part of initial evaluation. The only exception is when other life-threatening injuries take precedence. CT is not routinely indicated for minor HI. Similarly, if CT is going to be undertaken, there is no indication for plain skull radiographs.

Additional diagnostic evaluations such as MRI, cerebral angiography, and transcranial Doppler may be appropriate depending on clinical and/or CT findings.

Management

The management of minor HI is primarily directed toward a determination of the need for CT scanning and/or hospitalization for observation. Considerable effort has been expended to determine the risk of deterioration in this group of patients so that appropriate triage protocols might be established. A recent meta-analysis of a large number of series indicates that approximately 2.5% of patients presenting to emergency room with minor HI require neurosurgical intervention (16). This has led to current recommendations that only patients with a GCS score of 15 be discharged without prior CT scanning. Risk factors that must be taken into consideration when making this determination include palpable depressed skull fracture, seizures, extremes of age, persistent headache or vomiting, therapeutic anticoagulation, and suspected abuse. Unless there are significant associated extracranial injuries, it is rare for a minor HI to necessitate more than 24 hours of hospital observation.

Moderate HI is generally associated with significant symptoms and/or findings and necessitates CT scanning and hospitalization for serial neurologic monitoring. Repeat CT scanning is indicated if there is any deterioration in neurologic functioning. Delayed hematomas are occasionally seen after moderate HI. These usually represent bleeding into areas of contusion not well visualized initially and typically present 24 to 48 hours after injury (17).

A wide variety of potential sequelae must be considered after mild and moderate HI. Cochlear and vestibular dysfunction, delayed seizures, neuropsychologic impairments, and the postconcussion syndrome are examples. Persistent postconcussion symptoms have both a physiologic and a psychologic basis and include complaints such as headache, dizziness, difficulty concentrating, irritability, fatigue, and insomnia (18). Most of these problems can be dealt with by reassurance, education, and support. Occasionally, referral for rehabilitation services is appropriate.

The management of severe HI requires intensive support and monitoring. Since all of these patients are comatose, intubation and artificial ventilation is mandatory. Blood pressure monitoring and support is crucial. Monitoring via Swan-Ganz catheterization may be helpful. The first priority is complete and rapid physiologic resuscitation. Hypotension (systolic blood pressures less than 90 mm Hg) and hypoxia (Pa_{O_2} less than 60 mm Hg) should be avoided if possible, and corrected if present.

The institution of ICP monitoring remains somewhat controversial; however, ICP monitors are appropriate in this setting and provide the most reliable guide to treatment of the underlying brain injury. Additionally there are considerable data relating ICP to outcome (3,19). An appropriate threshold to begin aggressive ICP treatment appears to be 20 to 25 mm Hg.

Recently considerable interest has been focused on cerebral perfusion pressure (CPP) in treating severe HI (20). CPP is determined by subtracting the ICP from mean arterial blood pressure and represents the pressure driving cerebral blood flow. Thus, CPP and cerebral blood flow can be positively affected by either lowering ICP or elevating systemic blood pressure. It is generally felt that active attempts to maintain CPP above 70 mm Hg improve outcome.

The primary treatments for elevated ICP have traditionally included hyperventilation, diuretics, and, in extreme circumstances, barbiturates. If an ICP monitor is in place, the drainage of CSF may have significant therapeutic benefits. Care must be taken if hyperventilation is implemented as the cerebral vasoconstriction induced may produce ischemia. Thus Pa_{CO_2} levels lower than 25 mm Hg are rarely indicated. Mannitol is the primary diuretic used to control ICP. Effective doses range from 0.25 to 1.0 g/kg, typically given as intermittent boluses. Care must be taken to prevent hypernatremia and hyperosmolarity when giving frequent boluses.

High-dose barbiturate therapy is generally reserved for those situations in which ICP becomes refractory to other available therapies (21). There are, however, many potential complications, including cardiovascular instability, associated with barbiturate use, and extremely careful monitoring is absolutely necessary.

While steroids have been routinely used to treat severe HI, there are no data to support their use to either control ICP or impact on outcome (22). Their current use in this setting is thus discouraged.

Recent research has focused on attempting to identify neuroprotective agents to ameliorate secondary injury and thus improve outcome from severe HI. Two large-scale prospective randomized trials of the free radical scavengers Tirilazad and PEG-SOD (polyethelene glycol-superoxide dismutase) have been recently reported as showing no significant reductions in mortality or outcome. There are currently ongoing a number of trials with *N*-methyl-D-aspartate (NMDA)-receptor antagonists in an attempt to limit excitotoxicity.

PROGNOSIS

Minor HI is rarely associated with significant long-term sequelae. However, it is well established that a significant minority of patients will suffer chronic disability attributable to neurobehavioral sequelae (23). The exception to this is in sports-related minor HI in which death from the second impact syndrome or cognitive disability from cumulative concussions may occur. It has been well documented that

TABLE 24–3. *Guidelines for return to contact sports after minor head injury*

Concussion grade	First concussion	Second concussion	Third concussion
Grade 1—mild	May return when asymptomatic	May return in 3 weeks if asymptomatic for 1 week	Terminate season
Grade 2—moderate	May return when asymptomatic for 1 week	May return in 1 month if asymptomatic for 1 week	Terminate season
Grade 3—severe	May return in 1 month if asymptomatic for 1 week	Terminate season	

TABLE 24–4. *Current prognosis from severe head injury*

	Outcomes (%)				
Study	Good recovery	Moderate disability	Severe disability	Vegetative	Death
Tirilazad (n = 557)	44.8	19.6	14.4	21.4	
PEG-SOD (n = 162)	27	19	20	9	25

PEG-SOD, polyethelene glycol-superoxide dismutase.

fatal brain swelling may occur in the setting of one minor HI followed in short order by a second minor HI in athletes who are still symptomatic from the first injury (24). The cumulative effects of multiple minor HIs is recognized in boxing as the punch drunk syndrome; however, the occurrence of this type of syndrome in association with other sports is controversial.

For sports-related minor HI, it is thus important to establish firm guidelines such as those proposed by the Colorado Medical Society and promulgated by Cantu (25) for return to competition (Table 24-3).

Patients with moderate HI usually experience both cognitive and physical disabilities and typically require rehabilitation services after acute hospitalization. Nevertheless the incidence of severe long-term disability is small.

In contrast, few patients with severe HI recovery completely to their preinjury state. The most common system to rate recovery is the Glasgow Outcome Scale: good recovery (GR), moderate disability (MD), severe disability (SD), vegetative (V), and death (D) (26). The recently completed Tirilazad and PEG-SOD trials provide excellent information on current severe HI outcomes (Table 24-4).

REFERENCES

1. Miller JD, Becker DP. Secondary insults to the injured brain. *J R Coll Surg Edinb* 1982;27:292–298.
2. Chesnut RM, Marshall LF, Klauber MR, et al. The role of secondary brain injury in determining outcome from severe head injury. *J Trauma* 1993;34:216–222.
3. Marmarou A, Anderson RL, Ward JD, et al. Impact of ICP instability and hypotension on outcome in patients with severe head trauma. *J Neurosurg* 1991;75:S59–S66.
4. Hall ED, Yonkers PA, Andrus JK, et al. Biochemistry and pharmacology of lipid antioxidants in acute brain and spinal cord injury. *J Neurotrauma* 1992;19:S425–S442.
5. Braughler JM, Hall ED. CNS trauma and stroke. Biochemical considerations for oxygen radical formation and lipid peroxidation. *Free Radic Biol Med* 1989;6:289–301.
6. Siesjo B. The role of calcium in cell death. In: Price D, Aguayo A, Thoenen H, eds. *Neurodegenerative disorders: mechanisms and prospects for therapy.* London: Wiley, 1991:35–59.
7. Bullock R, Fujisawa H. The role of glutamate antagonists for the treatment of CNS injury. *J Neurotrauma* 19:S443–S46.
8. Lobosky JF. Epidemiology of head injury. In: Narayan R, Wilberger JE, Povlishok J, eds. *Neurotrauma.* New York: McGraw-Hill, 1996, 116–139.
9. Rimel RW, Giordani B, Barth JT. Disability caused by minor head injury. *Neurosurgery* 1981;9:221–229.
10. Masters SJ, McClean PM, Arcarese JS, et al. Skull x-ray examination after head trauma: recommendations by a multidisciplinary panel and validation study. *N Engl J Med* 1987;316:84–91.
11. Pang DA, Horton JA, Herron JM. Nonsurgical management of extradural hematomas in children. *J Neurosurg* 1983;59:958–971.
12. Seelig JM, Becker DP, Miller JD, et al. Traumatic acute subdural hematoma. Major mortality reduction in comatose patients treated within four hours. *N Engl J Med* 1981;304:1511–1518.
13. Wilberger JE, Harris M, Diamond DL. Acute subdural hematoma: morbidity, mortality and operative timing. *J Neurosurg* 1991;74:212–218.
14. Sprick C, Bettag M, Bock WJ. Delayed traumatic intracranial hematomas—clinical study of seven years. *Neurosurg Rev* 1989;12:228–230.
15. Wilberger JE, Rothfus W, Tabas J, et al. Tissue tear hemorrhages: CT and clinicopathologic correlations. *Neurosurgery* 1990;27:160–165.
16. Stein SC, Ross SE. Mild head injury: a plea for routine early CT scanning. *J Trauma* 1992;33:11–13.
17. Gudeman SK, Kishore PRS, Miller JD, et al. The genesis and significance of delayed traumatic intracerebral hematoma. *Neurosurgery* 1979;5:309–312.
18. Lishman WA. Physiogenesis and psychogenesis in the post concussional syndrome. *Br J Psychiatry* 1988;153:460–468.
19. Marshall LF, Gautile T, Klauber MR, et al. The outcome of severe closed head injury. *J Neurosurg* 1991;75:S28–S36.
20. Rosner MJ, Rosner SD, Johnson AH. Cerebral perfusion pressure: management protocol and clinical results. *J Neurosurg* 1995;83:949–962.
21. Eisenberg H, Frankowski R, Contant C, et al. High-dose barbiturate control of elevated intracranial pressure in patients with severe head injury. *J Neurosurg* 1988;69:15–23.
22. Braakman R, Schouten HJA, Blaauw-Van Dishoeck M, Minderhoud JM. Megadose steroids in severe head injury. *J Neurosurg* 1983;58:326–330.
23. Levin HS, Gary HE, Eisenberg HM, et al. Neurobehavioral outcome one year after severe head injury: experience of the traumatic coma data bank. *J Neurosurg* 1990;73:699–709.

24. Saunders RL, Harbaugh RE. The second impact in catastrophic contact sports head trauma. *JAMA* 1984;252:538–539.
25. Cantu RC. Guidelines to return to contact sports after cerebral concussion. *Phys Sports Med* 1986;14:79–82.
26. Jennett B, Snoek J, Bond MR, et al. Disability after severe head injury: observations on the use of the Glasgow Outcome Scale. *J Neurol Neurosurg Psychiatry* 1981;44:285–293.

SELECTED READINGS

Cooper PR. *Head injury,* 3rd ed. Baltimore: Williams & Wilkins, 1993.
Jordan BD, Tsairis P, Warren RF. *Sports neurology.* Rockville, MD: Aspen, 1989.
Narayan R, Wilberger JE, Povlishok J, eds. *Neurotrauma.* New York: McGraw-Hill, 1996.

Neurosurgical Issues in Otolaryngology: Principles and Practice of Collaboration,
edited by Moisés A. Arriaga and J. Diaz Day.
Lippincott Williams & Wilkins, Philadelphia © 1999.

CHAPTER 25

Facial Disassembly

Ivo P. Janecka

INDICATIONS

The seriousness of neoplastic involvement of the cranial base warrants appropriate therapeutic measures. As with most tumors, the control of the primary site is one of the most important determinants of the ultimate outcome of treated patients. Three-dimensional tumor resection with histologically clear margins is the primary goal of cranial base oncologic surgery. For example, the paranasal sinuses and orbits have a well-defined bony perimeter that, in localized tumors, permits en bloc resection of anatomically contained neoplasms. This has to be balanced, however, with an acceptable functional and aesthetic morbidity. Gross central nervous system involvement or internal carotid encasement in a patient with poor collateral cerebral circulation is considered a relative contraindication to oncologic surgery. However, numerous technical advances continually refocus our indications for surgery. Growth outside the natural bony margins of the primary neoplastic site poses great surgical challenges and is an indication of greater biologic aggressiveness of the tumor. The possibility of incorporating a normal cranial base as an additional tumor margin in such cases increases the possibility of surgical control of the primary tumor.

Two basic principles, well utilized in other surgical areas, are applicable to cranial base surgery: (a) *Simplicity.* Even in complex cranial base surgery, simplicity and proper sequential logic of the procedural steps should be a high priority. The surgical approach, tumor extirpation, and defect reconstruction must be anatomically as well as physiologically related to achieve the best result. (b) *Exposure.* It is essential that adequate surgical access to the skull base lesion be achieved to allow complete tumor removal or defect correction with preservation of uninvolved anatomic structures. In particular, the blood supply to the overlying skin and surrounding muscles has to be respected during exposure and tumor resection in order to have adequate and viable soft tissue available for reconstruction. The cranial nerves, if free of the neoplastic growth, are preserved or reconstructed following tumor removal.

Many questions can be raised regarding the indications for cranial base oncologic surgery and how it compares to major head and neck surgery:

- Is the biology of malignant tumors involving the cranial base different from those in the subcranial head and neck territory? At this time, there does not appear to be any difference. Sisson et al. (1) reported results with multimodality treatment of 60 patients with paranasal sinus cancer not treated with craniofacial resections (53% squamous cell carcinoma). Their 5-year survival was 49%. Our results with cranial base surgery for paranasal sinus cancer (2), at 40 months mean follow-up, showed survival of 74% and no evidence of disease (NED)/DOC (dead of other causes) status of 64%. This improvement likely reflects only technical factors (better control of posterior and superior margins) available with cranial base surgery and not different biology of neoplasms.
- Are complications more prevalent with cranial base surgery than with other head and neck procedures? The answer is probably no. Girod et al. (3) reported 63% incidence of complications with clean-contaminated head and neck cases (oropharynx-neck), which is higher than the complication rate with cranial base surgery.
- Is cranial base surgery beneficial as an oncologic treatment modality? The answer is still evolving, but the evidence to date suggests its benefits. Eibling et al. (4) reviewed the literature on outcomes in anterior skull base resections for squamous cell and undifferentiated carcinoma. They found 96 articles on craniofacial resection with a total of 425 patients. The 2-year disease-free survival in 89 eligible patients was 64%. The current results described in the literature support this finding with even longer follow-up (65% NED status at 5 years) (5).

I. P. Janecka: Harvard Medical School, Boston, Massachusetts 02115.

The evolutionary changes in indications for skull base surgery have been reflected in the expansion of surgical approaches to the skull base. The oncologic results have seen corresponding significant evolution. We have looked at the evolutionary record of cranial base surgery as related specifically to the indications and outcomes as reported in the literature (5).

We reviewed the results reported in the literature over the past 40 years in order to analyze the evolution of cranial base surgery and its contribution to the treatment of carcinomas and sarcomas. We have designated three periods of time that reflect the advancing indications and impact of skull base surgery and have summarized the outcomes of the major contributors in each era. The pioneers of the first period (1960s–1970) achieved 3- and 5-year survivals of 52% and 49% while attempting resection of tumors without intracranial or pterygopalatine extension. In the second period (1970s–1980), improved surgical techniques allowed resection of more extensive tumors including intracranial invasion, and 3-year survivals rose to 57% to 59% with limited reports of 5-year survivals in the range of 49%. The third period of cranial base surgery (1980s–1995) brought further expansion of indications and refinement of techniques. It also introduced the concept of a coordinated multispecialty approach. This combination resulted in increased 5-year survivals of 56% to 70%.

The combined transcranial approaches to tumors encroaching on the skull base arose from previous inadequate attempts at surgical extirpation using only extracranial or intracranial procedures. The standard lateral rhinotomy provided sufficient exposure to perform maxillectomy, partial ethmoidectomy, and even orbital exenteration to resect nasal or paranasal sinus tumors encroaching on the skull base. Those procedures, however, did not permit complete and safe resection of tumors breaching the cribriform and fovea ethmoidalis. Classic attempts at surgical removal of such tumors often left residual disease. Cranial base surgery attempted to provide a safer and complete three-dimensional en bloc resection.

The combined cranial base approaches incorporate modifications of neurosurgical and head and neck procedures. The result is not only a more rational treatment from an oncologic viewpoint, but also a safer procedure in that direct visualization of the tumor and intracranial contents is achieved. This team concept of combined surgical procedures goes beyond traditional boundaries of the head and neck surgeon and neurosurgeon. It necessitates the creation of multispecialty teams that also include the radiologist, anesthesiologist, plastic and reconstructive surgeons, pathologist, and radiation oncologist. Since the beginning of cranial base surgery, substantial progress from a diagnostic and operative standpoint has occurred. Improved diagnostic imaging with computed tomography (CT) (6) and magnetic resonance imaging (MRI) (7) has provided specific and anatomically detailed views of skull base bony structures such as the cribriform plate and neural foramina and allows assessment of dural and intracranial tumor extension. These valuable radiographic data enable the surgeon to accurately plan the extent of surgical resection. It also provides important prognostic information that can be discussed with the patient preoperatively so that realistic expectations and the possible need for adjuvant therapy can be established.

To achieve the en bloc goal that is fundamental to surgical oncology, the skull base surgeon may need to resect anatomic units. For example, the anterior skull base resection may include the cribriform plate, bilateral ethmoid labyrinths, frontal sinus, the involved dura and brain, and the anterior aspect of the sphenoid sinus (8). The orbit and maxillary sinus are often incorporated into the specimen as well (9). Although the combined intra- and extracranial approach allows such resections in a controlled fashion, the procedure is not complete without adequate reconstruction of the remaining defect. The cranial base surgeon needs to address the open communication between the intra- and extracranial compartments as well as the loss of facial skeleton and bony orbital support for the eye. Previously, skull base reconstruction and facial restoration entailed multistaged operations over many months, which may have prevented timely use of radiation or other adjuvant therapy and added substantial psychologic stress to the patient and family (10). The development of a one-stage approach to reconstruction with the option of using the pericranial, temporal muscle, and free tissue flaps has substantially improved the reconstructive efforts and decreased the associated morbidity of skull base procedures (10–13).

This chapter discusses the evolution of cranial base surgery from its inception to the current level of thought and techniques. The surgical and overall treatment results from the representative authors of the early, middle, and current eras (designated first, second, and third periods) have been categorized and standardized for comparison. Throughout the eras, greater indications, improved outcomes, and reduced morbidity have emerged. These advances correlate with the establishment of the team approach to solid tumors of the skull base. Also, the contraindications, limitations, and complications of the evolving procedures are discussed along with an emphasis on the importance of adequate primary tumor resection and reconstruction.

We reviewed the literature over the past 40 years to identify representative publications on surgery for malignant tumors of the cranial base. We then defined the three periods of advancement in skull base surgery and constructed summary tables for comparison of the most representative studies of each period.

Our focus was on skull base surgery for carcinomas and sarcomas. The publications that predominantly described other tumors such as esthesioneuroblastoma were excluded from this review (14,15). The contribution from these authors, however, is substantial and the reader is encouraged to review them. Also, studies that did not emphasize cranial base procedures were not considered. Nine publications describing the results of treatment on 466 patients were selected and the appropriate data was extracted from each of these papers for analysis.

FIRST PERIOD (1960s TO 1970)

After analyzing several of the initial reports of combined intra- and extracranial approaches to malignant skull base tumors, we found that Ketcham and Van Buren's team (16–18) emerged as the pioneers. A summary of their evolving experience with 54 patients from 1956 to 1973 is depicted in Table 25-1. The predominant tumors were squamous cell cancer (SCCA) and sarcoma, with smaller numbers of adenocarcinoma and adenoid cystic carcinoma. In this first period, tumors were designated inoperable if they extended intracranially or into the pterygopalatine fossa and were excluded from the reports. The extent of cranial base resection as a salvage procedure ranged from 47% to 68% in their earlier reports to an overall 78% in their final summary. Positive margins post–cranial base resection were reported to be as high as 47%.

It was difficult to accurately discern whether radiation was given as a primary modality for cure versus planned combined therapy; thus, for standardization of the data in all the tables, the number of patients receiving radiation includes primary, preoperative, and postoperative treatment collectively. Radiation was utilized in 61% of the patients in this period.

The number of complications in the first period was high. The most significant complications were selected for discussion and included infections, cerebrospinal fluid (CSF) leak, major bleeding, cerebrovascular accident (CVA), and mortality. Overall infection rate during this time frame was 54%, with 15% derived from meningitis or intracranial abscess and 19% derived from bone flap infection (4 of 10 patients required debridement and bone removal). CSF leak occurred in approximately one-third of all patients in this period; bleeding or CVA occurred in 11% of patients, and the overall perioperative mortality was reported as 4%.

In reviewing the outcome for this early period, 50% of patients displayed NED at a minimum of 30 months follow-up. Local control was reported at last follow-up, which ranged from 3 to 109 months (no mean stated) and was achieved in approximately 66% of patients. Distant metastases were not reported in the latest update by Ketcham and Van Buren, but their results from 1956 to 1968 listed a 34% incidence of distant metastasis. Three-year survival was estimated at 52%, but survival dropped somewhat to 49% upon following patients for 5 years.

SECOND PERIOD (1970s TO 1980)

The frequency and scope of cranial base surgery expanded in this second period. The experience of Van Tuyl and Gussack (19), Sisson et al. (20), and Cheesman and Lund et al.

TABLE 25–1. *First period (1960s–1970)*

	Ketcham and Van Buren et al. 1963		Ketcham and Van Buren et al. 1956–1968		Ketcham and Van Buren et al. 1973	
Number of patients	19		32		54	
Histology						
SCCA	7	37%	7	22%	17	31%
Sarcoma	7	37%	10	31%	14	26%
Adenocarcinoma	0	0%	3	9%	6	11%
Adenoid cystic CA	1	5%	0	0%	2	4%
Surgery						
Primary	6	32%	17	53%	12	22%
Salvage	13	68%	15	47%	42	78%
Margins positive	9	47%	N/A		17	31%
Radiation therapy	10	53%	N/A		33	61%
Complications						
Infections	4	21%	13	41%	27	54%
Meningitis/abscess	2	11%	4	13%	8	15%
Bone flap	1	5%	9	28%	10	19%
CSF leak	0	0%	15	47%	17	31%
CNS	1	5%	1	3%	6	11%
Deficit/bleeding perioperative mortality	1	5%	2	6%	2	4%
Results						
NED (30-month F/u)	(*n* = 17) 9	53%	(*n* = 30) 10	33%	27	50%
Local control at first F/U	13	68%	21	66%	N/A	
Distant metastases	6	32%	11	34%	N/A	
DOC	2	11%	2	7%	8	15%
Survival						
3 years	53%		56%		52%	
5 years	N/A		N/A		49%	

SCCA, squamous cell cancer; CA, cancer; CSF, cerebrospinal fluid; CNS, central nervous system; NED, no evidence of disease; F/U, follow up; DOC, died of other causes; N/A, not applicable.

TABLE 25–2. *Second period (1970s–1980)*

	Van Tuyl and Gussack 1979–1989		Sisson et al. 1970–1985		Cheesman et al. and Lund et al. 1978–1987	
Number of patients	21		60		92	
Histology						
SCCA	8	38%	32	53%	7	8%
Sarcoma	3	14%	4	7%	14	15%
Adenocarcinoma	2	10%	5	8%	25	27%
Adenoid cystic CA	0	0%	10	17%	9	10%
Surgery						
Primary	18	86%	58	97%	31	34%
Salvage	3	14%	0	0%	61	66%
Margins positive	N/A		N/A		N/A	
Radiation therapy	21	100%	53	85%	40	44%
Complications			N/A			
Infections	10	48%			4	4%
Meningitis/abscess	4	19%			2	2%
Bone flap	6	29%			2	2%
CSF leak	4	19%			3	3%
CNS	0	0%			5	5%
Deficit/bleeding perioperative mortality	1	5%			4	4%
Results						
NED (30-month F/U)	12	57%	22	37%	46	50%
Local control at first F/U	12	57%	28	47%	58	63%
Distant metastases	8	38%	3	5%	7	8%
DOC	0	0%	N/A		0	0%
Survival						
3 years	57%		N/A		59%	
5 years	N/A		49%		N/A	

(21,22) is summarized in Table 25-2. The major point of advancement in this era comes from the fact that surgeons operated on more extensive tumors than in the first period while maintaining similar complication rates and outcomes. Tumors with significant intracranial and even intracerebral extension as well as those entering the pterygopalatine fossa that were previously designated inoperable were now being resected. The most common histology again was SCCA, except in the English series (Cheesman and Lund) where adenocarcinoma predominated in a large population of woodworkers. Also, approximately 10% of the lesions in Cheesman and Lund's craniofacial series were benign, and the results of these specific cases could not be separated from the overall reported results. This factor must be considered when objectively interpreting their results as a representation of their experience with malignant tumors.

Salvage surgery in this period ranged from 0% to 66% and the extent of positive margins after surgical resection was not addressed. Radiation therapy was delivered at some point during the overall treatment in 44% to 100% of the patients.

Complications were not reported in Sisson's complete update, but his earlier studies on only eight patients receiving craniofacial resection reported infections in 50% of the patients with 38% requiring surgical bone debridement (23). Van Tuyl and Gussack also reported a high incidence of infections (48%), and CSF leaks occurred in 19% of their patients. Cheesman and Lund, however, reported much lower infection and CSF leak rates (4% and 3%) than the other authors in this period. Perioperative mortality was similar to that in the first period (4%–5%).

In a minimum 30-month follow-up exam, patients with NED ranged from 37% to 57%, and local control of disease at last follow-up ranged from 47% to 63%. The incidence of distant metastases varied widely from 5% to 38%. Three-year survival was reported at 57% to 59%, and only the series by Sisson et al. reported follow-up to 5 years with a survival of 49%.

THIRD PERIOD (1980s TO 1995)

In considering carcinomas of the skull base, the representative authors of the third period continued to approach more extensive malignant tumors, and a summary of their results is depicted in Table 25-3 (2). The skull base experience for malignant tumors for Janecka et al. contained mostly SCCA and sarcoma with smaller numbers of adenocarcinoma and adenoid cystic carcinoma. The experience of Shah et al. was composed of the above malignant histology in 54% of the cases, with the remaining patients having a mixture of malignant and benign tumors.

Salvage surgical procedures ranged from 44% to 63% and positive margins were noted in 21% to 43% of the cases. The use of radiation therapy at any time in the treatment course ranged from 66% to 100%. Complications in this third period dropped substantially. There was a 28% inci-

TABLE 25-3. *Third period (1980s–1995)*

	Shaw and Strong et al. 1974–1990		Janecka and Sekhar et al. 1987–1991		Janecka and Sekhar et al. 1994	
Number of patients	71		118		50	
Histology						
SCCA	11	15%	36	31%	13	26%
Sarcoma	15	21%	37	31%	18	36%
Adenocarcinoma	10	14%	7	6%	4	8%
Adenoid cystic CA	3	4%	16	14%	7	14%
Surgery						
Primary	40	56%	43	36%	23	46%
Salvage	31	44%	75	63%	27	54%
Margins positive	15	21%	51	43%	11	22%
Radiation therapy	47	66%	118	100%	50	100%
Complications						
Infections	20	28%	5	4%	0	0%
Meningitis/abscess	1	1%	1	1%	0	0%
Bone flap	9	13%	0	0%	0	0%
CSF leak	2	3%	5	4%	1	2%
CNS	4	6%	5	4%	3	6%
Deficit/bleeding perioperative mortality	2	3%	3	2%	0	0%
Results						
NED (30-month F/U)	37	52%	70	60%	30	60%
Local control at first F/U	50	70%	99	84%	41	82%
Distant metastases	18	25%	29	25%	5	10%
DOC	1	1%	7	6%	1	2%
Survival						
3 years	N/A		67%		74%	
5 years	56%		65%		70%	

dence of infection reported by Shah et al., and a 0% to 4% incidence of infection in the series by Janecka et al. Of the 239 patients in this last period, only two developed meningitis or intracranial abscess. The incidence of CSF leak ranged from 2% to 4%, bleeding or CVA occurred in 4% to 6%, and perioperative mortality diminished to 0% to 3% of the patients.

On last follow-up, the patients who maintained NED status ranged from 52% to 60% and local control was seen in 70% to 84% of cases. This improvement in local control is also reflected in the overall increased 3-year survival of 67% to 74% and 5-year survivals of 56% to 70%.

Over the last 40 years significant progress has been made in the field of cranial base surgery. The histology and extent of disease, approaches and surgical techniques, and levels of prior treatment vary among reports. However, an overall evolution of the outcomes is evident upon reviewing the representative series for each of three periods. In an attempt to standardize the reported results and allow comparison, we have categorized each of these series into three periods of advancement. We have tabulated the histology, surgical procedures, complications, and clinical results from the data that focused on carcinomas and sarcomas of the skull base. Based on this compilation of data, a template for recording cranial base cases and treatment outcomes (Table 25-4) has been designed and may be used by clinicians in their practice.

As depicted by the tables, the number of patients receiving cranial base procedures is growing substantially; however, the proportion of salvage and primary surgery has remained about the same. The overall incidence of primary surgery is approximately 50%, and this is unfortunate because the greatest benefit from cranial base surgery is as a primary oncologic treatment. Although not necessarily defined by the data presented in this work, the senior author's experience collectively demonstrates better outcomes after primary surgical resections of malignant skull base tumors (2).

The extent of reported positive margins and the clinical outcome in each of the papers reviewed do not necessarily correlate. This is likely a result of technical problems in assessing cut margins of fixed surgical specimens. Cranial base surgery involves a three-dimensional resection and usually contains multiple fragments or segments of bone. It is therefore very difficult for a pathologist to interpret margins in such a specimen. In general, the adequacy of oncologic margins must be interpreted clinically at the time of resection by the primary surgeon. In an attempt to incorporate a team approach and improve the accuracy of margin assessment, we now ask the pathologist to come to the operating suite, and we orient the specimen and review the surgical defect together.

It is difficult to interpret the usefulness of radiation because the majority of salvage cases had received radiation as part of the original primary treatment. The response to radiation therapy in the salvage cases must therefore be inter-

TABLE 25–4. *Cranial base case record*

Patient initials/SS or ID#:										
Follow-up	1 yr	2 yr	3 yr	4 yr	5 yr	6 yr	7 yr	8 yr	9 yr	10 yr
Histology (circle one)										
SCCA										
Sarcoma										
Adenocarcinoma										
Adenoid cystic CA										
Other										
Surgery date										
Primary										
Salvage										
Margins: positive/negative										
Adjuvant Therapy										
Preop radiation										
Postop radiation										
Chemotherapy										
Complications										
Infections										
Meningitis/abscess										
Bone flap										
CSF leak										
CNS deficit/bleeding										
Perioperative mortality										
Results										
NED										
Recurrence										
Local										
Regional										
Distant										
Died other causes										
Died of disease										
Survival summary										

Notes:

preted as a failure. The use of radiotherapy as a combined modality versus surgery alone was not specifically and objectively addressed by any study and so no conclusions can be drawn with respect to efficacy. Until controlled, randomized trials on the use of radiation in the treatment of cranial base solid tumors are performed, the true benefit will remain unclear.

There has been a trend toward lower complications in cranial base surgery especially when considering the incidence of meningitis, bone flap infections, and the occurrence of postoperative CSF leaks. We postulate that improved reconstructive techniques and the use of well-vascularized local flaps (pericranial, temporalis muscle) or microvascular flaps are the reasons for this decrease. The incidence of neurologic complications such as CVA and intracranial bleeding as well as perioperative mortality has remained about the same to slightly decreased despite the resection of more advanced and invasive disease as reported in the third period.

The number of patients with no evidence of disease and who have local tumor control has also improved in the recent reports with the more aggressive surgical resections. In the designated third period of cranial base surgery, 70% to 84% of patients achieved local control of their disease, and this benefit is reflected in the substantially higher survival rates. The need for adequate surgical resection and local control of the tumor is thus not only important to reduce mortality, but also imperative to extend survival.

The concept of contraindications for performing cranial base surgery has also changed over the past 40 years. Initially, tumors extending intracranially or into the pterygopalatine regions were designated unresectable (16–18,24). With improved surgical techniques and the formation of a surgical team, intracranial and infratemporal fossa invasion are now not considered contraindications to surgery (24–26). However, there are levels of disease that warrant reconsideration of surgical intervention. Tumor involvement of the carotid artery is in itself not a contraindication, but specifically the invasion into or surrounding the dominant carotid system should preclude surgical attempts in most cases. Currently, general contraindications include bilateral optic nerve or chiasm involvement and substantial invasion into the dominant temporal lobe.

The histology of the tumors is also very important when making a decision on resectability. For aggressive tumors such as squamous cell carcinomas, undifferentiated tumors, sarcomas, and melanomas, the need for adequate surgical margins is well known, and so involvement of critical intracranial structures such as the cavernous sinus should still be considered contraindications to surgery. However, a tumor such as adenoid cystic carcinoma is generally perceived to be slower growing with associated longer survivals even in the presence of recurrent or persistent disease. Surgical resections of such tumors that may result in close margins in the cavernous sinus or around critical cranial nerves may provide longer survival and improved morbidity.

The age and overall health of the patient is also critical when determining the extent of surgery. The elderly population, for example, has difficulty in tolerating deficits in the lower cranial nerves (27), and thus possible corrective procedures such as thyroplasty or arytenoid adduction should be incorporated into the surgical plan (28,29). Overall, the extent of surgery and the resulting CNS deficits must be balanced with the anticipated remaining quality of life.

Cranial base surgery is an important oncologic modality for the treatment of solid tumors at the skull base. Although the reported results to date are encouraging, future investigation into the effects of radiation therapy including brachytherapy or the gamma knife may further improve surgical results. As operative techniques are refined and new modalities of adjuvant therapy are studied, the frontiers of cranial base surgery should continue to advance.

TECHNIQUE

The facial translocation approach to the skull base is a valuable technique in skull base surgery, permitting partial or total facial disassembly. It has undergone a significant evolution since its original description in 1989 (30,31). Due to its modular design it permits great versatility and accommodates the surgical needs for limited as well as complex procedures at the skull base. The operative manipulation of cranial base anatomy and pathology, critical for oncologic surgery, can be tailored even more precisely to a specific skull base tumor. Maximum preservation and functional/aesthetic reconstruction of craniofacial anatomy is emphasized.

The intimate relationship of the skull base to the cranial as well as facial structures requires tissue displacement of one or both of these compartments to reach the desired section of the skull base. It is important to consider the effects of surgery on the normal but surgically manipulated tissues in order to select the most optimal approach. Any operative tissue displacement produces alterations in the anatomy and physiology of affected structures. Such changes have frequently variable consequences when they occur in the neural or facial viscerocranium. For example, facial swelling is usually self-limiting with minimal long-term consequences for the patient. Similar edema, however, may be very deleterious when it involves the neurocranium.

The current underlying principle of skull base approaches is to minimize brain retraction while maximizing skull base visualization. This concept facilitates three-dimensional tumors resection, tumor margin verification, and functional reconstruction with appropriate aesthetic concerns. The facial translocation approach to the skull base through its great versatility contributes to this goal.

In general, surgical treatment of lesions located anterior to the neuroaxis should be done through an anterior approach. This requires selection of a transfacial approach because of the anteroinferior anatomic relationship of the facial viscerocranium to the cranial base.

In the past, several surgeons worked on achieving additional oncologic exposure of the facial viscerocranium. Barbosa (32) expanded exposure for the treatment of maxillary sinus cancer and Altemir (33) did the same for the nasomaxillary area access.

Modular craniofacial disassembly is the principle of the facial translocation approach to the skull base (Fig. 25-1). It is based on creation of composite facial units that are designed along key neurovascular anatomy and aesthetic lines. The individual units merge into larger composites without compromising their function. It is possible to attach eponyms to the technical variations of facial translocation for ease of communication and comparison. Thus we can recognize "mini," "standard," "expanded" (vertically, medially, posteriorly), and "bilateral" facial translocation procedures. Complementary craniotomies or craniectomies are added to these approaches as necessary to assist with three-dimensional tumor resection.

Mini–facial translocation—central is designed to reach the medial orbit, sphenoid and ethmoid sinus, and the inferior clivus. The port of entry is through the displaced ipsilateral nasal bone, the nasal process of the maxilla, and the medial orbital rim (with an attached medial canthal ligament, the lacrimal duct, and skin). The skin incision is made along the lateral aspect of the nose and the inferior aspect of the eyebrow with triangular design at the level of the medial canthal ligament. Osteotomies create a rectangular pattern with a lateral extent being just medial to the inferior orbital nerve. The entire unit is displaced laterally for surgical exposure. Closure is accomplished with replacement of this composite unit (skin, bone, mucosa). Rigid fixation of the bone is accomplished with microplating. The perimeter of this approach can be further augmented with endoscopic instrumentation.

Mini–facial translocation—lateral opens the infratemporal fossa. The incisions run from the inner canthus horizontally in the inferior fornix of the eyelid through the lateral canthus to the preauricular area. Here it joins vertical temporal and preauricular incisions. The frontal branches of the facial nerve are temporarily disconnected. The temporalis muscle is reflected inferiorly following displacement of the zygomatic arch/malar eminence. The head of the mandible may be either displaced or resected.

Standard facial translocation achieves surgical access to

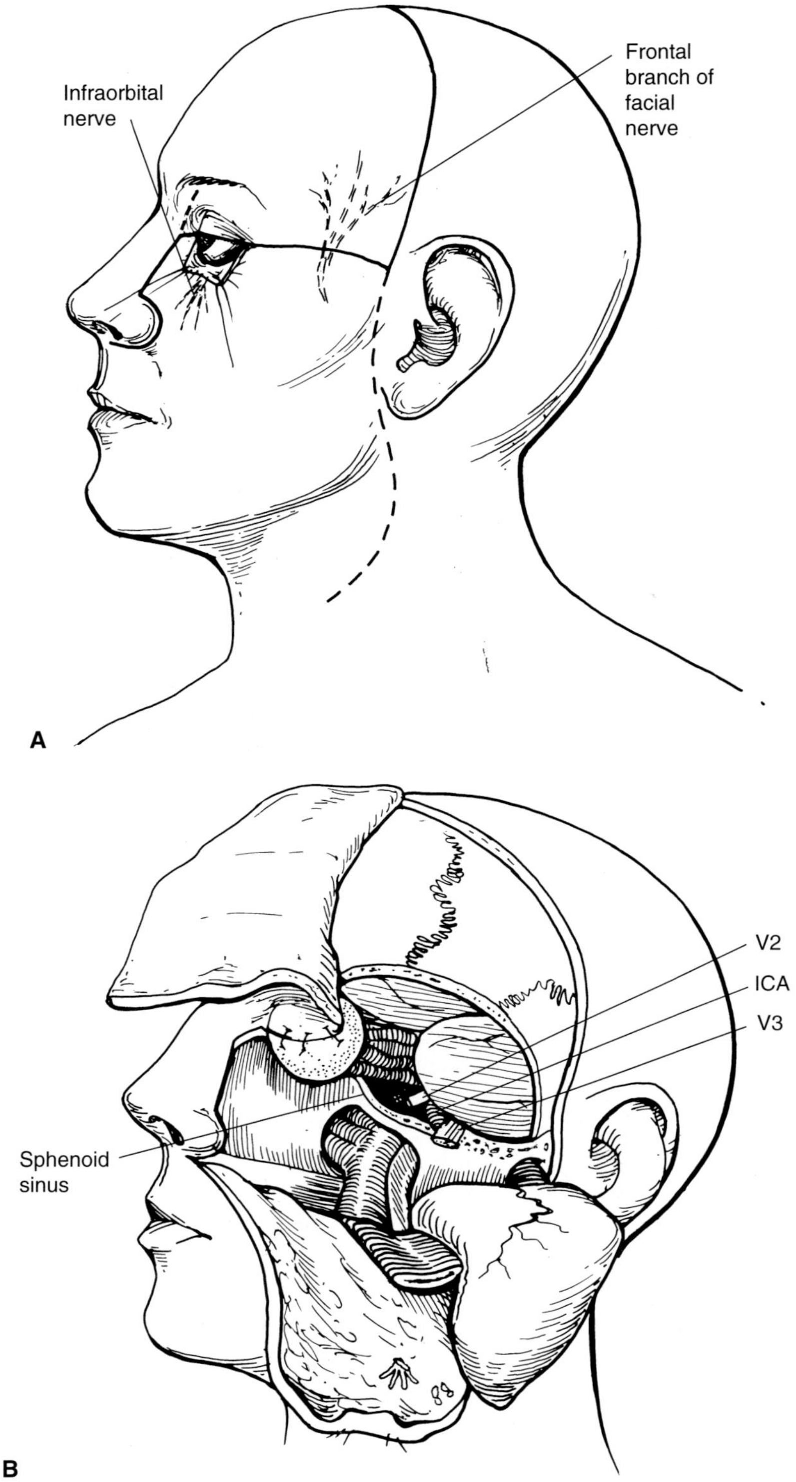

FIG. 25-1. **A**: Schema of standard facial translocation approach to skull base. **B**: Outline of surgical field.

the anterolateral skull base. The ipsilateral facial skin (including the lower eyelid) is displaced laterally and inferiorly with the underlying maxilla (with or without the hard palate). The nasal incision may extend inferiorly to include an upper lip split. The superior incision continues from the nose to the inferior fornix of the lower eyelid, and again through the lateral canthus horizontally to the preauricular area. In some cases (more anterior tumors) it is possible to conclude the horizontal incision about 1.5 cm beyond the lateral orbital rim after identifying and preserving the most anterior frontal branch of the facial nerve. This point then serves as the point of rotation of the displaced composite unit, which gives sufficient surgical space for some paracentral tumors. When the entire extent of the horizontal temple incision is needed, the frontal branches of the facial nerve are identified with a nerve stimulator, placed in silicone tubings and transected. During the reconstruction, these transected tubings are reconnected and the continuity of the facial nerve branches is reestablished. Osteotomies correlate to Le Fort I–II or the midpalatal lines when the entire maxilla is being displaced. The inferior orbital nerve is electively sectioned along the floor of the orbit, tagged, and repaired at the end of the procedure. Rigid fixation is achieved with mini- and microplates. With this technique of facial translocation, good exposure of the anterolateral skull base is achieved especially when the infratemporal fossa is involved as well.

Extended facial translocation—medial incorporates the standard translocation unit plus midfacial translocation unit (Fig. 25-2), the nose, and the medial half of the opposite face (up to the infraorbital nerve) with midline or paramedian incisions. It can be rotated at the Le Fort I level or include the ipsilateral palate and upper lip split. The skin incisions are similar to the standard technique, except that the paranasal incision is made on the contralateral side. The surgical exposure includes the ipsilateral infratemporal fossa and central and paracentral skull base bilaterally. The entire clivus is accessible as are the optic nerves, both precavernous internal carotid arteries, and the nasopharynx. The wide communication with the infratemporal fossa allows the placement of the temporalis muscle flap for vascularized reconstruction of the skull base defect. Bony fixation of craniofacial osteotomies is done with miniplates and a lag screw for the palate. The occlusal plane is reestablished with the help of an orthognathic splint. A palatal splint is attached to the maxillary dentition for additional stability and protection of the palatal incision. Temporary silicone intranasal stents are inserted as are bilateral lacrimal stents.

Extended facial translocation—medial and inferior includes the above procedure with an inferior extension via mandibular split. The lower lip incision is performed in a zigzag fashion to conform to the tension lines of the skin with an extension horizontally into the upper neck. Mandibular osteotomy is performed just medial to the mental foramen. Usually an interdental space is found wide enough to permit placement of a reciprocating saw for the osteotomy. This is performed is a step fashion, which then permits more stable reconstructive reapproximation of the bone. Prior to the osteotomy it is wise to select an appropriate miniplate for eventual fixation, contour it to the mandible, and create drill holes. This assists in the postoperative reestablishment of a normal occlusion. This extended translocation procedure adds a significant inferior as well as upper cervical surgical access.

Extended facial translocation—posterior incorporates the ear, temporal bone, and the posterior fossa into its surgical access. The horizontal temple incision of the standard translocation is extended posteriorly just above the external ear and curves inferiorly over the occipital bone to the neck. This provides access to the anterior as well as posterior aspect of the temporal bone with control of the key neurovascular structures.

Bilateral facial translocation combines complete right and left basic translocation units with or without palatal split. The exposure incorporates both infratemporal fossae, and the central and the entire paracentral skull base. Both distal cervical internal carotid arteries are in view as is the full clivus. The palatal split permits a reach to the level of C2-3. If further inferior extension is needed, a mandibular split can be added so a vertical reach to C3-4 is accomplished. A single temporalis muscle flap is sufficient for the coverage of the surgical defect at the skull base.

ADVANTAGES AND DISADVANTAGES

The advantages of transfacial approaches include the following:

1. Facial anatomy has developed through the embryonic fusion of nasofrontal, maxillary, and mandibular processes. Normally, the fusion takes place in the midline or in the paramedian region, thus logically presenting optimal lines of separation of facial units for a surgical approach, permitting the least traumatic displacement.
2. The primary blood supply to the facial units is through the external carotid system, which also has a lateral-to-medial direction of flow, thus ensuring viability of displaced surgical units.
3. The midface contains multiple hollow anatomic spaces (oronasal cavity, nasopharynx, paranasal sinuses) that facilitate the relative ease of surgical access to the central skull base.
4. Displacement of facial units for an approach to the cranial base offers much greater tolerance of postoperative surgical swelling, as opposed to similar displacement of the contents of the neurocranium.
5. Reestablishment of the normal anatomy, following repositioning of the facial units during the reconstructive phase of surgery, has a high degree of functional as well as aesthetic achievement.

Transfacial approaches also have disadvantages:

1. Contamination of the surgical wound with oropharyngeal bacterial flora.

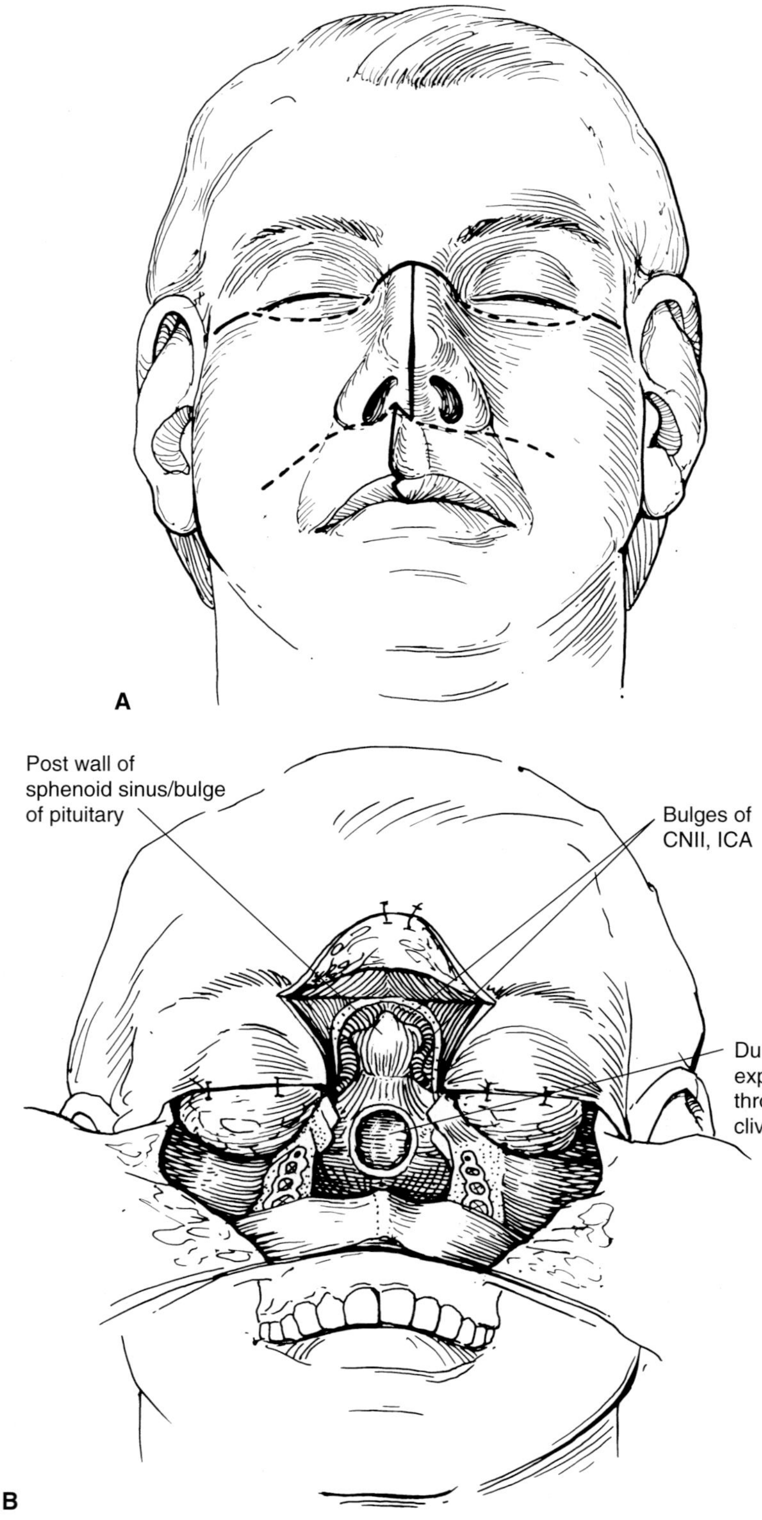

FIG. 25-2. A: Schema of midfacial split approach to skull base. **B**: Outline of surgical field.

2. The need for facial incisions with subsequent scar development.
3. Emotional considerations for the patient relate to surgical facial disassembly and the potential need for supplementary airway management (postoperative endotracheal intubation, temporary tracheostomy).

Postoperatively any potential complication may occur. Modular, fully vascularized disassembly adds considerable tolerance to the manipulated tissue. As composite (skin, bone, etc.) flaps/units, tissue has enhanced ability to heal and withstand postoperative adjuvant treatment. The full inclusion of the entire lacrimal draining system in the displaced tissue allows high probability of postoperative functioning system through the replanted nasolacrimal duct.

CONCLUSION

Facial disassembly through the translocation approach to the skull base has a modular design with composite facial units, which allows for systematic craniofacial disassembly. An improved oncologic visualization at the skull base is complemented by functional and aesthetic reconstruction.

ACKNOWLEDGMENTS

This chapter was adapted with permission from refs. 5,34–37.

REFERENCES

1. Sisson GA, Toriumi DM, Atiyah RA. Paranasal sinus malignancy: a comprehensive update. *Laryngoscope* 1989;99:143–150.
2. Janecka IP, Sen C, Sekhar L, Curtin H. Treatment of paranasal sinus cancer with cranial base surgery: results. *Laryngoscope* 1994;104: 553–555.
3. Girod DA, McCulloch TM, Tsue TT, Weymuller EA. Risk factors for complications in clean-contaminated head and neck surgical procedures. *Head and Neck* 1995;17(1):7–13.
4. Eibling DE, Janecka IP, Snyderman CH, Cass SP. Meta-analysis of outcome in anterior skull base resection for squamous cell and undifferentiated carcinoma. *Skull Base Surg* 1993;3(3):123–129.
5. O'Malley BW Jr, Janecka IP. Evolution of outcomes in cranial base surgery. *Semin Surg Oncol* 1995;11:221–227.
6. Curtin HD, Williams R, Johnson J. CT of the perineural tumor extension: pterygopalatine fossa. *AJR* 1985;144:163–169.
7. Som PM, Dillion WP, Sze G, et al. Benign and malignant sinonasal lesions with intracranial extension: differentiation with MR imaging. *Radiology* 1989;172:763–766.
8. Schramm VL, Myers EN, Maroon JC. Anterior skull base surgery for benign and malignant disease. *Laryngoscope* 1979;89:1077–1091.
9. Graamans K, Slootweg PJ. Orbital exenteration in surgery of malignant neoplasms of the paranasal sinuses. *Arch Otolaryngol Head Neck Surg* 1989;115:977–980.
10. Bridger GP, Baldwin M, Gonski A. Craniofacial resection for paranasal sinus cancer with free flap repair. *Aust NZ J Surg* 1986;56:843–847.
11. Johns ME, Winn HR, McLean WC, Cantrell RW. Pericranial flap for the closure of defects of craniofacial resection. *Laryngoscope* 1981; 91:952–955.
12. Stiernberg CM, Bailey BJ, Weiner RL, et al. Reconstruction of the anterior skull base following craniofacial resection. *Arch Otolaryngol Head Neck Surg* 1987;2:466–469.
13. Janecka IP, Sekhar LN. Reconstruction of base of skull surgical defects. In: Jackson CG, ed. *Surgery of skull base tumors*. New York: Churchill Livingstone, 1991:251–272.
14. Levine PA, Scher RL, Jane JA, et al. The craniofacial resection—eleven year experience at the University of Virginia: problems and solutions. *Otolaryngol Head Neck Surg* 1989;101:665–669.
15. McCaffrey TV, Olsen KD, Yohanan JM, et al. Factors affecting survival of patients with tumors of the anterior skull base. *Laryngoscope* 1994;104:940–945.
16. Ketcham AS, Wilkins RH, Van Buren JM, Smith RR. A combined intracranial facial approach to the paranasal sinuses. *Am J Surg* 1963; 10:698–703.
17. Van Buren JM, Ommaya AK, Ketcham AS. Ten years' experience with radical combined craniofacial resection of malignant tumors of the paranasal sinuses. *Neurosurgery* 1968;28:341–350.
18. Ketcham AS, Chretien PB, Van Buren JM, et al. The ethmoid sinuses: a re-evaluation of surgical resection. *Am J Surg* 1973;126:469–476.
19. Van Tuyl R, Gussack GS. Prognostic factors in craniofacial surgery. *Laryngoscope* 1991;101:240–244.
20. Sisson GA, Toriumi DM, Atiyah RA. Paranasal sinus malignancy: a comprehensive update. *Laryngoscope* 1989;99:143–150.
21. Cheesman AD, Lund VJ, Howard DJ. Craniofacial resection for tumors of the nasal cavity and paranasal sinuses. *Head Neck Surg* 1986;July/ Aug:429–435.
22. Lund VJ, Harrison DFN. Craniofacial resection for tumors of the nasal cavity and paranasal sinuses. *Am J Surg* 1988;156:187–190.
23. Sisson GA, Bytell DE, Becker SP, Ruge D. Carcinoma of the paranasal sinuses and cranial-facial resection. *J Otolaryngol Laryngol* 1976;90: 59–68.
24. Donald PJ. Recent advances in paranasal sinus surgery. *Head Neck Surg* 1981;4:146–153.
25. Sekhar LN, Moller AR. Operative management of tumors involving the cavernous sinus. *J Neurosurg* 1986;64:879–889.
26. Sekhar LN, Burgess J, Atkin O. Anatomical study of the cavernous sinus emphasizing operative approaches and related vascular and neural reconstruction. *Neurosurgery* 1987;21:806–816.
27. Poe DS, Jackson G, Glasscock ME, Johnson GD. Long-term results after lateral cranial base surgery. *Laryngoscope* 1991;101:372–378.
28. Netterville JL, Vrabec. Unilateral palatal adhesion for paralysis after high vagal injury. *Arch Otolaryngol Head Neck Surg* 1994;120: 218–221.
29. Netterville JL, Civantos FJ. Rehabilitation of cranial nerve deficits after neurotologic skull base surgery. *Laryngoscope* 1993;103:45–54.
30. Janecka IP. A new approach to the cranial base. In: *Proceedings of the XIV World Congress of Otolaryngology, Head and Neck Surgery,* Madrid, Spain, September 10–15, 1989. Amsterdam: Kugler & Ghedini, 1990.
31. Janecka IP, Sen CN, Sekhar LN, Arriaga M. Facial translocation: a new approach to the cranial base. *Otolaryngol Head Neck Surg* 1990; 103:413–419.
32. Barbosa J. Surgery of extensive cancer of paranasal sinuses. *Arch Otolaryngol* 1961;73:129.
33. Altemir FH. Transfacial access to the retromaxillary area. *J Maxillofac Surg* 1986;14:119–182.
34. Janecka IP. Surgical approaches to the skull base. In: *Neuroimaging clinics of North America: the base of skull.* Weber AL, ed. WB Saunders. Philadelphia: November 1994, 639–657.
35. Janecka IP. Transfacial approaches to the skull base. In: Myers EN, ed. *Operative otolaryngology.* Philadelphia: WB Saunders, 1997.
36. Janecka I. Classification of facial translocation approach to the skull base. *Otolaryngology Head Neck Surg* 1995:112, 579–585.
37. Janecka IP. Cranial base surgery: results. *Otolaryngology Head Neck Surg* 1994:110, 539–546.

Neurosurgical Issues in Otolaryngology: Principles and Practice of Collaboration,
edited by Moisés A. Arriaga and J. Diaz Day.
Lippincott Williams & Wilkins, Philadelphia © 1999.

CHAPTER 26

Optic Nerve Decompression

Joseph D. Ciacci and James P. Chandler

Ever since biblical times, when making the blind see was considered a divine intervention, healers have been called on to treat those who are losing their vision. Nothing is more terrifying to a patient than the loss of vision. The restoration or preservation of vision is the goal of surgical optic nerve decompression. The otolaryngologist frequently coordinates the care for these patients. The etiology of the compression of the optic nerve frequently involves intracranial extension or superomedial compression in the canal or orbit. In these cases, the neurosurgeon can assist the otolaryngologist in achieving the exposure necessary to accomplish adequate decompression. It must be stressed that exposure of the entire optic nerve may be necessary to ensure adequate decompression, and that this is best achieved via a combined approach.

ANATOMY

The optic nerve courses through anatomic territory that brings together several surgical subspecialties. It is not uncommon that a team including an ophthalmologist, otolaryngologist, plastic surgeon, and neurosurgeon participates in an optic nerve decompression procedure.

From the chiasm, the optic nerve travels intracranially in the subarachnoid space for about 15 mm and then into the orbit via the optic canal. The optic canal roof is formed by the lesser wing of the sphenoid bone. The inferolateral border of the canal is formed by the optic strut. The sphenoid sinus and ethmoid air cells form the medial border of the canal. The length of the optic canal ranges from 4 to 10 mm with a width of approximately 4.5 mm and a height of about 5 mm. The orbit is a pyramid whose apex is the optic canal and the superior orbital fissure. The frontal bone is the orbital roof and its floor is formed by the maxilla and zygoma. The maxilla, ethmoid bone, and lacrimal bone form the medial border. The lateral border is formed by the greater wing of the sphenoid and the zygoma (Figs. 26-1–26-3). In the orbit, the optic nerve is covered by pia arachnoid and dura. The annulus of Zinn loops around the nerve and in a portion of the apex forms the oculomotor foramen. The optic nerve is vascularized predominantly by the ophthalmic branch of the internal carotid artery. The ophthalmic artery enters the orbit via the optic canal traveling inferolateral to the nerve in the canal. In the orbit, the optic nerve is vascularized by pial ciliary arteries.

J. D. Ciacci: Department of Neurological Surgery, The Johns Hopkins Hospital, Baltimore, MD 21229.

J. P. Chandler: Department of Neurological Surgery, Northwestern Memorial Hospital, Chicago, Illinois 60611.

CLINICAL WORKUP

Compression of the optic nerve throughout its course can be the result of a variety of pathologies. The common denominator in terms of symptomatology is loss of visual acuity. The nature of the pathology determines the acuity of onset of visual loss, as well as associated symptoms. A thorough history and physical examination frequently directs the physician to the optic nerve as the anatomic location of the pathology along the visual pathway. The appropriate imaging studies such as magnetic resonance imaging (MRI) and computed tomography (CT) then elucidate the precise location of a lesion compressing the optic nerve. The nature of the lesion and its location along the nerve determine the indications for optic nerve decompression and define the appropriate surgical approach.

ETIOLOGY

Trauma

> Dimness of vision occurs in injuries to the brow.
> —Hippocrates.

Closed head injuries and maxillofacial trauma can cause visual loss by compression of the optic nerve by bone fragments, hematoma, and/or edema. Traumatic optic neuropa-

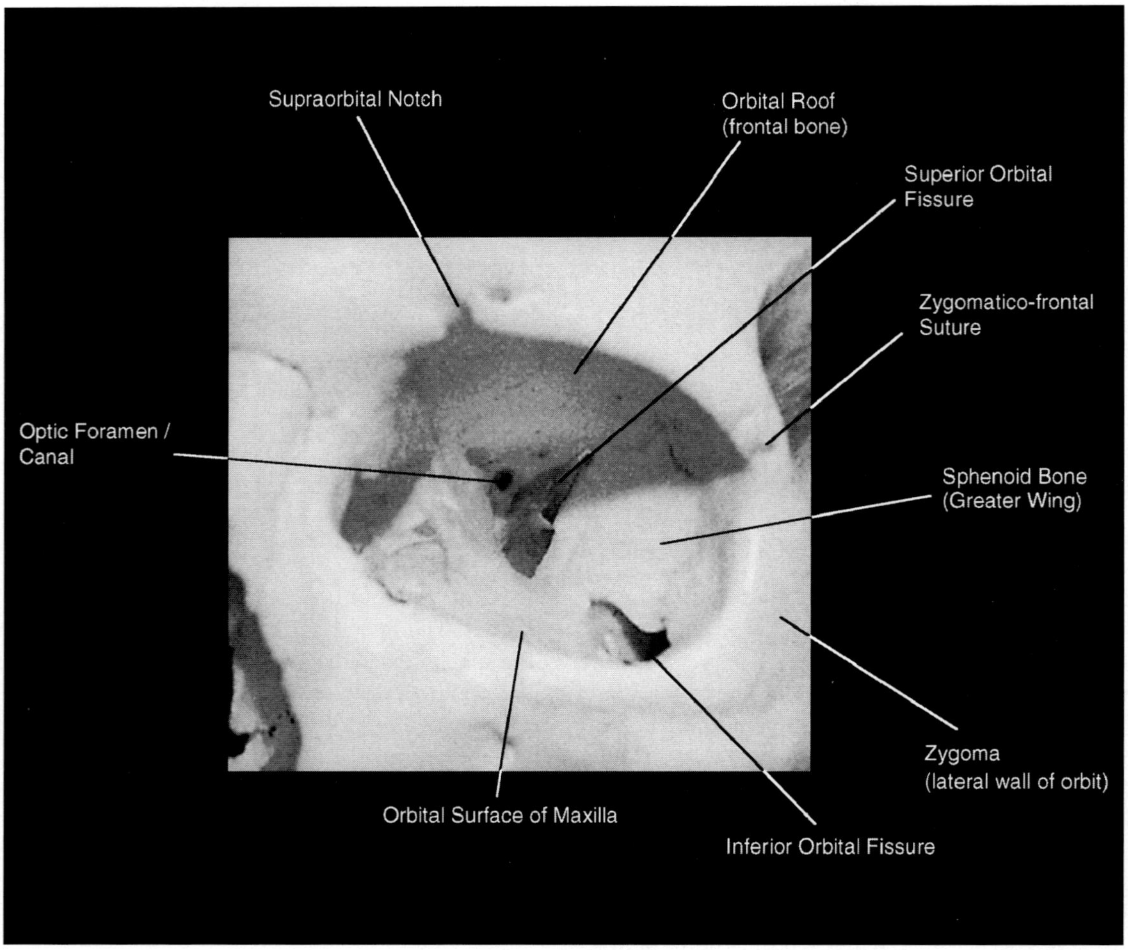

FIG. 26-1. Anatomy of the bony orbit.

thy is an infrequent but significant sequela of head trauma. Between 2% and 4% of patients with head trauma present with traumatic optic neuropathy. Most frequently this involves injury to the intracanalicular portion of the optic nerve. Management of these injuries by surgical optic nerve decompression is controversial. Early treatment with high-dose steroids is often recommended as the treatment of choice (1–6).

Indications

Once again the history and physical exam are indispensable in defining the role for surgical decompression. The finding of an afferent pupillary defect with a normal funduscopic exam points to the optic nerve as the site of injury in trauma. Imaging studies then can help confirm compression at the optic canal. The rapidity of onset and extent of visual loss are important factors. Some authors suggest that patients with instantaneous and complete loss of vision at the time of injury have a poor prognosis regardless of intervention. Surgical decompression is indicated in patients with compressive lesions in whom loss of vision progresses despite steroids.

Approach

The otolaryngologist is frequently on the front line in facial trauma. Not infrequently, these traumas involve facial fractures and isolated optic nerve compression in the optic canal without associated intracranial injury. The otolaryngologist has in his armamentarium several transfacial/transnasal approaches to the optic canal for optic nerve decompression. They include the transethmoid, lateral facial approach, and combined transconjunctival/intranasal endoscopic approach. These approaches are briefly mentioned here; they have been elegantly described in detail in the otolaryngology literature (7–9).

These approaches are accomplished without craniotomy and the associated morbidity. Exposure is limited; therefore, preoperative assessment and imaging is critical. If the pathology extends beyond the medial optic canal and/or intracranially, the transcranial approaches are indicated.

Once the decision has been made to attempt surgical decompression, the surgical approach must be carefully selected. Factors that influence this choice include location and severity of associated injuries, anatomic location of the compression, and the experience of the team of surgeons.

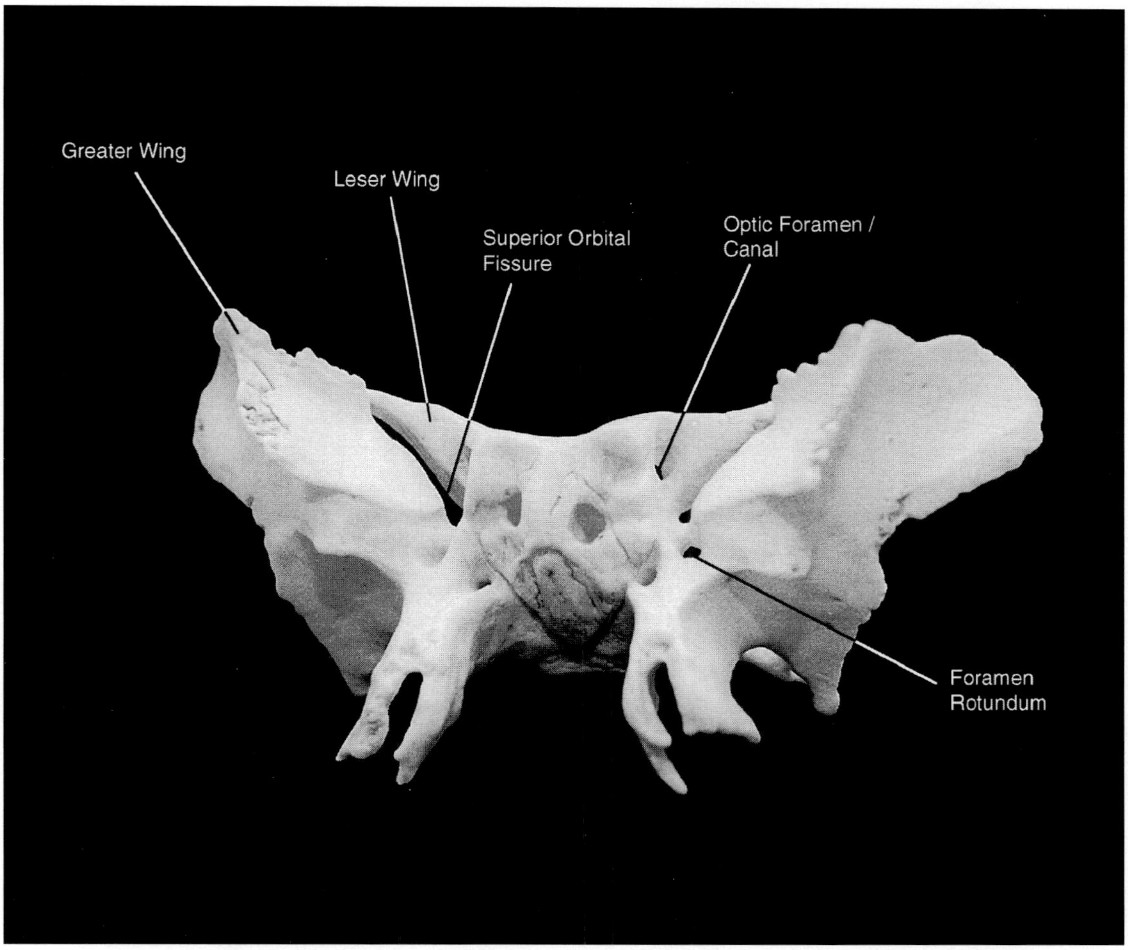

FIG. 26-2. The sphenoid bone.

The presence of associated intracranial injuries such as hematomas, contusions, and depressed fractures may indicate the need for neurosurgical intervention and craniotomy.

Tumors

Tumors frequently cause optic nerve compression and affect visual acuity. They most commonly arise from the optic nerve itself or from structures in and around the orbit and optic canal. These tumors may also present with exophthalmos and/or cranial nerve III, IV, and VI palsy-related diplopia. Anatomically, tumors causing optic nerve compression are usually located within the muscle cone or within the optic canal (Table 26-1).

Indications

Thorough history and physical examination will usually exclude nonneoplastic etiologies of visual loss. Imaging with CT and MRI helps define anatomically the presence of a mass lesion. From a technical standpoint, the vast majority of tumors causing optic nerve compression can be reached via the surgical approaches described in this chapter. Acuity of onset and extent of visual loss are important considerations in surgical decision making. Pathology and prognosis, when known, are important considerations. The availability of effective adjuvant therapies such as chemotherapy, radiation, and radiosurgery is relevant as well. Steroids are often an effective medical adjunct in the management of patients with neoplasm.

Approach

In the case of neoplasms perhaps more than any other etiology of optic nerve compression, the neurosurgeon can be an indispensable ally to the otolaryngologist. These tumors may involve intracranial extension and/or direct involvement of central nervous system elements. With tumors, the goals of surgery must include maximum cytoreduction as well as decompression. The extended exposure obtained by a collaborative effort between the otolaryngologist and the neurosurgeon is well suited for this purpose.

FIBROUS DYSPLASIA

Fibrous dysplasia is a congenital disorder of bone metabolism that can affect the anterior cranial base, resulting in

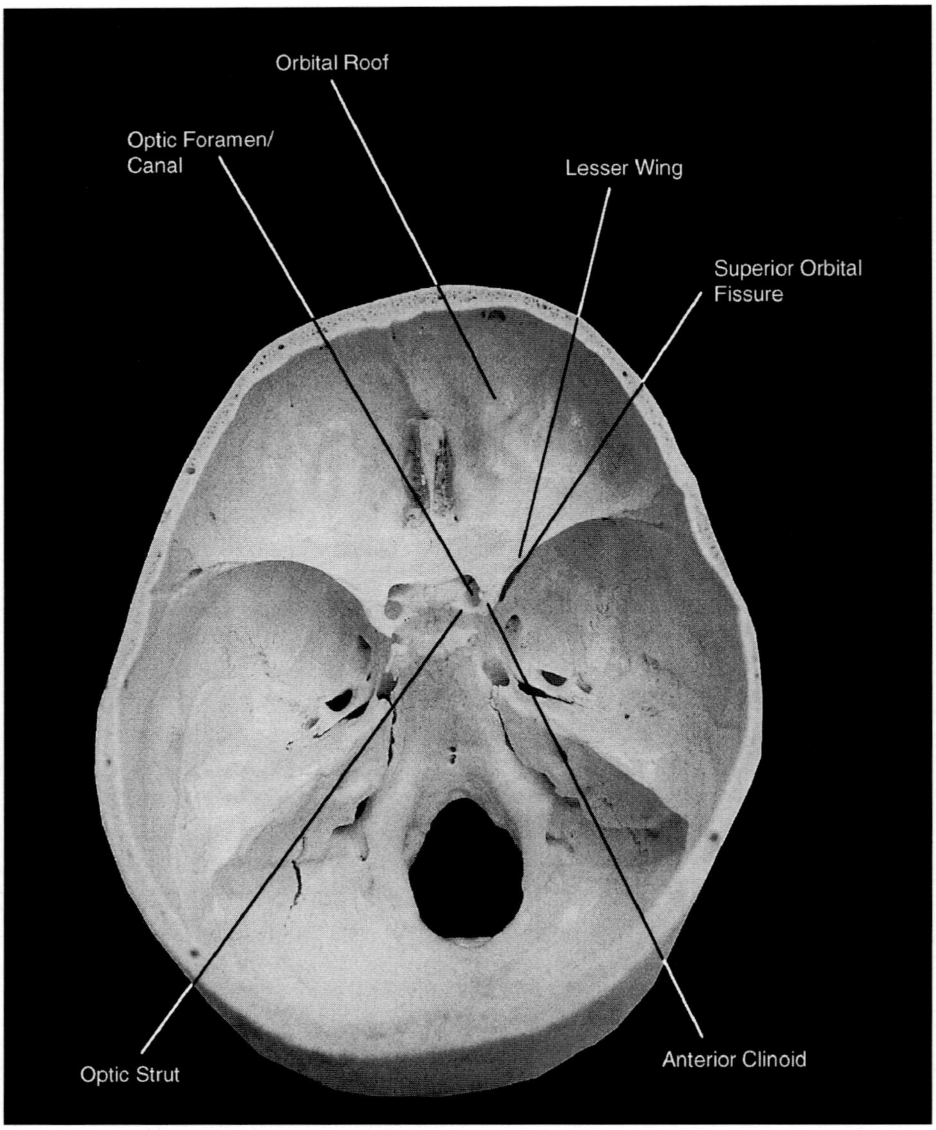

FIG. 26-3. The orbital roof and optic canal as viewed from the transcranial perspective.

mass effect on the optic nerve in the orbit and optic canal. Surgical optic nerve decompression has been performed in cases where this bony overgrowth has resulted in loss of vision (10,11).

Indications

Progressive fibrous dysplasia involving the optic canal compresses the optic nerve, causing loss of visual acuity.

TABLE 26–1. *Tumors most commonly associated with optic nerve compression*

Glioma	Neurofibroma
Meningioma	Rhabdomyosarcoma
Metastatic tumor	Craniopharyngioma
Pituitary adenoma	Giant cell tumors

Patients with known sphenoid fibrous dysplasia presenting with loss of vision secondary to bony overgrowth should be offered surgical optic nerve decompression. Some controversy exists regarding the timing of surgery, with some authors advocating prophylactic decompression.

Approach

Again, it is the nature of the pathology and its anatomic location that determines the surgical approach. Fibrous dysplasia can be progressive and behave as a neoplasm, sometimes undergoing malignant degeneration. Fibrous dysplasia that causes optic nerve compression is not usually limited to the optic canal. The anterior cranial base, sphenoid bone, and bony orbit may all be involved. Therefore, a team approach is recommended with a combined intracranial and intraorbital exposure. Through collaboration between the otolaryngologist and neurosurgeon, a safe maximum resection and adequate reconstruction can be achieved.

OSTEOPETROSIS

Osteopetrosis is sometimes referred to as "marble bone disease." It is a group of genetic disorders characterized by an increase in skeletal density with frequent involvement of the cranial base. The most common neurologic presentation on osteopetrosis is visual loss secondary to optic nerve compression in the bony canal. The indications and approach follow the same guidelines as for fibrous dysplasia with a combined intracranial/intraorbital approach providing the optimal exposure for decompression and reconstruction (12).

PSEUDOTUMOR CEREBRI

Pseudotumor cerebri, or so-called benign intracranial hypertension is an entity that presents with clinical signs of elevated intracranial pressure in the absence of a mass lesion. Patients with pseudotumor cerebri present with papilledema that may ultimately progress to a loss of visual acuity.

Indications

Pseudotumor cerebri that is unresponsive to medical therapy with diuretics and carbonic anhydrase inhibitors, which inhibit cerebrospinal fluid (CSF) formation, may lead to progressive loss of vision. These patients require surgical decompression. Surgical options include CSF shunting procedures and optic nerve sheath fenestration (13).

Approach

A medial or lateral orbitotomy approach may be used to gain access to the optic nerve sheath. A series of fenestrations or slits is then made in the sheath to permit communication with the subarachnoid space and decompression of the nerve.

SURGICAL APPROACHES

Transcranial/Cranial Base

The fronto-orbitozygomatic craniotomy and pterional craniotomy approaches with cranial base dissection are well suited to lesions located medial to the optic nerve in the orbital apex or in the optic canal and to lesions with intracranial extension.

Fronto-orbitozygomatic Craniotomy

The patient is positioned in the Mayfield head holder in the supine position with the head rotated approximately 30 degrees away from the pathology. We prefer a bicoronal skin incision made behind the hairline without shaving. The incision extends from the ipsilateral zygoma just anterior to the tragus to the opposite superior temporal line (Fig. 26-4). The scalp is reflected with subperiosteal dissection to the orbital rim where the supraorbital nerve is preserved and elevated in this plane. If the nerve is surrounded in a bony foramen rather than lying in a notch, an osteotome is used to free it. The dissection is extended in this plane into the orbit where the periorbita is continuous with the pericranium. The pericranium is elevated separately to be used as a graft in the reconstruction of the skull base. The periorbita is separated from the orbital roof and the zygomatic bone. A no. 15 blade is used to make an incision along the outer temporalis fascia, just along the superior margin of the zygomatic arch, extending from approximately the frontozygomatic attachment to the temporal attachment. Blunt dissection toward the inner fascial layers is then performed using the caudal dissector. The intervening fat pad, through which branches of the frontalis nerve will course, is then elevated anterolaterally off of the surface of the frontozygomatic process. The temporalis muscle is then incised posteriorly along the posterior margin of the scalp incision and the entire muscle reflected anterolaterally to expose the pterygopalatine fossa anteriorly and the temperozygomatic root posteriorly.

A frontal temporal craniotomy is then performed through a single burr hole in the region of the pterion (Fig. 26-4B). A Midas Rex with a B-1 attachment should be used to perform the craniotomy, taking care to bring the anterior cut as close to the superior orbital rim as possible. Frequently, the frontal sinus will be invaded with this cut, and prior to proceeding with the dissection the frontal sinus mucosa should be exenterated and the sinus packed with antibiotic-soaked fat, muscle, or Gelfoam. Next, an oscillating saw and osteotomes are used to make cuts through the superior orbital rim and roof to a depth of approximately 3 cm. The assistant should gently depress the periorbita for direct view of the saw blade as the orbital cuts are being performed. Laterally, a cut is performed in a similar manner to the level of the inferior orbital foramen and through the frontozygomatic process. The zygoma is additionally cut posteriorly, approximately 1 cm anterior to the temporozygomatic root. Osteotomes are then used to perform the final release and the orbital zygomatic rim is removed en bloc. Small tears in the periorbita can be repaired primarily with 4.0 Neurolon suture. Similarly, any tears in the dura should be repaired prior to proceeding with the exposure, so as to prevent any inadvertent CSF leakage. The remaining roof and lateral wall of the orbit can then be drilled down with a diamond drill bit to the point of transparency. Using microcurettes, the optic canal is completely unroofed and the lateral superorbital fissure completely skeletonized. If necessary, the anterior clinoid process is drilled extradurally and resected with fine-tipped bone rongeurs. Bone wax should be applied to the base of the anterior clinoid, as well as the residual medial wall of the orbit, to reduce the risk of a CSF leakage through the ethmoid sinus.

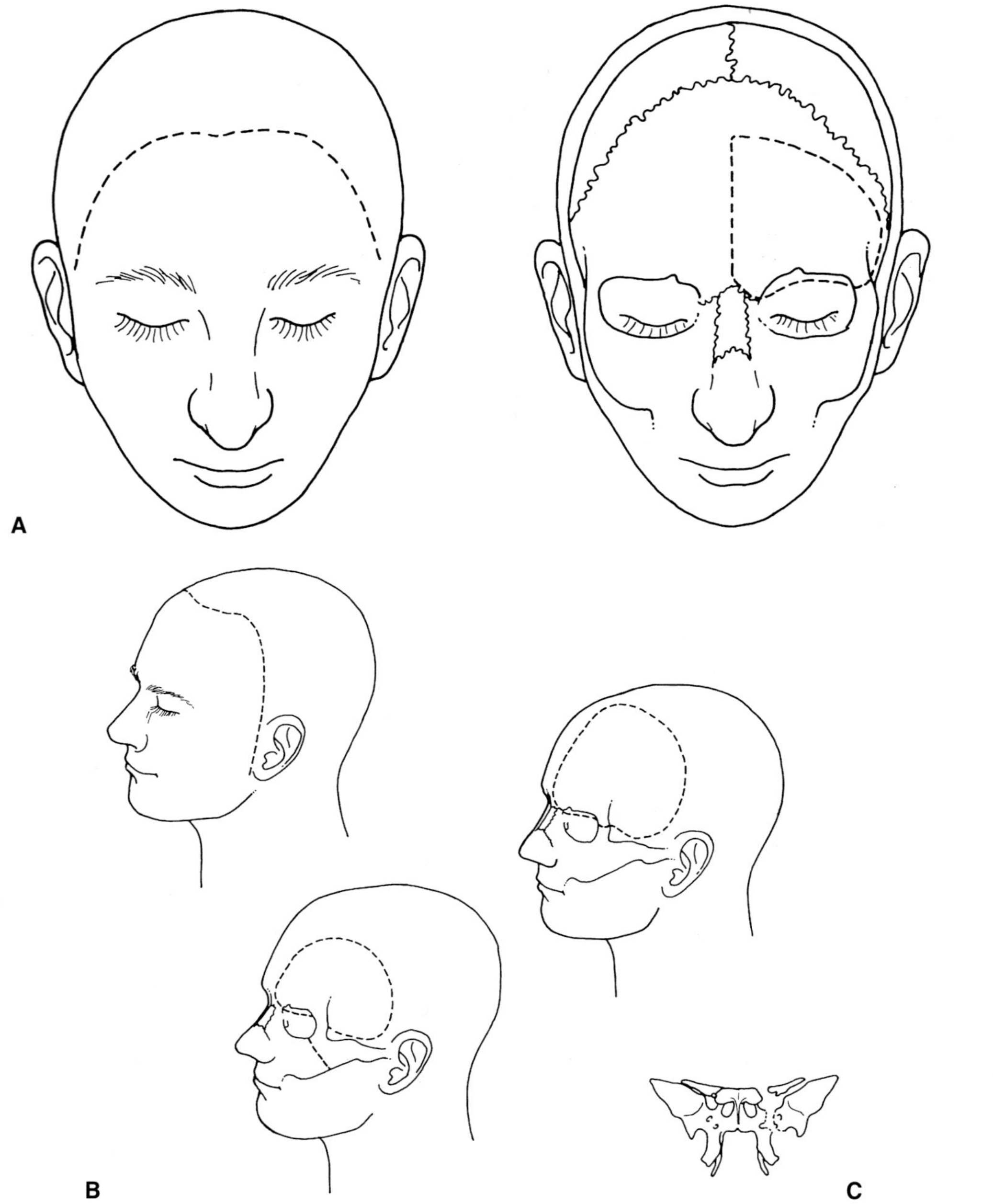

FIG. 26-4. Incision and bone flap for transcranial/cranial base approaches. **A:** Fronto-orbito-zygomatic craniotomy. **B:** Pterional. **C:** Schematic of skull base dissection of sphenoid bone that exposes superior orbit fissures and optic canal.

The resulting exposure allows excellent anatomic visualization of the optic apparatus beginning at the chiasm through the canal and into the orbit (Fig. 26-5). If necessary, the dura overlying the optic canal can be opened, as can the periorbita. Pericranium should be employed to repair any dural defects. Additionally, a pericranial flap should be brought down over the frontal sinus and secured to the dura prior to replacement of the bone flaps. The temporal bone flap is initially replaced and secured into position with miniplates. The orbitozygomatic piece is then replaced, with care taken to make certain that all bone edges align appropriately so as to enhance the cosmetic result (Fig. 26-6).

Pterional

The standard pterional craniotomy can be modified with a skull base dissection to expose the optic nerve from the chiasm intracranially through the optic canal and into the orbit. The greater and lesser sphenoid wings are exposed and an extradural skull base dissection is performed. Using a high-speed drill, the sphenoid wings are thinned down and bone is carefully removed (Figs. 26-2 and 26-4B,C). The superior orbital fissure is identified and its lateral wall is removed, exposing the pterygomaxillary fossa. The anterior clinoid process is resected extradurally with the high-speed

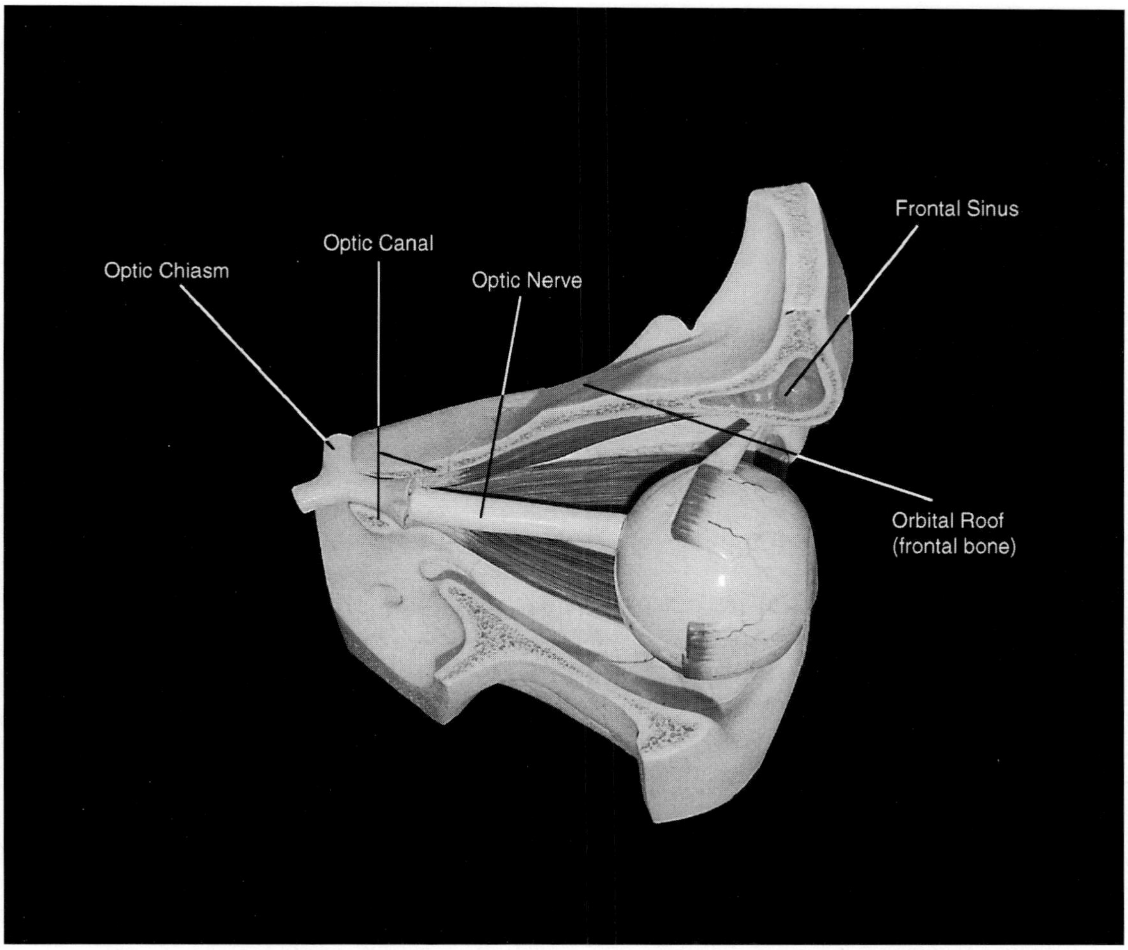

FIG. 26-5. View of the optic nerve along its entire course (from the chiasm through the canal and in the orbit) that can be achieved via transcranial/skull base approach.

drill, permitting approach to the orbital roof and the optic canal. Decompression of the optic canal can be performed by careful drilling with a high-speed drill and microcurettes. It is safest to thin the bone overlying the nerve until it is transparent and then to peel the shell away from the nerve. Depending on the nature of the pathology, the dura is opened and the optic nerve can be visualized from the chiasm through the canal and into the orbit. The dura is repaired primarily or with a graft if necessary. It is unnecessary to repair the bony orbital roof. The pterional bone flap is replaced in the usual fashion (Fig. 26-7).

Lateral Orbitotomy

A skin incision is made beginning at the lateral canthus and extended posteriorly to the temple (Fig. 26-8). The temporalis fascia is incised and access to the subperiosteal plain is gained via incision through the periosteum of the frontozygomatic bone. Subperiosteal dissection is used along the zygoma to elevate the periorbital fascia and temporalis muscle. The orbital rim is cut in two places with the reciprocating saw while the intraorbital contents are protected with a retractor and cottonoids. The orbital rim is then separated posteriorly from its attachment to the sphenoid wing with rongeurs. A high-speed drill can be used to remove addition bone from the greater wing of the sphenoid, exposing the deep orbital apex and the proximal optic nerve as well as the dura of the frontal and middle fossae. The periorbital fascia is incised, and a self-retaining orbital retractor can be used to displace the periorbital fat and muscle, permitting good visualization of the optic nerve (Fig. 26-9).

Following the decompression, the fascia is closed and the orbital rim is reconstructed with miniplates if necessary.

Medial Orbitotomy

Lesions medial to the optic nerve can be reached via a medial orbitotomy approach. The patient is prepared in the usual fashion for ophthalmic procedures. The cornea is incised and the medial rectus muscle is freed medially from its insertions (Fig. 26-10). A self-retaining orbital retractor is inserted to retract the globe laterally while holding the rectus medially, permitting access to the medial orbital compartment. Under the microscope the dissection is carried

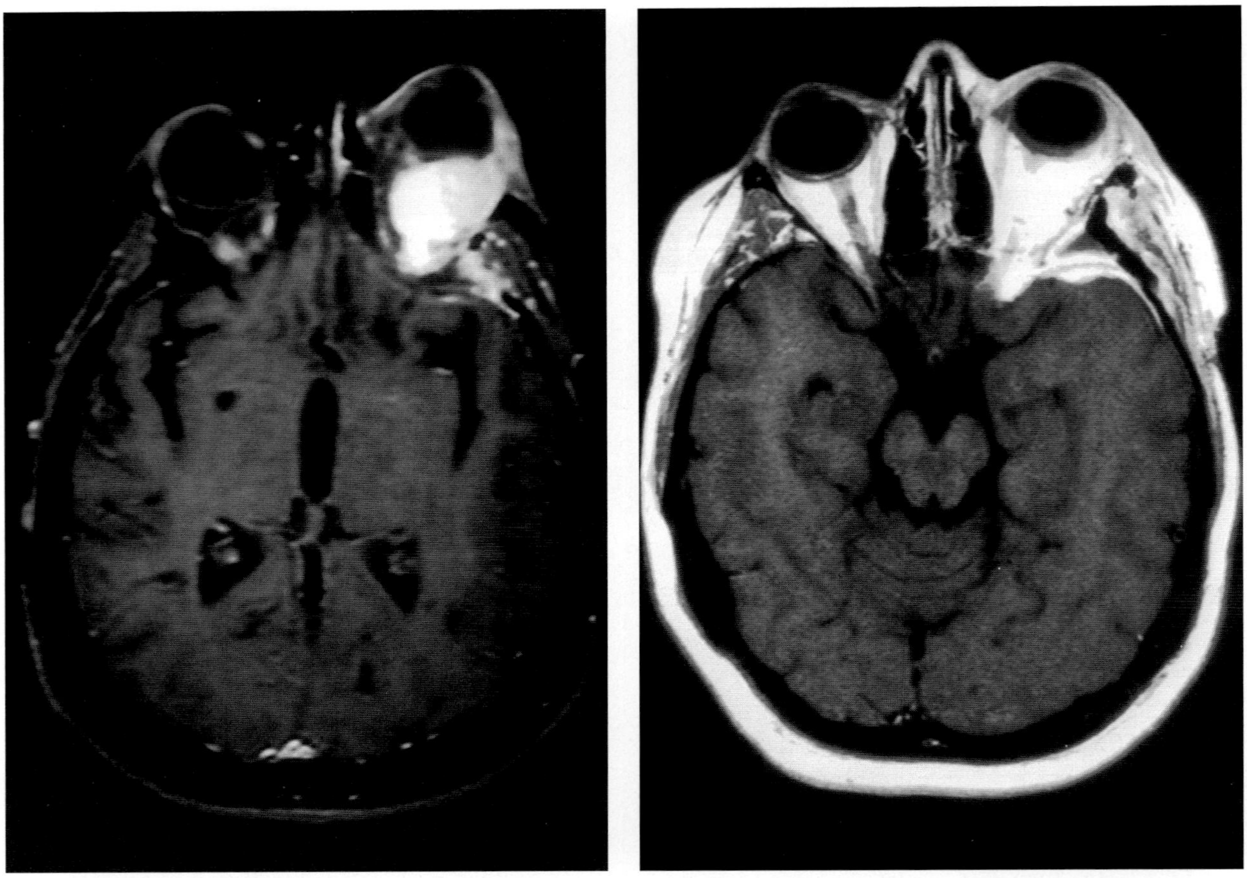

A B

FIG. 26-6. Axial magnetic resonance imaging (MRI) view of a 32-year-old woman with a 3-month history of progressive proptosis ophthalmolplegia and a severely impaired visual acuity of 20/300. **A:** Axial MRI images revealed a left orbital mass (osteosarcoma). **B:** Following a fronto-orbital osteotomy and decompression of her optic nerve, her visual acuity improved to 20/40 and her extraocular function normalized.

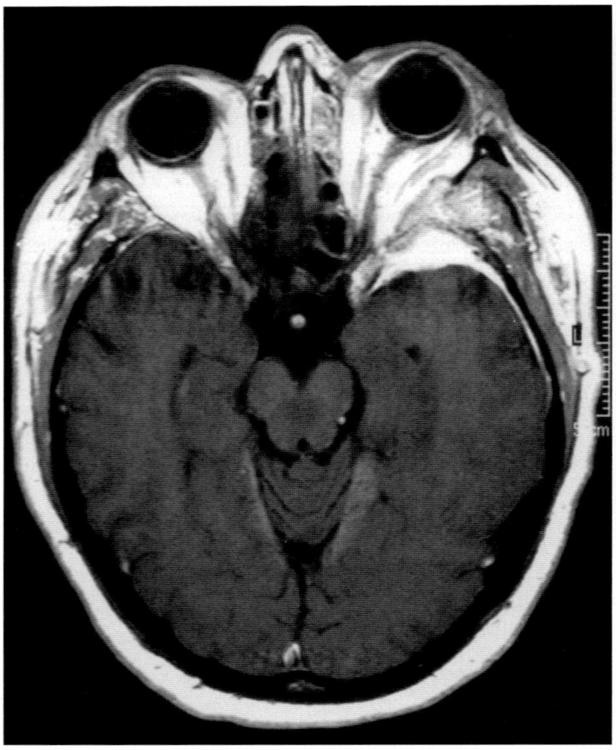

A

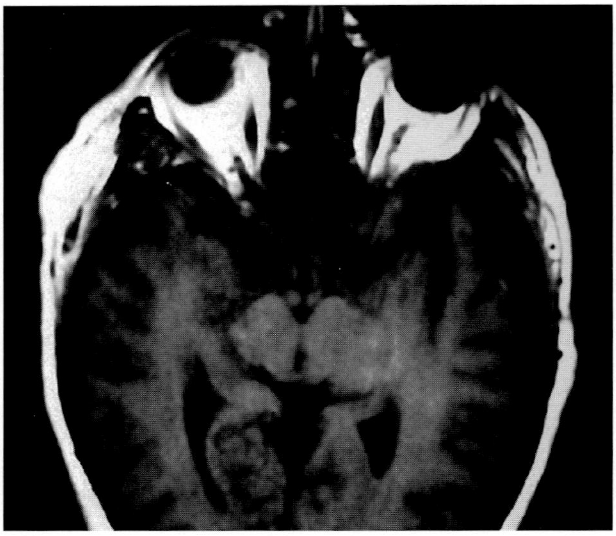

B

FIG. 26-7. A: Axial MRI images of a 50-year-old woman with a left ossifying sphenoid wing meningioma causing symptomatic compression of the optic canal and superior orbit fissure. **B:** Similar view 6 months following fronto-orbital craniotomy with complete resection of orbital roof, lateral wall, and tumor. Methyl methacrylate was utilized to re-create a portion of the lateral orbital wall and a large temporal defect.

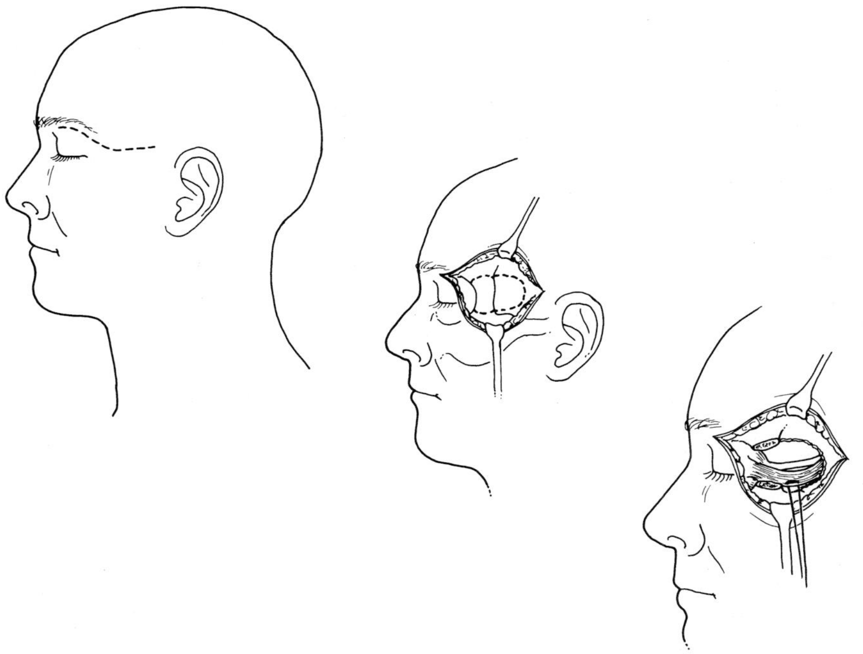

FIG. 26-8. Lateral orbitotomy approach.

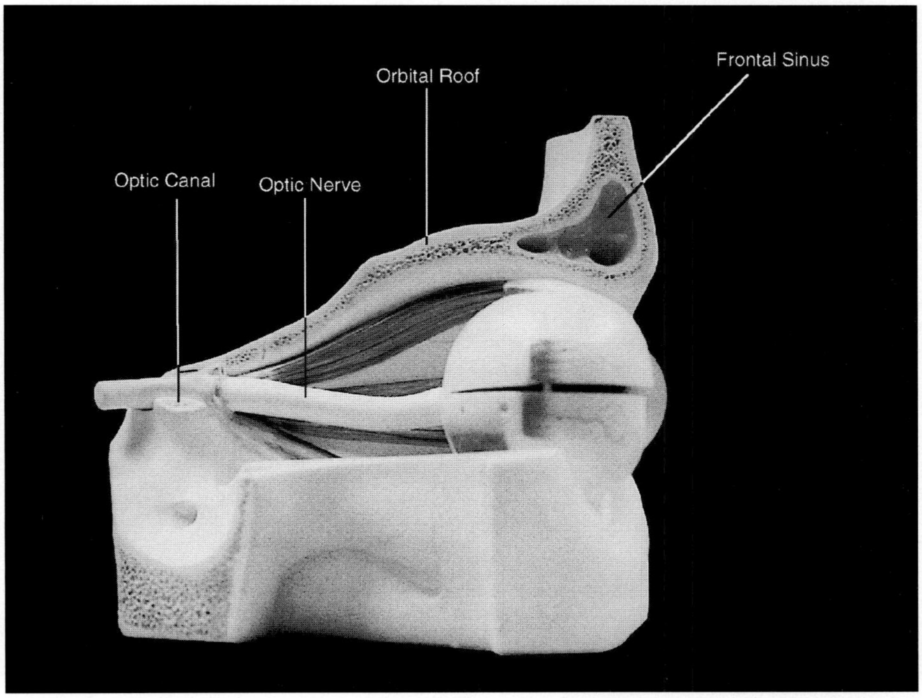

FIG. 26-9. Lateral exposure of a portion of the optic nerve can be achieved via lateral orbitotomy. This may be combined with transcranial approaches to achieve exposure of the optic canal and medial and superior optic nerves.

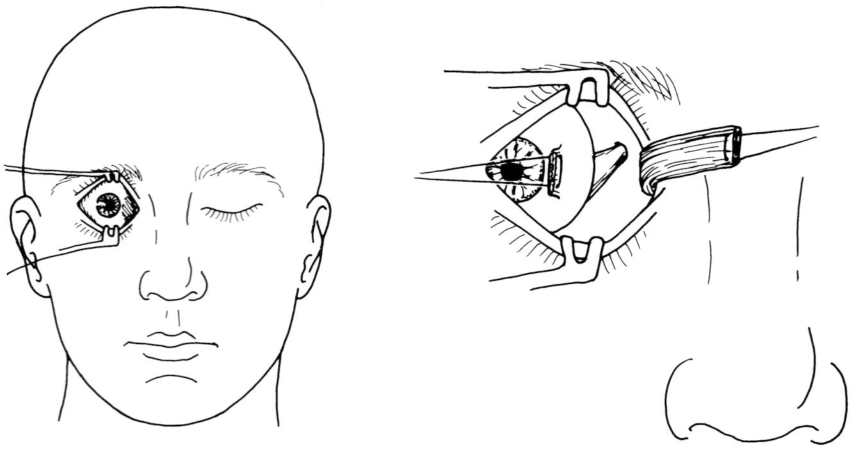

FIG. 26-10. Medial orbitotomy approach.

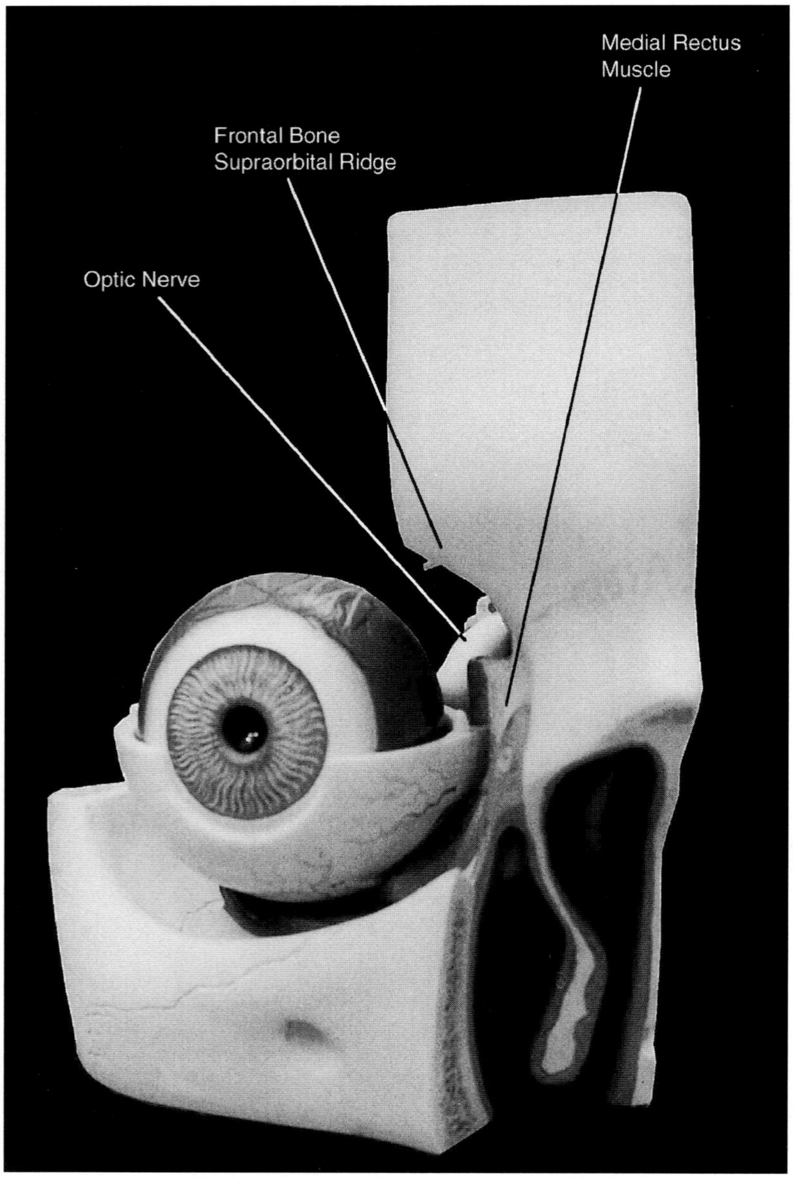

FIG. 26-11. Schematic view of limited exposure of optic nerve outlined via medial orbitotomy without bony removal. However, for appropriate lesions, this less invasive approach is preferred.

through the orbital fat with bipolar cautery and microinstruments. The retractors are repositioned as the optic nerve and pathology are exposed (Fig. 26-11). This exposure can be augmented with a lateral orbitotomy as indicated. Following optic nerve decompression, the medial rectus is reattached and the conjunctiva is closed. The eye is patched as in simple extraocular muscle surgery. As there is no bony dissection or significant muscle dissection, morbidity is minimal following this procedure.

CONCLUSION

Orbital pathology resulting in optic nerve compression is an uncommon and potentially serious medical and frequently surgical problem. Generally, swift and definitive intervention is required for the preservation of vision. Solid knowledge of orbital anatomy is a prerequisite to any of the standard orbital decompression procedures. The approach selected should provide the surgeon with maximal working room with as minimal brain retraction as possible. Commonly, these approaches require a combined effort between the ophthalmologists, the otolaryngologist, and the neurosurgeon. Provided the decompressive procedures are performed in a timely fashion and meticulous microsurgical technique is implemented, a favorable outcome is frequently achieved.

REFERENCES

1. Osguthorpe JD, Sofferman RA. Optic nerve decompression. *Otolaryngol Clin North Am* 1988;21:155–169.
2. Jorissen M, Feenstra L. Optic nerve decompression for indirect posterior optic nerve trauma. *Acta Otorhinolaryngol Belg* 1992;46:311–24.
3. Kurimoto M, Endo S, Onizuka K, Akai T, Takaku A. Optic nerve decompression. *Neurol Med Chir Tokyo* 1996;36:102–105.
4. Girard BC, Bouzas EA, Lamas G, Soudant J. Visual improvement after transethmoid-sphenoid decompression in optic nerve injuries. *J Clin Neuroophthalmol* 1992;12:142–148.
5. Maniglia AJ, Kronberg FG, Culbertson W. Visual loss associated with orbital and sinus diseases. *Laryngoscope* 1994;94:1050–1059.
6. Papay FA, Morales L Jr, Flaharty P, et al. Optic nerve decompression. *J Craniofac Surg* 1995;6:5–10.
7. Tandon DA, Thakar A, Mahapatra AK, Ghosh P. Trans-ethmoidal optic nerve decompression. *Clin Otolaryngol* 1994;19:98–104.
8. Knox BE, Gates GA, Berry SM. Optic nerve decompression via the lateral facial approach. *Laryngoscope* 1990;100:458–462.
9. Kuppersmith RB, Alford EL, Patrinely JR, Lee AG, Parke RB, Holds JB. Combined transconjunctival/intranasal endoscopic approach to the optic canal in traumatic optic neurology. *Laryngoscope* 1997;107: 311–315.
10. Chen YR, Fairholm D. Fronto-orbito-sphenoidal fibrous dysplasia. *Ann Las Surg* 1985;15:190–203.
11. Chen YR, Breidahl A, Chang CN. Extradural optic nerve decompression for fibrous dysplasia with a favorable visual outcome. *Plast Reconstr Surg* 1997;99:22–30.
12. Al Mefty O, Fox JL, Al Rodhan N, Dew JH. Optic nerve decompression in osteopetrosis. *J Neurosurg* 1988;68:80–84.
13. Sergott RC. Optic nerve sheath decompression: history, techniques, and indications. *Int Ophthalmol Clin* 1991;31:71–81.

Neurosurgical Issues in Otolaryngology: Principles and Practice of Collaboration,
edited by Moisés A. Arriaga and J. Diaz Day.
Lippincott Williams & Wilkins, Philadelphia © 1999.

CHAPTER 27

Head and Neck Neoplasms with Skull Base Involvement

Daniel W. Nuss and Peter L. Rigby

OVERVIEW

A wide variety of neoplasms originating in the head and neck can extend rostrally to involve the skull base, and many of these tumors require special diagnostic and therapeutic considerations for optimal management. For the purposes of this discussion, we employ the phrase *head and neck* in its conventional use, to describe tumors that originate in the regions treated by otorhinolaryngologists; as such, it includes pathologies of the sinonasal tract and upper airway, the upper digestive tract, the auditory apparatus and temporal bone, the salivary glands, the cranial nerves, the orbits, the facial skeleton and its supporting soft tissues, and the contents of the visceral compartments of the head (infratemporal fossa, masticator space, pterygopalatine fossa, and parapharyngeal space). By definition, then, such lesions are considered as distinct from lesions that arise within the cranium and neuraxis.

It is useful to consider head and neck neoplasms separately because they exhibit unique features that differ considerably from the intracranial pathologies, despite the fact that both may involve the very same portions of the skull base. Just as the tissues of origin differ, so too do the patterns of neoplastic development, local invasiveness, and tendency for metastatic spread. It is therefore critical for both the neurosurgeon and the otolaryngologist, as members of the skull base team, to appreciate these biologic features of head and neck tumors so that optimal collaborative management strategies can be formulated.

As one considers the distinctive biologic characteristics of head and neck lesions as opposed to neurosurgical lesions, it is also important to be mindful of the differences in oncologic perspectives as they have been traditionally taught and practiced in the two disciplines, otolaryngology and neurosurgery. Whereas neuro-oncologic resections—because of proximity of critically important structures—must often necessarily be carried out with very close margins, most head and neck tumor resections allow for, and in fact require, significantly wider margins. Patterns of head and neck tumor spread often mandate en bloc rather than incremental resections, and frequently call for regional lymph node dissection, which is not a concern for most primary neurogenic tumors. These differences in oncologic approaches between the specialties must be reconciled through collaborative preoperative planning to achieve the philosophical and procedural accord that is so crucial to successful tumor management. Thus, as the two disciplines come together to treat skull base tumors of head and neck origin, the oncologic modus operandi will sometimes have to be adjusted to suit the particular pathology at hand.

This chapter reviews the strategies of combining head and neck resections with intracranial procedures, and reviews the head and neck tumors that can involve the skull base. The material is intended to familiarize the neurosurgeon with important neoplasms of the head and neck, paying special attention to the features of these lesions that influence the neurosurgical and collaborative aspects of their management. A brief historical perspective, an overview of the advantages of collaboration in skull base surgery, indications for surgery for head and neck tumors, relevant technical issues, potential pitfalls, and management of complications are also addressed.

HISTORICAL MANAGEMENT

For the first three-fourths of the 20th century, most head and neck tumors that invaded the skull base were regarded as inoperable. When surgery was considered, technical prob-

D. W. Nuss and P. L. Rigby: Department of Otolaryngology—Head and Neck Surgery, Louisiana State University Medical Center, New Orleans, Louisiana 70112-2234.

lems imposed major limitations. Inadequate diagnostic imaging made it difficult to accurately assess the tumor extent and to know what important structures were involved; thus, preoperative planning was quite unsophisticated compared with today's standards. Skull base surgical approaches (aside from the purely neurosurgical and purely otolaryngologic routes) were few in number, and the available instrumentation was inadequate for safe tumor visualization and manipulation. Reconstructive options for patients undergoing complex resections were limited as well, and wound complications were commonplace and often devastating. Perioperative support in critical care environments was not widely available. Morbidity and mortality rates were prohibitive.

Beyond technical limitations, conceptual problems also impeded progress in treatment of head and neck tumors at the skull base. As alluded to above, oncologic management strategies were different between neurosurgeons and otolaryngologists by virtue of their exposure to different kinds of pathologies. In addition, traditional training in both specialties fostered the implicit acceptance of the concept of a no-man's-land with regard to the skull base, and the boundaries of each of the specialties, for all practical purposes, essentially halted at the basicranium. Interdisciplinary teams were practically nonexistent.

Fortunately, a number of important developments occurred in a relatively short time to make skull base surgery both feasible and safe. One of the most important of these was the quantum leap in imaging technology that came with the advent of computed tomography (CT) in the 1970s, and magnetic resonance imaging (MRI) scans in the 1980s, making preoperative assessment far more accurate. The ability to know preoperatively the full extent of a tumor—something now taken very much for granted—introduced an element of predictability to skull base operations that was previously not possible.

A renaissance of interest in skull base anatomy followed, and the intricate anatomic relationships of the skull base were redefined from a contemporary surgical perspective. Refinements in surgical microscopes with better illumination, and development of microsurgical instruments, helped make it possible to remove tumors with greater precision. Progress in craniofacial reconstructive surgery for congenital deformities, using elective cranial and facial osteotomies, translated into a new conceptual approach for oncologic application, namely that of craniofacial disassembly, through which safe exposure of large portions of the cranial base could be reliably achieved by traversing the facial region instead of using transcranial routes alone (1–5). Improved understanding of regional vascular anatomy, particularly of the pericranium, the galea, and the temporalis muscle and fascia, brought a new level of dependability to skull base reconstruction (6–10). The advent of microvascular transfer of tissues from other parts of the body made it possible to safely reconstruct even very large cranial base defects, helping to reduce infectious, functional, and aesthetic complications (11–14). Advances in neuroanesthesia and perioperative critical care made it possible to sustain patients through lengthy procedures and difficult postoperative courses.

This convergent evolution of technology from a number of sources ushered in an era of intense interest in surgical treatment of skull base tumors by both neurosurgeons and otolaryngologists. In the 1980s, the concept of skull base teams gained acceptance, with its emphasis on interdisciplinary collaboration. Such teams have now evolved to a point where they include specialists from neurosurgery and otolaryngology, as well as plastic and reconstructive surgery, diagnostic and interventional radiology, neuroanesthesia, nursing, critical care medicine, neurophysiology, radiation oncology, medical oncology, dental oncology, oral and maxillofacial surgery, speech and swallowing therapy, maxillofacial prosthedontics, rehabilitational medicine, social services, psychology, and psychiatry.

In the last few decades, a truly remarkable number of innovative surgical approaches have been introduced for removal of skull base tumors (15–51). Pioneers in both specialties contributed to the development of these approaches, which have been refined to the extent that now there is essentially no part of the skull base that is inaccessible. Most of these approaches have been the result of collaboration, which has been so fruitful that interdisciplinary skull base societies have been organized in countries around the globe, as have a variety of international forums for scientific and collegial exchange on all topics relating to cranial base disease. These observations underscore the value of collaboration in dealing with cranial base tumors to obtain optimal results for our patients.

ADVANTAGES OF COLLABORATIVE SURGERY

For skull base tumors that originate from *subcranial* (as opposed to *intracranial*) sites, collaboration offers several important advantages. The participation of both the otolaryngologist and the neurosurgeon in the planning and execution of a skull base operation increases the margin of safety. This increase in safety is attributable to the fact that, in collaborative surgery, two (or more) concerned physicians each contribute their expertise, increasing the likelihood that all appropriate concerns will be properly addressed. More than just a second-opinion reevaluation, the different perspective from which each team member views the situation subjects the problem at hand to a more critical review, and takes into consideration the cross-disciplinary needs of the patient.

Let us take as an example a patient with a temporal bone tumor that extends intracranially. Such a patient, in the neurosurgical evaluation, will have a comprehensive neurologic examination and careful review of imaging studies to determine the extent of intracranial pathology and to assess whether there are any contributing factors that will influence the tumor treatment. Special attention will be given to issues such as which is the dominant cerebral hemisphere, where is the dominant venous drainage, whether the tumor appears to be extradural or intradural, whether the tumor derives its blood supply from any vital intracranial vessels, whether any coincident intracranial pathology or anomaly exists, and whether there is any associated hydrocephalus secondary to tumor.

Evaluated by the otolaryngologist, this patient will then have a careful head and neck exam that includes thorough assessment of all of the temporal bone structures. Otologic examination is complemented by audiometric studies such as pure-tone hearing thresholds, speech-reception thresholds, acoustic reflex testing, otoacoustic emissions testing, or auditory brainstem response testing, which are obtained as needed to fully investigate all aspects of hearing. Vestibular function (or dysfunction) can be quantified if necessary using electronystagmography, posturography, and other techniques. Facial nerve function (or dysfunction) is assessed, and may be quantified, photographically or electromyographically. Inspection of the naso-oropharynx, hypopharynx, and larynx will assess the status of cranial nerves IX, X, and XII. All of this information assumes importance not only for surgical planning and patient counseling, but also to aid in postoperative planning for short-term recovery as well as long-term rehabilitation.

At surgery, technical collaboration between the specialties enhances the safety of the procedure as well as the margin of oncologic control. As another example, let us consider a patient with a large malignancy of the anterior cranial base. With the neurosurgeon designing the intracranial approach, and the otolaryngologist designing the extracranial approach, each can provide the safest avenue for access to the tumor and nearby important structures. At the time of tumor resection, the neurosurgeon protects the brain, pituitary, and intracranial portions of the carotid arteries, while the otolaryngologist protects the eye, optic nerve, and extracranial portions of the carotid arteries, and both surgeons enjoy optimal visualization of the tumor margins, which allows the widest possible resection with the least morbidity.

Thus, the combination of the neurosurgical and the otolaryngologic inputs yields a truly comprehensive preoperative evaluation, a surgical resection that is likely to be safer and oncologically more effective, and a postoperative outcome that maximizes function and quality of life.

Given the theme of this chapter, certain aspects of the otolaryngologist's role as a member of the skull base team warrant emphasis. The otolaryngologist brings to the team a variety of skills that are vital to optimal management of head and neck tumors that invade the skull base, beginning at the time of diagnosis and lasting the duration of the long-term follow-up.

From a diagnostic perspective, otolaryngologists are well versed in the recognition of critical signs and symptoms of skull base tumors, and they are often the first to be consulted by patients with such tumors because of common presenting complaints affecting hearing, balance, taste, smell, nasal respiration, facial sensation, mastication, and the like (see Tables 27-3, 27-4, and 27-5). Otolaryngologists are also involved in the recognition and initial management of a variety of cranial nerve disorders, including but not limited to facial nerve, auditory nerve, and vagus nerve lesions, and their role in documenting and quantifying such deficits is well established. Otolaryngologists routinely perform upper airway endoscopy, otomicroscopy, audiologic testing, tumor staging procedures such as panendoscopy, and fine-needle aspiration biopsies, all of which can be important in the workup of a suspected skull base tumor (especially those originating from head and neck regions). This familiarity with the signs and symptoms of skull base tumors, and with the techniques employed in definitive diagnosis, facilitates an orderly diagnostic approach and ensures that appropriate information is gathered in a timely way.

From an oncologic standpoint, otolaryngologists are knowledgeable regarding the local and regional considerations relevant to treatment of head and neck cancer. Issues such as when to dissect regional lymph nodes in the neck and parotid regions, when to use pre- or postoperative radiation therapy and chemotherapy, and how best to coordinate adjuvant treatments are all within the scope of treatment of head and neck tumors. These concerns must be assiduously addressed so that local recurrences and regional and distant metastases can be avoided or controlled.

From a technical viewpoint, it is fundamental to note that successful surgical approaches through the orbits, nasal cavity, paranasal sinuses, maxillofacial skeleton, temporal bone, infratemporal fossa, oral cavity, and neck are only possible when the surgeon has a thorough, in-depth command of the related anatomy. The otolaryngologist therefore plays a major role in many skull base operations because of his/her familiarity with the extracranial anatomy. In addition, the otolaryngologist's experience in management of the secondary manifestations of skull base tumors (e.g., obstructive sinusitis, serous otitis media, epistaxis, hearing loss, dysequilibrium, dysphagia, etc.) makes it possible to minimize morbidity by providing any needed treatment for such manifestations before or at the time of the definitive skull base operation.

Following resection, the otolaryngologist has much to contribute in the reconstructive phase of the operation as well. Proficiency in designing composite tissue flaps comes from experience in head and neck reconstruction, which is a major part of the otolaryngologist's training. Understanding such concepts as angiosomes and vascularized territories of the extracranial tissues that are commonly employed in head and neck tumor surgery makes it possible to use reconstructive flaps and grafts intelligently when the need arises in skull base reconstruction. Well versed in the indications for, and limitations of, a variety of vascularized local flaps (including temporalis muscle flaps, temporoparietal fascial flaps, galeal and pericranial flaps, septal and turbinal mucosal flaps, pharyngeal flaps, pectoralis and trapezius flaps, and even local skin and scalp flaps), the otolaryngologist often is the primary reconstructive surgeon for skull base defects. Further, experience acquired from management of facial trauma, the performance of facial cosmetic surgery, and the use of biomaterials and facial prosthetic devices gives the otolaryngologist an optimal sense of how best to repair a given craniofacial defect to achieve both functional and aesthetic goals.

The postoperative management of skull base surgery patients frequently demands the attention of the otolaryngologist as well. Such patients are at risk for significant and potentially life-threatening functional deficits. Aspiration, dysphagia, and vocal cord paralysis are among the most serious of these, in that they can result in respiratory insufficiency, malnutrition, and airway compromise. Less critical but nonetheless important deficits include facial paralysis, deafness, dysequilibrium, tinnitus, and facial pain syndromes. Appropriate and timely otolaryngologic intervention can hasten recovery, and improve the patient's quality of life.

SURGICAL TECHNIQUE

General Considerations

As an introduction to the technical portion of this chapter, it is important to begin with a foundation concerning what needs to be accomplished in cranial base tumor surgery. Regardless of tumor type, there are always four specific goals that must be realized (Table 27-1) (5,52):

1. Extirpation of disease. An effective skull base surgical approach must provide access sufficient to allow for complete extirpation of the tumor.
2. Protection of vital structures. The surgical approach must be selected with safety and preservation of functionally important structures in mind. In some cases the approach has to be expanded not for access to the tumor, but for access to—and control of—nearby vital structures, such as the carotid artery, brain, cranial nerves, orbital contents, etc. It is this "control of the surgical perimeter" (as Janecka has described it), this management of the area beyond the tumor, that in many cases makes it possible to reduce postoperative morbidity. This need for protection of vital structures presents one of the strongest of all the arguments in favor of collaboration between the specialties. Often in skull base surgery, the tumor problem per se is predominantly manageable by either the neurosurgeon or the otolaryngologist alone, but the other specialist's expertise becomes essential in providing the needed margin of safety on the "other side" of the tumor. In this way, for example, the neurosurgeon protects the brain while the otolaryngologist resects the tumor during anterior craniofacial resection; the otolaryngologist isolates and protects the carotid artery, jugular vein, and lower cranial nerves while the neurosurgeon resects the intracranial portion of a glomus tumor, and so forth.
3. Restoration of critical anatomic barriers. The so-called critical anatomic barriers of the skull base include the dura, the bony basicranium, and the underlying soft tissues that separate the neurocranium from the visceral compartments. These barriers, in the absence of pathology, serve to contain the cerebrospinal fluid (CSF), to separate the cranial vault from the contaminated spaces below, and to insulate the carotid artery from septic exposure. Many skull base operations disrupt these barriers, either for oncologic reasons or to achieve optimal access. It is imperative that these barriers be restored in order to prevent serious sequelae including CSF fistula, ascending infection, and carotid artery rupture (see Management of Complications, below). One way to assure restoration of critical barriers is to address it in the planning, so that the surgical approach will not unnecessarily violate them, or at least will avoid damaging regional tissues that are important in replacing them, such as the temporalis muscle, galea, and pericranium. "Beginning with the end in mind" (53) is excellent advice in this regard. If the tumor resection or preexisting circumstances (previous surgery or radiation) will render it impossible to use regional tissues for reconstruction, then provisions must be made preoperatively for free tissue transfer.
4. Functional and aesthetic reconstruction. Survival data notwithstanding, removal of a skull base tumor can only be judged successful if the patients recover what they would consider a reasonable quality of life. This goal, though difficult to define, can usually be met if the members of the surgical team exercise care in planning and executing the approach, and especially in the reconstruction. Proper placement of facial incisions, respecting the "aesthetic units" of the face, along with careful wound closure following principles of plastic surgery, can minimize scars. Normal facial contour can be preserved in most cases if osteotomies are performed carefully and if the craniofacial bone segments are replaced accurately. Indeed, it is possible to completely dismantle large segments of the craniofacial anatomy, providing excellent surgical exposure of the skull base, with superb results, as long as the disassembly is done correctly and the reconstruction is meticulous.

TABLE 27–1. *Goals of cranial base surgery*

Goals
Extirpation of disease
Protection of vital structures
Restoration of critical anatomic barriers
Functional and aesthetic reconstruction

From ref. 5, with permission.

Functional outcomes are usually best when the nerves, muscles, other soft tissues, and skeletal structures have been preserved intact; when this is impossible for oncologic reasons, reconstruction must attempt to either simulate the lost tissues or compensate in other ways for their functional loss. Generally it is fairly straightforward to replace resected structural components (using bone grafts, muscle, and other soft tissue flaps, etc.) but very difficult to restore normal function after loss of a cranial nerve or end-organ. Even in such cases, however, compensatory procedures can give gratifying results. For example, the vagus nerve when sacrificed cannot currently be replaced, but by performing vocal cord medialization, aspiration pneumonia can usually be prevented, and speech and swallowing can be much more readily rehabilitated, affording an excellent functional outcome.

In patients with advanced skull base tumors, fulfillment of the above four goals becomes a complex endeavor. Collaboration between the neurosurgeon and the otolaryngologist, combining intracranial procedures with classic head and neck or facial tumor resections, facilitates the process immeasurably.

Regional Anatomic Considerations

The cranial base is usually described as having three anatomic regions—anterior, middle, and posterior—each named for its relation to the overlying cranial fossa. Although this conceptual division is somewhat arbitrary (tumors do not always respect the boundaries), it is useful because the operative approaches to these regions, despite their diversity, share certain anatomic and clinical concerns.

Just as each of the three cranial base regions is named for its relation to the overlying cranial fossa, each can also be thought of in terms of its relation to the underlying extracranial compartments and their respective contents. It is important to view them in this way and to understand the anatomic relations well, because the extracranial compartments assume tremendous importance in the management of head and neck tumors that invade the cranial base.

Why are the extracranial compartments so important? First, the majority of head and neck tumors invade the cranial base by direct progression from one compartment to the next, generally following predictable patterns. Second, choosing a route for access to the cranial base involves deciding which compartments will be traversed along the way. Knowledge of the contents of each of the compartments helps one to assess both the utility and the likely morbidity of the approaches that go through them. An overview of the unique anatomic features of each cranial base region and the corresponding potential morbidity of traversing them is presented in Table 27-2.

Key Issues in Surgical Collaboration

A collaboration may be variously defined as a cooperative endeavor, a pooling of resources, a concurrence of opinion, an agreement to proceed, and a consortium of trust. All of these define well the interaction that takes place in successful surgery for head and neck neoplasms that invade the skull base. It is with these definitions in mind that we examine the techniques of collaboration.

So abundant now are the number of skull base techniques that it would require an atlas of considerable scope to do them justice; the reader is referred to several excellent resources for details (54–61). Rather than reviewing a variety of surgical techniques, the remainder of this section illustrates, using one familiar surgical approach examined in some detail, the key issues involved in surgical collaboration for management of head and neck tumors.

The anterior skull base resection (anterior craniofacial resection) illustrates well the collaborative process for management of head and neck tumors (Fig. 27-1). This operation is typically carried out for sinonasal or orbital malignancies that have extended to or through the skull base. It nearly always involves the combination of a frontal craniotomy with some form of transfacial tumor resection (e.g., en bloc ethmoidectomy, maxillectomy, orbital exenteration, etc.). In this operation—and indeed in any skull base operation for a head and neck tumor—the major technical points requiring collaboration can be divided into the following elements: (a) allocation of tasks, (b) sequencing of the operative steps, (c) management of the airway, (d) patient positioning and head fixation, (e) other preoperative issues, (f) selection of the incisions, (g) soft tissue dissection, (h) craniofacial osteotomies, (i) tumor resection, and (j) reconstruction.

Allocation of Tasks

Before surgery, it behooves the surgeons to delineate the various responsibilities clearly so the procedure can progress smoothly. Having the tasks well understood, agreed upon, and mapped out in advance helps each surgeon organize and focus his/her thoughts and efforts regarding the case. [Aside from the ergonomic advantage, there is also a pragmatic reason for delineating tasks clearly: the *Physicians' Current Procedural Terminology* code book (CPT) (62), widely used as a guide for medical documentation and reimbursement, recommends specific skull base surgery codes that recognize just three components: operative approach, definitive resection, and reconstruction. Appropriate use of these CPT codes requires that the surgeons agree on who does what, and also mandates documentation to that effect.]

Sequencing of the Operative Steps

Just as the division of tasks is important, agreeing on the proper sequence of events has a significant impact on the outcome as well. With head and neck neoplasms, it is usually prudent to execute the extracranial part of the operation first. This offers two main advantages: (a) Since these tumors take their origins in the extracranial compartments, their primary blood supplies are usually vulnerable through these compartments as well. Putting the extracranial approach first thus allows a stepwise exposure of the tumor's perimeter, usually giving the opportunity for control of its feeding vessels. (b) It is desirable to minimize the time of exposure of cranial contents to contaminated spaces below. If the intracranial work were done first, followed by several hours of extracra-

TABLE 27–2. *Anatomic features of the cranial base regions with clinical implications*

Region	Related extracranial compartments	Significant anatomic structures	Potential postoperative morbidity
Anterior cranial base	Paranasal sinuses	Frontal sinus	Sinusitis, mucocele
		Ethmoid sinus	Meningitis
		Sphenoid sinus	CSF fistula
Anterior cranial base	Nasal cavity	Cribriform plate and olfactory apparatus	CSF fistula
			Anosmia
		Nasal septum and turbinates	Nasal obstruction
			Epistaxis
			Crusting
			Infection
Anterior cranial base and middle cranial base	Orbits	Bony orbital walls	Enophthalmos
			Pulsatile exophthalmos
		Lacrimal apparatus	Epiphora
			Dacryocystitis
		Globe and optic nerve	Visual loss
		Superior orbital fissure and extraocular muscles	Diplopia
			Corneal anesthesia
		Inferior orbital fissure and V2	Facial numbness
Middle cranial base	Sphenoid sinus	—	Sinusitis, mucocele
	Upper and mid-clivus	—	CSF fistula
	Nasopharynx	Eustachian tube	Serous otitis, hearing loss
Middle cranial base	Pterygopalatine fossa	Pterygoid muscles	Difficulty chewing, trismus
		V2 (maxillary nerve)	Oral/facial numbness
Middle cranial base	Infratemporal fossa and masticator space	Internal maxillary artery and branches	Compromised blood supply to temporalis muscle
		V3 (mandibular nerve)	Oral/facial numbness and difficulty chewing
		Temporalis, pterygoid muscles	Trismus, difficulty chewing
Middle cranial base	Parapharyngeal space	Carotid artery	Stroke, hemorrhage, death
		Jugular vein	Thrombosis, hemorrhage
		Cranial nerves 9, 10, 11	Dysphagia, aspiration
			Hoarseness
			Shoulder dysfunction
		Parotid gland	Facial nerve paralysis
Middle cranial base and posterior cranial base	Temporal bone	Cochlea and cranial nerve 8	Hearing loss, deafness
			Tinnitus
		Vestibular apparatus	Dysequilibrium
		Facial nerve	Facial paralysis
		Carotid artery	Stroke, hemorrhage, death
		Jugular vein and sigmoid sinus	Thrombosis, hemorrhage
		Cranial nerves 9, 10, 11	Dysphagia, aspiration
			Hoarseness
			Shoulder dysfunction
		Mastoid and middle ear	Conductive hearing loss
			CSF fistula, meningitis
		Mandibular (condylar) fossa	Trismus, difficulty chewing, malocclusion
Posterior cranial base	Foramen magnum	Vertebral arteries	Stroke, hemorrhage, death
	Occiput	Paravertebral muscles	Chronic postoperative pain
	Lower clivus	Spinal cord	Variable neurologic deficits

CSF, cerebrospinal fluid.

nial dissection, the opportunity for ascending infection would likely increase. Most teams prefer to keep the duration of intracranial exposure to a minimum.

Occasionally in skull base surgery the issue of performing the operation in two separate stages is worth considering. This can be useful if the procedure will be very lengthy, or if the patient is better suited to tolerate two moderate anesthetic exposures instead of a single prolonged one. Staging of operations is not often necessary in anterior skull base surgery but can be helpful in other cases, e.g., when extensive temporal bone dissection or brainstem tumor dissection will be required. For staging to be practical, there must be a sensible point at which to terminate the procedure on day 1, and to resume on day 2, without compromising patient safety or oncologic principles. Usually this point is reached when the approach is completed but before tumor removal begins. The

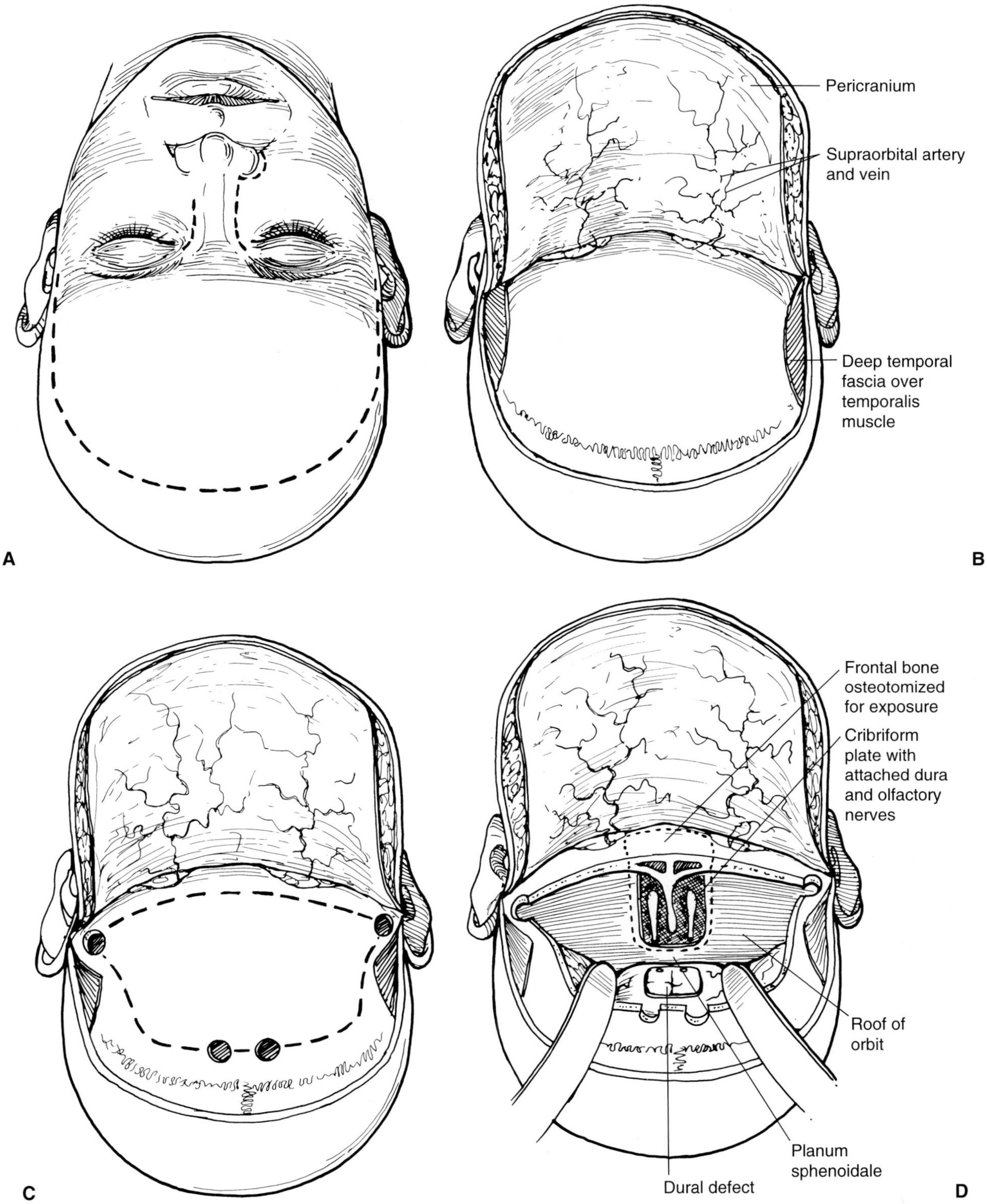

FIG. 27-1. Anterior craniofacial resection. **A:** Incisions. High bicoronal scalp incision is used for cranial access, while transfacial access is usually accomplished via lateral rhinotomy, with or without contralateral Lynch incision, depending on tumor location (see text). **B:** Dissection of scalp flap. Pericranium has been released from its attachments to deep temporal fascia; supraorbital vascular pedicles have been carefully preserved to maintain vascularity to the pericranial flap (see text). **C:** Bifrontal craniotomy is outlined. Note burr hole placement in temporal fossae and above hairline, away from visible portions of forehead, to minimize postoperative aesthetic deformity. **D:** Intracranial exposure. Frontal lobes have been retracted, and dura over anterior cranial fossa floor incised, to obtain the necessary margin around tumor. Resection osteotomies, the precise placement of which are determined in each case by tumor extent, are marked around cribriform plate. Additional exposure osteotomies of anterior frontal skull are designed to provide improved access. *(Continued.)*

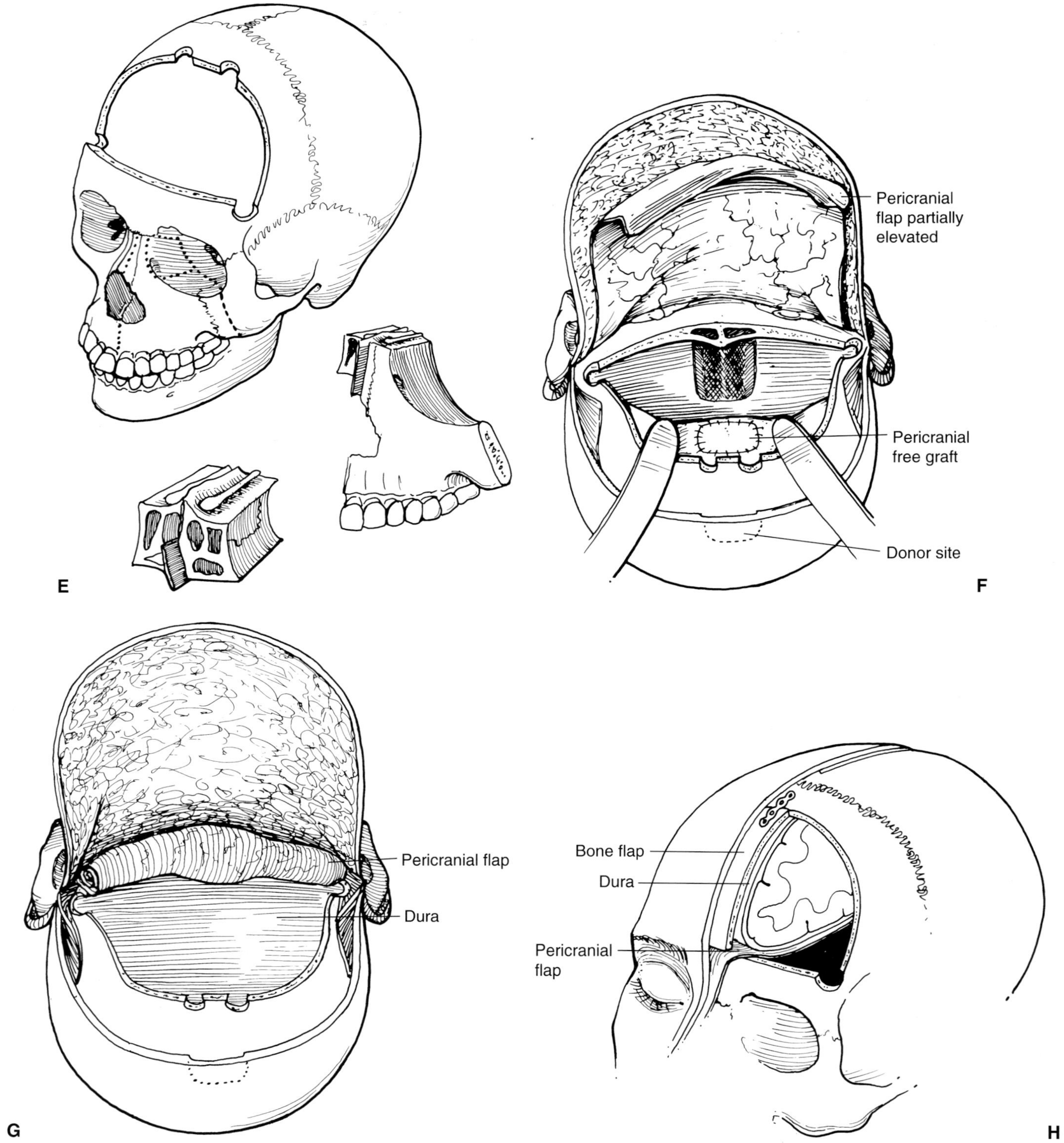

FIG. 27-1. *Continued.* **E:** Facial osteotomies. En bloc ethmoidectomy results in specimen as shown at *bottom left.* Extension to include maxillectomy (with or without orbital exenteration), results in specimen as shown at *bottom right.* Note that in either case, resection encompasses part of anterior cranial fossa floor. **F:** Operative defect and preparation for closure. Large communication between anterior cranial fossa and nasal cavity will be closed by inset of vascularized pericranial flap (shown partially elevated from galea). Dural defect created by resection of olfactory nerves and surrounding dura has been closed with free graft of pericranium taken from posterior scalp (*dotted lines*). Frontal sinuses have been stripped of mucosa and will be filled with autogenous fat after obliterating frontonasal ducts. **G:** Cranial base defect repaired. Pericranial flap has been inset intracranially along anterior cranial fossa floor. **H:** Cutaway view of final closure showing position of pericranial flap relative to brain. Note that frontal bone flap is secured so as to avoid compressing base of pericranial flap. (Adapted from ref. 102, with permission.)

advantage is that in stage two, the team is fresh and optimally prepared for a challenging resection. Staging is most appropriate for benign tumors whose removal is likely to require prolonged tedious microdissection. Oncologically, staging may be inappropriate for malignancies.

Management of the Airway

Agreement concerning the most appropriate method of securing the airway is of considerable importance. A dislodged airway during a lengthy skull base procedure can be disruptive or even disastrous. The need to change the position of the patient's head, or to have access to the nasal or oral cavities during tumor dissection, may influence the decision for oral versus nasal intubation, or tracheotomy. Dialogue regarding operative airway management as well as the need for postoperative airway diversion (see Management of Complications, below) should take place before the procedure begins, and must not be arbitrary.

Patient Positioning and Head Fixation

Proper patient positioning and stable fixation of the head can be crucial to achieving a good result, but the needs of the team members are frequently at variance. In executing a maxillectomy as part of craniofacial resection, the otolaryngologist must view the operative field from a variety of perspectives, which makes it desirable to be able to freely turn the head during the surgery. In contrast, absolute stability of the head in pins might be needed during microneurodissection. Usually there is room for compromise, but the needs of each case are unique, and therefore these issues must be agreed upon in advance.

Other Preoperative Issues

Decisions regarding anesthetics, the use or avoidance of neuromuscular blockers, and electrophysiologic monitoring strategies should also be agreed upon by the team members prior to the beginning of the surgery. These issues can play a major role in bringing about a successful neurologic outcome.

Sometimes even the most minor details can become obstacles to a satisfactory end. Despite the fact that this is the enlightened era of skull base surgery, the surgical world is still a fairly ritualistic one, and surgeons have particular preferences about their style of operating. Whether or not to shave the patient's head, the manner of laying out the sterile drapes, and other related tasks may not be of any real scientific consequence, and yet it is still true that in skull base surgery attention to small details can sometimes set the tone of an operation that can make the difference between success and failure. In these matters collaboration sometimes means compromising on the lesser issues and focusing on the overall outcome.

Selection of the Incisions

Incision placement for craniofacial resection (and for skull base surgery in general) can be highly consequential and is never a minor issue. Poor incision design can restrict the operative exposure or compromise blood supply to adjacent tissues, both of which can be problematic and sometimes dangerous. At the very least, a poor incision may produce a disappointing aesthetic result.

In designing incisions, the question is frequently asked: What incision will give the best access? Optimal placement of incisions, however, must take into consideration more than just the question of access. The ideal incision (a) provides needed access to underlying structures, (b) does not unnecessarily interrupt blood supply to useful regional tissues, and (c) does not "burn any bridges" in the event that future surgeries become necessary. In dealing with head and neck neoplasms, it is well to remember the clinical dictum, "Once a tumor patient, always a tumor patient." Despite our best efforts, tumors do indeed recur, and it is therefore prudent to employ incisions that will be utilitarian for the present as well as the future. A final condition: (d) the ideal incision also leaves a satisfactory aesthetic result.

A variety of incisions can be used to expose the frontal skull, including browline, midforehead, hairline, hemicoronal, and bicoronal incisions. For anterior skull base surgery, the most utilitarian of these is the bicoronal incision (see Fig. 27-1). It gives unrestricted access to both frontotemporal regions (as well as the zygomatic and orbital areas), it facilitates development of a pericranial flap with a generous length, it serves equally well for reoperation, and it gives a good aesthetic result.

In contrast to the scalp, many different incisions can be used on the face with good result (lateral rhinotomy, Lynch, Weber-Fergusson, facial degloving, and others). More so than for the scalp incision, the choice of facial incision is influenced by the tumor's extracranial extent. The same overall criteria for incision placement apply.

Soft Tissue Dissection

The soft tissue dissection (i.e., the mobilization of single-layer, composite, or full-thickness units of the face and scalp) is also an extremely important aspect of skull base surgery, because if it is not well planned and executed, it can jeopardize the success of the entire operation. In anterior craniofacial resection, probably the most crucial aspect of soft tissue dissection is that related to the pericranial flap. Since the pericranial flap is the workhorse flap for anterior skull base reconstruction (7–9), elevation of the scalp from the skull must be carried out cautiously so as to preserve the pericranium with its vascularity intact.

There are several methods for developing the pericranial flap. Some surgeons favor a subgaleal plane of dissection (within the loose areolar connective tissue) for reflecting the scalp forward, leaving the pericranium attached to the skull.

The pericranium is then elevated from the skull and laid back over the galea, where it remains until time for reconstruction. This technique has the advantage of being fast and simple, since the areolar tissue readily gives way to blunt dissection. Unless done very carefully, however, this method often results in inadvertent stripping or perforation of the pericranium, and may thus compromise the utility of the flap.

Another method (more reliable in the authors' experience) is to undermine the scalp in a subpericranial plane, leaving the pericranium attached to the galea until the reconstructive phase of the operation, when it can be readily dissected with minimal difficulty and with less chance of injury (Fig. 27-1F–H). The importance of dissecting this flap carefully cannot be overemphasized, because it serves as the chief protection against ascending infection from the nasal cavity to the cranium. Either of the two methods can be effective, but the neurosurgeon and the otolaryngologist must be cognizant of the flap's pivotal role in preventing disastrous complications, and both must guard against injury to the flap during all phases of the operation.

Craniofacial Osteotomies

Another crucial aspect of the surgery is the placement of osteotomies to complete the process of craniofacial disassembly. There are many ways of dismantling the skull and facial skeleton, and the number of possible combinations of osteotomy sites is infinite. The purpose here is not to recommend one pattern or another; quite the contrary—the recommendation is to avoid using one standard method and instead to always place osteotomies where they make the most sense in each particular case; guidelines for optimal placement follow.

One should distinguish between osteotomies made for exposure and those made as part of the tumor resection. *Exposure osteotomies* are designed to temporarily displace healthy bone segments for the purpose of achieving better access, while *resection osteotomies* constitute the actual resection margins necessary to effect complete tumor removal from the base of the skull (Fig. 27-1C–E). While there is a great deal of flexibility in choosing where to place the exposure osteotomies, the placement of resection osteotomies is dictated solely by the extent of the tumor. Collaboration regarding osteotomy placement begins with mapping out the tumor extent, which in turn dictates the placement of resection osteotomies; exposure osteotomies are then adapted to optimize access. Extremely helpful in this regard is the concomitant use of CT and MRI scans, anatomic diagrams, and model skulls, so that both the surgeons have a clear picture of what the resection and disassembly plan will be.

Technically, exposure osteotomies should be made as precisely as possible, and in as few pieces as possible, avoiding the tendency to simply "nibble away" with rongeurs at bone that obstructs access. By preserving as much bone as possible in its natural contour, reconstruction can be more accurate, minimizing the need for bone grafting and reducing the number of potential sites for nonunion. This is crucial when disassembling the orbital walls, where even small discrepancies in reconstruction can lead to diplopia or dystopia that can be very difficult to correct.

Even very extensive disassembly is safe if done carefully. The adage that "bone removal is better than brain retraction" merits repeating. Exposure osteotomies should be used liberally, as opposed to working through restricted openings in the skull and having to retract the brain. Similarly, it is better to disassemble the orbital framework than to vigorously retract against the globe and orbital contents.

An important related factor to consider is the postoperative milieu for bone healing. If the patient has had prior radiation therapy, preexisting bone disease, or osteitis (often seen with chronic infection caused by obstructing tumors), there is an increased risk of postoperative bone infection, which can be a devastating reconstructive problem because it usually requires removal of the affected bones. In these cases, disassembly should be designed in such a way as to preserve blood supply to the osteotomized bones. The frontal bone can be pedicled on the temporalis muscle (Fig. 27-2), and the facial bones can be mobilized using a variety of vascularized flap designs. Vascularized bone flaps are much more resistant to postoperative infection. Again, this is a situation in which planning is vital.

Tumor Resection

Definitive tumor resection is the point when the collaborative effort reaches its zenith. Both the neurosurgeon and the otolaryngologist have completed their approaches to the tumor, and established a perimeter around it. Tumor removal is now a complex three-dimensional exercise in which each member of the team depends on the other to provide continuous feedback regarding the accuracy of the cuts, the adequacy of the margins, and the safety of the nearby vital structures, until the specimen is ultimately removed.

Reconstruction

With the tumor out, both team members work to establish hemostasis and if necessary to submit appropriate specimens from the margins for histologic study. Prompt closure of the dura is usually the next priority. Discussion then focuses on the best method for repairing the cranial floor to isolate the sinonasal tract from the intracranial space (nasocranial separation). Generally, the bony cranial floor need not be replaced with bone unless the defect is quite large, provided that a suitable soft tissue barrier is placed. Most often, this will be accomplished with the pericranial flap (Figs. 27-1F–H and 27-3). (In other areas of the skull base, the issue is the same: isolating the cranium from the contaminated spaces below. The temporalis muscle flap is the workhorse of the middle and posterior skull base regions; other alternatives exist depending on the situation.)

A key issue at this point is the management of the frontal

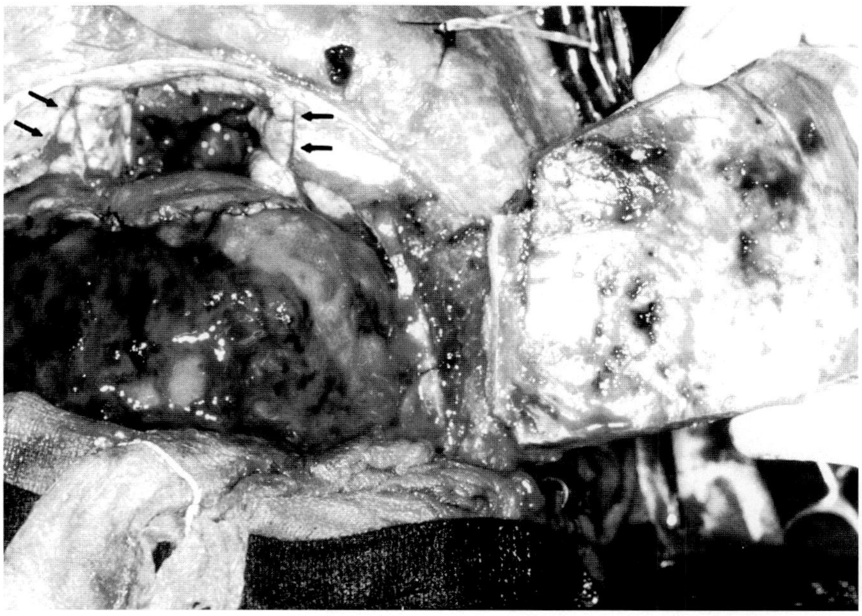

A

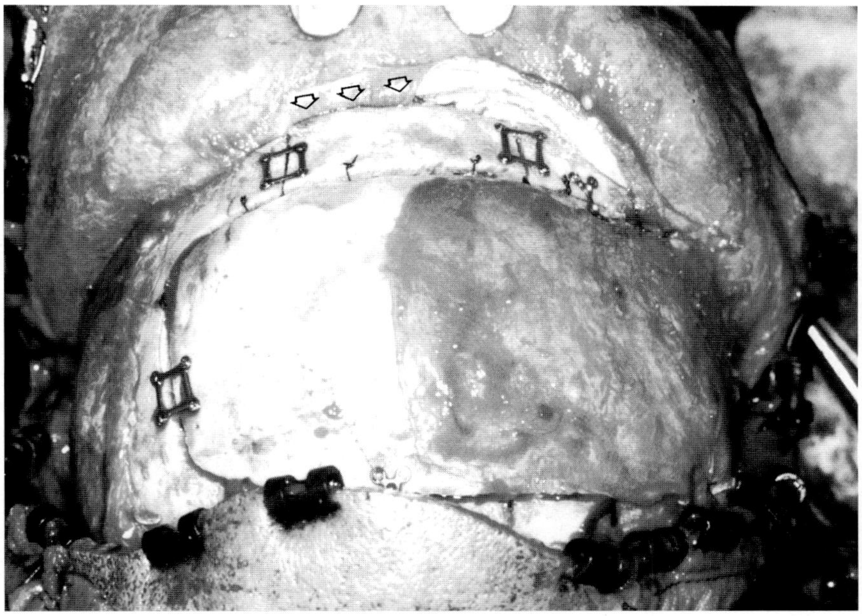

B

FIG. 27-2. Vascularized frontal craniotomy bone flap. **A:** The frontal bone (held in surgeon's hand at *right*) has been osteotomized in such a way as to preserve soft tissue attachment to right temporalis muscle and fascia. Note active bleeding from internal surface of bone at multiple sites. Additional exposure osteotomies of the orbital rims and nasion have been made (*arrows*), improving access to frontobasal area and orbits (see also Fig. 27-1D). **B:** Bone flap replaced and secured, showing generous fascial attachment to right temporal region. A pericranial flap based unilaterally on the left supraorbital vascular pedicle has been inserted through the more inferior exposure osteotomy site (*open arrows*). (Courtesy of Dr. Roger D. Smith.)

sinus. If the sinus has been transected by the osteotomies, it must be completely stripped of all mucosa (to eliminate all traces of epithelium) and isolated from the nasal cavity. The nasofrontal ducts must be obliterated (usually packed with fat or muscle), and the remainder of the sinus can be managed either by cranialization (removing the posterior wall) or by obliteration (filling it with fat or muscle) (Fig. 27-1F–H). Failure to do so will render it a dead space, which can lead to osteomyelitis, loss of the frontal bone flap, meningitis, or epidural abscess. Frontal sinus management is an extremely important detail demanding the attention of both teams.

The otolaryngologist then makes sure that the remaining paranasal sinuses are adequately opened so that no isolated potentially septic spaces remain. Although this portion of the reconstruction (actually it is more of a renovation) does not require collaboration per se, it is crucial for the neurosurgeon to understand the importance of devoting extra time at this point to verify that all the remaining sinuses are indeed well opened and easily accessible through the nose for postoperative suctioning and cleaning, which is vital for healing.

It should be reemphasized here that no matter which part of the skull base is being addressed, the team must exercise great diligence in definitively separating the cranial vault from the pneumatized and mucosalized compartments below.

Once the nasocranial separation phase of reconstruction has been completed, the cranial and facial bone segments are replaced. Soft tissue flaps are now meticulously replaced and closed with precision. Fine details such as fixation of

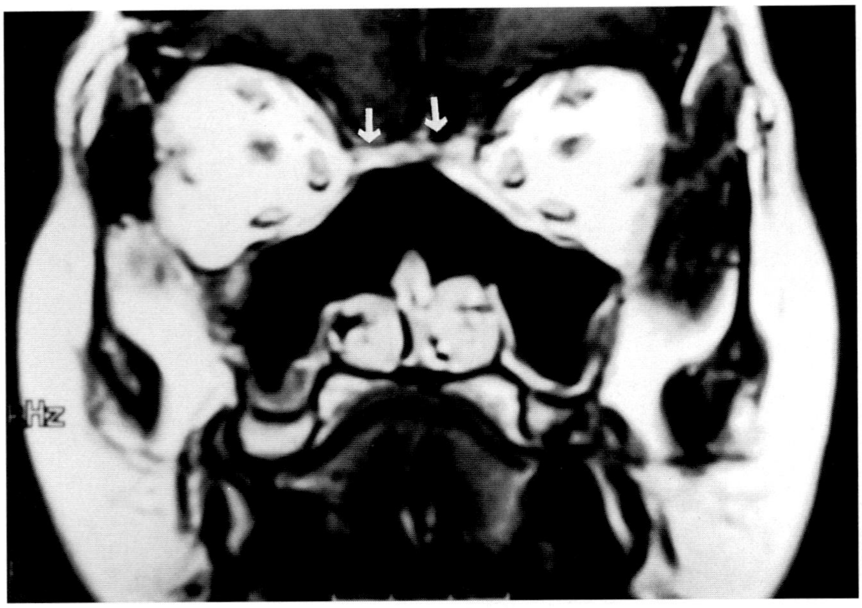

FIG. 27-3. Coronal MRI after craniofacial tumor resection, demonstrating pericranial flap (*arrows*) as it separates cranial vault from sinonasal cavity below. No bone graft has been used to reconstruct the cranial floor. Extensive resection of ethmoid and maxillary sinuses as well as medial orbital walls has been carried out.

the medial canthal ligament, stenting of the lacrimal drainage system, and accurate approximation of key aesthetic units are executed. Whenever possible, burr holes in the skull are filled in or covered with circular plates; bone flaps should be replaced as accurately as possible to minimize visible ridges, and all fixation hardware should be low profile, so as to avoid an irregular forehead contour.

The preceding description of the collaborative process, as it unfolds relative to anterior craniofacial resection, illustrates the interactions between neurosurgeon and otolaryngologist in the management of a head and neck tumor invading the skull base. The scheme is very much the same whether the operation involves the anterior, middle, or posterior cranial base, though the specifics change by region (see Table 27-2). Whatever the region, the process is ideally one in which there is a step-by-step, side-by-side, thoughtfully planned and cautiously executed sequence of events, conducted by individuals who have a vested mutual interest in the patient's welfare; its culmination is successful tumor removal, with good outcome. This is in sharp contrast to the ''relay-race'' notion of ''experts taking turns'' without significant overlap or engagement.

HEAD AND NECK TUMORS WITH SKULL BASE INVOLVEMENT

There is remarkable diversity in the kinds of head and neck tumors that can involve the skull base. This diversity reflects the many tissue types that compose the region: cartilage, bone, muscles, fasciae, and connective tissues; epithelial coverings and sensory surfaces (mucosa, skin, olfactory, auditory, vestibular, and gustatory receptors); glandular structures (lacrimal, mucous, and salivary) and their ductal systems; blood vessels, nerves, lymphoreticular tissue, and others. The abundance of tumor types mandates an understanding of the clinical behavior of each, so that treatment planning can be tailored appropriately.

Before discussing specific tumors, a few general observations are in order. First, the signs and symptoms of head and neck tumors involving the cranial base are different from those of tumors that arise intracranially. A brief review of the most common clinical manifestations of these tumors is presented in Tables 27-3, 27-4, and 27-5. Tables 27-6 and 27-7 list the most common head and neck tumors affecting the skull base.

Second, the role of surgery is well defined in the treatment of head and neck tumors that involve the skull base. On a general basis, surgery is the treatment of choice for virtually all the benign tumors, and for most of the malignant tumors as well (often in conjunction with adjuvant treatments). Having acknowledged that general rule, however, it is important to point out that each patient needs to be evaluated according to specific criteria before surgery is recommended.

TABLE 27–3. *Clinical manifestations of head and neck tumors involving the anterior skull base*

Sign/symptom	Cause
Nasal obstruction, mucorrhea	Mass effect
Epistaxis	Mucosal erosion
Anosmia	CN I involvement
Decreased visual acuity	CN II involvement
Proptosis, diplopia	Mechanical displacement of ocular globe
Epiphora	Lacrimal duct obstruction
Sinusitis	Obstruction of ostia
CSF rhinorrhea	Destruction of anterior fossa floor
Facial pain, swelling	Direct extension of lesion

CSF, cerebrospinal fluid; CN, cranial nerve.
Modified from ref. 52, with permission.

TABLE 27–4. *Clinical manifestations of head and neck tumors involving the middle skull base*

Sign/symptom	Cause
Ocular gaze palsy	Involvement of CN III, IV, or VI at superior orbital fissure or within cavernous sinus
Facial numbness, pain	Involvement of CN V1, V2, V3, or all
Trismus, difficulty in chewing	Involvement of CN V3
Serous otitis media and conductive hearing loss	Eustachian tube obstruction
Endocrinopathies	Direct involvement of sella turcica or interference with its blood supply
Facial swelling	Extension of lesion into buccal soft tissues from infratemporal fossa

Modified from ref. 52, with permission.

TABLE 27–5. *Clinical manifestations of head and neck tumors involving the posterior skull base*

Sign/symptom	Cause
Facial palsy, hemifacial spasm	Involvement of CN VII
Hearing loss, tinnitus	Involvement of CN VIII or cochlea
Dysequilibrium, vertigo	Involvement of CN VIII or vestibular apparatus
Glossopharyngeal neuralgia	Involvement of CN IX
Aspiration, cough	Involvement of CN IX, X
Hoarseness, vocal cord paralysis	Involvement of CN X
Shoulder weakness	Involvement of CN XI
Tongue weakness, atrophy	Involvement of CN XII
Weakness of limbs	Compression of descending motor tracts in ventral brainstem
Ataxia, paralysis of conjugate gaze	Advanced compression of brainstem and cerebellum

Modified from ref. 52, with permission.

TABLE 27–6. *Benign head and neck tumors affecting the skull base*

Inverting papilloma
Angiofibroma
Pleomorphic adenoma
Schwannoma
Neurofibroma
Paraganglioma (glomus tumor)
Osteoma
Chondroma
Fibrous dysplasia*
Cholesteatoma (epidermoid cyst)*
Cholesterol granuloma*

* Nonneoplastic lesions that behave like benign tumors.
Modified from ref. 52, with permission.

TABLE 27–7. *Malignant head and neck tumors affecting the skull base*

Squamous cell carcinoma
Adenoid cystic carcinoma
Adenocarcinoma
Mucoepidermoid carcinoma
Chondrosarcoma
Osteogenic sarcoma
Rhabdomyosarcoma
Esthesioneuroblastoma
Melanoma
Lymphoma
Nasopharyngeal carcinoma
Chordoma
Metastatic tumors

Modified from ref. 52, with permission.

What are those criteria? Three key questions must be answered in each case (52): Is the tumor resectable? Is the patient operable? Is the situation curable?

Resectability is in most cases a fairly straightforward technical question that is best addressed using information from the physical examination and the imaging studies, as outlined in Surgical Technique, above. The term *unresectable* in this context would mean that for technical reasons, the tumor simply cannot be satisfactorily removed.

Operability is a more difficult question that goes beyond, and should be kept separate from, the technical issue of resection. This term has been used to describe the patient's ability to undergo (and recover from) the operation that would be needed to achieve tumor resection (52). Being *inoperable* would imply that the patient is not a candidate for the resection for reasons not related to technical tumor removal. These reasons may be objective and medical, e.g., the patient is too infirm to undergo the operation; or they may be subjective and individual, e.g., the patient is unwilling to agree to an operation that has a high risk of stroke, severe neurologic injury, deafness, or blindness.

Curability is a question best answered with a combination of pathologic and clinical information. If a lesion is histologically benign, and its clinical behavior is benign, then the probability of cure with surgery is good. If a lesion is histologically malignant, but its clinical course is indolent, the probability of surgical cure may still be good. If, however, a lesion exhibits an aggressive, destructive clinical course—regardless of its histology—the probability of cure may be poor despite the surgeons' best efforts (see Potential Pitfalls, below). This is not to imply that surgery is only done for the purpose of providing a cure; there are many instances in which cure is not possible but palliation is a reasonable goal. Nevertheless, there should be a realistic assessment of the probable outcome before proceeding.

Specific Neoplasms

The following discussion of head and neck tumors that affect the skull base is organized by region. The discussion begins with lesions of the anterior cranial base (sinuses, nasal cavity, and orbits), and then progresses to middle cranial base (nasopharynx, clivus, pterygopalatine fossa, parotid gland, infratemporal fossa, and parapharyngeal space), and posterior cranial base (ear, temporal bone). Some of the lesions occur in more than one compartment, and to the extent that their management changes, appropriate mention will be made with regard to each site.

Anterior Cranial Base: Paranasal Sinuses, Nasal Cavity, and Orbits

The anterior cranial base is the region most commonly involved by malignancy originating extracranially. Because presenting symptoms (Table 27-3) are at first mild and nonspecific, tumors in these areas typically go unrecognized for long periods; thus they often present in advanced stages.

Squamous Cell Carcinoma

From 70% to 90% of malignant tumors arising in the nasal cavity and paranasal sinuses are squamous cell carcinomas (SCCs). This tumor is most frequent in men over the age of 50; the most common presenting complaint is unilateral nasal obstruction. Fifteen percent of patients have a history of chronic sinusitis or nasal polyps. A history of smoking is common, but it is not as clearly linked to sinonasal SCC as it is to other respiratory cancers. On examination, 86% have an identifiable mass, with pain or bleeding present in over half of cases. The early extension of sinonasal SCC into adjacent compartments, including the skull base, the orbits, and the oral cavity, is testimony to its aggressive behavior (63).

SCC of the paranasal sinuses most often originates in the maxillary, followed by the ethmoid, sphenoid, and frontal sinuses. Almost all cases demonstrate erosion through at least one of the bony walls that separate the nasal and paranasal spaces; thus bone erosion is an important diagnostic sign radiographically. Regardless of the site of origin, all of these tumors have ready access to the cranial base because of the thin bony partitions at the anterior cranial floor (Fig. 27-4).

Surgical resection is the treatment of choice for SCC, usually in conjunction with radiation. The extent of resection depends on the extent of the tumor. SCC of the sinuses involves the walls of the orbit in up to 60% of cases, but does not breach periorbita in half of those cases, making globe preservation possible without compromise to overall survival (64). If the periorbita has been penetrated, orbital exenteration is usually recommended, because of the high risk of recurrence. Involvement of the pterygoid plates is noted in 10% of cases; this is important because it mandates extending the resection to include the pterygopalatine fossa, part of the infratemporal fossa, and part of the sphenoid bone itself.

Ten percent of patients with SCC have cervical lymph nodal metastases at the time of presentation, with another 15% to 20% developing neck disease during their subsequent course. Thus, careful attention must be paid to evaluation of the neck both clinically and radiographically, and neck dissection plays an important role in the management of this disease. The neck must also be evaluated carefully at each postoperative visit to identify treatable metachronous metastases. Similarly, the neck is usually included in the postoperative radiation fields.

Five-year survival for SCC of the sinonasal region has historically been reported in the range of 20% to 50% depending on stage and histologic grade. Recent reports indicate that outcomes have improved with modern skull base techniques, to 67% to 70% (65–68).

Inverting Papilloma

Inverting papilloma (IP) of the sinonasal tract is a benign but dangerous neoplasm. Papillary overgrowth of nasal mucosa becomes progressively disorganized and the epithelial cells ''invert'' into the basement membrane, giving an invasive appearance that is similar to that seen with well-differentiated SCC. Interestingly, SCC occurs in association with IP in 10% to 15% of cases, and IP must therefore be treated as a premalignant lesion (69).

IP typically arises in the lateral nasal wall and secondarily involves adjacent sinuses as well as the orbit; it is locally very destructive, often eroding bone. Intracranial invasion may occur, even in the absence of malignant degeneration (Fig. 27-5). Treatment for IP is exclusively surgical, and wide margins of resection are needed to eradicate the tumor. Skull base resection is justified whenever tumor is in contact with the anterior fossa floor.

Glandular Tumors of the Nose and Sinuses

Adenoid cystic carcinoma (ACC) is the most common cancer of minor salivary gland tissue, which can appear throughout the nasal cavity and paranasal sinuses. This is one of the most interesting and frustrating of all head and neck neoplasms because of its characteristic perineural spread. The neurotropism nearly always involves proximal extension (toward the central nervous system); distal extension is observed less often. The perineural invasion may span long distances, and affected nerves must be resected with generous margins if the disease is to be eradicated. Thus, cranial nerve invasion and proximal spread are the hallmarks of ACC, and these features significantly influence operative management. Like SCC, treatment of ACC is primarily surgical, paying special attention to neural margins.

Postoperative radiation therapy is often used although the tumor is not highly radiosensitive.

The biologic course of ACC is one of relentless progression, local invasion, and recurrence following attempts at surgical removal (70). Unlike most head and neck tumors, the risk of recurrence remains high years after treatment, with recurrences appearing even 10 to 20 years later. Lym-

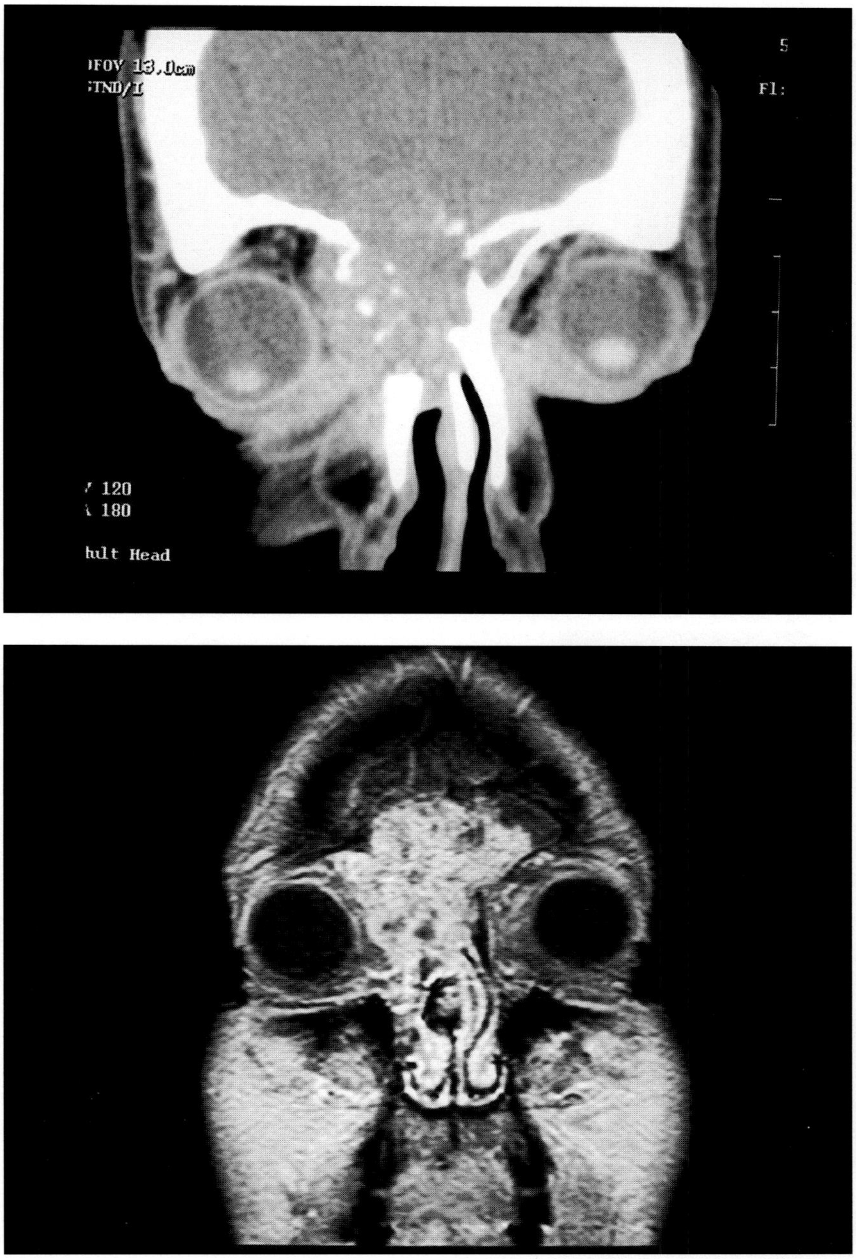

A

B

FIG. 27-4. Squamous cell carcinoma (SCC) of frontal and ethmoid sinuses. **A:** Coronal computed tomography (CT) scan showing extensive destruction of anterior cranial fossa floor and right medial orbital wall. **B:** Coronal magnetic resonance imaging (MRI) scan demonstrating irregular borders of tumor mass in orbit and brain, suspicious for invasion rather than simple displacement. This invasive appearance is typical of SCC.

phatic metastasis is infrequent, with only approximately 14% involving regional lymph nodes. Vascular dissemination is more common, with distant metastases in nearly 40% of patients, mainly affecting lung, bone, and brain. Distant metastases in this disease tend to follow a more indolent course than with other cancers, accounting for only 10% of deaths, and surgical resection of isolated metastases may be beneficial. Recurrent local growth is by far the more common cause of death. Unfortunately, recurrences after skull base resection tend to involve proximal portions of the cranial nerves and the brainstem, and re-resection is not often beneficial (Fig. 27-6).

Adenocarcinoma arises from minor salivary glands, and it often develops in the superior nasal cavity and ethmoids, making skull base involvement likely. Three forms of adenocarcinoma are recognized: papillary, sessile, and alveolar-mucoid. Of the three, papillary has a better prognosis, partly because it metastasizes less often. The papillary form has been linked with occupations involving the leather-tanning, woodworking, and furniture-finishing industries, implicating a possible chemical carcinogen. Cervical lymph nodal metastases occur in less than a third of adenocarcinomas, and the incidence of distant metastases is significantly lower than with ACC. Otherwise, clinical behavior is similar to that of SCC, as is treatment.

Mucoepidermoid carcinoma most frequently involves the maxilla and nasal cavity, with extension into the skull base occurring late. Histologically, these tumors are divided into

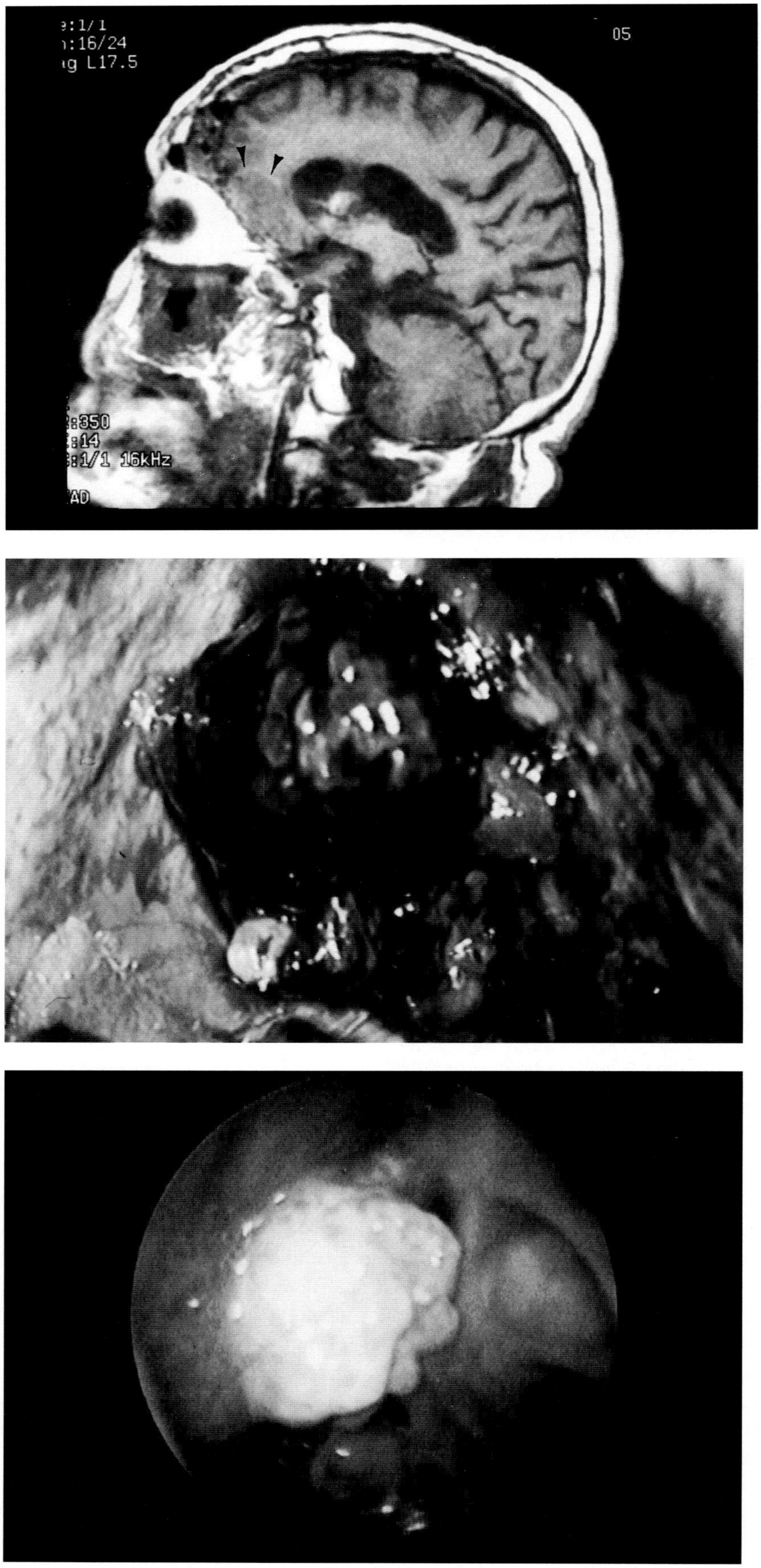

A

B

C

FIG. 27-5. Recurrent inverting papilloma with intracranial invasion. **A:** Parasagittal MRI showing inverting papilloma (*arrowheads*) invading brain. **B:** Magnified intraoperative view of anterior cranial fossa floor, showing intradural tumor after dissection from surrounding brain. **C:** Transnasal endoscopic view of same tumor at superolateral nasal wall.

A

B

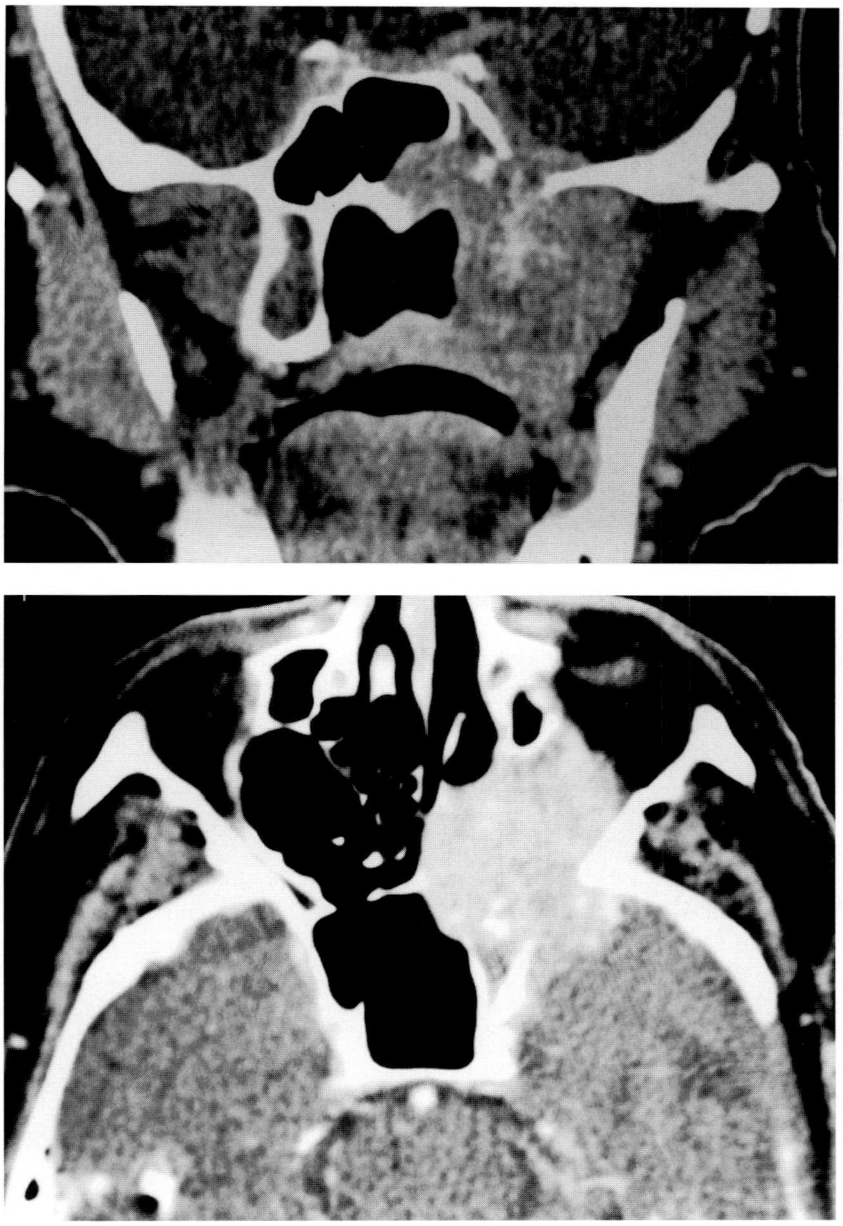

FIG. 27-6. Adenoid cystic carcinoma (ACC), originally arising in maxillary sinus, recurrent after craniofacial resection. **A:** Coronal CT scan shows tumor destroying pterygoid process of sphenoid bone and sphenoid sinus, and invading region of cavernous sinus and Meckel's cave. Patient presented with progressive facial numbness. **B:** Axial view of same patient, showing invasion of orbital apex and temporal lobe. Given the neurotropic pattern of spread of ACC, this recurrence likely followed the infraorbital nerve proximally.

low, intermediate, and high grade based on their degree of cellular differentiation. Low-grade tumors have a reasonably good prognosis, but survival for intermediate- and high-grade tumors is much worse. Aggressive resection is the mainstay of treatment, as these tumors are not often sensitive to radiation therapy; still, radiation is used in the adjuvant role for all but low-grade lesions. The management of these tumors is similar to that for adenocarcinoma and SCC.

Sarcomas

Chondrosarcomas (CSs) are typically slow-growing but very aggressive neoplasms that have a high propensity to recur. They are evenly distributed between the nasal septum, the maxilloethmoidal complex, the sphenoid sinus, and the nasopharynx. They occur in patients from 30 to 50 years of age, with equal gender distribution. Symptoms are related to progressive sinonasal obstruction (congestion, mucorrhea, sinusitis). CS tends to displace local structures prior to invading them, but can be eventually quite destructive, often involving orbits and the cranium (Fig. 27-7).

Histologically, chondrosarcomas can be confused with benign chondroma because of the hypocellular appearance of most cartilaginous neoplasms. Unlike chondromas, however, CS often grows to substantial size. Thus any cartilaginous tumor of the anterior skull base region that is larger than 2 cm should be considered probable CS, and treated as such (70). Radiographically, CS demonstrates characteristic curvilinear calcifications, seen in conjunction with diffuse erosion of the skull base at the tumor margins (71).

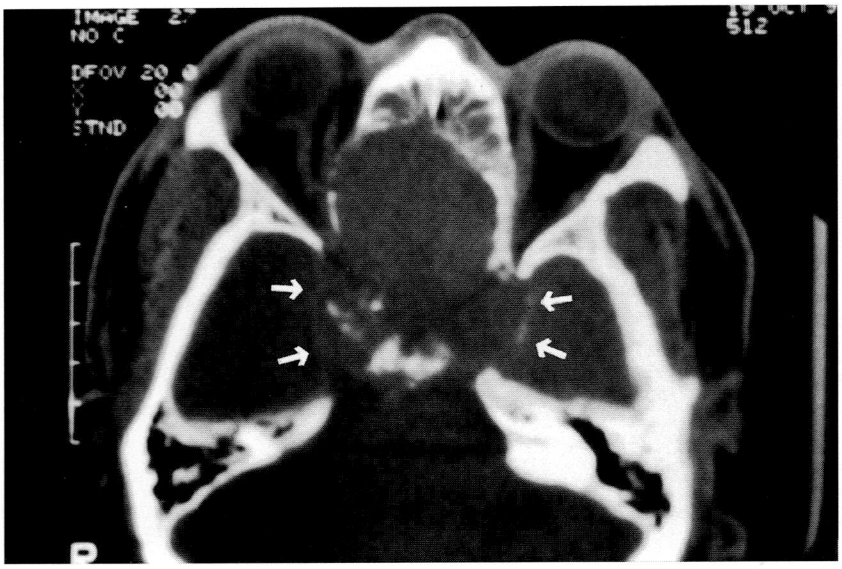

FIG. 27-7. Axial CT scan of chondrosarcoma originating in nasal cavity showing considerable skull base destruction, including invasion of right orbit and extension into clivus as well as both middle cranial fossae (*arrows*). Note at the periphery small scattered calcifications, which are typical of this tumor.

CS is minimally radiosensitive, so surgical resection must be complete. Survival depends on adequacy of resection, location, and histologic grade. Tumors growing posteriorly to involve the central skull base (nasopharynx, sphenoid sinus, clivus) have a poorer ultimate prognosis, because it becomes technically much more difficult to achieve negative margins in these areas as compared with the anterior skull base. Metastases are uncommon, occurring in less than 10% of cases, whereas local recurrence is the rule. Though 5-year survival is 50% to 60%, a significant number of early survivors ultimately succumb to late recurrences (63).

Osteogenic sarcoma (OS) of the head and neck is a rare disease that most often affects the mandible. Of OSs that involve the cranial base, the maxilla and orbit are the most common sites of origin (Fig. 27-8). The mean age of incidence for facial osteosarcomas is in the fourth decade of life, making OS a disease of young adults. Predisposing conditions include prior irradiation, trauma, or preexisting bone disorders, including Paget's disease and fibrous dysplasia (72,73). OS of the orbits and anterior skull base is an unfortunately common occurrence in young adults who have received successful radiation treatment for childhood retinoblastoma.

OS of the maxilla usually presents with facial pain and swelling, and less commonly, facial numbness, loose teeth, trismus, or nasal obstruction. Delay in diagnosis is common not only because of the nonspecific initial complaints, but because the index of suspicion for tumors is typically low in this young age group. The single most effective therapeutic measure for OS is radical resection. Metastases are usually hematogenous; the incidence of cervical metastasis is low.

Rhabdomyosarcoma (RMS) accounts for about 45% of

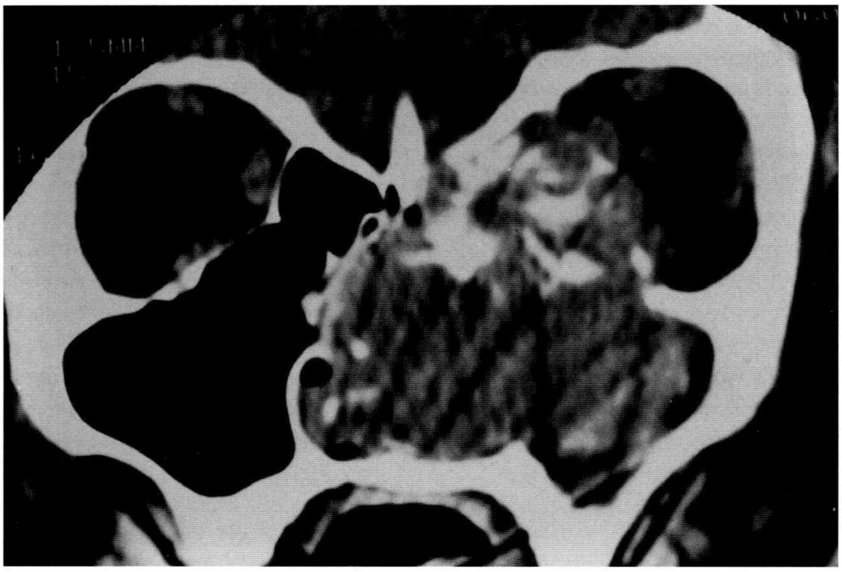

FIG. 27-8. Osteogenic sarcoma of left maxilla and orbit, involving cribriform plate. Osteoblastic activity has produced large areas of new bone within the tumor.

all sarcomas involving the head and neck (73). These tumors are most frequent in the orbit, where they occur in young children and have a fairly good prognosis. The prognosis is worse for RMS in the nasal and paranasal (also infratemporal and middle ear/mastoid) areas, which are classified as cranial-parameningeal sites, because of an increased tendency to spread intracranially from these locations. Presenting findings in the orbit usually include rapidly progressive proptosis, visual loss, and palpable orbital mass. In the nasal/paranasal areas, presentation is similar to other mass lesions. In the middle ear/mastoid areas, RMS frequently masquerades as a smoldering infection, with purulent otorrhea, bleeding, and hearing loss.

Treatment of RMS has evolved in recent years, and is now usually multimodal, including surgery (either for biopsy alone or for nonradical resection), radiation, and multidrug chemotherapy. Much of what we know about RMS comes from studies of the pediatric population, where the tumor is much more common than in adults (74). In children, surgical resection is recommended when it can be accomplished without producing major functional morbidity, especially if removal of tumor will either obviate or reduce the need for postoperative radiation, a major concern in the typically young RMS patient. In the orbits, surgery is usually restricted to biopsy alone, since the functional morbidity of resection is high, and because the results of radiation and chemotherapy at this site are quite good (75–77).

Because patients with parameningeal RMS are at highest risk for recurrent or persistent disease, skull base resection is an option that has been the subject of some debate, and one that needs further study (78). Many adult patients with RMS are still treated with primary surgical resection, followed by radiation and chemotherapy (79). Shah and colleagues (67), however, no longer recommend initial surgery for RMS, treating patients instead with radiation and chemotherapy, and reserving surgery for isolated resectable, persistent disease.

Other Tumors

Esthesioneuroblastoma (ENB) is an unusual (3% of all intranasal neoplasms) but important nasal malignancy arising from olfactory neuroepithelial cells lining the upper nasal septum, the cribriform plate, and the superior turbinate (Fig. 27-9A). Its site of origin at the nasal roof renders it an exemplar for anterior skull base tumors, for it virtually always requires collaborative multidisciplinary surgical management. ENB has been known by a variety of synonyms, including *olfactory neuroblastoma*, *esthesioneurocytoma*, *neuroesthesioma*, and *olfactory esthesioneuroblastoma*.

The typical friable reddish-gray polypoid lesions of ENB can be multifocal and are often bilateral at the time of diagnosis. As one would expect from the usual site of this tumor, penetration of the cribriform plate occurs early in the disease, and both orbital and intracranial invasion can be extensive (Fig. 27-9B). Most patients are young adults, with a slight male predominance (80). Symptoms can precede definitive diagnosis by years; they include rhinorrhea, obstruction, epistaxis, anosmia, and headache.

ENB is a tumor of neural crest origin that may be difficult to differentiate histologically from other small round-cell tumors, such as undifferentiated carcinoma, lymphoma, melanoma, plasmacytoma, metastatic neuroblastoma, and embryonal rhabdomyosarcoma. Thus, a battery of cell surface markers and/or electron microscopy may be necessary to correctly identify ENB. Similar to other neuroendocrine tu-

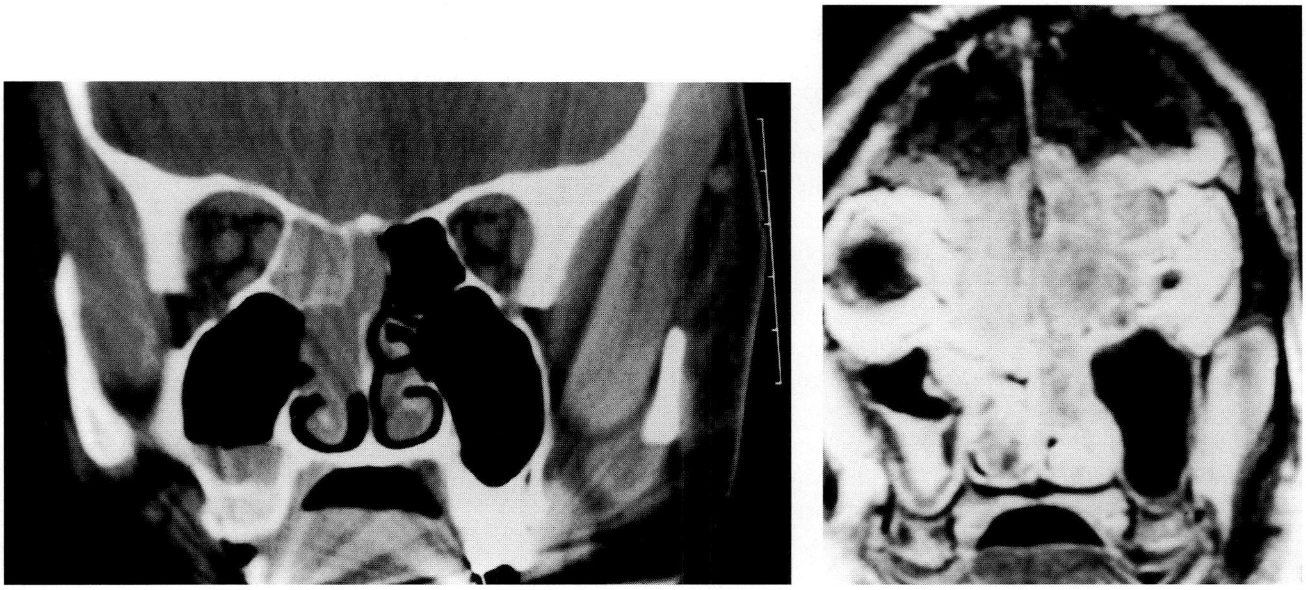

A B

FIG. 27-9. Esthesioneuroblastoma. **A:** Coronal CT scan of early lesion involving upper nasal septum, cribriform area, and ethmoid. **B:** Coronal MRI of advanced lesion showing large intranasal tumor with extensive invasion of anterior cranial fossa and both orbits.

mors, these tumors stain positive on immunohistochemical study for neuron-specific enolase (NSE), chromogranin, and synaptophysin. Carcinoma and mesenchymal and lymphoreticular tumors are excluded by negative staining for epithelial membrane antigen, desmin, myoglobin, S-100 protein, HMB 45, and leukocyte common antigen (70).

Because of the difficulty of diagnosis of a small round-cell tumor (especially on frozen section), and because the differential diagnosis includes several lesions for which the definitive treatment would be quite different (lymphoma, plasmacytoma, metastatic neuroblastoma), it is extremely important to try to confirm the diagnosis prior to undertaking skull base resection (see Potential Pitfalls, below). Usually this is possible via transnasal biopsy; if initial biopsy is insufficient, it should be repeated.

ENB has been reported to show good initial response to chemotherapy and radiation therapy without surgery, but if surgery is feasible it should be performed. Shah et al. (67) have noted that in their series and in Levine et al.'s (81), all patients who underwent craniofacial resection were long-term survivors (most also received radiation), and Shah suggested that adjuvant chemotherapy is unjustifiable in ENB. In these two series, ENB treated with skull base resection had a better prognosis than did any other malignant tumor. Clear surgical margins strongly correlate with prognosis (20% vs. 60% mortality for clear vs. positive margins).

Metastases from ENB occur in 20% of cases, with cervical lymph nodes most common, followed by lungs and long bones. Metastases have shown good initial response to radiotherapy, though they remain the leading cause of mortality in those patients with recurrence (80).

Melanoma accounts for approximately 3% of all malignant neoplasms in the nasal and paranasal spaces. The peak age incidence is between the fifth and eighth decades with no gender predilection. Inspection of the nose may disclose a sessile mass, polyp, or large obstructing tumor, which may or may not appear pigmented.

Radical surgical resection, usually followed by radiation, is the treatment of choice. Even with aggressive treatment, the prognosis is poor for mucosal melanoma, with average survival following diagnosis of 2.3 years, and only 11% survival at 5 years. As with ACC, the risk of recurrence does not appear to decline over time; the 20-year survival rate is only 0.5%. These tumors are noted for early local recurrences with frequent metastases, both to regional lymph nodes and to distant sites. Prophylactic neck dissection is not indicated, but therapeutic neck dissection is recommended when adenopathy is present.

Lymphoma may involve the skull base via the nasal cavity, paranasal sinuses, or orbit. A variety of clinicopathologic terms have been applied to a spectrum of sinonasal diseases now believed to be consistent with lymphoma, including *lethal midline granuloma*, *polymorphic reticulosis*, *midline destructive granuloma*, and *lymphomatoid granulomatosis*. With lymphomas of the skull base, as with lymphomas elsewhere in the body, immunohistochemical, genetic, and molecular testing of carefully handled biopsy material is crucial for determining the tumor subtype and for ruling out other tumor types.

Lymphomas often present as necrotizing lesions of the midline nasal cavity, septum, and adjacent areas. They nearly always produce bleeding, nasal crusting, pain, and irritation; secondary infection is common. Once histologic confirmation is complete, optimal treatment can be determined. Radiation alone cures approximately 50% of patients with low-grade lymphomas; controversy exists as to whether chemotherapy improves this result. For intermediate-grade lymphomas, chemotherapy is now clearly the treatment of choice, and the role of radiation has become controversial. For high-grade lymphomas (Burkitt's and lymphoblastic lymphoma), aggressive chemotherapy is the only treatment (82).

Lymphoma is one of the small round-cell neoplasms that are easily misdiagnosed; this should serve as a reminder that a definitive pretreatment diagnosis is worth pursuing aggressively, to avoid performing an unwarranted skull base resection. Surgical resection for lymphoma is not indicated; the only role for the surgeon—albeit an important one—is in retrieving diagnostic material.

Middle Cranial Base: Nasopharynx, Clivus, Pterygopalatine Fossa, Parotid Gland, Infratemporal Fossa, and Parapharyngeal Space

Nasopharyngeal Carcinoma (NPC)

NPC actually represents a spectrum of cancers that occur in the nasopharynx. Several putative factors have been implicated in the genesis of these tumors, including the Epstein-Barr virus (EBV) and inhalational and dietary agents. NPC is more common in patients of Chinese lineage; it predominates in males by 3:1. The average age at onset is 45 years. Epistaxis, serous otitis and hearing loss (from eustachian tube obstruction), and the presence of a neck mass (from metastasis) are the most frequent initial symptoms.

Diagnosis of NPC usually comes late because of the seemingly trivial initial symptoms in young, otherwise healthy patients. The location of the nasopharynx at the midline skull base provides these tumors with ready access to intracranial structures via nearby foramina and fissures, and it is not unusual for patients to have multiple cranial nerve palsies at presentation (Fig. 27-10) (83). The highly infiltrative nature of the tumor and the rich vascular and lymphatic network surrounding the nasopharynx are additional factors that predispose to tumor progression.

Classification of NPC has important prognostic and therapeutic implications. The World Health Organization (WHO) has recognized three types of NPC: type 1, a keratinizing squamous cell carcinoma; type 2, a nonkeratinizing but differentiated carcinoma; and type 3, an undifferentiated carcinoma. Type 1 behaves like SCC elsewhere in the head and neck, with a resistance to radiotherapy and a generally poor prognosis. Types 2 and 3 have been associated with EBV, are radiosensitive, and have a better prognosis (84).

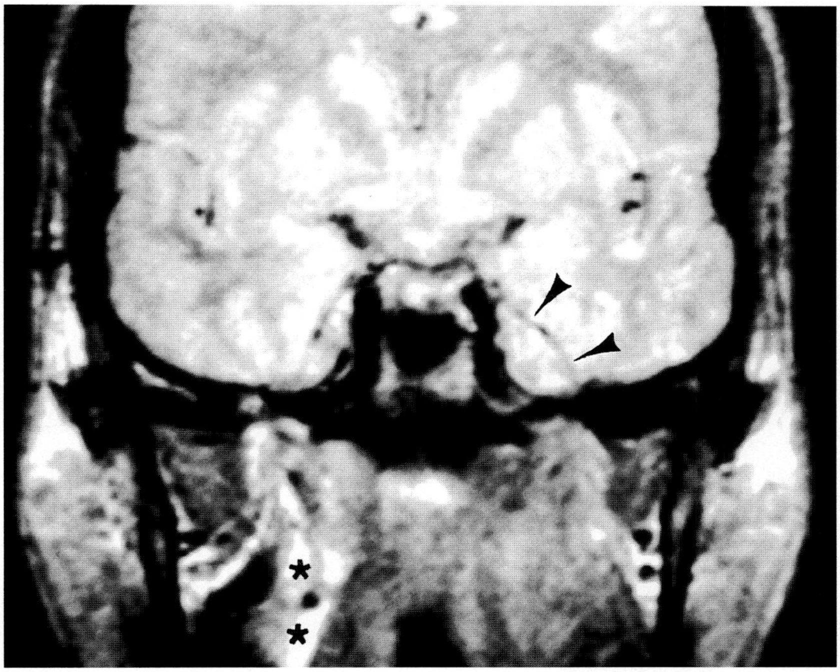

FIG. 27-10. Coronal MRI of patient with nasopharyngeal carcinoma, showing tumor involving left cavernous sinus (*arrowheads*). Note fullness of cavernous sinus as well as concavity of medial temporal lobe, as compared with opposite side. This patient presented with facial pain and sixth nerve palsy. Extracranially, the normal fat planes surrounding the pterygoid muscles have been obliterated by tumor on the left side, but remain intact on the right (*asterisks*).

The mainstay of treatment for NPC of all subtypes is high-dose (60–70 Gy) external beam radiation therapy. Intracavitary, interstitial, and stereotactic radiation have been used successfully for treating recurrent tumors. Anatomic and biologic limitations have traditionally restricted surgical treatment of NPC except for very limited primary lesions or for cervical metastases, in which neck dissection plays an important role. As skull base surgery has evolved, surgical treatment has occasionally been employed as salvage therapy with good results (85,86). Surgical therapy warrants consideration in selected cases, especially in radio-unresponsive WHO type-1 tumors, for which the 5-year survival is expected to be less than 10% (87). Prospective evaluations will be needed before skull base resection can be recommended on a broader basis for NPC.

Juvenile Nasopharyngeal Angiofibroma (JNA)

JNA is a benign but destructive tumor that originates in or near the nasopharynx and nearly always affects adolescent males. These tumors are highly vascular (composed of immature blood vessels) and often signal their presence by severe and sometimes life-threatening epistaxis. Other common symptoms are nasal obstruction and conductive hearing loss.

The diagnosis is based on the highly characteristic clinical scenario of a nasal mass occurring in a teenage boy who has a history of nosebleeds. Biopsy of JNA is dangerous due to the extreme vascularity. Angiography is diagnostic and allows for embolization (Fig. 27-11) prior to surgery, which is the definitive treatment. (Embolization has only a temporary effect, but it facilitates surgery by diminishing the blood supply to the tumor.) Antiandrogenic hormonal manipulation and radiation therapy have been used as alternatives or adjuncts to surgery, but both present serious unwanted side effects.

JNA may recruit vascular supply from any nearby branches of the external or internal carotid system, and although the primary blood supply usually comes from the internal maxillary artery, there are almost always multiple feeders. JNA readily penetrates the skull base and most often gains access through the pterygopalatine fossa, into the orbit, and into the cavernous sinus. There it usually remains extravascular but can sometimes invade, recruiting blood supply from the cavernous portion of the internal carotid artery. Preoperative analysis of the angiogram is extremely important in anticipating this event.

With preoperative embolization and collaborative surgery, most of these tumors are curable. Selection of a surgical approach is individualized according to tumor extent and vascular patterns (88), but for most JNA lesions penetrating the skull base, some combination of transfacial and transcranial exposure is required.

Chordoma

Chordoma arises from remnants of the notochord along the craniospinal axis; 30% to 40% of all chordomas affect the skull base. They are most familiar in the region of the clivus, but may occur anywhere along the skull base, including the anterior cranial floor, orbits, parasellar area, sphenoethmoid region, petroclival region, basiocciput, and also the upper cervical spine. Symptoms vary with location.

Most chordomas appear histologically bland, but their clinical behavior is malignant; these tumors are frequently described as relentless. Chordoma destroys bone and often

A

B

C

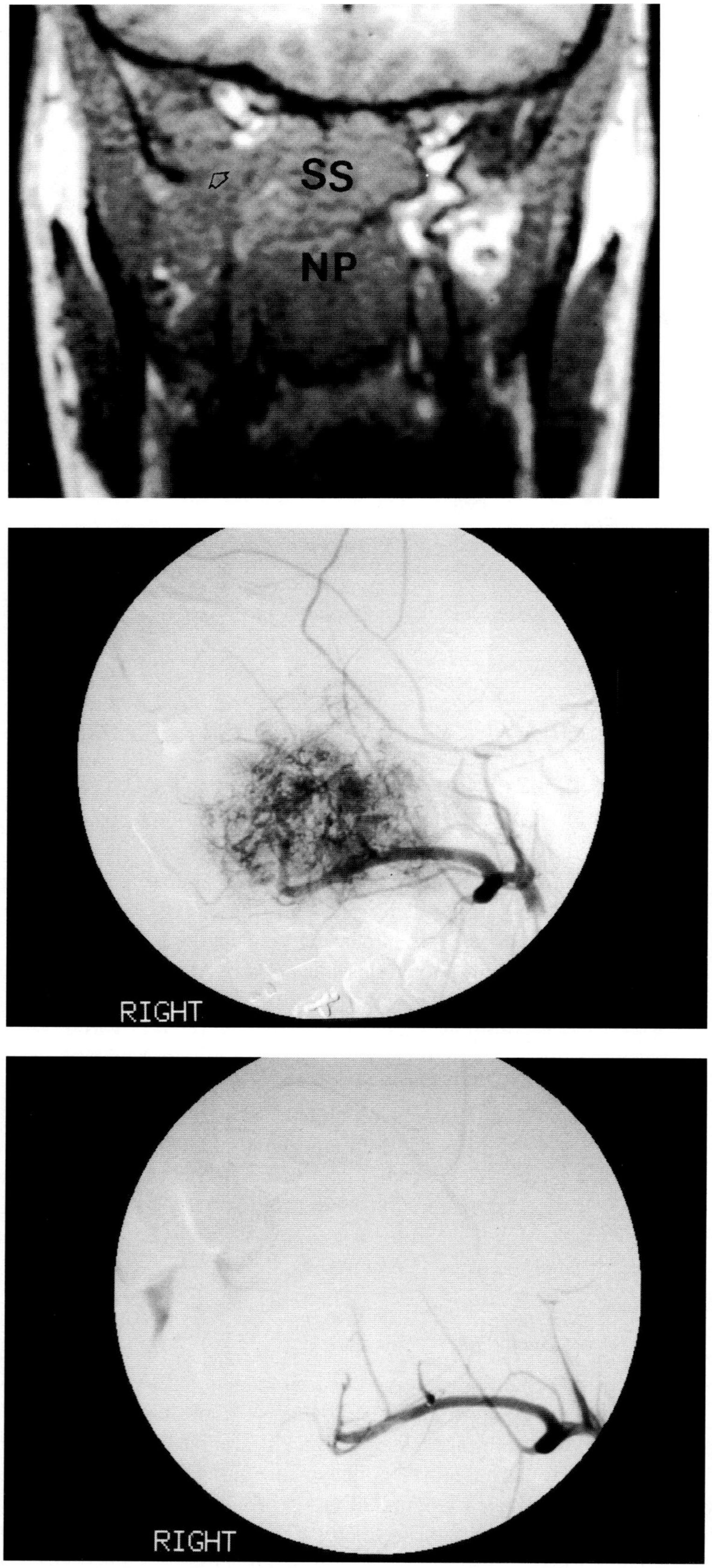

FIG. 27-11. Juvenile nasopharyngeal angiofibroma. **A:** Coronal MRI showing tumor filling sphenoid sinus (SS) and nasopharynx (NP), and extending through the right inferior orbital fissure to enter middle cranial fossa (*open arrow*). Note that tumor has obliterated the normal high-signal fat within the infratemporal fossa, which is well demonstrated on the normal (*left*) side. **B:** Lateral external carotid angiogram demonstrating characteristic tumor blush, prior to embolization. **C:** Following embolization, in preparation for surgical resection.

causes cranial nerve palsies. It typically affects patients between 20 and 40 years of age. A pattern of local recurrence, repeated surgery, and ultimately, death from unresectable tumor is the rule. Although these tumors may remain extraaxial for some time (Fig. 27-12A), invasion of dura and brainstem is often the limiting technical factor that prohibits complete resection of recurrences (Fig. 27-12B). Radiation is frequently recommended for unresectable tumor despite the fact that traditional external beam therapy is largely ineffective in this disease. Studies of proton-beam radiation for chordoma are encouraging but indications for its use are not yet clear.

Chordoma has been classified into two subtypes: typical and chondroid. In the past, the chondroid variant was believed to have a better prognosis, but current information suggests no significant difference in outcomes for the two subtypes. The majority of patients eventually succumb to local recurrence (70).

Despite the almost uniformly dismal course of chordoma, skull base surgery plays a critical role in extending both the time of survival and the quality of life in affected patients (72,89). Aggressive resection can delay symptomatic recurrence, in some cases for years.

Salivary Gland Tumors

Tumors of salivary gland origin can involve the skull base either by arising in the parotid gland (one of the major salivary glands) or by arising in minor salivary gland tissue that occurs microscopically throughout the soft tissues of the sinonasal tract, the infratemporal fossa, and the parapharyngeal space. The most important of the malignant salivary

A
B

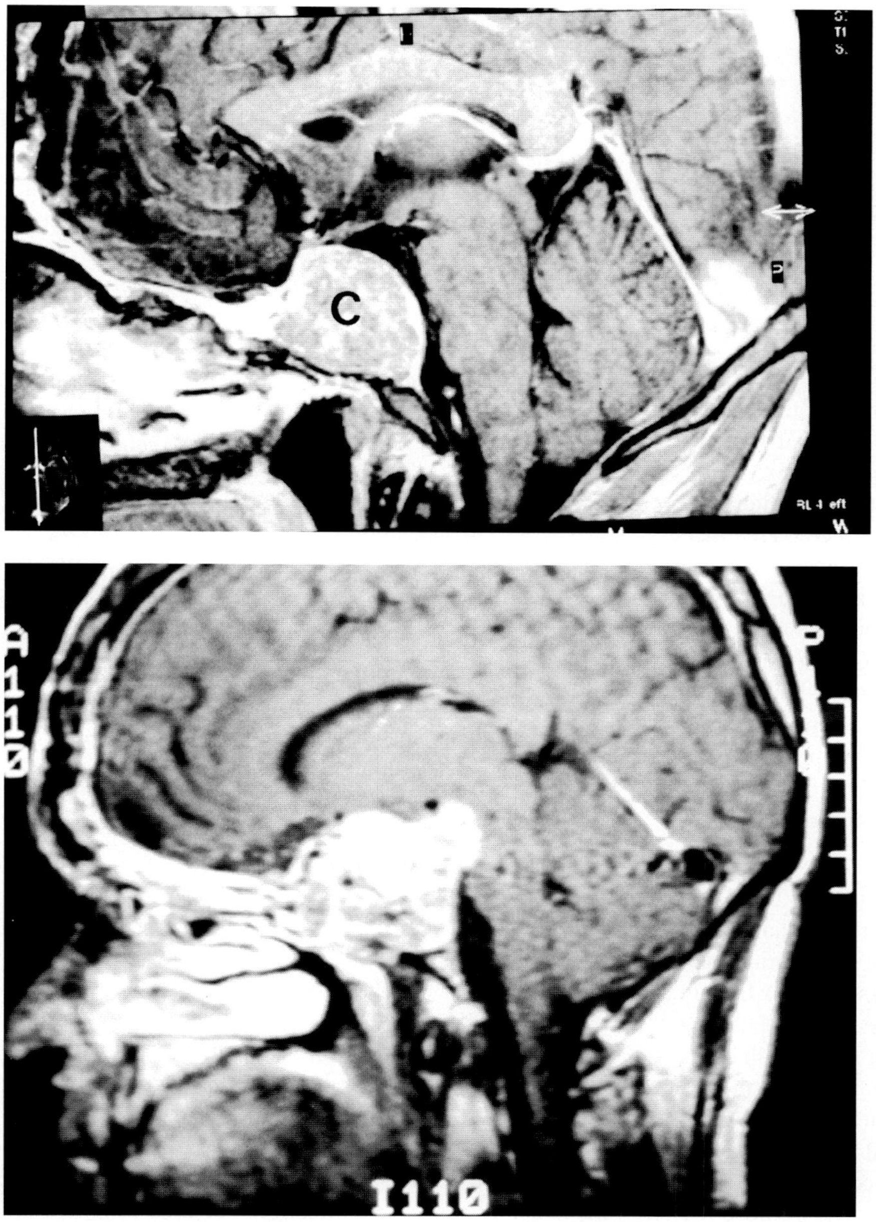

FIG. 27-12. Chordoma, as seen in sagittal MRI scans. **A:** First-time recurrence of clival chordoma (*C*). The clivus has been replaced and expanded by tumor, but the tumor is still extradural. **B:** Recurrent chordoma in same patient 4 years later, showing invasive tumor with involvement of brainstem.

gland tumors have been described above in conjunction with sinonasal tumors.

For practical purposes, management of major and minor salivary tumors differs only with respect to location and the structures that must be manipulated. The parotid gland poses the special technical obstacle of dealing with the facial nerve; this nerve is preserved whenever possible but should be resected if invaded by malignancy. This is especially true when adenoid cystic carcinoma is present.

Statistically, a major salivary gland tumor is more likely to be benign, while in minor salivary tissue, malignancy is the rule. The most common benign salivary neoplasm is *pleomorphic adenoma* (commonly referred to as benign mixed tumor). This lesion, though benign, has a propensity for local recurrence in the parotid gland, and occasionally exhibits aggressive growth that may necessitate resection of adjacent compartments including the infratemporal fossa and parapharyngeal space. Pleomorphic adenoma is notorious for recurrence if the tumor is violated (spilled) during the original surgical resection; thus, every attempt is made to remove it in a monobloc. This tumor occasionally undergoes malignant transformation, in which case it is referred to as carcinoma ex pleomorphic adenoma. Treatment is similar to that for other salivary malignancies.

The parotid gland sometimes is resected as part of the treatment for nonsalivary neoplasms as well, since it contains intraparotid lymph nodes that can be at risk for metastases from cancers in the facial skin, orbit, sinuses, and scalp.

Neurogenic Tumors

Schwannoma and *neurofibroma* occur in various locations throughout the head and neck, with the potential for great morbidity. Much attention has been focused on these lesions in both the neurosurgical and the otolaryngologic literature, so the pathologic details are not reviewed here. Treatment for schwannomas and for solitary neurofibromas is surgical excision. For neurofibromas that occur in the setting of generalized neurofibromatosis, surgery is reserved for palliation in those instances in which the lesion causes severe deformity or dysfunction, since the condition itself is incurable. Skull base approaches are often necessary to eradicate these tumors, because they commonly involve the proximal segments of the cranial nerves, making resection difficult from either the intracranial or the extracranial approach alone.

Parapharyngeal Space Tumors

Parapharyngeal space (PPS) tumors are especially challenging in head and neck surgery, because this region is anatomically complex, and its pathology diverse (90,91). Briefly, the PPS is a potential space (fascial compartment) lateral to the pharynx and posterior to the masticator space, with its lateral border at the mandible and its posterior border at the prevertebral muscles. It takes the shape of an inverted pyramid that has its base at the skull and its apex at the hyoid bone. It is divided into prestyloid and poststyloid compartments.

The prestyloid compartment contains fat and the deep portion of the parotid gland, and it is in contact with the masticator muscles, the mandibular division of the trigeminal nerve (V3), and branches of the internal maxillary artery. Because tumors seldom arise in the nonsalivary structures of this area, the majority of tumors of the prestyloid compartment are of salivary gland origin.

The poststyloid compartment contains the carotid artery, jugular vein, cranial nerves IX to XII, and lymphatic tissue. Thus, it can give rise to tumors of vascular, neurogenic, or lymphoid origin, and because these lymph nodes serve as drainage routes for the pharynx, sinuses, and other areas of the head, this space can also be the site of metastatic cancers from a variety of sources.

Eighty percent of PPS tumors are benign. Many are not discovered until they are quite large and displace the pharyngeal structures medially or the parotid gland laterally. Symptoms vary with the tissue of origin. The common PPS tumor types (salivary gland and neurogenic neoplasms), have been discussed above in relation to other regions. The chief remaining PPS tumor, paraganglioma, is reviewed here.

Paraganglioma is a term used to describe tumors that arise from neuroectodermal tissue (glomus tissue) that normally resides in the PPS along the neurovascular structures. Tumors may originate along the the jugular vein, vagus nerve, or carotid artery. Depending on location, a variety of terms are used to refer to specific paragangliomas, including *glomus jugulare, glomus vagale, carotid paraganglioma (carotid body tumor)*, and others. (*Glomus tympanicum* is the term applied to this tumor when it arises in the middle ear.) Paragangliomas are highly vascular, often destructive, and may be metabolically active, secreting catecholamines that can complicate perioperative management (90). Paragangliomas are sometimes multifocal (up to 10%) and occasionally familial.

Symptoms of paragangliomas relate to their size, location, and cranial nerve involvement. Angiography is diagnostic and serves to define tumor extent. The preferred treatment is surgical resection. When this is not feasible, radiation can arrest tumor growth. Resection for extensive paragangliomas frequently involves combined intracranial-extracranial approaches. When the carotid artery is involved, preoperative balloon occlusion testing and cerebral blood flow studies may be helpful in determining the safest course of action (44).

Posterior Cranial Base: Temporal Bone

SCC is the most frequent head and neck malignancy to affect the posterior skull base. It usually originates in the pinna or ear canal, but occasionally may develop in the middle ear or mastoid. The clinical characteristics of SCC have been reviewed with tumors of the anterior cranial base, but a few observations specific to the temporal bone are warranted.

In the temporal bone, SCC is often a lethal malignancy. It tends to be diagnosed late, in part because it is commonly mistaken for chronic ear infection. The presenting symptoms are essentially those of chronic infection, including otorrhea, hearing loss, bleeding, and pain. To complicate matters further, many patients with SCC of the ear canal and middle ear have a history of chronic otitis media or otitis externa, and are treated on that basis until it becomes obvious that a more serious problem has developed. On the pinna, sun exposure is the likely carcinogen; in the ear canal, middle ear, and mastoid, chronic infection may play an etiologic role.

SCC of the pinna alone is manageable by resection, radiation, or electrodesiccation, with cure rates in excess of 90%. Once the external ear canal is involved, however, the situation becomes far more serious. SCC easily penetrates through the thin skin of the ear canal to the periochondrium and periosteum, where it gains ready access to the parotid gland (via the fissures of Santorini), the middle ear space, and the mastoid (Fig. 27-13). Once in the middle ear and mastoid, it has access to the eustachian tube, carotid artery, jugular bulb, and facial nerve, all within a short distance. Thus, cancer of the external ear canal can be a treacherous disease.

Patients with SCC in or medial to the ear canal experience intense deep, boring pain, and often present with facial weakness or paralysis. Typically a friable mass with foul or bloody discharge is noted. Biopsy confirms the diagnosis. Staging is extremely important for surgical planning (92). High-resolution CT is essential to define tumor extent within the temporal bone; MRI may provide complementary information about extratemporal extension, especially intracranially.

Surgery is the only effective treatment for cancer in the

A

B

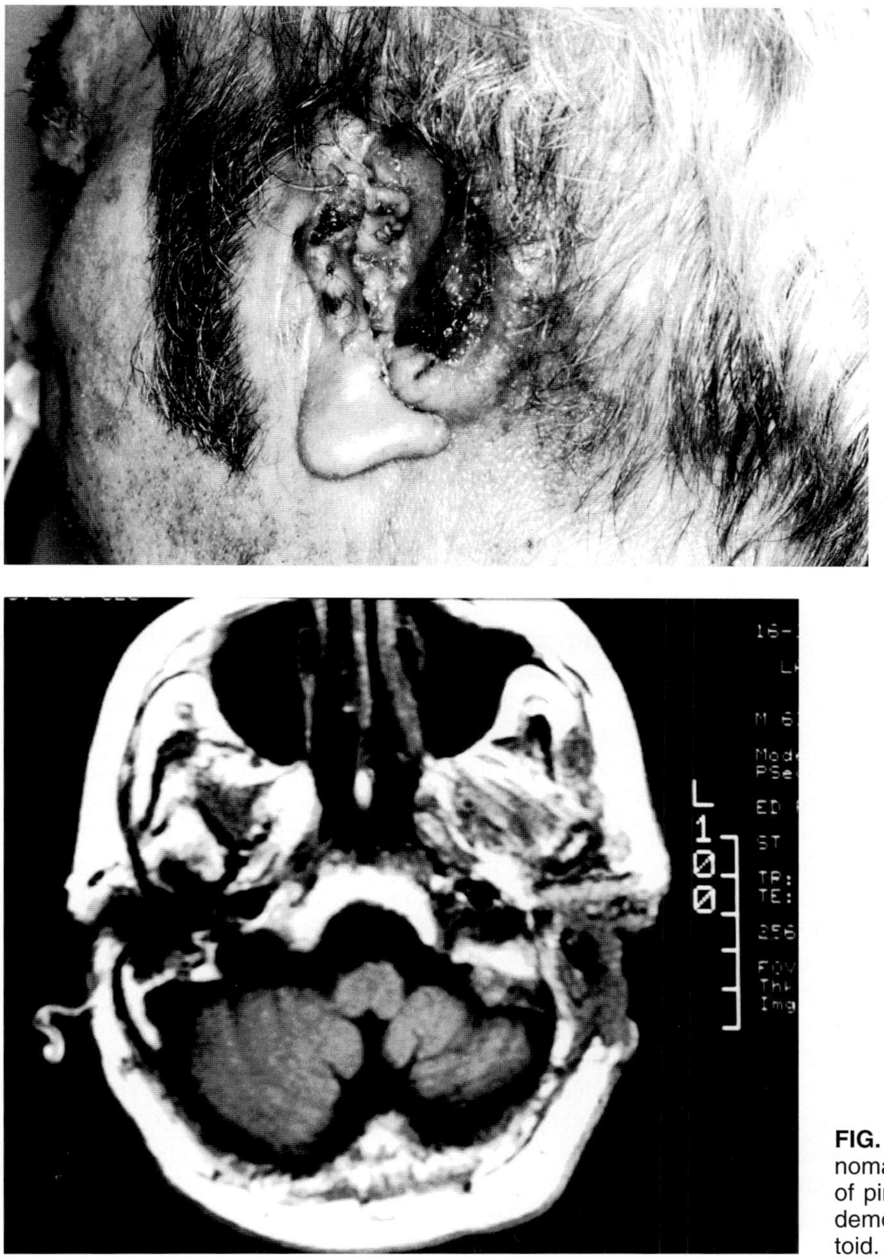

FIG. 27-13. Advanced squamous cell carcinoma of external ear. **A:** Extensive destruction of pinna and surrounding skin. **B:** Axial MRI demonstrating tumor deeply infiltrating mastoid.

temporal bone. Radiation alone is ineffective, although it is useful as an adjuvant. As with SCC elsewhere, partial resection is of no benefit. Therefore, to be effective, the surgery must be en bloc and sufficiently radical. Because of the need for en bloc resection, collaborative surgery by the skull base team is often required.

Temporal bone resection (TBR) can be classified as lateral, subtotal, or total. *Lateral TBR* removes the external ear canal, the tympanic membrane, and the malleus and incus. *Subtotal TBR* removes those structures plus the otic capsule (cochlea, labyrinth, and vestibule). *Total TBR* encompasses all of the above plus the petrous apex. The extent of the lesion dictates which operation is most appropriate.

Total temporal bone resection is one of the most formidable of all skull base operations because of the importance of the structures that adjoin or traverse that portion of the skull, including cranial nerves V and VII through XII, internal carotid artery, jugular vein, sigmoid sinus, and petrosal sinuses (93–95). Carotid artery involvement is a special concern that requires careful preoperative evaluation and meticulous intraoperative management if the patient is to survive the surgery. Reconstruction of the defect usually requires a large regional flap or free tissue transfer. Postoperative rehabilitation for multiple cranial nerve deficits must attempt to compensate for paralysis of the face, vocal cord, and tongue in particular.

Temporal bone resection also has its place in the management of tumors that invade the temporal bone secondarily, such as ACC of the parotid gland, basal cell carcinoma of the facial skin, and others. Whenever TBR is performed for malignancy, consideration should be given to simultaneous neck dissection and parotidectomy to address the regional lymph nodes if the primary tumor is prone to nodal metastasis or if adenopathy is present. TBR is usually not considered appropriate for treatment of metastatic disease to the temporal bone from remote (non–head and neck) primary cancers.

POTENTIAL PITFALLS

In the management of head and neck tumors with skull base involvement, the most significant potential pitfalls lie in the planning process. This is fortuitous because in most cases, with adequate preparation, they can be avoided.

One of the most serious potential pitfalls in skull base surgery is when an *unexpected histologic diagnosis* is discovered intraoperatively, and the surgical plan has not adequately prepared for it. This disturbing ordeal is avoidable. Because the variety of head and neck tumor pathologies that can involve the skull base is vast, and because the surgical options are complex, it helps a great deal to have, whenever possible, histologic confirmation prior to surgery. Luckily, unlike intracranial tumors, the majority of head and neck tumors are readily accessible for direct inspection, biopsy, or both. For most, preoperative biopsy can be safely obtained either directly (through the nose, sinuses, oral cavity, or ear) or indirectly (via transcutaneous or transmucosal fine-needle aspiration, with or without CT guidance). Careful study of the histologic material almost always yields a definitive diagnosis, or at least narrows the range of possibilities considerably. Preoperative knowledge that a tumor is malignant rather than benign mandates a more aggressive surgical approach, and this kind of information helps the team to prepare decisively, and to avoid the potential oncologic compromise that occurs when a tumor is thought to be benign but is unexpectedly found to be otherwise.

Similarly, accurate preoperative assessment can prevent another dangerous pitfall: *underestimation of tumor extent.* Optimal preoperative "reconnaissance" involves integration of the findings from the physical examination with the findings from the imaging studies. Accordingly, three axioms apply: (a) the physical exam must be thorough, (b) the imaging studies must be fully adequate, and (c) both must be timely in relation to the surgery.

How are these axioms addressed? For skull base tumor patients being cared for by multidisciplinary teams, a thorough physical exam should be a given, as outlined in Advantages of Collaborative Surgery, above. The adequacy of imaging studies warrants emphasis because, in skull base surgery, the role of imaging studies is really twofold: to provide a diagnosis, and to serve as a navigational map during surgery. Often patients are referred to skull base surgery centers as soon as an initial imaging study has yielded a diagnosis of a probable skull base tumor. These initial studies, adequate for diagnosis, may or may not be adequate for surgical planning. It is incumbent upon the skull base team to see to it that diagnostic imaging has been as complete as necessary to map out the tumor's full extent, and not to simply proceed on the basis of preliminary radiographs. This is a subtle point but not a minor one.

The need for *timely acquisition of preoperative information* may seem obvious, but this can become a significant logistical challenge. Because skull base surgery is usually only practiced in tertiary centers, and many affected patients see several physicians before being referred for specialized care, there is almost always a lapse of days or weeks between initial diagnosis and definitive treatment. Depending on the tumor biology, significant growth can take place during this referral interval, and if the preoperative studies are not current, they will underestimate the tumor—sometimes substantially. It may be wise, then, in some cases to repeat parts of the diagnostic sequence just before surgery if the interval has been long.

Another critical potential pitfall is the *failure to appreciate limitations imposed by a tumor's biologic behavior.* As outlined in Head and Neck Tumors with Skull Base Involvement, above, the biology of head and neck tumors varies widely between tumor types. It also varies from patient to patient. Thus, not every patient with SCC of the anterior cranial base will experience the same clinical course. The danger is that a complex, demanding, and potentially morbid surgical procedure can be performed, and everything can go technically well, only to have the patient develop recurrence within a month or two, or die of metastatic disease within a few months. There are few experiences more profoundly disappointing to surgeon and patient alike.

There is no formulaic approach to this difficult problem; nor is there a reliable way of predicting which tumors will behave in this way. However, there are sometimes signs of extraordinarily aggressive behavior that may alert one to the possibility. For example, when a patient presents with malaise or constitutional symptoms out of proportion to the obvious disease, or when a tumor exhibits an unusually fast growth pattern, or if the patient develops rapidly progressive local symptoms beyond what would normally be expected for that tumor type, the surgical team should pause and reevaluate its initial treatment recommendation. In such cases, consideration may be given to using radiation or chemotherapy as the first treatment, either in lieu of or in preparation for surgery. The surgeon should in these cases be willing to postpone or withhold surgery in the patient's best interest, even if the standard recommendation would be operative treatment.

Another significant pitfall in collaborative surgery is *failure of collaboration*. Strategies for collaboration were reviewed in previous sections, but a few aspects are worth reprising here. To have a successful outcome, there must be advance discussion with mutual agreement regarding all phases of care, including the necessary diagnostic workup, the delineation of responsibilities, the surgical approaches, oncologic techniques, reconstructive methods, postoperative management, and planned adjuvant therapy when appropriate.

One more comment regarding pitfalls: with skull base surgery, the "house-of-cards" analogy has often been applied. These are complex operations that often require many successive steps, most of which are intrinsically challenging, and which when taken in aggregate may become extraordinarily difficult. The analogy infers that the higher the house of cards is built, the more likely it is to fall. To some extent, the analogy is correct, at least to the degree that the success of each consecutive step depends on the successful completion of the preceding step. Thus, failure to complete each step to the requisite degree of perfection represents one of the unseen pitfalls in skull base surgery. The surgery requires many levels of effort, and most of them require both intellectual and technical work. That work can be made simpler by diligent attention to preparation.

MANAGEMENT OF COMPLICATIONS

Complications in skull base surgery can run the gamut from minor aggravations to fatal events. A comprehensive discussion of complications relative to the full scope of skull base surgery has been presented in Chapter 8. This section focuses on a select few complications that are especially relevant and consequential in patients who undergo skull base surgery for head and neck tumors.

Cerebrospinal Fluid Leakage, Pneumocephalus, and Ascending Infection

Among the most dreaded complications in skull base surgery is the spectrum of problems that includes CSF leakage, pneumocephalus, and ascending infection. The reader is referred to Chapter 1, which reviewed this subject in detail. A discussion of these problems, however, is particularly pertinent in the context of head and neck neoplasms, and it is presented here from that perspective.

The skull base approaches required by head and neck tumors, by virtue of their subcranial dimensions, create substantial defects in the basicranium and supporting structures, providing potential avenues for fistula formation and increasing the risk that a fistula will occur. As previously alluded to, the best management is prevention, which is best accomplished by following these basic principles:

1. Reconstruction must be meticulous, achieving watertight closure of dura and bolstering the dural closure with additional soft tissue to insulate the cranial vault from the compartments below (see restoration of critical anatomic barriers in Surgical Techniques, above).
2. In most cases, the best materials for this reconstruction are autogenous and, when possible, vascularized tissues (e.g., pericranial, galeal, temporalis flaps) because these characteristics enhance the likelihood of healing *per primum*, without having to rely on the delayed healing by secondary intention that attends the use of nonautogenous or nonvascularized grafts (96). While there are certainly situations in which other materials can be beneficial, the optimal choice usually calls for autogenous and vascularized tissues.
3. If the patient has any preexisting circumstance that will make a CSF fistula more likely (chronic infection, increased intracranial pressure, poor wound-healing profile, morbid obesity, respiratory conditions that cause chronic cough, gastrointestinal conditions that cause chronic constipation, and others), those contributing factors must be taken into account and additional precautionary measures must be instituted accordingly (96).

When a postoperative CSF fistula becomes manifest, two aspects of treatment should be considered. First, many postoperative fistulas can be fixed (if conservative measures fail) via extracranial routes. That is to say, the approach to the fistula need not necessarily recapitulate the original skull base resection approach. Often fistulas can be safely approached and successfully rectified by the otolaryngologist using otologic or rhinologic methods alone, eliminating the need for extensive reopening of the entire surgical field (96).

Second, when treating a CSF fistula following skull base surgery, one should consider diverting the airway definitively, either by tracheal intubation or tracheotomy. Why? Normal (undiverted) respiration through the nose can lead to undesired insufflation of air into the skull base wound, increasing the likelihood of pneumocephalus and bacterial contamination. The use of nasal packing and nasopharyngeal airways does not always reliably prevent this problem. Intubation or, better still, tracheotomy definitively reroutes airflow away from the fresh wound, eliminating this part of the problem (97). Normal breathing can be restored once the fistula has been resolved.

Carotid Artery Rupture

Another formidable complication in skull base surgery that is prone to occur in head and neck tumor patients is rupture of the carotid artery (carotid ''blowout''). Most skull base surgeons are well versed in methods for intraoperative control of the carotid, which have been reviewed elsewhere in detail (44,98). It is the postoperative rupture of the vessel that presents the special concern for head and neck tumor patients. Many of these patients undergo extensive dismantling of the skull base, which may uncover, and in some cases extensively mobilize, the carotid at one or more of the following sites: in the parapharyngeal space, at the entrance to the carotid canal, within the petrous portion of the temporal bone, in the cavernous sinus, or intracranially. Often this results in exposure of the artery to adjacent contaminated spaces such as the pharynx, middle ear, petrous apex, nasopharynx, and sphenoid sinus. Contamination leads to weakening and subsequent rupture, which is usually sudden and catastrophic. Desiccation of the artery can have similar effects.

Like CSF fistulas, carotid rupture is more likely to occur in certain specific scenarios. Risk factors include wound-healing problems related to previous radiation treatment, diabetes mellitus, or steroid use; preexisting infection in the area; extensive manipulation of the artery at surgery, especially if arteriotomy or repair has been required; and prolonged time of exposure of the artery intraoperatively. Prevention therefore includes delicate handling of the vessel; keeping it moist to avoid desiccation; keeping it free of sinonasal, oral, and mucous secretions by frequent irrigation with topical antibiotic solution; and using appropriate systemic antibiotic coverage. Reconstruction must focus on insulation of the artery from contaminated spaces, preferably using autologous, vascularized tissues.

Carotid rupture demands immediate and drastic intervention if the patient is to survive. Application of pressure on the artery at and proximal to the ruptured segment is the first measure. If the bleeding is coming from the nose following a sinonasal approach, tamponade can be accomplished quickly by inserting and inflating a Foley catheter or epistaxis balloon in the nose and nasopharynx. If bleeding is coming from the ear or neck wound following a lateral facial, cervical, or temporal approach, direct pressure on the wound is applied. Digital pressure on the artery in the neck may be helpful. Aggressive fluid replacement takes place simultaneously. Definitive management involves emergent surgical exploration with ligation, repair, or grafting; endovascular management with intraarterial balloon placement; or combinations of surgery and endovascular management, depending on the site of bleeding and on the neurologic status of the patient.

Radiation-Related Complications

The majority of head and neck malignancies that are managed by skull base resection, by virtue of their skull base extension, require adjuvant radiation therapy. Certain benign lesions benefit from radiation as well. Radiation thus plays a pivotal role in the oncologic scheme, but it also unfortunately figures significantly in the genesis of complications. A few words about radiation therapy for head and neck tumors are therefore appropriate.

The therapeutic considerations for administering external beam radiation to the facial and cervical regions are different from those for irradiating the brain. (Note: stereotactic radiation is addressed in Chapter 30.) The variability in regional tissue tolerances for radiation in the different subcranial compartments is substantial (Table 27-8) (99), and the radiation oncologist must weigh the need for tumoricidal dosimetry against the need to protect adjacent functionally sensitive structures. To achieve oncologic control, a significant risk of serious long-term complications must often be conceded, including major complications such as visual loss, hearing loss, craniofacial osteoradionecrosis, and pituitary dysfunction, and less major complications (which are not necessarily minor) such as xerostomia, xerophthalmia, and soft tissue fibrosis.

Short-term radiation complications are equally dangerous, and in some ways worse. For most head and neck tumors, it is has been shown that in order to realize the maximal biologic efficacy of radiation, treatments must commence within 6 weeks of the surgery. Unfortunately, after extensive disassembly of the craniofacial region, healing is often incomplete within this short window of opportunity. Thus

TABLE 27–8. *Tolerance doses for fractionated radiotherapy for selected key tissues of importance in the treatment of head and neck cancer*

Organ system	Complication	$TD_{5/5}$–$TD_{50/5}$ (Gy)[a]
Lens	Cataract	6–12
Cornea	Keratitis	50–60
Retina	Retinitis	55–70
Middle ear	Serous otitis	50–70
Vestibular apparatus	Meniere's syndrome	60–70
Salivary gland	Xerostomia	30–45
Spinal cord (10 cm)	Myelopathy	50–60
Brain (25%)	Encephalopathy	70–80
Thyroid gland	Hypothyroidism	45–150
Mucosa	Ulceration	65–75
Mature bone	Fracture	65–75

Listed radiation doses are approximate.

[a] TD 5/5 refers to the 5% probability of occurrence within 5 years; TD 50/5 refers to the 50% probability of occurrence within 5 years.

Data from refs. 100 and 101, with permission.

competing goals of achieving optimal wound healing on the one hand, and getting the radiation started in a biologically timely way on the other, sometimes make it necessary to begin radiation at a time when healing may be imperfect. The deleterious effects of radiation on healing tissues may lead to wound complications that would be unlikely or less likely in the absence of radiation.

Acute radiation effects on mucosal surfaces are such that the nasal cavity and paranasal sinuses (and, to a lesser extent, the temporal bone) are particularly prone to problems. Radiation's effect on mucus glands and epithelial cells is a reduction in the volume of secretions, and a severe delay in mucociliary clearance. This leads to stagnation of sinonasal secretions, which then become inspissated due to the drying effect of nasal respiratory airflow. Inspissated secretions accumulate and harden into scab-like crusts, which can be remarkably tenacious. This creates an ideal environment for secondary bacterial infection, increasing the risk of wound breakdown and intracranial infection. For these reasons, patients at risk must be seen by the otolaryngologist frequently during radiation therapy. Treatment consists of humidification (using room humidifiers), hydration, mucolytic agents (e.g., guaifenesin), nasal irrigations with saline and sometimes antibiotic solutions, cautious debridement when necessary, and systemic antibiotics when indicated.

Tumor-Related Complications

From the patients' viewpoint, tumor recurrence may be the most dreaded complication of all because it reinitiates them into the unpleasant and frightening process of treatment. From the surgeon's point of view, recurrence—like other complications—is a frustrating, disappointing, but nevertheless sometimes unavoidable fact of life.

The best strategy for management of tumor recurrence is to approach it in the same way as the team approaches other complications of skull base surgery: (a) *prevention* to the greatest extent possible, (b) *vigilance* so that if it does happen it can be recognized early, and (c) *aggressive and timely intervention.*

Prevention of recurrence has been discussed in the form of techniques for optimal tumor management that have been presented throughout this book. Aggressive and timely intervention has also been stressed elsewhere, and should be self-evident. It is the vigilance that should be underscored and amplified here, because head and neck tumor patients do indeed require some unique kinds of follow-up that differ from that of patients who have skull base tumors of intracranial origin.

Vigilance in the follow-up of head and neck tumor patients is vital for early detection of recurrences. Early detection is crucial because the best chance to intervene effectively is at the earliest opportunity. For this reason, patients who have had treatment for head and neck tumors should always receive periodic surveillance that is commensurate with the biologic characteristics of their original tumors. For most patients who have had skull base involvement, this will mean lifelong follow-up. ("Once a tumor patient, always a tumor patient.")

The optimal timing of follow-up clinical examinations varies with the tumor type, the tumor's original extent, and the patient's overall progress in the posttreatment period. The first few postoperative visits take place within a few weeks of the surgery, and the main purpose of these early visits is to ensure that recovery from surgery is proceeding as expected. Beyond these early visits, the focus shifts away from issues of wound healing and toward oncologic surveillance.

What is appropriate oncologic surveillance? No single answer applies in all cases. With tumors of the head and neck, however, it is generally accepted that patients should have a clinical follow-up examination approximately every 2 months in the first year, every 3 months in the second year, every 4 months in the third year, and then every 6 to 12 months thereafter. This graduated schedule takes into account the observation that for most (not all) head and neck tumors, the risk of recurrence is highest in the first year, declines significantly over the next 2 to 3 years, and then reaches a plateau. This schedule should be adapted to the patient's particular needs.

Each clinical follow-up visit should consist of a thorough head and neck examination, a neurologic examination, and a general oncologic assessment. The head and neck examination is crucial because of the subcranial site of origin of the index tumor. It includes thorough inspection (and, when applicable, palpation) of the head and face as well as all accessible mucosal surfaces, including the mouth, pharynx, nasal cavity, larynx, and hypopharynx. The use of flexible fiberoptic telescopes to inspect the roof of the nasal cavity, frontal and ethmoid sinuses, nasopharynx, and sphenoid region allows a direct viewing of portions of the cranial base, which can facilitate detection of local recurrences readily and in a cost-effective manner. Similarly, otoscopy and otomicroscopy can detect recurrences in the external and middle ear spaces. The head and neck exam also includes palpation of the regional lymph nodes in the parotid gland as well as in the neck. This helps to identify regional metastases.

The neurologic exam includes assessments of the status of the patient's cognitive/intellectual functions, cranial nerves, motor and sensory systems, cerebellar functions, and reflexes. This can be helpful in detecting intracranial recurrences.

The general oncologic assessment for patients who have had head and neck malignancies includes an assessment of their overall performance status and a careful review of systems to identify possible signs of metastases to lungs, liver, and bone, three of the most common sites of distant spread from the head and neck. For these patients, a yearly chest x-ray, complete blood count, and serum chemistries (especially hepatic enzymes, alkaline phosphatase, and calcium) are recommended. When appropriate, other blood tests may also be helpful, depending on the original tumor type (e.g., EBV titers in the follow-up of NPC).

The timing of follow-up imaging studies is another key concern. Regular imaging studies play an extremely important role in posttreatment surveillance for skull base tumors, and they should be employed as often as necessary. As a general rule, imaging for initial tumor follow-up should be obtained approximately 3 months after surgery. (Imaging studies obtained sooner tend to be less useful for tumor surveillance because of the acute postoperative changes that occur and evolve within the first few months.) These initial studies serve as a tumor-surveillance benchmark with which to compare all future imaging studies. Like the clinical exam, the imaging should then be repeated at intervals that reflect the biologic characteristics of the original tumor. Again, for most (not all) head and neck tumors, the risk of recurrence is highest within the first few years, and it diminishes and levels off thereafter. A reasonable schedule for imaging would be to establish the baseline at 3 months and then repeat the imaging study at every other clinical follow-up visit, or roughly half as often as clinical checkups. Certainly, any suspicious new signs or symptoms discovered clinically should trigger new imaging studies as soon as they are noted.

The question of what is the ideal follow-up imaging study has been the subject of some debate; guidelines for skull base imaging have been reviewed in Chapter 9. For many tumors, a simple CT scan, carefully performed and interpreted in comparison with previous studies, yields sufficient information to determine tumor status. Specific skull base imaging protocols, as opposed to sinus, orbit, or brain protocols, should be employed to maximize the sensitivity of the studies. For other tumors, MRI scans offer specific advantages. In every case, collaboration with the radiologist helps to optimize the diagnostic power of the study.

Much of the preceding discussion regarding tumor recurrence focused on malignant tumors. Benign tumors of the skull base are followed in much the same way because of their propensity to be ''malignant by position.'' The major difference is that with benign lesions, metastatic surveillance is not a concern.

SUMMARY

Neoplasms originating in the subcranial structures of the head and neck may invade the skull base in complex ways that require diagnostic and therapeutic approaches that are different from those employed for intracranial tumors. Historical limitations in the management of these tumors have given way to modern collaborative strategies and technical improvements, so that these tumors can now be effectively treated with surgery. By virtue of their proficiency in dealing with head and neck disorders, otolaryngologists play an important role in the skull base surgical team, complementing the neurosurgeon's skills in a variety of ways.

Characteristics of some of the most important head and neck tumors have been reviewed, emphasizing aspects that influence key decisions made by the skull base team. Technical precepts regarding the collaboration required to bring about successful surgical management have been presented, and potential pitfalls and complications have been outlined.

Through interdisciplinary collaboration in the diagnosis, preoperative planning, surgical treatment, and follow-up phases, the challenges of treating head and neck tumors with skull base involvement can be successfully met.

ACKNOWLEDGMENT

The authors gratefully acknowledge Mrs. Dorothy H. Neill for her assistance in the preparation of this manuscript.

REFERENCES

1. Tessier P, Guiot G, Rougerie J, Delbet JP, Pastoriza J. Osteotomies cranio-naso-orbitales hypertelorism. *Ann Chir Plast* 1967;12: 103–118.
2. Tessier P. Osteotomies totales de la face: syndrome de Crouzon, syndrome d'Apert, oxycephalies, scaphocephalies, turricephalies. *Ann Chir Plast* 1967;12:273–286.
3. Tessier P, Guiot G, Derome P. Orbital hypertelorism. II: definite treatment of orbital hypertelorism by craniofacial or by extracranial osteotomies. *Scand J Plast Reconstr Surg* 1973;7(1):39–58.
4. Jackson IT, Marsh WR, Bite U, Hide TA. Craniofacial osteotomies to facilitate skull base tumour resection. *Br J Plast Surg* 1986;39: 153–160.
5. Nuss DW, Janecka IP, Sekhar LN, Sen CN. Craniofacial disassembly in the management of skull base tumors. *Otolaryngol Clin North Am* 1991;24(6):1465–1497.
6. Abul-Hassan HS, Ascher GVD, Acland RD. Surgical anatomy and blood supply of the fascial layers of the temporal region. *Plast Reconstr Surg* 1986;77(1):17–24.
7. Johns ME, Winn HR, McLean WC, Cantrell RW. Pericranial flap for the closure of defects of craniofacial resection. *Laryngoscope* 1981; 91:952–959.
8. Jackson IT, Adham MN, Marsh WR. Use of the galeal frontalis myofascial flap in craniofacial surgery. *Plast Reconstr Surg* 1986;77: 905–910.
9. Snyderman CH, Janecka IP, Sekhar LN, Sen CN, Eibling DE. Anterior cranial base reconstruction: role of galeal and pericranial flaps. *Laryngoscope* 1990;100:607–614.
10. Antonyshyn O, Gruss JS, Birt BD. Versatility of temporal muscle and fascial flaps. *Br J Plast Surg* 1988;41(2):118–131.
11. Jones NF, Sekhar LN, Schramm VL. Free rectus abdominis muscle flap reconstruction of the middle and posterior cranial base. *Plast Reconstr Surg* 1986;78:471–477.
12. Jones NF, Schramm VL, Sekhar LN. Reconstruction of the cranial base following tumor resection. *Br J Plast Surg* 1987;40:155–162.
13. Shestak KC, Jones NF, Ramasastry SS. Microvascular reconstruction of the cranial base. In: Sekhar LN, Janecka IP, eds. *Surgery of cranial base tumors*. New York: Raven Press, 1993:427–433.
14. Urken ML, Catalano PJ, Sen CN, Post K, Futran N, Biller HF. Free tissue transfer for skull base reconstruction: analysis of complications and a classification scheme for defining skull base defects. *Arch Otolaryngol Head Neck Surg* 1993;119:1318–1325.
15. House WF. Surgical exposure of the internal auditory canal and its contents through the middle cranial fossa. *Laryngoscope* 1951;71: 1363–1365.
16. Smith RR, Klopp CT, Williams JM. Surgical treatment of cancer of the frontal sinus and adjacent areas. *Cancer* 1954;7:991–994.
17. Wilson CP: Observations on surgery of the nasopharynx. *Ann Otol Rhinol Laryngol* 1957;66:5–40.
18. Fairbanks-Barbosa J. Surgery of extensive carcinoma of the paranasal sinuses. *Arch Otolaryngol* 1961;73:129–138.
19. Fang HS, Ong GB. Direct anterior approach of the upper cervical spine. *J Bone Joint Surg [Am]* 1962;44:1588–1604.
20. Ketcham AS, Wilkins RH, Van Buren JM, Smith RR. A combined

intracranial facial approach to the paranasal sinuses. *Am J Surg* 1963; 106:698–703.
21. House WF. Middle cranial fossa approach to the petrous pyramid: report of 50 cases. *Arch Otolaryngol* 1963;78:460–469.
22. Parkinson D. A surgical approach to the cavernous portion of the carotid artery: anatomical studies and case report. *J Neurosurg* 1965; 23:474–483.
23. Hitselberger WE, House WF. A combined approach to the cerebellopontine angle: a suboccipital/petrosal approach. *Arch Otolaryngol* 1966;84:267–285.
24. Fisch U. Transtemporal extralabyrinthine surgery of the internal auditory canal. *Arch Klin Exp Ohren Nasen Kehlkopfheilkund* 1969; 194(2):232–243.
25. Terz JJ, Alksne JF, Lawrence W. Craniofacial resection for tumors invading the pterygoid fossa. *Am J Surg* 1969;118:732–740.
26. Hakuba A, Greenberg A. Surgery for large glomus jugular tumors: the combined suboccipital transtemporal approach. *Arch Otolaryngol* 1971;90:227–231.
27. Ketcham AS, Chretien PB, van Buren JM, Hoye RC, Beazley RM, Herdt JR. The ethmoid sinuses: a re-evaluation of surgical resection. *Am J Surg* 1973;126:469–476.
28. House WF, Hitselberger WE. The transcochlear approach to the skull base. *Arch Otolaryngol* 1976;102:334–342.
29. Sisson GA, Bytell DE, Becker SP, Ruge D. Carcinoma of the paranasal sinuses and cranial-facial resection. *J Otolaryngol Laryngol* 1976; 90(1):59–68.
30. Rhoton AL Jr. Microsurgical removal of acoustic neuromas. *Surg Neurol* 1976;6:211–219.
31. Yasargil MG, Gasser JC, Hodosh RM, Rankin TV. Carotid-ophthalmic aneurysm: direct microsurgical approach. *Surg Neurol* 1977;8: 155–165.
32. Derome PJ. The transbasal approach to tumors invading the base of the skull. In: Schmidek HH, Sweet WH, eds. *Current techniques in operative neurosurgery*. New York: Grune & Stratton, 1977:223–245.
33. Fisch U. Infratemporal fossa approach to tumours of the temporal bone and base of skull. *J Laryngol Otol* 1978;92:949–967.
34. Glasscock ME, Hays JW, Jackson CG, Steenerson RL. A one-stage combined approach for the management of large cerebellopontine angle tumors. *Laryngoscope* 1978;88(10):1563–1576.
35. Glasscock ME, Miller GW, Drake FD, Kanok MM. Surgery of the skull base. *Laryngoscope* 1978;88(6):905–923.
36. Fisch U, Pilsbury HC. Infratemporal fossa approach to lesions in the temporal bone and base of skull. *Arch Otolaryngol* 1979;105:99–107.
37. Schramm VL, Myers EN, Maroon JC. Anterior skull base surgery for benign and malignant disease. *Laryngoscope* 1979;89:1077–1091.
38. Biller HF, Shugar J, Krespi Y. A new technique for wide-field exposure of the base of the skull. *Arch Otolaryngol* 1981;107:698–702.
39. Jane JA, Park TS, Pobereskin LH, Winn HR, Butler AB. The supraorbital approach: technical note. *Neurosurgery* 1982;11:537–542.
40. Dolenc V. Direct microsurgical repair of intracavernous vascular lesions. *J Neurosurg* 1983;58:824–831.
41. Krespi YP, Sisson GA. Transmandibular exposure of the skull base. *Am J Surg* 1984;148:534–538.
42. Crockhard HA. The transoral approach to the base of the brain and upper cervical cord. *Ann R Coll Surg Eng* 1985;67:321–325.
43. Sekhar LN, Møller AR. Operative management of tumors involving the cavernous sinuses. *J Neurosurg* 1986;64:879–889.
44. Sekhar LN, Schramm VL, Jones NF. Operative exposure and management of the petrous and upper cervical carotid artery. *Neurosurgery* 1986;19:967–982.
45. Sekhar LN, Burgess J, Atkin O. Anatomical study of the cavernous sinus emphasizing operative approaches and related vascular and neural reconstruction. *Neurosurgery* 1987;21:806–816.
46. Sekhar LN, Schramm VL, Jones NF. A subtemporal-preauricular infratemporal approach to large lateral and posterior cranial base neoplasms. *J Neurosurg* 1987;67:488–499.
47. Sekhar LN, Janecka IP, Jones NF. Subtemporal-infratemporal and basal subfrontal approach to extensive cranial base tumors. *Acta Neurochir (Wien)* 1988;92:83–92.
48. Al-Mefty O, Smith R. Surgery of tumors invading the cavernous sinus. *Surg Neurol* 1988;30:370–381.
49. Janecka IP, Sen CN, Sekhar LN, Arriaga M. Facial translocation: a new approach to the cranial base. *Otolaryngol Head Neck Surg* 1990; 103:413–419.
50. Cocke EW, Robertson JH, Robertson JT, Crook JP. The extended maxillotomy and subtotal maxillectomy for excision of skull base tumors. *Arch Otolaryngol Head Neck Surg* 1990;116(1):92–104.
51. Sekhar LN, Nanda A, Sen CN, Snyderman CH, Janecka IP. The extended frontal approach to tumors of the anterior, middle and posterior cranial base. *J Neurosurg* 1992;76:198–203.
52. Nuss DW, Janecka IP. Current indications for skull base surgery. *Adv Otolaryngol Head Neck Surg* 1992;6:63–91.
53. Covey S. *Seven habits of highly effective people*. New York: Simon & Schuster, 1989.
54. Sekhar LN, Janecka IP, eds. *Surgery of cranial base tumors*. New York: Raven Press, 1993.
55. Jackson CG, ed. *Surgery of skull base tumors*. New York: Churchill Livingstone, 1991.
56. Janecka IP, Tiedemann K, eds. *Skull base surgery: anatomy, biology, and technology*. Philadelphia: Lippincott-Raven, 1997.
57. Al-Mefty O, ed. *Surgery of the cranial base*. Boston: Kluwer Academic, 1989.
58. Sen CN, Chen CS, Post KD. *Microsurgical anatomy of the skull base and approaches to the cavernous sinus*. New York: Thieme, 1997.
59. Fisch U, Mattox D. *Microsurgery of the skull base*. New York: Thieme, 1988.
60. Jackler RK. *Atlas of neurotology and skull base surgery*. St. Louis: Mosby-Year Book, 1996.
61. Sekhar LN, Schramm VL, eds. *Tumors of the cranial base: diagnosis and treatment*. Mt. Kisko, NY: Futura, 1987.
62. American Medical Association. *Physicians' current procedural terminology*. Chicago: AMA, 1998.
63. Rice DH, Stanley RB. Surgical therapy of nasal cavity, ethmoid sinus, and maxillary sinus tumors. In: Thawley SE, Panje WR, Batsakis JG, Lindberg RD, eds. *Comprehensive management of head and neck tumors*. Philadelphia: WB Saunders, 1987:368–389.
64. Perry C, Levine PA, Williamson BR, Cantrell RW. Preservation of the eye in paranasal sinus cancer surgery. *Arch Otolaryngol Head Neck Surg* 1988;114:632–634.
65. Janecka IP, Sen C, Sekhar L, Curtin H. Treatment of paranasal sinus cancer with cranial base surgery: results. *Laryngoscope* 1994;104: 553–555.
66. Catalano PJ, Hecht CS, Biller HF, et al. Craniofacial resection: an analysis of 73 cases. *Arch Otolaryngol Head Neck Surg* 1994;120(11): 1203–1208.
67. Shah JP, Kraus DH, Bilsky MH, Gutin PH, Harrison LH, Strong EW. Craniofacial resection for malignant tumors involving the anterior skull base. *Arch Otoloaryngol Head Neck Surg* 1997;123:1312–1317.
68. Jackson IT, Bailey MH, Marsh WR, Juhasz P. Results and prognosis following surgery for malignant tumors of the skull base. *Head Neck* 1991;13:89–96.
69. Becker SP, Berktold RE, Sisson GA. Controversy in the management of tumors of the nasal cavity and paranasal sinus. In: Thawley SE, Panje WR, Batsakis JG, Lindberg RD, eds. *Comprehensive management of head and neck tumors*. Philadelphia: WB Saunders, 1987: 445–458.
70. Barnes L, Kapadia SB, Nemzek WR, Weissman JL, Janecka IP. Biology of selected skull base tumors. In: Janecka IP, Tiedeman K, eds. *Skull base surgery: anatomy, biology, and technology*. Philadelphia: Lippincott-Raven, 1997:263–289.
71. Rassekh CH, Nuss DW, Kapadia SB, Curtin HD, Weissman JL, Janecka IP. Chondrosarcoma of the nasal septum: skull base imaging and clinicopathologic correlation. *Otolaryngol Head Neck Surg* 1996; 115(1):29–37.
72. Calcaterra TC, Wang MB, Sercarz JA. Unusual tumors. In: Myers EN, Suen JY, eds. *Cancer of the head and neck*. Philadelphia: WB Saunders, 1996:644–669.
73. Kapadia SB, Bumpous JM, Janecka IP. Cancer of the orbit. In: Myers EN, Suen JY, eds. *Cancer of the head and neck*. Philadelphia: WB Saunders, 1996:184–203.
74. Raney RB, Tefft M, Newton WA, et al. Improved prognosis with intensive treatment of children with cranial soft tissue sarcomas arising in nonorbital parameningeal sites: a report from the Intergroup Rhabdomyosarcoma Study. *Cancer* 1987;59(1):147–155.
75. Wharam M, Foulkes M, Lawrence W, et al. Soft tissue sarcoma of the head and neck in childhood: nonorbital and nonparameningeal sites. *Cancer* 1984;53(4):1016–1019.
76. Wharam M, Beltangady MS, Heyn RM, et al. Pediatric orofacial and

laryngopharyngeal rhabdomyosarcoma. *Arch Otolaryngol Head Neck Surg* 1987;113(11):1225–1227.
77. Anderson GJ, Tom LWC, Womer RB, Handler SD, Wetmore RF, Potsic WP. Rhabdomyosarcoma of the head and neck in children. *Arch Otolaryngol Head Neck Surg* 1990;116(4):428–431.
78. Healy GB, Upton J, Black PM, Ferraro N. The role of surgery in rhabdomyosarcoma of the head and neck in children. *Arch Otolaryngol Head Neck Surg* 1991;117(10):1185–1188.
79. Stern SJ, Hanna E. Cancer of the nasal cavity and paranasal sinuses. In: Myers EN, Suen JY, eds. *Cancer of the head and neck.* Philadelphia: WB Saunders, 1996:205–233.
80. Batsakis JG. Other neuroectodermal tumors and related lesions of the head and neck. In: Batsakis JG, ed. *Tumors of the head and neck.* London: Williams & Wilkins, 1982:334–349.
81. Levine PA, Debo RF, Meredith SD, Jane JA, Constable WC, Cantrell RW. Craniofacial resection at the University of Virginia (1976–1992): survival analysis. *Head Neck* 1994;16:574–577.
82. Rodriguez MA, Hong WK. Diagnosis and management of lymphomas in the head and neck. In: Myers EN, Suen JY, eds. *Cancer of the head and neck.* Philadelphia: WB Saunders, 1996:670–678.
83. Neel HB. Nasopharyngeal carcinoma: diagnosis, staging, and management. *Oncology* 1992;6:87–95.
84. Sham JST, Wei WI, Nicholls J, Chan CW, Choy D. Extent of nasopharyngeal carcinoma involvement inside the nasopharynx: lack of prognostic value on local control. *Cancer* 1992;69:854–859.
85. Yumoto E, Okamura H, Yanagihara N. Transmandibular transpterygoid approach to the nasopharynx, parapharyngeal space, and skull base. *Ann Otol Rhinol Laryngol* 1992;101:383–389.
86. Fisch U. Infratemporal fossa approach. Part IV: applications. In: Fisch U, Mattox D, eds. *Microsurgery of the skull base.* New York: Thieme, 1988:368–386.
87. Nuss D, Janecka IP. Carcinoma of the nasopharynx. *Crit Rev Neurosurg* 1992;2:332–342.
88. Draf W. Juvenile angiofibroma. In: Sekhar LN, Janecka IP, eds. *Surgery of cranial base tumors.* New York: Raven Press, 1992:485–496.
89. Sen CN, Sekhar LN, Schramm VL, Janecka IP. Chordoma and chondrosarcoma of the cranial base: an 8-year experience. *Neurosurgery* 1989;25(6):931–940.
90. Myers EN, Johnson JT, Curtin HD. Tumors of the parapharyngeal space. In: Myers EN, Suen JY, eds. *Cancer of the head and neck.* Philadelphia: WB Saunders, 1996:562–585.
91. Carrau RL, Myers EN, Johnson JT. Management of tumors arising in the parapharyngeal space. *Laryngoscope* 1990;100:583–589.
92. Arriaga M, Curtin H, Hirsch B, Takahashi H, Kamerer D. Staging proposal for external auditory meatus carcinoma based on preoperative clinical examination and computed tomography findings. *Ann Otol Rhinol Laryngol* 1990;99:714–721.
93. Graham M, Sataloff R, Kemink J, Wolf G, McGillicuddy J. Total en bloc resection of the temporal bone and carotid artery for malignant tumors of the ear and temporal bone. *Laryngoscope* 1984;94:528–533.
94. Kinney SE, Wood BG. Malignancies of the external auditory canal and temporal bone: surgical techniques and results. *Laryngoscope* 1987;97:158–164.
95. Lewis JS. Squamous carcinoma of the ear. *Arch Otolaryngol* 1973; 97:41–42.
96. Nuss DW, Costantino PD. Diagnosis and management of cerebrospinal fluid fistulas. *Adv Otolaryngol Head Neck Surg* 1994;8:247–274.
97. Nuss DW. Prevention of intracranial complications in anterior skull base surgery. *Insights Otolaryngol* 1992;7(6):1–12.
98. Linskey ME, Sekhar LN, Sen CN. Cerebral revascularization in cranial base surgery. In: Sekhar LN, Janecka IP, eds. *Surgery of cranial base tumors.* New York: Raven Press, 1992:45–68.
99. Laramore GE. General principles of radiation therapy for head and neck cancer. In: Myers EN, Suen JY, eds. *Cancer of the head and neck.* Philadelphia: WB Saunders, 1996:768–781.
100. Laramore GE. *Radiation therapy of head and neck cancer.* Berlin: Springer-Verlag, 1989.
101. Rubin P, Siemann DW. Principles of radiation oncology and cancer radiotherapy. In: Rubin P, McDonald S, Qazi R, eds. *Clinical oncology: a multidisciplinary approach for physicians and students,* 7th ed. Philadelphia: WB Saunders, 1993;71–90.
102. Schramm VL. Craniofacial resection. In: Sasaki CT, McCabe BF, Kirchner JA, eds. *Surgery of the skull base.* Philadelphia: JB Lippincott, 1984;43–61.

Neurosurgical Issues in Otolaryngology: Principles and Practice of Collaboration, edited by Moisés A. Arriaga and J. Diaz Day. Lippincott Williams & Wilkins, Philadelphia © 1999.

CHAPTER 28

Anterior Skull Base: The Neurosurgical Perspective

Ghassan Bejjani, Donald C. Wright, and Laligam N. Sekhar

OVERVIEW

A number of specialized medical and surgical disciplines are often required to effectively manage various clinical problems localized to the junction of the basal neurocranium and anterior viscerocranium, which is collectively referred to as the anterior skull base (ASB) (Fig. 28-1). Recognizing the difficulties in treating resistant neoplasms, penetrating trauma, and serious infections (e.g., fungal abscess, mucocoele, etc.) surgeons and other specialists applied their combined skills fostering the development of skull base surgery as a recognized specialty. Indeed, one of the major nontechnical advances in skull base surgery has been the recognition by a diverse group of specialists (otolaryngology, head and neck, maxillofacial, ophthalmology, plastic surgery, neurosurgery, radiology, and radiation oncology) of the need to pool the collective skills and experience in a coordinated team-based approach and apply it to advance the care of patients with complex skull base problems.

Historically, neurosurgery was constrained by the potentially septic paranasal sinuses and the serious consequences of cerebrospinal fluid (CSF) fistula and ascending infection if these areas were transgressed during surgery. In a similar manner, specialists treating problems of the oropharynx, paranasal sinuses, and orbit were obliged to respect the basal dura and parenchymal surfaces of the brain due to the high morbidity arising when crossing these anatomic boundaries.

Various lesions occur along the ASB, mostly tumoral (Table 28-1). The tumors of the ASB can arise within the dura, from the bone or from the nasal cavity and sinuses. The most commonly encountered intradural mass is meningioma, although giant pituitary adenoma may extend into the ASB. Tumors arising from the bony elements of the ASB are chondromas, chondrosarcomas, chordomas, fibrous dysplasia, ossifying fibromas, and osteogenic sarcoma. Metastasis can be seen to the bony ASB or to the adjacent elements. Esthesioneuroblastomas, lymphomas, squamous cell carcinomas, juvenile angiofibromas, adenoid cystic carcinomas, and inverted papillomas take origin from the nasal cavity and adjacent sinuses. Approaching these lesions can be done via an exocranial or an endocranial route or through a combination of both.

This chapter presents an overview of the neurosurgical approach to management of ASB problems and emphasizes the management philosophy over specific technical aspects of various surgical approaches.

ANATOMIC CONSIDERATIONS

The ASB encompasses a region of complex anatomy with elements of the nervous and endocrine systems, aerodigestive tract, vascular supply, and myocutaneous and osseous elements. The somewhat arbitrary confines of the anterior cranial base defined below reflect the practical considerations of the many structures and areas that must be managed and the tendency for pathologic processes to extend across anatomic boundaries to involve multiple compartments. A convenient, though arbitrary classification approach to problems of the ASB is to place the origin or epicenter of the pathologic process into one or another of two fundamental categories: exocranial (e.g., orbit, paranasal sinuses, nasopharynx, sphenoclival, etc.), and endocranial (e.g., olfactory epithelium, meninges, neuroendocrine, etc.). The more stringent boundary of the ASB includes the endocranial and exocranial components along the median plane beginning with the frontal sinuses to the floor of the sphenoid sinus and the

G. Bejjani: Department of Neurosurgery, Allegheny University Hospitals, Pittsburgh, Pennsylvania 15212-4746.

D. C. Wright and L. N. Sekhar: Department of Neurosurgery, Center for Cranial Base Surgery, George Washington University Medical Center, Washington, DC 20037.

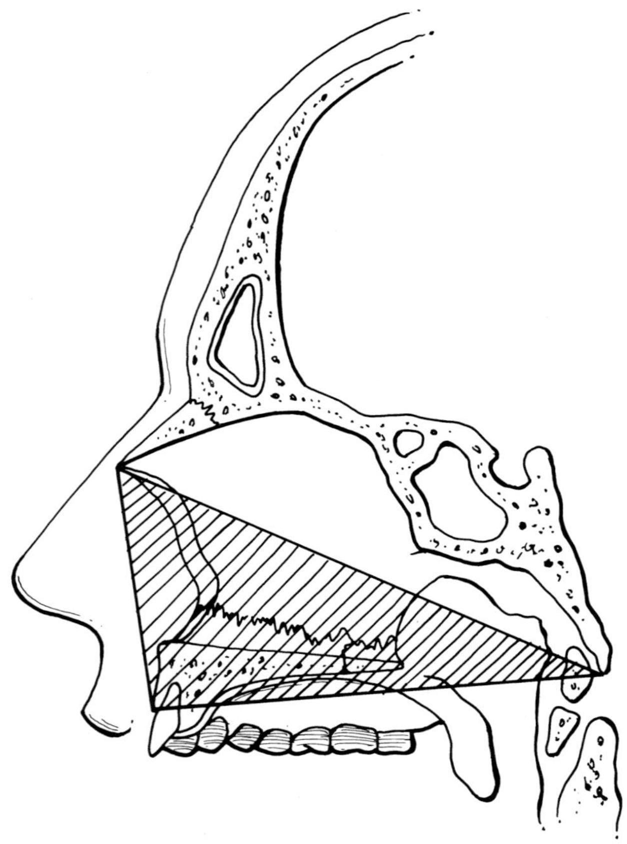

FIG. 28-1. Sagittal section of the skull outlining the anterior skull base. Adapted from Wright DC, Sekhar LN. Management of anterior cranial base tumors. In: Tindall GT, Barrow DC, Cooper PR, eds. *The practice of neurosurgery.* Baltimore: Williams & Wilkins, 1995:949–962.

TABLE 28–1. *Differential diagnosis of anterior cranial base tumors*

Benign	Malignant
Papilloma (inverting)	Squamous cell carcinoma
Benign mixed salivary tumors	Minor salivary gland carcinomas
Angiofibroma (juvenile)	Adenoid cystic carcinoma
Meningioma	Adenocarcinomas
Neurogenic neoplasms	Mucoepidermoid carcinoma
Neuroma	Undifferentiated carcinoma (SNUC)
Neurofibroma	Acinous cell carcinoma
Granular cell tumors (myoblastomas)	Carcinoma expleomorphic adenoma
Pituitary adenoma (invasive)	Oncocytoma
Fibro-osseous lesions	Nasopharyngeal carcinoma
Osteoma	Melanoma
Osteoid osteoma	Lymphomas
Osteoblastoma	Leukemias (pediatric)
Chondroma	Chondrosarcoma
Fibrous dysplasia	Chordoma
Ossifying fibroma	Plasma cell dyscrasia
Orbital tumors	Multiple myeloma
Lymphomas	Plasmacytoma
Leukemias	Rhabdomyosarcoma (pediatric)
Capillary hemangioma	Osteogenic sarcoma
Cavernous hemangiomas	Metastases
Lymphangiomas	Lung
Schwannoma	Breast
Neurofibroma	Prostate
Retinoblastoma	Kidney
Miscellaneous	Other
Giant cell tumor of bone (sphenoid)	
Sarcoid (tuberculum/optic foramen)	
Craniopharyngioma	
Ossifying myxoma	
Fibrous histiocytoma	
Hemangiopericytoma	
Hemangioma	
Radiation necrosis	
Eosinophilic granuloma	
Paget's disease	

Adapted from Wright DC, Sekhar LN. Management of anterior cranial base tumors. In: Tindall GT, Barrow DC, Cooper PR, eds. *The practice of neurosurgery.* Baltimore: Williams & Wilkins, 1995:949–962.

outer orbital walls laterally. A broader definition, subscribed to by the authors and many others, includes all the anterior paranasal sinuses (maxillary, frontal, ethmoid, sphenoid), the perioptic region (sellar turcica, planum, tuberculum, and optic canals), central and lower clivus, occipital condyles, atlas, dens, and the retropharyngeal space and upper pharynx (Figs. 28-1 and 28-2).

PHILOSOPHY OF MANAGEMENT: BENIGN VERSUS MALIGNANT LESIONS

Neurosurgeons, by necessity, are less inclined to heed the well-established oncologic principles of radical resection with wide margins in comparison to specialists treating patients with malignant tumors originating in other organs. This oncologic concept derives from experience treating tumors with inadequate or partially effective adjuvant therapy originating in other anatomic compartments (e.g., peritoneum, chest) where sacrifice of surrounding tissues does not result in appreciable morbidity for the patient. Piecemeal or morsellation techniques are common in neurosurgery to minimize morbidity, and wide margins are rarely possible. It is unproven that this approach results in a higher rate of recurrence, but the principle is widely held in treating malignant tumors, since they are frequently a regional rather than a generalized problem. Patients with highly malignant tumors should be subjected to aggressive ASB approaches and resection only if a complete removal (en bloc if feasible) is possible. Sacrifice of neurologic function (e.g., vision) is warranted if this can maximize the patient's chances of long-term survival. Palliative treatment, or partial removal of malignant lesions is rarely indicated and restricted to situations where the patient will enjoy at least short-term benefit.

Benign lesions should be subjected to surgical resection with the paramount goal of complete resection with preservation (or improvement) of neurologic function. It is incum-

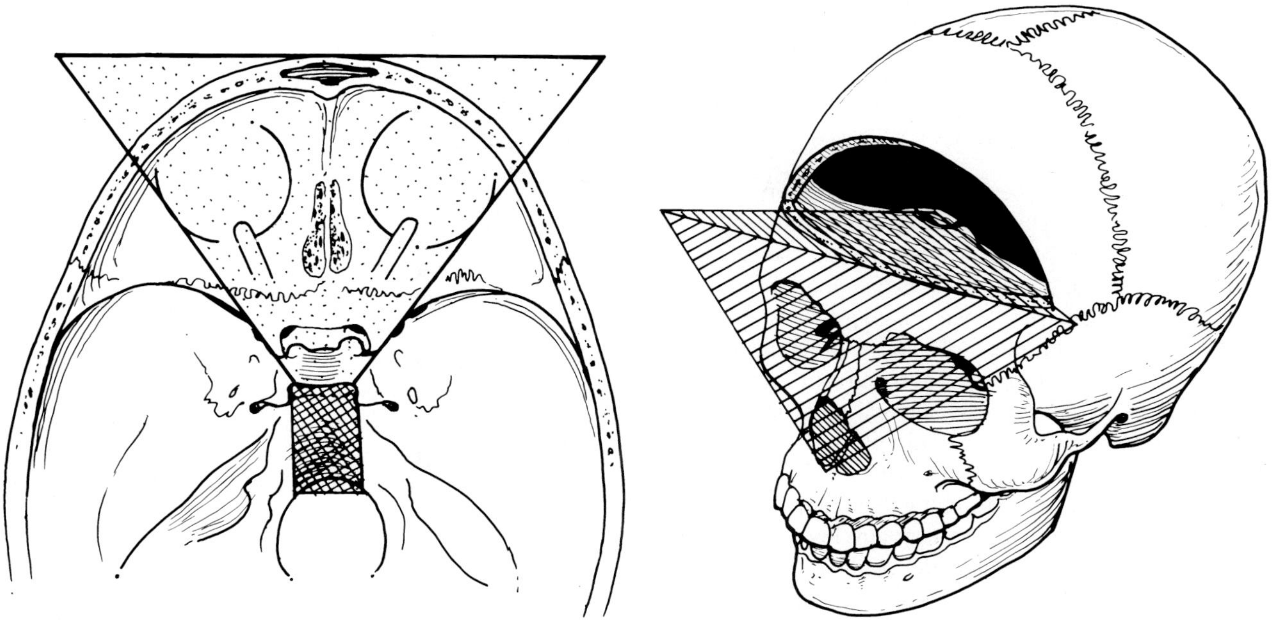

FIG. 28-2. Axial and oblique lateral views of the pyramidal anterior cranial fossa. Adapted from Wright DC, Sekhar LN. Management of anterior cranial base tumors. In: Tindall GT, Barrow DC, Cooper PR, eds. *The practice of neurosurgery.* Baltimore: Williams & Wilkins, 1995:949–962.

bent upon the surgeon to carefully weigh the benefits of a complex procedure applied to the removal of a benign, though potentially dangerous, lesion. It is our preference to intercept crucially located benign lesions with progressive enlargement prior to the production of a potentially irreversible deficit.

HISTORICAL MANAGEMENT

Skull base approaches to ASB lesions are a combination of cranial and facial approaches. In a combined effort of neurosurgeons and maxillofacial surgeons or ear, nose, and throat (ENT) surgeons, craniofacial osteotomies are added to more conventional craniotomies to improve exposure of lesions located under the basal aspect of the forebrain. It has been demonstrated that the angle of the field of view is increased by 73% from 11 to 19 degrees when an orbital osteotomy is added to a pterional craniotomy (1). These osteotomies were described in the early 20th century. MacArthur (2) in 1912 and Frazier (3) in 1913 advocated removal of part of the orbital rim to improve exposure of the pituitary gland and sellar area. Ray and McLean (4) were the first to describe a combined transcranial and transfacial approach to orbital tumors in 1943. It was Smith et al. (5) in 1954 who reported the use of combined approaches for paranasal sinus tumors. Later series were published with long-term follow-up of these combined approaches to paranasal sinus tumors. In 1972 Derome et al. (6–8) described the subfrontal transbasal approach in which a bifrontal craniotomy is made down to the orbital rim and extensive ethmoidal and sphenoidal lesions approached extradurally, after decompression of the optic nerves and orbital roof removal. This technique allows approach to the anterior cranial fossa, the sphenoid sinus, and the clivus. Cophignon et al. (9) added an orbital osteotomy to the bifrontal craniotomy; thus the term *extended transbasal approach.*

ADVANTAGES OF TEAM SURGERY

Before the days of combined approaches, when the maxillofacial surgeons would attempt removal of ASB tumors via facial approaches, many problems would arise. En bloc total resection was not possible except in very small tumors (10). Extension of tumors into the ethmoidal sinus and the impossibility of removing it en bloc transfacially led Frazell and Lewis (11) to warn in 1963 that the entire cribriform plate can rarely be resected without creating cerebral complications. Dural tears are hard to repair transfacially, and frontal lobe injury may occur when aggressive removal is attempted transfacially. Transcranial approaches have the advantage of exposing the dura and frontal lobe, reducing the risk of injury and facilitating repair. The main disadvantage of these approaches is the brain retraction required to access subfrontal lesions. This may become a serious issue when prolonged retraction is needed, such as during resection of extensive tumors involving delicate neurovascular structures; the addition of facial access improves exposures and lessens retraction.

There are more advantages of team surgery than just combining technical skills. These advantages come from the fact that each team is more familiar with its territory and more accustomed to preventing and dealing with complications related to that territory. Neurosurgeons are more apt to handle possible neurosurgical complications such as CSF leak and brain edema. Maxillofacial surgeons are experienced in reconstructing the face to obtain the best cosmetic results and in oncologic techniques of total exenteration.

DIAGNOSTIC EVALUATION

Accurate preoperative localization is a necessary prelude to successful surgery. The routine use of computer-based imaging has been a revolutionary advance in the management of complex cranial base lesions. Computed tomography (CT) and magnetic resonance imaging (MRI) are complementary exams, defining the bony structure of the paranasal sinuses, anterior fossa floor, and exit foramina of cranial nerves (CT) and the parenchymal or neurovascular involvement (MRI) by the pathologic process. Specialized algorithms (three-dimensional reconstruction, fat-saturation/suppression techniques, etc.) further extend the utility of CT and MRI. Angiography is essential in any lesion involving the proximal vascular supply of the skull base. It is also useful in assessing the adequacy of the cerebral circulation and in selective embolization of highly vascularized tumors. Diagnostic biopsy of accessible lesions can be important in surgical planning in terms of a preoperative diagnosis, consistency, and vascularity of the lesion. Advances in endoscopic techniques and instrumentation have simplified this procedure and reduced the risk of obtaining tissue for histologic analysis (12–14).

POTENTIAL PITFALLS

In assessing risk, preoperative localization is of primary importance. Many pathologic processes affecting the ASB with an extradural or exocranial epicenter are effectively blocked by the meninges and represent relatively low risk if a purely extradural approach is possible. The risk of parenchymal or cranial nerve injury and CSF fistula increases substantially if a lesion requires a combined intra- and extradural approach. The prototypic lesion requiring such an approach is the esthesioneuroblastoma, which characteristically spans the cribriform and posterior nasopharyngeal regions. Most benign lesions and slow-growing malignancies (e.g., chordomas, chondrosarcomas) do not tend to cross the dura, and have lower relative risk.

Involvement of critical neural structures (e.g., optic nerves, internal carotid arteries, brain parenchyma) by these processes requires careful management to limit or avoid permanent neurologic deficits. In like manner, management of functional and aesthetic aspects of the facial skeleton and aerodigestive tract are equally important to minimize the morbidity of the surgical procedure. While many of the highly malignant lesions of the ASB still resist treatment, in many cases anticipation and avoidance of complications or the successful management of complications determines the ultimate long-term outcome of the patient.

The paranasal sinuses form a convenient anatomic entry portal to the anterior cranial base and are accessed in many surgical approaches. This relative ease in access when utilizing the paranasal sinuses is tempered by serious potential complications if the normal barriers between the intracranial compartment and the aerodigestive are not restored. ASB surgery remains, to some extent, true to its high-risk heritage due to this proximity to the paranasal sinuses, and other factors, although substantial reduction in the morbidity of surgery has been achieved.

The ASB can be considered an inverted pyramid–shaped region with the roof approximating an equilateral triangle that stands on a tapering base (Fig. 28-2). The roof outlines the orbits, frontal sinus, cribriform plate, planum, tuberculum, sella turcica, and dorsum sellae. The base includes the remaining paranasal sinuses, central and lower clivus, occipital condyles, retropharyngeal space, upper pharynx, and craniocervical junction. In practical terms, risk increases as one approaches the posterior and inferior limits of the ASB (optic foramen, sella, clivus) and the surgeon must employ progressive care to avoid injuring neurovascular structures. Lesions located within the more anterior and inferior portions of the triangle are generally amenable to removal with lower morbidity to the brain, optic nerves, pituitary gland, and internal carotid arteries, although CSF fistula and secondary infection remain serious complications of surgery in this area.

SURGICAL APPROACHES

The goals of any surgical approach to a lesion of the ASB are wide surgical exposure, preservation of function, and low morbidity. Numerous surgical approaches to the central skull base have been described and utilized successfully for a variety of specific tumors and locations (6,15–28). The authors employ an "extended" frontal or transbasal approach (26,27) with modifications or in combination with other approaches for the majority of lesions of the ASB. This approach is suitable for tumors and tumor-like conditions affecting the areas defined by the ASB from the frontal sinuses to the anterior tip of the lower clivus, with or without dural transgression and limited lateral extension. Lesions extending beyond the lateral aspect of the superior orbital fissure, cavernous sinus, or hypoglossal canals require anterolateral or lateral approaches, in combination with the transbasal approach as indicated. Specific details of the approach are beyond the scope of this chapter and have been described elsewhere (6–8,15,18,26,27,29–35). An abbreviated description of the complete procedure includes a bifrontal craniotomy, biorbital osteotomy with or without olfactory preservation, sphenoethmoidectomy, and removal of planum and tuberculum sellae, medial and superior walls of the optic foramen, and anterior sella wall, and clivectomy to the anterior foramen magnum and laterally to the hypoglossal foramen. Drilling of the medial wall of the carotid canal is performed as necessary, allowing bony removal to the anterior tip of the petrous apices in selected cases. Many lesions do not require the full complement of bony removal described here, and the approach can be tailored to the lesion as necessary. The standard reconstruction employs a watertight dural closure (if transgressed) and a vascularized pericranial flap (36), which completely isolates the bifrontal cranial plate

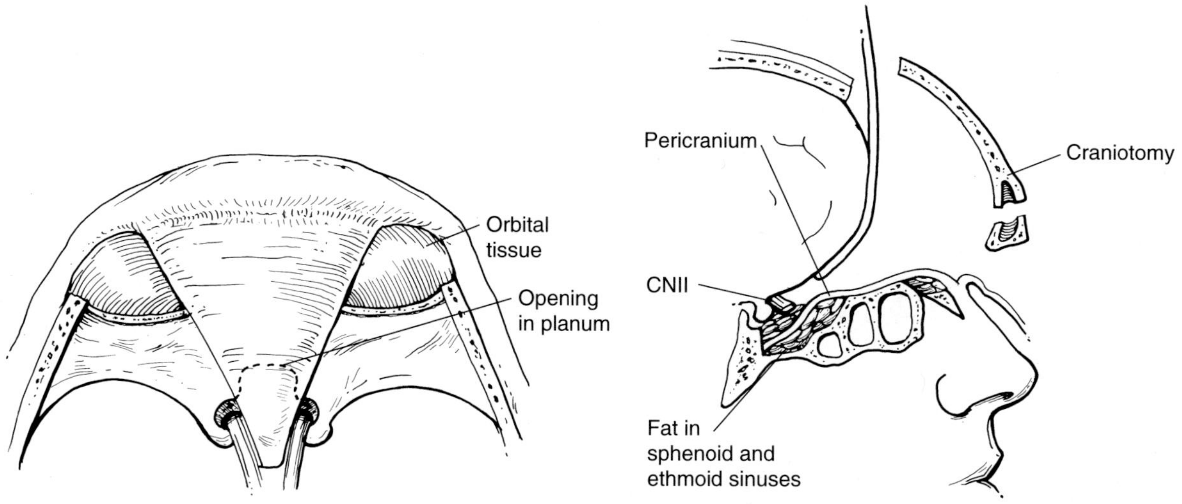

FIG. 28-3. Axial and sagittal view of the reconstruction after tumor resection. Adapted from Wright DC, Sekhar LN. Management of anterior cranial base tumors. In: Tindall GT, Barrow DC, Cooper PR, eds. *The practice of neurosurgery.* Baltimore: Williams & Wilkins, 1995:949–962.

and biorbital osteotomy segments from the nasal cavity (Fig. 28-3).

The advantages of the procedure include wide exposure with reduced retraction of the brain, ease in combination with anterolateral and lateral approaches to improve access, and simplified single-stage reconstruction. It is readily combined with anterior transfacial procedures for en bloc resection of malignant tumors. Potential disadvantages include olfactory denervation and creation of epidural dead space over the frontal pole(s) when cranialization of the frontal sinus is done. Those patients requiring a transcranial-transdural approach with intraoperative communication of the extradural and intradural compartments have an increased risk of CSF fistula and meningitis, but the surgical approach per se does not add to this risk if proper reconstruction is done (Figs. 28-4, 28-5, and 28-6).

COMPLICATION AVOIDANCE AND MANAGEMENT (TABLE 28-2)

Cerebrospinal Fluid Leak

CSF leaks occur because of extensive drilling of the frontal base and wide excision of involved segments of the dura. Virtually all ASB procedures should be approached with the expectation that the dural boundary will be transgressed either by necessity in order to achieve a complete resection or as a result of the surgical approach and inadvertent dural laceration. The proximity of the nasal sinuses and nasal cavity makes the presence of CSF leak a very dangerous situation, leading easily to meningitis. This complication is prevented by adequate reconstruction. Preoperative preparation and planning for repair of the dura should be made to restore the integrity of this crucial anatomic boundary. As indicated, this can encompass simple watertight resuture of a small fenestration, patch-grafting of the dura using free fascial material, or, in large defects, patch-grafting with reinforcement and dead-space obliteration using vascularized pericranium, free microvascular tissue grafts (e.g., radial forearm, rectus abdominis), or regional vascularized flaps (5,36–48). The latter approach is used when patients have had prior therapy

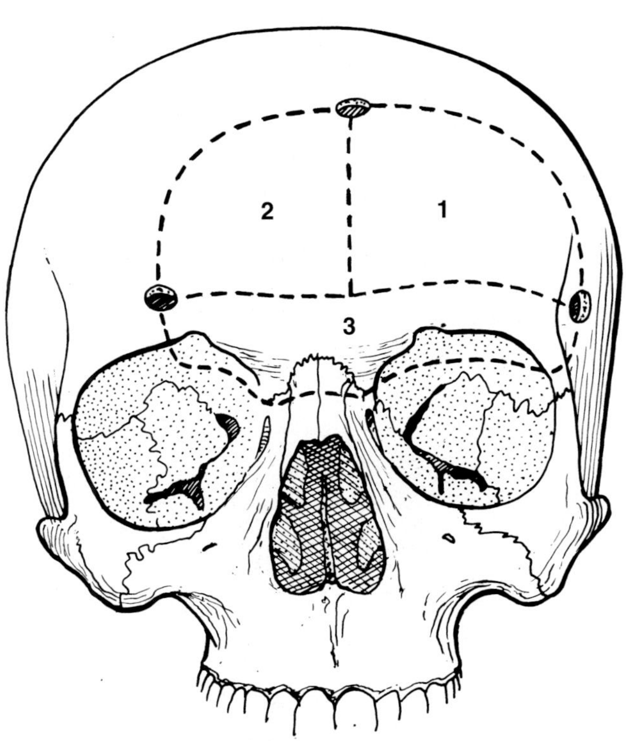

FIG. 28-4. Bony segments removed to expose the anterior skull base. Adapted from Wright DC, Sekhar LN. Management of anterior cranial base tumors. In: Tindall GT, Barrow DC, Cooper PR, eds. *The practice of neurosurgery.* Baltimore: Williams & Wilkins, 1995:949–962.

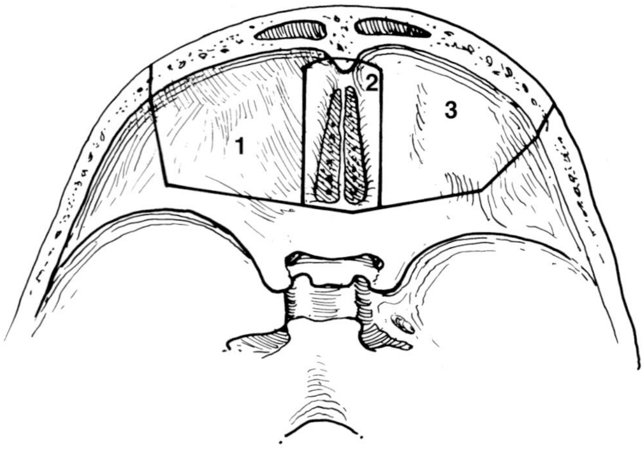

FIG. 28-5. Axial view of the biorbital osteotomy (1). Isolating the cribriform plate makes it possible to preserve olfaction. Adapted from Wright DC, Sekhar LN. Management of anterior cranial base tumors. In: Tindall GT, Barrow DC, Cooper PR, eds. *The practice of neurosurgery.* Baltimore: Williams & Wilkins, 1995:949–962.

TABLE 28–2. *Potential risks of anterior skull base surgery*

Event	Comment
Parenchymal injury	
Direct	Retraction injury, hematoma formation
Indirect	Arterial/venous injuries
Cranial nerve injury	
Olfactory	Preservation possible using special techniques
Optic	Compressive/thermal injury (drilling), vascular injury
Superior orbital fissure	CN III, IV, VI; $V_{ophthalmic}$
Foramen rotundum	$V_{maxillary}$
Cerebrospinal fistula	
Hydrocephalus	Can aggravate or promote CSF fistula
Meningitis	Unrecognized/untreated fistula
Abscess formation	Epidural, subdural, parenchymal
Osseous problems	
Periorbital	Enophthalmus, proptosis, dystocia
Resorption	
Infection	
Aesthetic problems	
Telecanthus	Loss of bony support at medial canthus
Bone loss	Necrosis, infection
Scalp	Necrosis, frontalis palsy

CSF, cerebrospinal fluid.
Adapted from Wright DC, Sekhar LN. Management of anterior cranial base tumors. In: Tindall GT, Barrow DC, Cooper PR, eds. *The practice of neurosurgery.* Baltimore: Williams & Wilkins, 1995:949–962.

(surgery/radiation) or other factors (infection) making scalp pericranium unsuited or unavailable for reconstruction and requiring these surgical adjuncts. Biocompatible tissue adhesives such as fibrin glue are useful, but only as an adjunct to a technically sound dural closure (32). If it is not possible to directly repair the dura in a watertight fashion, reinforcement of the wound with vascularized flaps is necessary. The use of free fat grafts or other tissue to reinforce a dural boundary without a watertight suture line will ultimately fail with CSF collection or fistula as a consequence.

The risk of CSF leak has been estimated at 4% to 14%, and it varies with the extent of surgical resection and the patient population (26,49,50). The leak may show as clear or serosanguineous fluid leaking through the nose, or less often the patient may report fluids over the back of the throat. A reservoir sign maneuver helps elicit the fluid leak. This is best performed in the morning after a full night with the patient in the supine position. The patient is asked to sit up and lean his head forward. Usually the patient reports the feeling of a hot fluid coursing through the nose (similar to the feeling that occurs after a nose bleed). Moments later the fluid will be seen leaking through the nares. If the fluid is serosanguineous, looking for a halo sign may be helpful to discern

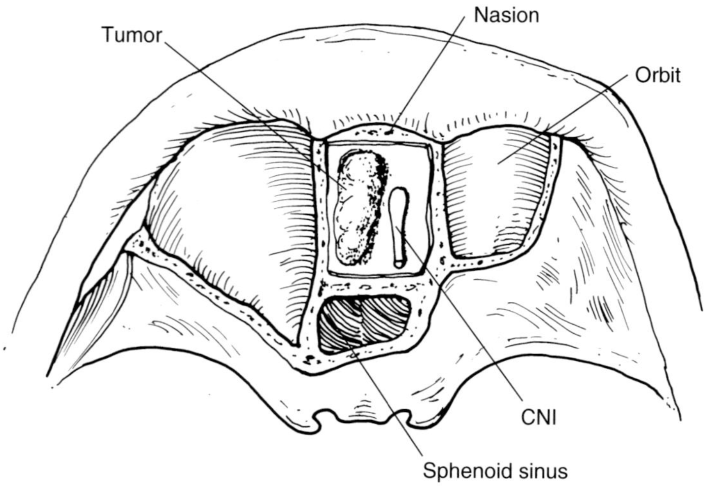

FIG. 28-6. Axial view of a tumor invading the dura of the anterior cranial base. The invaded dura is left attached to the tumor. Adapted from Wright DC, Sekhar LN. Management of anterior cranial base tumors. In: Tindall GT, Barrow DC, Cooper PR, eds. *The practice of neurosurgery.* Baltimore: Williams & Wilkins, 1995:949–962.

the serous component. β_2-Transferrin assay can be also helpful in delineating the origin of the fluid as it is a specific test for CSF. Postoperative pneumocephalus, persistent or delayed, is another indicator of CSF leak. The leak may occur early (<5 days) or late (>7 days) after surgery.

CSF fistula must be promptly recognized and aggressively treated to avoid ascending meningitis, epidural abscess, subdural empyema, or brain abscess formation. Early leaks are usually treated with CSF diversion (lumbar or ventricular drainage). Depending on the initial closure, most will resolve after a few days of drainage. However, if they do not resolve, then direct surgical obliteration may be required. Late CSF leaks may require permanent CSF diversion [lumbar peritoneal shunt (LPS) or ventricule peritoneal shunt (VPS)] or direct surgical obliteration, depending on the presence of associated hydrocephalus. In high-volume fistulae, CSF diversion may worsen hydrocephalus and should not be used until after direct surgical repair. Pneumocephalus can be encountered when spinal drainage is excessive postoperatively, leading to air trapping in the epidural space. It manifests with mental status change. Using lumbar drainage sparingly and draining by volume prevents pneumocephalus.

Infection

The risk of infection is relatively high (0%–23%), mainly because of the proximity of the approach to the aerodigestive tract (39,51). A short period of postoperative antibiotic prophylaxis, previous irradiation, postoperative dead space, and fluid collections are some of the risk factors (51). The infection can manifest with either meningitis or epidural abscess formation. Meningitis is usually secondary to CSF fistulae and requires prompt antibiotic treatment. The CSF leak also should be promptly addressed. Abscesses should be surgically drained.

Neural Tissue Injury

Direct parenchymal or cranial nerve injuries are normally an avoidable complication in the absence of contributing factors (tumor invasion, coagulopathy, acute hydrocephalus, etc.). Brain swelling or contusion may be seen. Such injuries usually reflect excessive retraction of the brain. They should not occur with increasing surgical experience and more liberal use of orbital osteotomies, reducing the amount of frontal lobe retraction. Direct cranial nerve injuries are associated with removal of bone over exit foramina [optic foramen, superior orbital fissure (SOF), foramen rotundum], or dissection injury in the subarachnoid space. Anosmia is an expected postoperative occurrence of this approach. Unilateral approach may preserve smell as well as some technical variations advocated by some authors. Spetzler et al. (28) described a technical variation that should theoretically preserve smell. The osteotomy cuts are made circumferentially around the cribriform plate. The nasal mucosa is left attached to the bone and the ethmoid trabeculae are cut individually with scissors. The olfactory nerves are not severed and the cribriform plate is elevated with the frontal dura. But to perform this osteotomy, the orbital osteotomy must extend posteriorly to allow the posterior cut of the ethmoidal osteotomy to be made through the planum sphenoidale. The optic nerve can be also injured during the bony removal. This may occur during the osteotomy cuts if carried too posteriorly, or if the orbital roof is prematurely cracked, leading to a fracture line through the optic canal. The nerves of the SOF are usually more resilient and rarely injured by the approach itself. Rather, they are injured by the intradural work. Frontal anesthesia results from the sacrifice of the supraorbital nerves when pericranial flaps are used, or if the nerves are subject to excessive traction in their foramina before releasing them. Releasing the supraorbital nerve anteriorly from its foramina will protect it from injury.

Indirect injuries arising from vascular injury lead to ischemic or congestive infarction of the parenchyma or nerves and can be obscure or unrecognized until manifested in the postoperative period. Elective or unplanned occlusion of the internal carotid results in minor or major infarction of the brain in 10% to 45% of patients (regardless of age and adequacy of collateral circulation) and should be avoided in almost all circumstances.

Aesthetic and Functional Complications

Aesthetic and functional problems include airway patency, sinus obstruction with mucocele formation, osteonecrosis of facial or cranial bones, and orbital (dystocia, proptosis, enophthalmos, telecanthus) and scalp problems (frontalis palsy, necrosis). Prior or planned therapy (surgery or radiation) can affect healing and the final cosmetic result in such patients and threaten the success of an otherwise uncomplicated procedure. Such complications, though rarely life threatening, frequently have a disproportionate effect on the psychologic adjustment of the patient and can impede or prolong recovery to functional activity.

Osseous reconstruction of the floor of the ASB is only occasionally indicated, but routine reconstruction of bone defects over the cranium and periorbital regions (particularly orbital roof) are done for aesthetic and functional concerns. Extensive rongeuring of the roof of the orbit may lead to postoperative enophthalmos. It is wise to include as much as needed of the orbital roof in the orbital osteotomy rather then rongeuring it. Defects in the periorbita are carefully closed or covered with fascial grafts to reduce herniation of orbital fat and subsequent atrophy. Preservation of the periorbita and orbital fat is a factor in avoiding enophthalmos, and equal in importance to preserving or reconstructing the bony orbital walls. An acquired telecanthus may result from removing the bony insertion of the medial canthal ligament. This complication can be prevented by restoring the canthal ligament with absorbable suture or wire (16). Scalp flap necrosis may occur when galeal-pericranial flaps are used in previously radiated and operated cases by reducing the blood supply to the skin. Alternative flaps should be used in these cases.

The key to complication avoidance and management of

complications is anticipation of potential problems and rapid, effective therapy if and when they occur.

SUMMARY

An interdisciplinary approach utilizing the combined skills and experience of multiple specialists can overcome many of the hurdles in treating complex lesions of the ASB. Accurate preoperative localization, careful surgical planning, adherence to specific surgical goals, anticipation of potential complications, and meticulous surgical technique has benefited patients with ASB lesions and increased the likelihood of complete resection with low morbidity.

REFERENCES

1. Alaywan M, Sindou M. Frontotemporal approach with orbito-zygomatic removal: surgical anatomy. *Acta Neurochir* 1990;104:79–83.
2. MacArthur LL. An aseptic surgical access to the pituitary body and its neighbourhood. *JAMA* 1912;58:2009–2011.
3. Frazier CH. An approach to the hypophysis through the anterior cranial fossa. *Ann Surg* 1913;57:145–150.
4. Ray BS, McLean JM. Combined intracranial and orbital operation for retinoblastoma. *Arch Ophthalmol* 1943;30:437–445.
5. Smith RR, Klopp CT, Williams JM. Surgical treatment of cancer of the frontal sinus and adjacent areas. *Cancer* 1954;7:991–994.
6. Derome PJ, Guiot G. Surgical approaches to the sphenoidal and clival areas. *Adv Tech Stand Neurosurg* 1979;6:101–136.
7. Derome P, Akerman M, Anquez L. Les tumeurs sphenoethmoidales: possibilite d'exerese et de reparation chirurgicale. *Neurochirurgie* 1972;18(suppl):1–164.
8. Derome P. The transbasal approach to tumours invading the base of the skull. In: Schmidek HH, Sweet WH, eds. *Operative neurosurgical techniques: indications, methods, and results.* New York: Grune & Stratton, 1982:357–379.
9. Cophignon J, George B, Marchac D, Roux FX. Voie transbasale elargie par mobilisation du bandeau fronto-orbitaire median. *Neurochirurgie* 1983;29:407–410.
10. Sundaresan N, Shah JP. Craniofacial resection for anterior skull base tumors. *Head Neck Surg* 1988;10:219–224.
11. Frazell EL, Lewis JS. Cancer of the nasal cavity and accessory sinuses: a report of the management of 416 patients. *Cancer* 1963;16:1293–1301.
12. Becker SP, Atiyah RA. Nasal and paranasal malignancies: carcinoma of the paranasal sinuses. *Otolaryngol Clin North Am* 1985;18:491–497.
13. Lyons BM, Donald PJ. Radical surgery for nasal cavity and paranasal sinus tumors. *Otolaryngol Clin North Am* 1991;24:1499–1521.
14. Snyderman C, Janecka IP, Sekhar LN, Sen CN, Eibling DE. Anterior cranial base reconstruction: role of galeal and pericranial flaps. *Laryngoscope* 1990;100:607–613.
15. Al-Mefty O. The supraorbital-pterional approach to skull base lesions. *Neurosurgery* 1987;21:474–477.
16. Beals SP. Principles of craniofacial surgery. *BNI Q* 1986;2:10–15.
17. Cocke EWJ, H RJ, Robertson JH. The extended maxillotomy and subtotal maxillectomy for excision of skull base tumors. *Arch Otolaryngol Head Neck Surg* 1990;116:92–104.
18. Crockard HA. The transmaxillary approach to the clivus. In: Sekhar LN, Janecka IP, ed. *Surgery of cranial base tumors.* New York: Raven Press, 1993:235–244.
19. Jackson CG. *Surgery of skull base tumors.* New York: Churchill Livingstone, 1991.
20. Janecka IP, Sekhar LN. Anterior and anterolateral craniofacial resection. In: Sekhar LN, Janecka IP, ed. *Surgery of cranial base tumors.* New York: Raven Press, 1993:147–156.
21. Janecka IP, Sen CN, Sekhar LN, et al. Facial translocation: a new approach to the cranial base. *Otolaryngol Head Neck Surg* 1990;103:413–419.
22. Krespi YP, Har-El G. The transmandibular-transcervical approach to the skull base. In: Sekhar LN, Janecka IP, ed. *Surgery of cranial base tumors.* New York: Raven Press, 1993:261–265.
23. Samii M, Draf W. *Surgery of the skull base: an interdisciplinary approach.* Berlin: Springer-Verlag, 1989:525.
24. Samii M, Knosp E. *Approaches to the clivus.* Berlin: Springer-Verlag, 1992:169.
25. Sasaki CT, McCage BF, Kirchner JA. *Surgery of the skull base.* Philadelphia: JB Lippincott, 1984.
26. Sekhar L, Sen C, Jho HD, Janecka I. Surgical treatment of intracavernous neoplasms: a four-year experience. *Neurosurgery* 1989;24:18–30.
27. Sekhar LN, Nanda A, Sen CN, Snyderman CN, Janecka IP. An extended frontal approach to tumors of the anterior, middle, and posterior skull base. *J Neurosurg* 1992;76:198–206.
28. Spetzler R, Herman JM, Beals S, Joganic E, Milligan J. Preservation of olfaction in anterior craniofacial approaches. *J Neurosurg* 1993;79:48–52.
29. Al-Mefty O. *Surgery of the cranial base.* Boston: Kluwer Academic, 1989:356.
30. Jackson I, Laws E Jr, Martin R. A craniofacial approach to advanced recurrent cancer of the central face. *Head Neck Surg* 1983;5:474–488.
31. Persing JA, Jane JA, Levine PA, et al. The versatile frontal sinus approach to the floor of the anterior cranial fossa: technical note. *J Neurosurg* 1990;74:513–516.
32. Sekhar LN, Wright DC, Sen C. An extended frontal approach to tumors and aneurysms of the cranial base. In: Wilkins R, Rengachary, eds. *Neurosurgery.* McGraw-Hill, NY: 1994.
33. Soutar DS, Scheker LR, Tanner NSB, McGregor IA. The radial forearm flap: a versatile method for intraoral reconstruction. *Br J Plast* 1983;36:1–8.
34. Stevenson G, Stoney R, Perkins R, et al. A transcervical transclival approach to the ventral surface of the brain stem for removal of a clivus chordoma. *J Neurosurg* 1966;24:544–551.
35. Van Buren JM, Ommaya AK, Ketcham AS. Ten years' experience with radical combined craniofacial resection of malignant tumors of the paranasal sinuses. *J Neurosurg* 1968;28:341–350.
36. Johns ME, Winn HR, McLean WC, et al. Pericranial flap for the closure of defects of craniofacial resections. *Laryngoscope* 1981;91:952–959.
37. Baker SR. Closure of large orbito-maxillary defects with free latissimus dorsi myocutaneous flaps. *Head Neck Surg* 1984;6:828–835.
38. Bridges GP, Baldwin M, Gonski A. Craniofacial resection for paranasal sinus cancer with free flap repair. *Aust NZ J Surg* 1986;56:843–847.
39. Freije JE, Gluckman JL, Van Loveren H, McDonough JJ, Shumrick KA. Reconstruction of the anterior skull base after craniofacial resection. *Skull Base Surg* 1992;2:17–21.
40. Horowitz JH, Persing JA, Nichter LS, et al. Galeal-pericranial flaps in head and neck reconstruction: anatomy and application. *Am J Surg* 1984;148:489–497.
41. Jones NF, Schramm VL, Sekhar LN. Reconstruction of the cranial base following tumour resection. *Br J Plast Surg* 1987;40:155–162.
42. Pennington DG, Lai MF, Pelly AD. The rectus abdominis myocutaneous free flap. *Br J Plast Surg* 1980;33:277–282.
43. Price JC, Loury M, Carson B, Johns ME. The pericranial flap for reconstruction of anterior skull base defects. *Laryngoscope* 1988;98:1159–1164.
44. Schaefer SD, Close LG, Mickey BE. Axial subcutaneous scalp flaps in the reconstruction of the anterior cranial fossa. *Arch Otolaryngol Head Neck Surg* 1986;112:745–749.
45. Schramm VL, Myers EN, Maroon JC. Anterior skull base surgery for benign and malignant disease. *Laryngoscope* 1979;89:1077–1091.
46. Sekhar L, Burgess J, Akin O. An anatomical study of the cavernous sinus emphasizing operative approaches and related vascular and neural reconstruction. *Neurosurgery* 1987;21:806–916.
47. Shaffrey CI, Spotnitz WD, Shaffrey ME, Jane JA. Neurosurgical applications of fibrin glue: dural closure in 134 patients. *Neurosurgery* 1990;26:496–501.
48. Som PM. Sinonasal cavity. In: Som PM, Bergeron RT, eds. *Head and neck imaging.* St. Louis: Mosby Year Book, 1991:51–276.
49. Blacklock JB, Weber RS, Lee YY, et al. Transcranial resection of tumors of the paranasal sinuses and nasal cavity. *J Neurosurg* 1989;71:10–15.
50. Couldwell WT. Surgery of the anterior skull base. *Otolaryngol Clin North Am* 1993;4:673–693.
51. Carrau RL, Synderman C, Janecka IP, Sekhar L, Sen C, D'Amico F. Antibiotic prophylaxis in cranial base surgery. *Head Neck Surg* 1991;13:311–317.

Neurosurgical Issues in Otolaryngology: Principles and Practice of Collaboration,
edited by Moisés A. Arriaga and J. Diaz Day.
Lippincott Williams & Wilkins, Philadelphia © 1999.

CHAPTER 29

Vascular Lesions

Julian E. Bailes

Despite the numerous and profound advances in late 20th century medicine, stroke remains an important source of mortality, morbidity, and health care expenditure. The annual cost of stroke, including the extensive potential for long-term care and rehabilitation, is estimated at $40 billion in the United States. Many etiologies are responsible for stroke or cerebrovascular accidents (CVAs), with thrombotic occlusion secondary to atherosclerotic disease in the cerebral and carotid vessels being most common. Embolic CVA is next in frequency, usually from cardiac (e.g., atrial fibrillation) or cervical carotid artery bifurcation sources.

CVAs can also be characterized as bland (nonhemorrhagic) or hemorrhagic in nature. The most common type of hemorrhagic CVA results from hypertensive hemorrhage, ordinarily associated with many years of poorly controlled or uncontrolled blood pressure. It is believed that serial deleterious alterations occur, primarily in the small penetrating arteries of the brain. This degenerative process is termed lipohyalinosis. Progressive weakness occurs leading to sudden rupture, with acute intracerebral hematoma resulting. Most intracerebral hypertensive hemorrhages are located in deep brain locations, such as the basal ganglia, deep white matter, cerebellum, or brainstem.

Hemorrhagic events also occur as subarachnoid hemorrhage, which represents bleeding into the subarachnoid space. This is usually due to rupture of an intracranial aneurysm, although bleeding in this location may be caused by a ruptured arteriovenous malformation (AVM), bleeding dyscrasias, or another hemorrhagic malady. Intracranial berry aneurysms are present in perhaps up to 5% of the general population. However, they are ordinarily asymptomatic and unnoticed until they compress vital cranial nerves or spontaneously hemorrhage, the latter being the most common presentation. The rupture rate, however, is fortunately much lower than the aneurysm incidence, occurring in approximately 15 persons/100,000 population annually.

Patients with aneurysmal subarachnoid hemorrhage usually present with a major or "worst of my life" headache. It is associated with a spectrum of neurologic symptoms and presents with a graded expression of cerebral dysfunction. In addition to headache, other signs of meningeal irritation such as photophobia and nuchal rigidity may be present. Compression of cranial nerves, especially III, IV, VI, and the optic nerve, may occur. Various grading systems have been derived to assist in categorizing subarachnoid hemorrhage patients for treatment and prognostic purposes. Patients in grades I, II, and III are often referred to as good-grade patients, and generally respond well to treatment modalities including early surgical interventions. Patient in grades IV and V are poor grade and have a more difficult hospital course, related to diminished cerebral perfusion pressure, intracranial hypertension, and various medical and cardiac complications (1). Patients with subarachnoid hemorrhage also are in jeopardy of developing cerebral vasospasm, as a result of the released blood components irritating the arteries, causing a narrowing and diminished cerebral perfusion. This phenomenon is usually seen at days 7 to 11 following the hemorrhage and is somewhat proportional to the volume of extravasated blood.

AVMs represent abnormal persisting embryonic blood vessels, which ordinarily present in adulthood with symptoms resulting from their hemorrhage, mass effect, or irritation of surrounding brain tissue (i.e., seizures). The majority of AVMs are located supratentorially, in lobar, superficial, or deep white matter locations. These as well as cerebellar hemispheric AVMs are usually approached using standard operating techniques and procedures. Approximately 2% to 5% of intracranial vascular malformations are located in the brainstem and thus often require specialized skull base approaches for their removal (2).

AVMs located in the brainstem tissue usually present with a clinical syndrome due to mass effect or hemorrhage. Their

J. E. Bailes: 400 Celebration Place, Celebration, Florida 34747.

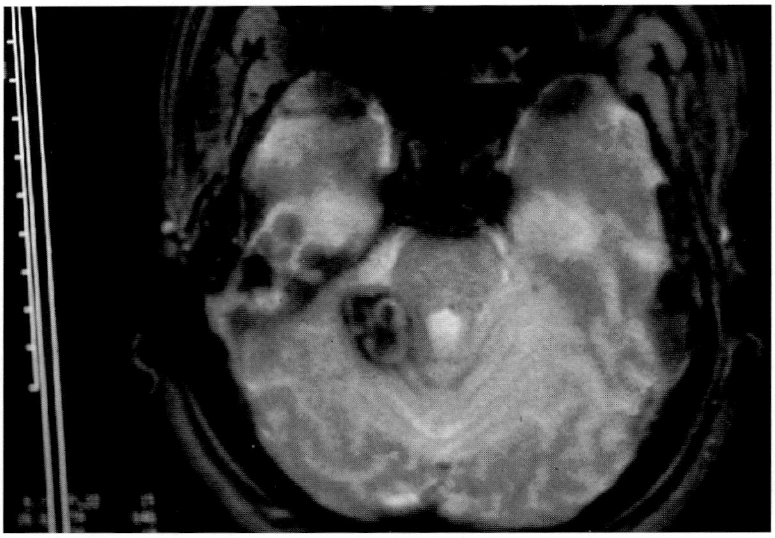

FIG. 29-1. Magnetic resonance imaging scan showing large cavernous malformation with brainstem involvement. These vascular malformations tend to undergo repetitive hemorrhage and usually necessitate operative resection. A combined petrosal approach was utilized to achieve total resection.

natural history is often that of repeated hemorrhages with resultant devastating clinical deficits (Fig. 29-1). Modern neuroradiologic imaging, and especially magnetic resonance imaging (MRI), has markedly improved upon our diagnostic acumen with these lesions, allowing accurate pinpointing of the pathologic entity and assisting in planning for surgical strategy (2,3). Standard operative approaches such as the infratentorial, supracerebellar, retromastoid suboccipital, and midline suboccipital are often employed for posterior fossa cerebellar and dorsal brainstem AVMs (4). However, those AVMs located in the ventral or lateral medulla, pons, or mesencephalon often are much more readily removed by using skull base approaches. Most surgicallly accessible brainstem AVMs, including cavernous malformations, are operated on once the patient is medically and neurologically stabilized. Because we now appreciate that brainstem vascular malformations tend to have a progressive and malignant course, almost all patients benefit from surgical resection.

Cerebrovascular surgery has undergone many refinements and innovations in the past 40 years. The resulting improved outcomes for surgery on patients with cerebral aneurysms have also paralleled the improvements in anesthesiology and critical care medicine. Early attempts at operative intervention were severely limited due to poor exposure, inadequate visualization and lighting, and lack of developed equipment and surgical instrumentation. Through the efforts of Yasargil et al. (5) and others, microsurgical techniques and instrumentation were advanced in the 1970s and 1980s, making successful surgical treatment of cerebrovascular conditions (aneurysms, AVMs, cavernous malformations) routine. Further refinements in more recent years have occurred in surgical microscope systems, diagnostic testing, intraoperative localization and navigation, anesthetic techniques, and instrumentation, which have marked improved management outcomes.

SURGICAL APPROACHES

Vascular lesions surrounding the cerebellum and brainstem have always been some of the most challenging operative endeavors for the neurosurgeon. The anterior circulation, supplied by the two carotid arteries, is the site of the majority, approximately 80%, of all intracranial aneurysms. The circle of Willis, where high-velocity blood flow is quickly diverted into major branch arteries, is where most aneurysms occur, coinciding with branch points in these vessels and at defects in the arterial tunica media. Using primarily a frontotemporal or pterional approach, there is usually adequate and ready access to the anterior circle of Willis and its major branches, the anterior and middle cerebral arteries, and the anterior and posterior communicating arteries, where the aneurysms of the anterior circulation predominate (Table 29-1).

The posterior circulation of the human brain, supplied by

TABLE 29–1. *Skull base approaches for cerebral aneurysms*

Paraclinoid aneurysms—anterior pericavernous approach
Cavernous aneurysms—transcavernous approach
Posterior circulation aneurysms
Basilar apex-pterional, pericavernous, "half and half" approaches
Low-lying basilar apex—subtemporal approach
High-lying basilar apex—transzygomatic or orbitozygomatic approach
P1, P2–subtemporal approach
Basilar trunk
Retromastoid, transsigmoid approach
Combined petrosal approach
VB junction—ELITE approach
Vertebral, PICA—lateral suboccipital approach

ELITE, extreme-lateral inferior transtubercular exposure; PICA, posterior inferior cerebellar artery; VB, vertebrobasilar.

the two vertebral arteries, which unite to form the basilar artery, is located in the relatively inaccessible posterior cranial fossa and ventral to the midbrain, pons, and medulla oblongata. The depth of the exposure overlying critical brain structures and the inability to retract adjacent brain tissue make surgical intervention most difficult on the vasculature composing the posterior circulation. It is in these locations where the talents of the neuro-otologist and neurosurgeon are often combined to improve access and anatomic exposure to deal effectively with cerebral aneurysms.

The neurosurgeon and neuro-otologist often have occasion to collaborate in dealing with aneurysms and AVMs arising from the posterior circulation. Vascular lesions of the posterior fossa present difficulty due to the limited avenues of approach, the associated vital brain, cranial nerve, and vascular structures, and the dire consequences of any brain injury to these areas. Cerebral ischemia is ill-tolerated by the posterior fossa structures, and numerous minute and critical perforating arteries make it unlikely that the patient can sustain any insult to brainstem or cerebellar tissues without incurring a significant neurologic deficit. Tremendous attention to detail, meticulous handling of all structures, and a thorough understanding of the microanatomy is therefore paramount to achieving success in operative intervention in this area.

Due to the aforementioned anatomic characteristics and the attendant complex bony anatomy of the skull base and otologic structures, a direct approach to the posterior circulation is prevented. Modifications in technique are always occurring, presenting the operative team with important choices to consider for virtually every patient. Several key operative approaches have evolved over the last 20 years, allowing us to safely and adequately access every region of the brain, and in particular the posterior fossa, for surgical treatment of cerebrovascular anomalies. The operative routes currently favored include the pterional approach, which gives the surgeon a superior-inferior viewing angle from the frontotemporal starting point for access to the top of the basilar artery. The other approaches available are the retrolabyrinthine-transsigmoid approach for exposure of the basilar artery trunk and related structures, the combined petrosal approach, for the mid- to upper basilar trunk, and the suboccipital, inferior approaches for access to the caudal basilar artery and its tributaries (Fig. 29-2). The majority of cerebral aneurysms can be exposed and clipped by standard craniotomy openings such as the frontotemporal (pterional), subtemporal, or far-lateral suboccipital. However, anatomically difficult aneurysms, giant aneurysms, basilar trunk, and vertebrobasilar junction lesions often require skull base approaches (Table 29-2).

SUPRATENTORIAL APPROACHES

The operative treatment of vascular lesions of the anterior circulation has been primarily based on the frontotemporal approach, which entails bone removal centered at the confluence of the frontal, temporal, and zygomatic bones, known as the pterion. This approach has been refined through the

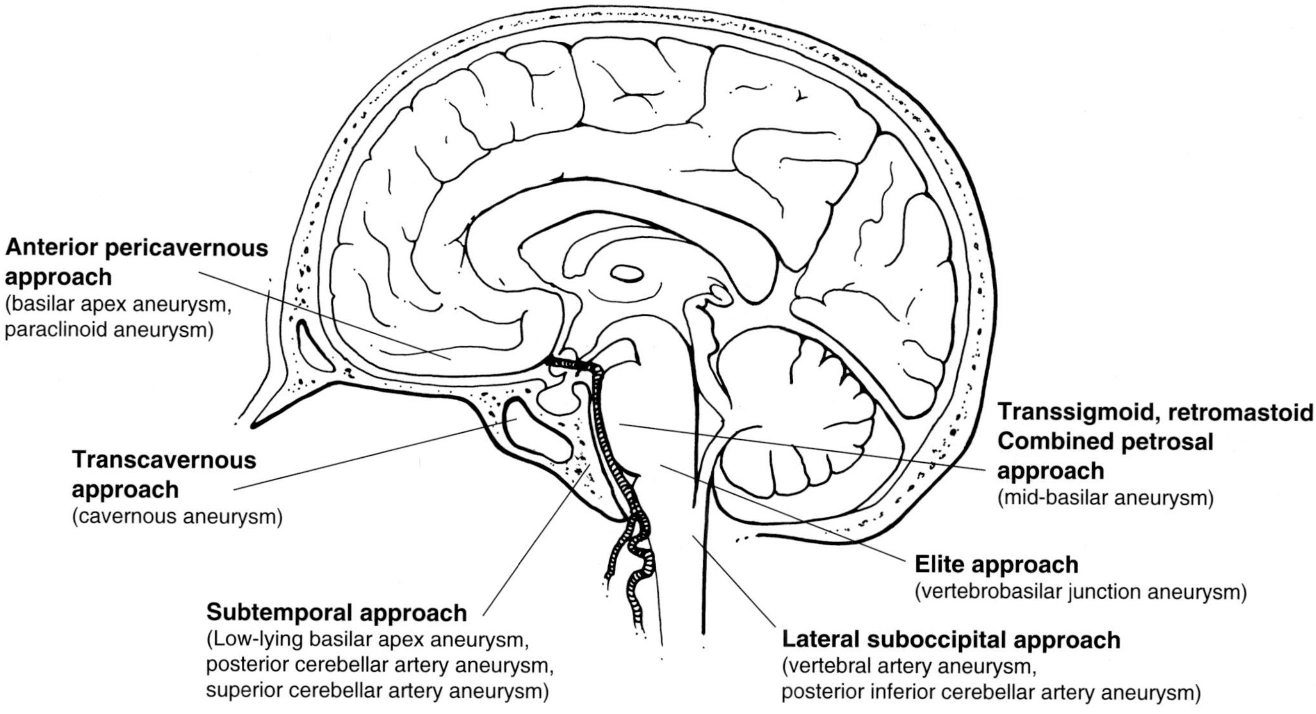

FIG. 29-2. The basic operative approaches for vascular lesions of the anterior and posterior circulation.

TABLE 29–2. *Selection of approaches—vertebrobasilar vascular lesions*

Upper basilar segment
Standard Pterional
Extradural, Temporopolar, Pericavernous
Orbitozygomatic
Subtemporal/Transtentorial
Anterior Transpetrosal (Kawase)
Mid-basilar trunk
Subtemporal/Transtentorial
Combined Petrosal
Retromastoid, Transsigmoid
Transoral
Vertebrobasilar junction and VA
Suboccipital, far lateral
ELITE—transcondylar, transtubercular
Retromastoid, transsigmoid
Transoral

VA, vertebral artery.

years and involves a frontal and temporal craniotomy flap, which is extended down low over the orbit to expose the lesser wing of the sphenoid bone. The latter is then drilled down, to near its junction with the superior orbital fissure, allowing a flat approach to enter the region of the carotid and optic cerebrospinal fluid (CSF) cisterns. The pterional approach was perfected over many years and was popularized by Yasargil et al. (5), who, with others, including Sugita et al. (6) and Sano (7), subsequently modified the approach to allow access to the basilar artery apex. Starting with a flat bony opening along the anterior cranial fossa, the carotid cistern is opened and dissection proceeds lateral to the carotid artery, following the posterior communicating artery posteriorly to its junction with the P1-P2 segment of the posterior cerebral artery. From this vantage point, the basilar artery apex is accessible, and excellent visualization is afforded of the upper basilar region and its associated neurovascular structures.

Modifications have been made to the basic pterional approach for an improved ability to operate on lesions in the vicinity of the upper basilar complex (Table 29-3). An extended pterional exposure has been made to gain greater access to this region, termed the extradural temporopolar approach (8). This technique begins with the patient in the supine position, with the head placed in 15 degrees of extension and rotated 30 degrees to the opposite side. An incision is made along the hairline and a routine frontotemporal craniotomy performed. After elevating the bone flap, the pterion is drilled down to the region of the superior orbital fissure. The dura is then elevated from the anterior and middle cranial fossae in the perisylvian region, and all bony prominences are flattened using the high-speed drill.

TABLE 29–3. *Anterior temporopolar pericavernous approach*

Standard pterional opening
Extradural, anterolateral removal of sphenoid wing, ACP, optic canal roof
Exposure of SOF, foramen rotundum
Transcavernous exposure ICA-fibrous ring
IIIn.—porus oculomotorius
Extradural retraction temporal pole
Removal PCP
Wide opening Sylvian fissure, retract ICA

ACP, anterior clinoid process; ICA, internal carotid artery.

The key to liberating this exposure is extradural removal of the anterior clinoid process. By using a rotating movement under the operating microscope, with constant cool saline irrigation, the anterior clinoid is hollowed out until only a thin halo of bone remains. The optic strut is integral to this bony architecture and must be removed, allowing the anterior clinoid to be excised in a single piece with a micropituitary rongeur, using a slow twisting motion. The optic canal is unroofed, again using great care to avoid any heat transfer from the drill to the optic nerve, accomplished by proper drilling technique including constant saline irrigation. Further bony exposure requires the skeletonization of the superior orbital fissure and foramen rotundum (8).

By utilizing sharp dissection, the plane between the dura propria, covering the temporal lobe, and the outer cavernous membrane is entered, allowing the brain to be protected. The dura is widely opened over the sylvian fissure and the optic nerve sheath. The carotid fibrous ring is next incised, providing the ability to safely retract and work lateral to the internal carotid artery. The oculomotor nerve is mobilized and protected by opening its dural sleeve, the porus oculomotorius. With medial movement of the carotid artery and lateral, gentle retraction of the third cranial nerve, the exposure thus expands to the region of the basilar tip. The posterior clinoid process and superior portions of the zygoma can likewise be removed if necessary, to provide more caudal and cephalad exposure, respectively.

A combined approach has also been used to effectively create greater access to the basilar artery bifurcation region. It is also known as the one-and-a-half procedure, in which the lateral bony opening of the pterional approach is extended to the floor of the temporal fossa (7,9). This will develop a flat plane extending from the pterion to the area of the middle cranial fossa. Combined with the traditional frontotemporal exposure, access can be obtained to the area of the basilar bifurcation through a pure transsylvian approach, or through a subtemporal approach by rotating the patient to the opposite side. A somewhat more lateral exposure can thus be seen, giving better access to the basilar artery than a mere anterior trajectory can offer. The entire middle cranial fossa floor is exposed, with retraction of the temporal lobe, and improved access is gained, which merges the advantages of the more traditional pterional and subtemporal exposures.

SUBTEMPORAL APPROACH

The subtemporal approach was used extensively by Drake (9) and others and has provided a reliable standard for which

TABLE 29–4. *Subtemporal approach—disadvantages*

Temporal lobe retraction
Edema
Hemorrhage
Infarction
Vein of Labbé
Petrous ridge obstructs view
Can't see opposite P1
Limited field

to gain necessary operative control and visibility of the upper basilar complex. The operation begins by placing the patient's head in a lateral position, either with a supine or lateral decubitus body position. A linear preauricular incision is made from in front of the tragus to the superior temporal line. After exposing the temporal bone, a quadrangular-shaped temporal craniotomy is performed and extended down flat with the temporal floor. After drilling all bony protruberances down, the dura is opened and temporal lobe elevated. This plane is followed medially until the tentorial hiatus is visualized and the midbrain is exposed. The tentorial free edge is either incised or retracted with stay sutures, the oculomotor nerve dissected on its medial side, and basal arachnoid cisterns opened to expose the neurovascular anatomy of the basilar apex region.

Although this approach has been widely used and is still a very satisfactory method of accessing routine lesions in this area, there remain several drawbacks to the procedure, especially if one is dealing with complex lesions. The significant limitations include the necessity to retract the temporal lobe, which can easily lead to temporal hemorrhage and/or edema, often an inability to visualize a high basilar region, and poor visualization of the opposite posterior cerebral artery (Table 29-4). We have had success by employing a modification of the subtemporal approach, including skull base techniques to widen the operative field. To accomplish this, extensive drilling is performed of the middle cranial fossa, including taking the bony removal as far medial as possible, usually to the foramen spinosum. The superior aspect of the zygoma is drilled down, giving an increased ability to "look up" for greater cephalad exposure. The porus oculomotorius is opened and third nerve mobilized, allowing a widespread dissection into the basilar cisterns, especially the perimesencephalic cistern. Further widening of this corridor is provided by placing multiple stay sutures in the free edge of the tentorium. There is much greater ability to see and operate in a cephalad and caudad direction, giving more rostral-caudal exposure along the neuroaxis and basilar artery using these modifications (Table 29-5).

TABLE 29–5. *Subtemporal pericavernous approach*

Extradural bony opening
4 × 4 cm temporal craniotomy
Extradural middle fossa flat trajectory, to V3, mma
Removal upper portion zygoma
Intradural exposure
Location tentorial hiatus
Open p. oculomot. to postcavernous sinus
Extensive arachnoid dissection
Multiple (3–7) stay sutures in tentorium
Identify IVn
Vascular dissection
Identify and follow ICA, p. comm, P2, P1, SCA, BA apex, opp IIIn
Go to BA proximal to SCA
Identify aneurysm, dissect neck
Identify perforators and dissect free

BA, basilar artery; mma, middle meningeal artery; SCA, superior cerebellar artery.

INFRATENTORIAL APPROACHES

Retrolabyrinthine-Transsigmoid Approach

This approach, described and modified by Giannotta and Maceri (10) in 1988, has provided many instances of excellent operative results based on proven tenets of surgical philosophy (Fig. 29-3). It gives a straight lateral to medial corridor to the vasculature ventral to the brainstem, in addition to minimizing the extent of necessary brain retraction. This procedure begins with the patient in the supine position with his head turned away from the side of the approach. A retroauricular scalp incision is made and the soft tissues are reflected anteriorly to expose the posterior aspect of the external auditory meatus. After performing a mastoidectomy and retrolabyrinthine exposure, the sigmoid sinus is skeletonized from its junction with the superior petrosal sinus to the jugular bulb. The sigmoid sinus can subsequently be ligated at those two junctions and the dura opened and retracted over the intact labyrinth. Once inside the dura, microscopic dissection of the subarachnoid space allows exposure of the upper vertebral artery, the vertebrobasilar junction (VBJ), and the lower portion of the basilar trunk to the anterior inferior cerebellar artery.

This method of exposure has provided greater access than a standard retrolabyrinthine technique achieves. It allows efficient entry to the midline vascular structures ventral to the brainstem and, for the more straightforward lesions less than 2 cm in size, an excellent placement of the surgeon at the basilar trunk and VBJ. To fully exploit this corridor of entry, it is often necessary to ligate the sigmoid sinus. This is done only after angiographic determination has been made of the presence of adequate collateral venous outflow, i.e., a patent contralateral sigmoid sinus. If there is any doubt concerning the functionality of the sinus ipsilateral to the procedure, an intraoperative test occlusion can be made using a temporary aneurysm clip, with an increase of less than 5 mm Hg signifying that it is probably safe to proceed with occlusion of that sigmoid sinus. The side of the approach is governed by the side to which the aneurysms point or originate, or, if the lesion is in a midline location, by the side of the nondominant or smaller sigmoid sinus.

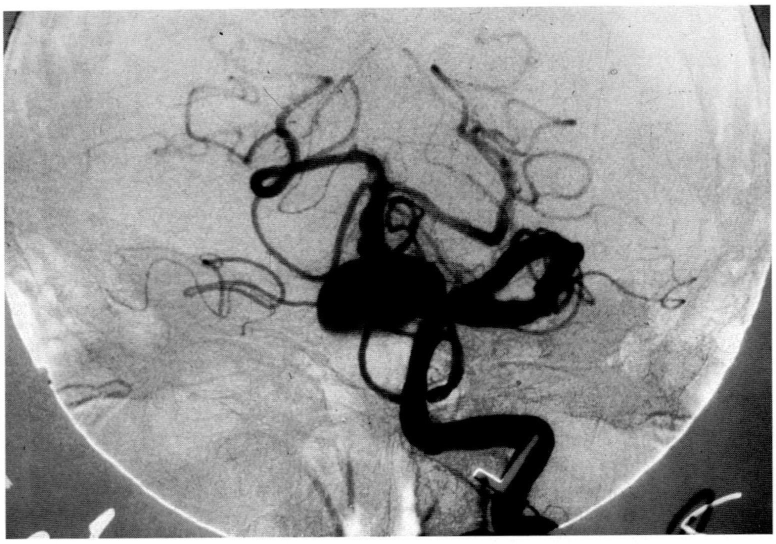

FIG. 29-3. Cerebral angiogram showing a giant basilar trunk aneurysm that presented with signs of brainstem compression. This lesion was successfully clipped using a retromastoid, transsigmoid approach.

Combined Petrosal Approach

The combined petrosal approach is a more complex surgical exercise that is employed when wider or more extensive exposure of the basilar trunk is mandated. It is most useful for large vascular or neoplastic lesions of the ventral brainstem (Fig. 29-4) (11,12). To perform the combined petrosal approach, begin with an incision 1 cm behind the mastoid body and 1 cm below the mastoid tip, extended superiorly 4.5 cm above the external auditory meatus, the latter portion corresponding to the height of the temporal squama. The incision extends with a question-mark shape around the ear, with the anterior limb in front of the tragus, toward the zygoma root along the preauricular line. The patient is best positioned three-quarter lateral, with the external auditory meatus and mastoid as the highest points (Table 29-6).

Four burr holes are placed: the first just posterior to the asterion over the transverse sinus, the second on the temporal squama in the midportion of the anterior limb of the scalp incision, the third just behind the mastoid body under the superior nuchal line, and the fourth 2.5 cm in distance from the third burr hole immediately superior to the supramastoid crest. To facilitate the completion of the craniotomy flap, a groove is drilled in an anterior subtemporal location to detach the anterior-inferior portion. Using small diamond burrs, the posterior margin of the sigmoid sinus is exposed by creating a retromastoid groove. This is next connected

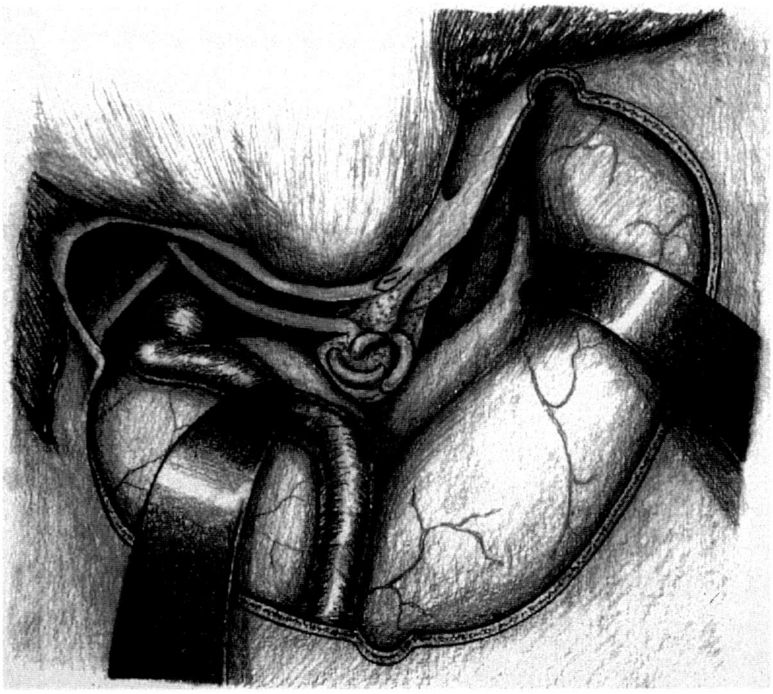

FIG. 29-4. The expansive exposure attained using the combined petrosal approach. For basilar trunk or clival lesions, this approach gives an unequaled view and working space with excellent exposure of the vasculature of the brainstem.

TABLE 29–6. *Combined petrosal approach—technique*

Cosmetic mastoid flap
Mastoidectomy
Skeletonize—sigmoid sinus to juglar bulb
Skeletonize—bony labyrinth and VII fallopian canal
Elevate middle fossa dura—GSPN, mma, V2, V3
Extradural petrous apex removal
Kawase triangle (enter between V and VII, VIII)
Ant: V ganglion
Post: Cochlea
Lat: Sphenopetrosal groove
Inf: IAC and ICA
Intradural dissection

IAC, internal auditory canal; GSPN, greater superficial petrosal nerve.

inferiorly as an L-shaped groove to a suboccipital groove, the latter extended medially to connect with the craniotomy flap previously sawed with the craniotome connecting the burr holes. Great care must be exercised when using the air drills around the sinuses.

The mastoid outer bony surface is removed with an oscillating or sagittal saw as a thin, triangular portion for later replacement as a cosmetic mastoidectomy. After the sigmoid sinus and the suboccipital and posterior subtemporal dura are elevated and protected with extradural self-retaining retractors, a complete mastoidectomy is performed. By removing the mastoid air cells and bone, the middle fossa dura, the sinodural angle, and the presigmoid dura are exposed. Following the skeletonization of the sigmoid sinus to the jugular bulb, the mastoid antrum is identified and extensively opened, revealing the compact bone of the lateral semicircular canal. Next, the bony labyrinth posterior, the superior semicircular canal, and the facial nerve lying within the fallopian canal are found. The exit site of the facial nerve is identified by using the digastric ridge as a landmark, which notes the stylomastoid foramen just medial to the anterior limit of this ridge. To optimize the exposure in the retrolabyrinthine approach, the posterolateral aspect of the bony labyrinth must be exactly defined by drilling the bony canal flat.

The arcuate eminence is found by elevating the posterior subtemporal dura along the petrous ridge. The geniculate ganglion is identified immediately anteromedially from the middle ear cavity (malleus head) and as a continuation of the greater superficial petrosal nerve. The middle fossa rhomboid is formed by the intersection of the trigeminal nerve V3 portion with the greater superficial petrosal nerve (GSPN), the geniculate ganglion, the arcuate eminence-petrous ridge, and the porus trigeminus. The middle meningeal artery is found and divided after careful coagulation. After the foramen ovale is skeletonized peripherally, the rhomboid area is widely drilled away to expose the internal auditory canal, the petrous carotid artery, and the clivus. Additional drilling is carried out inferiorly toward the deeper structures and anteriorly beneath the gasserian ganglion, thus removing the entire petrous apex. With the petrous tip removed, the ascending C5 portion of the carotid artery, the entire extent of the VI nerve, and Dorello's canal are exposed. This then provides the key anatomic opening for this exposure.

The middle and posterior fossae dura are then able to be opened, facilitated by ligation of the superior petrosal sinus near its entrance into the transverse and sigmoid sinuses. The lymphatic sac is closed to prevent leakage of endolymphatic fluid. The petrosal vein may also need to be ligated to facilitate exposure through posterior tentorial retraction.

The tentorium is incised to the incisura, allowing the sigmoid sinus and lateral cerebellar hemisphere to be retracted posteriorly. The inferior dura is opened minimally, protection thus being afforded for both the vein of Labbé and the temporal lobe. The arachnoid is next opened leading into the basal cisterns and providing a great view of the basilar artery trunk, the VBJ, and cranial nerves V through X, through a wide lateral and extensive rostral-caudal exposure (Fig. 29-4). The disadvantages of this approach are the prolonged operative time, the necessity of ipsilateral hearing sacrifice, and difficult watertight dural closure, which usually necessitates a dural graft.

Ultimately, this exposure gives a superior ability for vascular control of the basilar artery, with both proximal and distal basilar access. The lateral-to-medial and superior-to-inferior exposure is outstanding, resulting in an expansive, and at times, panoramic view of the brainstem and associated ventral structures. There is a resultant reduced need for brain retraction and no ligation of the sinus. At present, this exposure, which was an evolutionary concept with major contributions by Drake, Malis, Fukushima, and others, represents perhaps the most dramatic visualization of the basal cerebral anatomy (8,9,11,13,14).

SUBOCCIPITAL APPROACHES

Various surgical exposures have been developed throughout the history of neurosurgical practice to provide access to the inferior portion of the posterior cranial fossa. The basic suboccipital approach has been used for many years to gain entry into the lateral and midline structures of the posterior fossa, particularly the cerebellum and cerebellopontine angle. However, the suboccipital exposure was inadequate for access to most of the vascular lesions situated ventral to the medulla and at the craniovertebral junction. The far-lateral suboccipital approach requires the removal of bone lateral to the foramen magnum, signifying that the further lateral the bony opening is extended, the more inferior to superior visualization is afforded, especially underneath the brainstem (15). The vertebral artery, posterior inferior cerebellar artery, and VBJ are all accessible by such exposure, and it is reliable for non–giant lesions and especially those localized laterally.

The extreme-lateral inferior transtubercular exposure (ELITE) has been a further modification of the far-lateral suboccipital approach, extending it such that a superior view is obtained for selected extensive lesions or when more rostral exposure is desired (11). The patient is positioned in the lateral decubitus posture with placement of a lateral retromastoid incision carried down to the C-3 level. A lateral suboccipital craniotomy through the foramen magnum with a partial mastoidectomy are performed to expose the lower portion of the sigmoid sinus and jugular bulb. The exposure is then completed by removing the anterolateral rim of the foramen magnum including the posterior and medial third of the occipital condyle. Using the high-speed drill, the skull base is removed to expose the hypoglossal canal. The key element in this procedure is to next drill the bone down to and including the jugular tubercle, often at a depth of 2 cm from the foramen magnum, including the bone between the hypoglossal canal and the jugular bulb.

The dural opening is extended laterally to the inferior aspect of the sigmoid sinus. Subarachnoid dissection liberates the intracranial structures into view and allows a caudal-rostral visualization along the course of the intracranial vertebral artery up to the VBJ. Vascular and neoplastic lesions alike are readily approached using ELITE or a lesser modification in selected cases. It represents the high evolution of the original standard suboccipital exposures and provides outstanding visualization without brainstem retraction (Fig. 29-5). The lower cranial nerves are negotiated in this approach, and their attendant postoperative dysfunction remain the greatest concern with utilization of this method.

The concepts of skull base surgery exemplify the evolution of thought and experience of intracranial surgery, and attest to the brilliance and determination with which many surgeons have dealt with the most difficult of vascular and neoplastic lesions of the human body's most inaccessible location. The preferred operative approaches in current use attempt to employ several current tenets of microsurgical planning and technique. These have been discussed by many

A

B

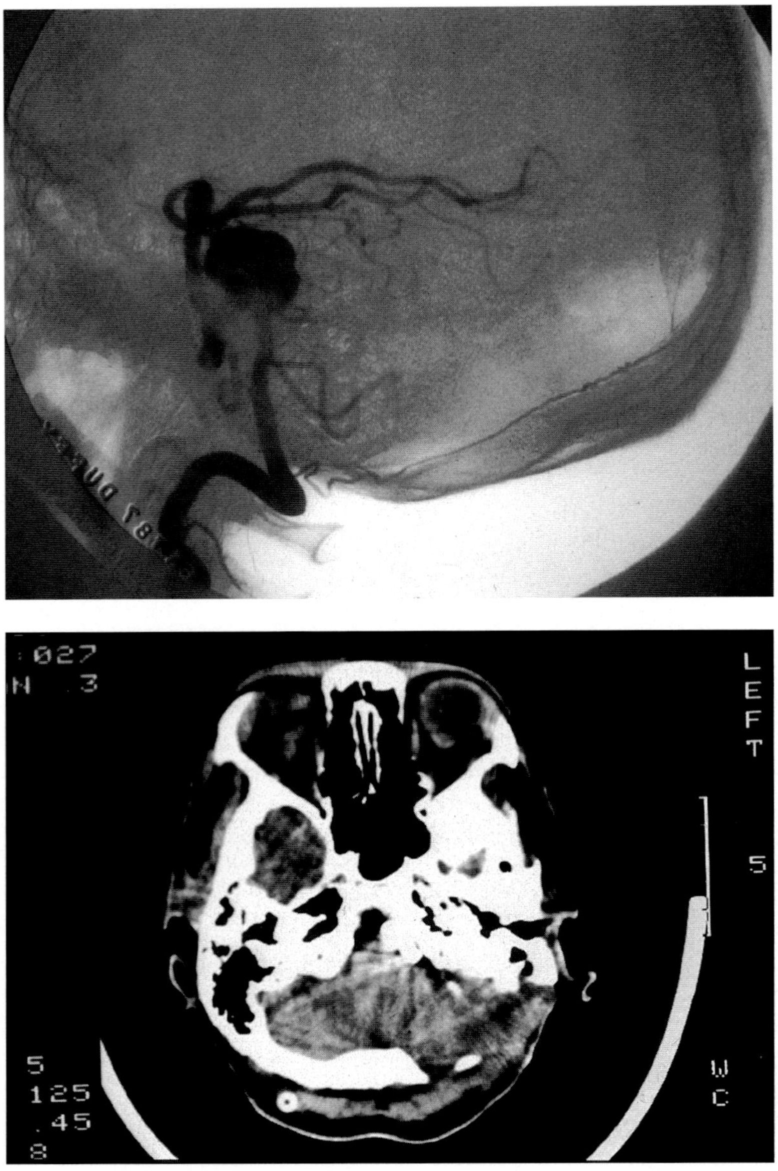

FIG. 29-5. A: The extreme-lateral inferior transcondylar exposure (ELITE) offers the best inferior to superior view of the ventral brainstem. It is ideally suited for approaching distal vertebral artery and vertebrobasilar junction aneurysms or for brainstem lesions. Here a giant basilar trunk aneurysm under the medulla is readily accessed using ELITE. **B:** Postoperative computed tomography scan showing the extent of suboccipital bone removal, including the lateral margin of the foramen magnum and jugular tubercle with the ELITE technique. Note the completely flat plane, allowing this aneurysm to be successfully clipped, with no bony obstacle within the line of sight to the ventral brainstem.

TABLE 29–7. *Principles of cranial base surgery*

Shortest trajectory to lesion
Bone removal in lieu of brainstem retraction
Maximize extradural exposure
CN preservation
Skeletonize, decompression, mobilization of CNs, vessels
Reconstruction of dural openings
Reconstruction of cranium

CN, cranial nerve.

and well summarized by Giannotta and Maceri (10) and others, explaining the basic objectives of achieving exposure to spare brain retraction and injury (Table 29-7). This anatomic exposure is gained at the expense of bony removal. These principles also include taking the shortest and most direct trajectory to the pathology, and maximizing the extradural exposure, in order to better protect the intradural contents, increase atraumatic technique, and open operative corridors. The cranial nerves and vascular structures are thus skeletonized to the greatest extent possible, providing decompression and visualization. Finally, careful reconstruction of all dural openings is necessary to restore CSF pathways and prevent fistula formation (11).

Posterior Fossa Dural Arteriovenous Fistula

Dural arteriovenous fistulas (AVFs) compose approximately 10% to 15% of all intracranial AVMs. These lesions consist of direct arteriovenous shunting, which occurs within the dural leaflets of venous sinuses. Cranial dural AVFs can be acquired (e.g., posttraumatic or postsurgical), idiopathic, or, in very rare cases, congenital. The acquired type of dural AVF has dural sinus thrombosis or venous thrombosis as an etiology. It is believed that with obstruction or thrombosis of a dural sinus, the venous channels that normally drain into the sinus develop thrombosis at the dural sinus point of entry. These venous channels establish alternative drainage pathways, either into the opposite sinus in cases involving the transverse or sigmoid sinuses, or retrograde into cortical leptomeningeal veins. Also, the thrombus in the sinus undergoes organization and vascularization through the hyperactivity of the angiogenic system triggered by the thrombosis, causing various arterial feeders to be recruited. The arterial supply of dural AVFs is usually derived from the dural contribution from the branches of the external carotid artery, such as the occipital artery, ascending pharyngeal artery, middle meningeal artery, and other meningeal arteries. Recruitment of branches of the internal carotid artery may also occur. Arterial supply from deep branches of the internal carotid artery is common with recurrent dural AVFs. Additionally, dural AVFs often recruit branches from contralateral arteries. The nidus of a dural AVF is located within the leaflets of the dura mater, thus distinguishing it from a cortical AVM. The majority of AVFs are located at the transverse and sigmoid sinuses; they may also involve the tentorial incisura (16).

For surgery, the patient with a dural AVF involving the transverse and sigmoid sinus is positioned in the lateral decubitus or three-quarter prone position. The head is positioned so that the neck is moderately flexed and rotated slightly toward the operating room floor with the vertex tilted slightly downward. To decrease the air emboli risk, the ear and mastoid process should be no higher than the level of the heart. A curvilinear incision is made that begins just anterior to the tragus of the ear at the level of the root of the zygoma, coursing superiorly anteriorly behind the hairline for approximately 45 mm. This incision is then made to curve posteriorly along the temporal squama until approximately 30 mm behind the tip of the ear, where it curves inferiorly and anteriorly to parallel the mastoid process. The scalp is incised down to the periosteum, which is incised with monopolar electrocautery. Once the scalp is retracted to expose the mastoid process, care is taken not to compromise the integrity of the external auditory canal. The bone can be very vascular, resulting in the potential for heavy blood loss during the bony opening. Having blood ready for transfusion at the beginning of the craniotomy is a useful precautionary measure. Monopolar electrocautery and bone wax can be utilized to control bleeding from the scalp and bone.

The craniotomy for AVF is made with a high-speed drill and rough diamond-tipped burr. A diamond-tipped burr is used without irrigation to prevent significant bleeding from the bone, as well as bone wax is applied. Care should be taken so as not to injure the nearby dural venous sinus and to expeditiously limit the bleeding that will occur from the bone. Usually four burr holes are used: at the junction of the inferior nuchal line and the mastoid process, at the supramastoid crest, 2 cm lateral to the inion and above the transverse sinus near the asterion, and in the superior temporal line. The digastric groove is drilled with the rough diamond-tipped burr, exposing the sigmoid sinus medial aspect. Using progressively smaller burrs, the burr holes are connected to produce an L-shaped bone flap. Finally the craniotomy is performed using diamond burrs instead of a craniotome to prevent inadvertent injury to the dural sinus, which could result in catastrophic hemorrhage. The edge of the craniotomy should be thoroughly waxed with bone wax.

There is often considerable bleeding from the dura once the bone flap is elevated. This bleeding can be controlled by placing thrombin-soaked Gelfoam on the dura and covering it with a large sponge. Bleeding vessels from the dura can then be slowly and individually meticulously coagulated. Once dural hemostasis is obtained, a cosmetic mastoidectomy is performed by removal of the outer cortical layer of the bone of the mastoid process with an oscillating saw. This is done to prevent a bony defect from the mastoidectomy due to the scalp sinking in with time, by replacing the cortical bone with titanium microplates at the operative closure. This mastoidectomy is completed with a high-speed drill and diamond-tipped burr. The sigmoid sinus is skeletonized by drilling out the bone over the sigmoid sinus until only a thin shell of bone remains. The mastoid antrum and the lateral semicircular canal are carefully exposed using the high-speed drill.

The dural venous sinus and the nidus of the dural AVF, which is within the dural leaflets, is then skeletonized. This is accomplished by making incisions above and below the transverse sinus and by placing cottonoid patties on the superior and inferior aspects of the tentorium. The transverse sinus is then ligated using a right-angled clamp on the distal transverse sinus. Gentle traction is applied to expose the tentorium. The tentorium is incised and any arterial feeding vessels are coagulated or occluded with vascular clips. The transverse sinus is incised and any arterial feeding vessels are likewise closed. The transverse sinus is skeletonized to the location of the thrombus, which fortunately is usually proximal to the vein of Labbé. The sinus is clamped distal to the thrombus and proximal to the vein of Labbé. The involved dural leaflet and dural sinus are then resected. The distal and proximal ends of the sinus are then sutured closed. In situations in which the vein of Labbé is thrombosed or is part of the retrograde leptomeningeal drainage of the dural AVF, the sinus can be ligated distal to the vein of Labbé and the vein of Labbé can be ligated, since there is no anterograde venous drainage of the temporal lobe by the latter.

SURGICAL ADJUNCTS

The development of special techniques in neurologic surgery has vastly improved our ability to treat vascular lesions, especially those of the cerebellum and brainstem. Many intraoperative methods now exist that enable us to more clearly approach and define the selected area of pathologic involvement. Principal among these is ability to choose the approach pathway and localization provided by image-guided stereotactic systems. This technology has rapidly advanced our ability to track safely and enter a region of the brain that may otherwise be fraught with anatomic and physiologic difficulties. A primary example is the brainstem region, in particular for brainstem AVMs. Whether a true AVM or angiographically occult AVM, such as a cavernous malformation, visualization of the lesion on the brainstem surface is often not possible, and exploration without accurate localization or image guidance is ill-advised. Several types of stereotactic guidance systems are available, whether computed tomography or MRI based, with the latter being the most accurate and most often used. New systems employ frameless methodology and allow very accurate precision for virtually every intracranial location. The most common usage involves localization for brainstem, pontine, or medullary AVMs, which have no surface expression but require resection due to prior hemorrhagic episodes or because of progressive neurologic deficits secondary to mass effect.

Intraoperative angiography has become a vital adjunct to cerebrovascular surgery in many instances, especially in cases where it is necessary to discern the exact anatomic detail to allow determination of the preservation of normal vascular structures (17). Several techniques have been utilized to allow the surgeon to determine the degree of obliteration of vascular lesions, which in the case of aneurysms, AVMs, and cavernous malformations must be totally resected in order to effect a cure (18). Intracranial aneurysms represent the most common lesion that must be dealt with, and are obliterated by aneurysm clip application. In accomplishing this task, two errors are commonly made: (a) leaving a remnant of the aneurysm, usually a portion of the aneurysm origin or neck, termed an aneurysm rest; (b) causing branch vessel or parent artery occlusion or compromise, which is often neurologically devastating. This usually leads to subsequent cerebral ischemia and infarction (Fig. 29-6).

The consequences of improper aneurysm clip placement can be severe and often are unpredictable. Using visual inspection alone of the operative field for evaluation of aneurysm obliteration and parent vessel patency has not proven to be effective in many cases. Recent efforts to ensure the patency of arteries have included the use of intraoperative angiography and electrophysiologic monitoring. The former has gained popularity at many large centers because of its relatively rapid evaluation of clip placement and its ability to guide appropriate changes in clip application. We have used a new, 1 mm diameter, 20 MHz, Doppler microprobe for direct intraoperative arterial flow assessment, finding it advantageous over intraoperative angiography. In our expe-

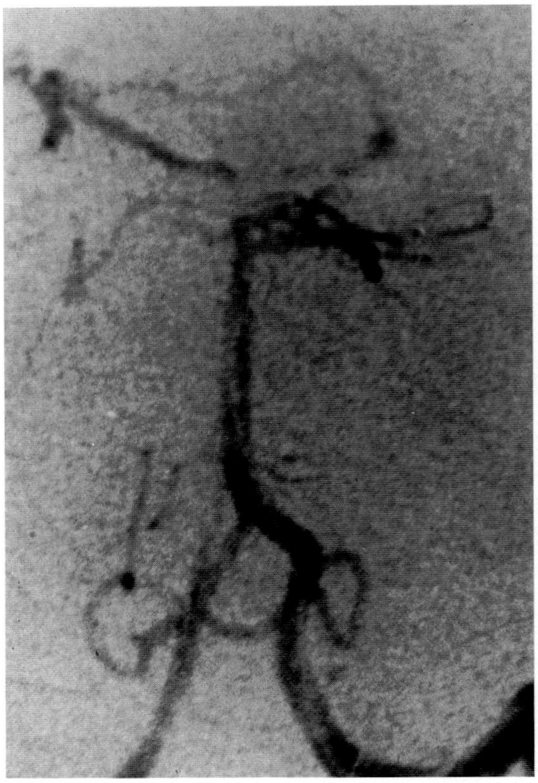

FIG. 29-6. Intraoperative anteroposterior projection angiogram initially demonstrated that this basilar artery apex aneurysm was incompletely obliterated, allowing the surgeon to reposition the clip for optimal occlusion.

rience of over 75 patients, intraoperative microvascular Doppler sonography was successfully used to guide clip placement in the treatment of cerebral aneurysms. Our reported series was the first to use a 1-mm microvascular Doppler probe, allowing insonation of all vessels in the operative field, including perforators. There was a 100% correlation of sonographic findings and intraoperative or postoperative angiographic findings, and there was no incidence of parent vessel occlusion or stenosis (19).

Although the resolution of intraoperative angiography does not allow for the evaluation of small perforating arteries such as thalamoperforators or the recurrent artery of Heubner, the microvascular Doppler probe is capable of reliably insonating perforating arteries in most cases. Complex vascular anatomy is better evaluated with Doppler sonography than with angiography, because of the tendency for vessels to be obscured by clip artifacts in areas where multiple clips are placed or where there is complex branching of vessels, such as is experienced in patients with aneurysms in close proximity to the middle cerebral artery trifurcation. Intraoperative microvascular Doppler sonography can be utilized during the dissection of aneurysms and related vessels and does not significantly add to the length of the operation. Evaluation of the vessels and aneurysm before and after clipping can be completed within 5 minutes in all cases. In fact, clip application is evaluated immediately, and any appropriate modifications to clip placement are made instantly. This compares favorably with the 30 minutes to 1 hour required for angiography. We found that the use of microvascular Doppler sonography has greatly reduced the length of the operation, compared with the use of intraoperative angiography, and there have been no risks of emboli, dissection, femoral artery occlusions, or contrast allergies as with angiography.

REFERENCES

1. Bailes JE, Spetzler RF, Hadley MN, Baldwin HZ. Management morbidity and mortality of poor-grade aneurysm patients. *J Neurosurg* 1990; 72:559–566.
2. Sisti MB, Stein BM. Arteriovenous malformations of the brain stem. *Neurosurg Clin North Am* 1993;4:497–505.
3. Solomon RA, Stein BM. Management of arteriovenous malformations of the brain stem. *J Neurosurg* 1986;64:857–864.
4. Solomon RA, Stein BM. Management of deep supratentorial and brain stem arteriovenous malformations. In: Barrow DL, ed. *Intracranial vascular malformations.* Park Ridge, IL: AANS, 1990:125–140.
5. Yasargil MG, Antic J, Laciga R. Microsurgical pterional approach to aneurysms of the basilar bifurcation. *Surg Neurol* 1976;6:83–92.
6. Sugita K, Kobayashi S, Shintani A, Mutsuga N. Microneurosurgery for aneurysms of the basilar artery. *J Neurosurg* 1979;51:615–620.
7. Sano K. Temporo-polar approach to aneurysms of the basilar artery at and around the distal bifurcation: technical note. *Neurol Res* 1980;2: 361–367.
8. Day JD, Giannotta SL, Fukushima T. Extradural temporopolar approach to lesions of the upper basilar artery and infrachiasmatic region. *J Neurosurg* 1994;81:230–235.
9. Drake CG. The treatment of aneurysms of the posterior circulation. *Clin Neurosurg* 1979;26:96–144.
10. Giannotta SL, Maceri DR. Retrolabyrinthine transsigmoid approach to basilar trunk and vertebrobasilar artery junction aneurysms: technical note. *J Neurosurg* 1988;69:461–466.
11. Day JD, Fukushima T, Giannotta SL. Cranial base approaches to posterior circulation aneurysms. *J Neurosurg* 1997;87:544–554.
12. Spetzler RF, Daspit CP, Pappas CTE. The combined supra- and infratentorial approach for lesions of the petrous and clival regions: experience with 46 cases. *J Neurosurg* 1992;76:588–599.
13. Drake CG. Surgical removal of arteriovenous malformations from the brain stem and cerebellopontine angle. *J Neurosurg* 1975;43:661–670.
14. Malis LI. Surgical resection of tumors of the skull base. In: Wilkins RH, Regachary SS, eds. *Neurosurgery,* vol 1. New York: McGraw-Hill, 1985:1011–1021.
15. Heros RC. Lateral suboccipital approach for vertebral and vertebrobasilar artery lesions. *J Neurosurg* 1986;64:559–562.
16. Tantuwaya L, Bailes JE. Surgical management of cranial dural arteriovenous fistulas. In: Rengachary SS, Wilkins RH, ed. *Neurosurgical operative atlas,* vol 6. Park Ridge, IL: AANS, 1997:75–83.
17. Barrow DL, Boyer KL, Joseph GJ. Intraoperative angiography in the management of neurovascular disorders. *Neurosurgery* 1992;30: 153–159.
18. Bailes JE, Deeb Z, Wilson JA, Jungreis CA, Horton JA. Intraoperative angiography and temporary balloon occlusion of the basilar artery as an adjunct to surgical clipping: technical note. *Neurosurgery* 1992;30: 949–953.
19. Bailes JE, Tantuwaya LS, Fukushima T, Schurman GW, Davis D. Intraoperative microvascular Doppler sonography in aneurysm surgery. *Neurosurgery* 1997;40:965–972.

Neurosurgical Issues in Otolaryngology: Principles and Practice of Collaboration, edited by Moisés A. Arriaga and J. Diaz Day. Lippincott Williams & Wilkins, Philadelphia © 1999.

CHAPTER 30

Stereotactic Radiosurgery

Felipe C. Albuquerque, Arun P. Amar, Cheng Yu, Zbigniew Petrovich, and Michael L. J. Apuzzo

The role of stereotactic radiosurgery in the treatment of skull base and intracranial lesions continues to evolve. As an alternative to open microsurgical techniques, radiosurgery offers several advantages (1,2). Technologic improvements in the last decade have revolutionized the field and increased its applicability to a number of disease states that once were addressed only through a surgical approach (1,2). The future will undoubtedly witness an even broader utility of this relatively nascent therapeutic modality.

Specific advantages of stereotactic radiosurgery over microsurgery include a lower rate of morbidity and virtually no risk of mortality. These benefits have allowed treatment of inoperable lesions and extended therapy to elderly and medically unfit patients who were once considered poor operative candidates (1,2). Technologic advances such as the switch from computed tomography (CT) planning methods to magnetic resonance imaging (MRI)-based modalities, the use of smaller irradiation beam diameters, and the implementation of rapid dose administration systems have furthered the utility and success of this technique. These improvements and advantages, however, must be viewed with recognition of the fact that the long-term sequelae and results of stereotactic radiosurgery have yet to be documented fully (1,2).

Regarding those intracranial lesions that come to the attention of both the neurosurgeon and otolaryngologist, knowledge of radiosurgical techniques and their applicability in specific clinical scenarios is invaluable when contemplating the optimal treatment plan. Specifically, acoustic neuromas (ANs), head and neck tumors, intracranial metastases, vascular anomalies, skull base meningiomas, perisellar lesions, and neurocompressive syndromes such as tic douloureux are pathologic conditions that are amenable to treatments that include microsurgery, radiosurgery, or a combination of the two. This chapter delineates which patients and what lesions are optimally managed through stereotactic radiosurgery.

ACOUSTIC NEUROMAS

Microsurgical results in the treatment of ANs are the standard against which radiosurgery is judged (3). Comparative series assess these results following the treatment of lesions that are typically less than 3 cm in diameter. A multitude of salient end points in the treatment of AN can be delineated and compared between the treatment modalities. These factors include the success of tumor resection or recession following treatment, the rate of hearing preservation, the percentage of facial nerve deficits, the incidence of injury to the brainstem and associated cranial nerves, the rate of operative complications such as wound infection and cerebrospinal fluid (CSF) leak, and the mortality rate.

The largest series of stereotactic gamma knife irradiation for the treatment of AN document results are comparable to microsurgery on a number of fronts (4–13). Reports from the Karolinska Institute and the University of Pittsburgh assert tumor control rates, after variable periods of follow-up, of approximately 90% (7,9,10). Preservation of hearing to any extent exceeds 70% in the immediate postoperative period, while the rate of useful hearing preservation typically declines with longer follow-up to the range of 30% to 40% (7,9,10). The coexistence of neurofibromatosis is associated with a higher incidence of hearing loss (7,9,10). The likelihood of facial and trigeminal neuropathies has decreased with improvements in technique to the range of 10% to 15% and 5% to 18%, respectively (7,9,10). The rate of facial and trigeminal neuropathies is higher with increasing tumor size and lower when a larger number of isocenters are employed.

Preservation of seventh and eighth nerve function in microsurgical cases varies with the approach employed and the size of the tumor resected (Fig. 30-1). Hearing preservation

F. C. Albuquerque, A. P. Amar, C. Yu, Z. Petrovich, M. L. J. Apuzzo: Department of Neurological Surgery, University of Southern California, Los Angeles, California 90033.

A
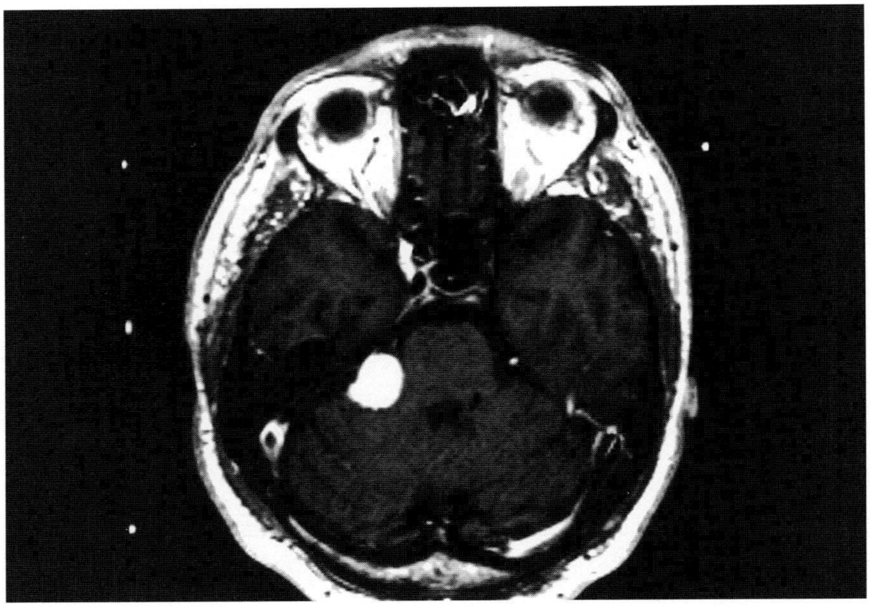

B
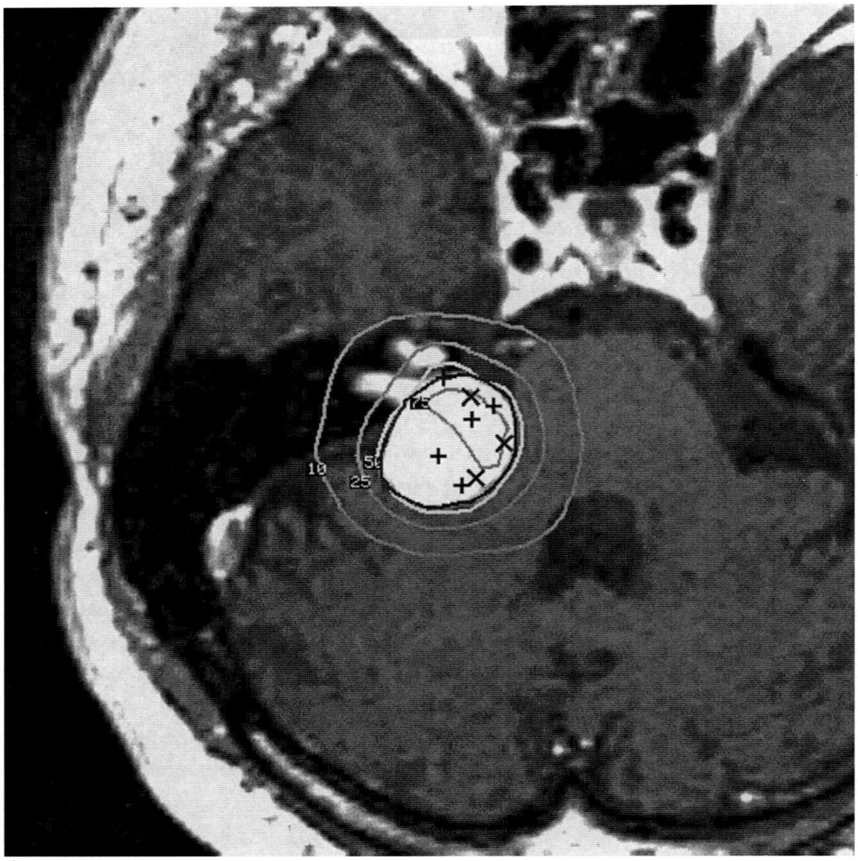

FIG. 30-1. This 59-year-old woman presented with a 1-year history of tinnitus and hearing loss. An axial magnetic resonance imaging (MRI) **(A)** reveals a 2-cm lesion centered at the internal auditory meatus. Treatment planning **(B)** reveals that 75% of the maximum dose is given to the center of the lesion, while 50% is given to the tumor's margin.

surgery through either the suboccipital (retrosigmoid) or the middle fossa approach is typically reserved for those patients with functional preoperative hearing and tumors less than 2.5 cm in diameter (3). In those centers performing the largest number of cases, anatomic preservation of the eighth nerve is effected in 80% to 90% of patients using either of the two approaches (3). Functional or serviceable hearing preservation, however, declines to less than 40% of cases operated upon via the suboccipital approach and from 50% to 60% of cases using the middle fossa approach. Anatomic preservation of the facial nerve typically varies from 80% to 100% but may fall to as low as 20% in patients with tumors greater than 3 cm in diameter. Normal facial function (House-Brackmann grade I), however, typically ranges from 70% to 80%

of patients (3). The middle fossa approach, in which the surgeon encounters the facial nerve early in the dissection, is associated with a higher incidence of seventh nerve injury than either the suboccipital or translabyrinthine approaches (3).

Specific advantages of stereotactic radiation include the fact that patients typically return to work or their preoperative daily routine more rapidly, their hospital stays are shorter and less costly, and patients avoid those complications only attendant to surgery such as CSF leak, wound infection, and perioperative mortality (8,13–15).

Factors typically associated with a higher incidence of cranial nerve injury include a longer expanse of irradiated nerve, increased tumor diameter and volume, higher radiation doses to the margin of the lesion, and use of the 18-mm collimator (6,9,11,12,16–18). Cranial nerves show marked variation in their susceptibility to radiation-induced injury, with the sensory nerves being less tolerant than motor nerves. In the cerebellopontine angle (CPA), the cochlear nerve is the most sensitive to radiation injury followed by the trigeminal nerve and then the facial nerve (6,8,9,11,16–18). This variation in radiosensitivity is possibly related to the type of myelin involved, since sensory nerves carry central rather than peripherally derived myelin. Other factors that mitigate cranial nerve injury include damage to the blood supply of these structures with resulting fibrosis and scarring of the nerves themselves, direct axonal radiation injury, and end-organ damage such as radiation-induced fibrosis and sclerosis of the cochlea (6,16–18). Older age, with its higher likelihood of microvascular disease, and larger tumor volumes compound the deleterious effects (16,17).

The efficacy of stereotactic radiation is assessed as therapeutic if the tumor either regresses in size or fails to grow (4,5,8,9). This result is the product of two types of injury. Direct cytotoxic damage to the cells' reproductive machinery is compounded by injury to the endothelial cells that support the tumor's vasculature. With hyalinization and thickening of the feeding vessels, ischemia generally ensues. Central necrosis follows while fibrosis typically occurs in the periphery. These processes begin as early as 2 weeks after stereotactic treatment and can continue throughout the second postoperative year. Single photon emission computed tomographic (SPECT) studies confirm a progressive decline in tumor vascular supply throughout this 2-year period.

Determining which patients should undergo stereotactic radiosurgery versus those better treated through microsurgery requires an assessment of the patients' preoperative health and an objective analysis of the potential end points of therapy.

Specific indications for stereotactic radiation include tumors smaller than 3 cm, poor preoperative health, recurrent tumor after microsurgery, tumor on the side of the only hearing ear, and bilateral tumors (4,5,8,9). Elderly patients are often preferentially treated with stereotactic radiation, although the obvious benefits of avoiding surgical morbidity must be weighed against a higher likelihood of cranial nerve injury. Tumor location may also favor radiosurgery, as small, intracanalicular tumors are associated with the least amount of radiation delivered to the fifth and seventh cranial nerves. Patients with tumors larger than 3 cm are less likely to have tumor control and more likely to suffer adverse sequelae from radiation. These patients are better served through an open approach. Brainstem compression from the tumor mass is another microsurgical indication. A combined therapy of microsurgery followed by radiosurgery may be employed in cases of subtotal resection (8,9). Stereotactic radiosurgery has been associated with tumor expansion and rupture in cases of large, cystic lesions, rendering microsurgery the best treatment for this subgroup of patients (19).

HEAD AND NECK TUMORS

Head and neck tumors constitute a group of cranial neoplasms that often come to the attention of both the neurosurgeon and otolaryngologist. The incidence of recurrence of these tumors, which typically invade the skull base and insinuate themselves near and around critical neurovascular structures, is high. Uncontrolled local growth produces significant morbidity from pain and cranial neuropathy and increases the likelihood of metastasis (20–26). Fractionated radiotherapy has proven a useful adjunct to surgical resection in the treatment of these neoplasms, although its utility is often limited to a single therapeutic course. In such cases, radiosurgery offers an alternative treatment that confers the advantage of delivering a high radiation boost to the tumor itself while reducing irradiation of surrounding normal tissues (26).

Although series of such patients treated with radiosurgery are small, a practical cohort of these patients includes those who have failed multiple resections and do not wish further aggressive therapy, as well those who are poor operative candidates or with recurrent lesions in proximity to critical structures (20–26). Treatment is typically reserved for those lesions smaller than 3.5 cm in diameter and for those patients who are able to function independently despite recurrence of their neoplasm.

Neoplasms of the head and neck are heterogeneous in their histology, location, and behavior. In the majority of cases, prognosis is tied to the extent of surgical resection (20–26). Tumors of this region include adenocarcinoma, adenoid cystic carcinoma, mucoepidermoid carcinoma, squamous cell carcinoma, chordoma, chondrosarcoma, paraganglioma, glomus jugulare tumor, malignant melanoma, and rhabdomyosarcoma (20–26) (Fig. 30-2). Typical sites of occurrence are the parotid gland, the paranasal sinuses, the tonsils, the alveolar ridge, the external auditory canal, the palatine fossa, the cranial base and its basilar canals, as well as the face (20–26). Invasion and recurrence can progress from the parotid gland to the jugular and hypoglossal canals, from the alveolar ridge to the cavernous sinus and peripon-

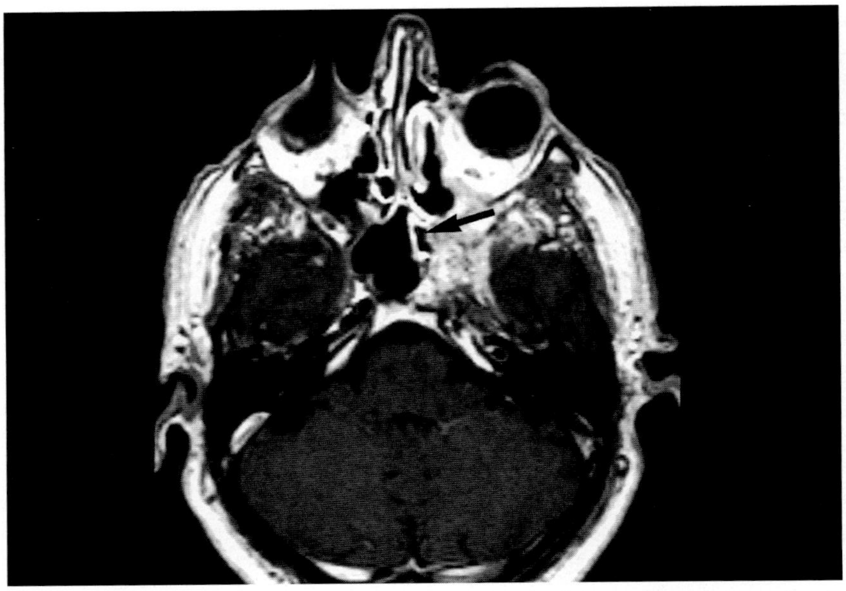

A

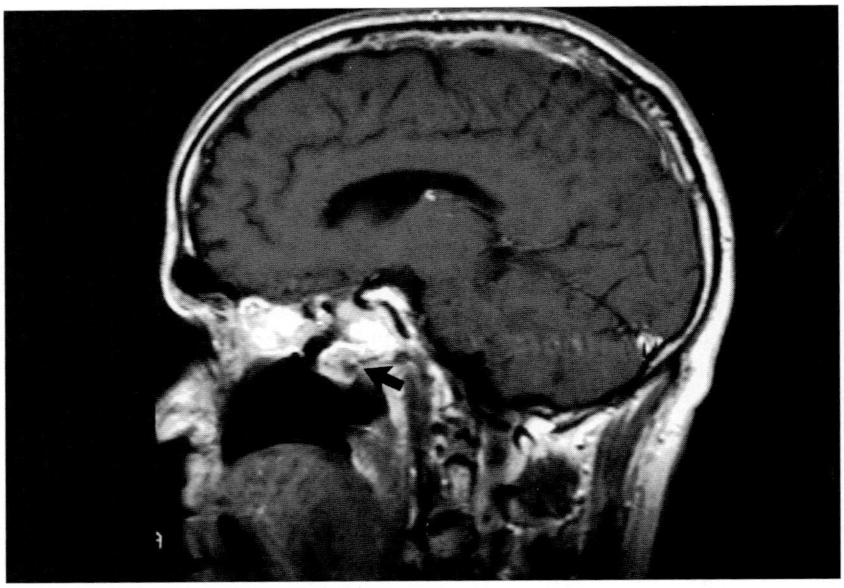

B

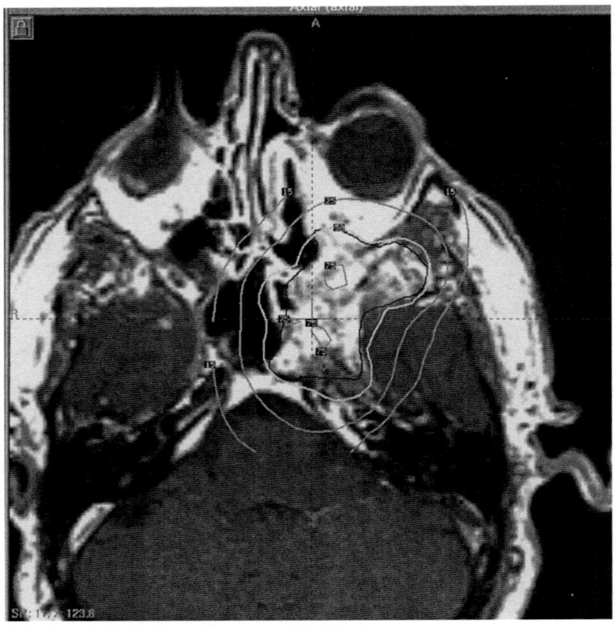

C

FIG. 30-2. This 65-year-old man had undergone endoscopic biopsy and resection of an adenocarcinoma of the ethmoid sinus. He presented 15 months later with recurrence **(A,B)**. Invasion of the sinus cavity is demonstrable on both the axial and sagittal images (*arrows*). Treatment planning **(C)** reveals a steep fall in dosage in the region of the optic nerve.

tine cisterns, from the infraorbital nerve to the cavernous sinus and orbit, from the tonsil to the jugular and hypoglossal canals, and from the maxillary sinus to the nasopharynx, middle cranial fossa, and orbit (20–26).

Because of the heterogeneity of these tumors and their points of origin, a consensus as to the response of each neoplasm to radiosurgery has not been delineated (Fig. 30-3). Results of the largest series document excellent tumor control rates for the majority of lesions, although follow-up is frequently variable in length. Despite control rates of greater than 90%, head and neck tumors are still associated with survival times under 1 year (20–26). This poor prognosis is secondary to the propensity of these tumors to metastasize. Chordomas and chondrosarcomas, which are unlikely to metastasize beyond the cranial base, demonstrate a better survival rate, although follow-up beyond 3 years has yet to be

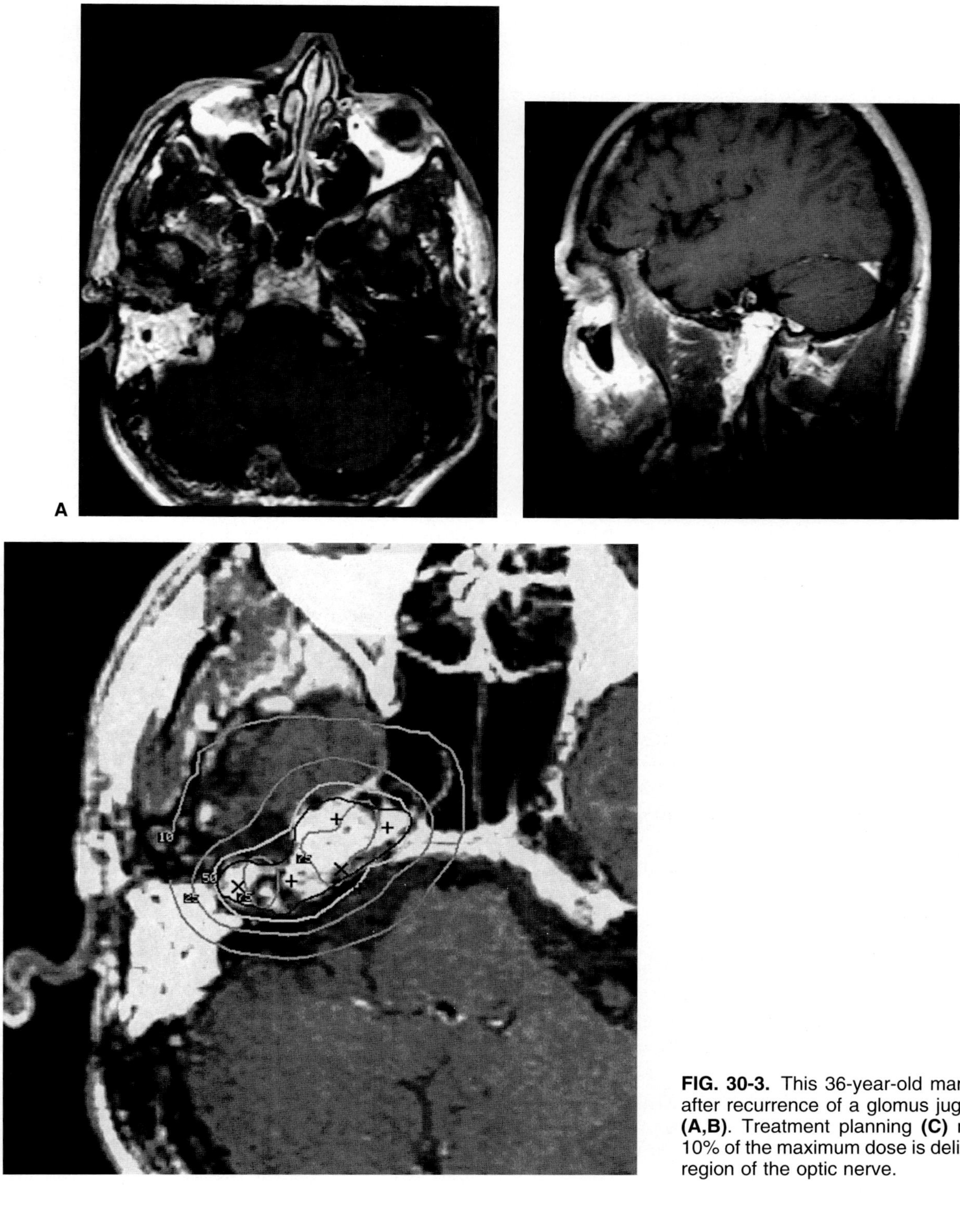

FIG. 30-3. This 36-year-old man presented after recurrence of a glomus jugulare tumor **(A,B)**. Treatment planning **(C)** reveals that 10% of the maximum dose is delivered to the region of the optic nerve.

reported. The arrest of progressive cranial neuropathy and pain occurs in more than 60% of patients following radiosurgery (20–26). This figure, however, must be viewed with caution as relatively few cases have been reported in the literature.

A number of technical adjuncts must be employed in the treatment of head and neck tumors using the gamma knife. Most importantly, the geometry of the collimators prevents treatment of neoplasms occurring below the foramen magnum (20–26). Angulation of the stereotactic frame is limited by the range of cervical flexion or extension, and by the orbits anteriorly. Because the target must remain within the coordinate system, the frame is often positioned anteriorly and inferiorly (20–26). Such is the case in the treatment of lesions originating in the nasopharynx and infratemporal region. Radiographic factors also play a critical role in treatment. Often, both MRI and CT scanning are required in treatment planning. While soft tissues are better visualized with MRI, bony invasion and air-tissue interfaces, such as the nasopharyngeal and mastoid areas, are more easily delineated with CT (20–25). The proximity to cranial nerves and critical neurovascular structures is another consideration in the use of stereotactic radiosurgery to treat head and neck neoplasms. Multiple isocenters and selective beam-blocking patterns are often employed. Finally, in cases of anteriorly located, extracranial lesions, treatment dosage must account for the passage of the posterior beams through two layers of skull (20–26). Recognition of the prior fractionated radiation field and dose also limits the likelihood of injury to vital structures.

Regional complications excluding cranial nerve and neurovascular injuries, which are discussed later in this chapter, include parotiditis, trismus, and delayed intratumoral hemorrhage (20,22–25).

ARTERIOVENOUS MALFORMATIONS

Arteriovenous malformations (AVMs) typically produce symptoms in young patients (less than 40 years of age) and account for nearly 4% of strokes. The combined risk of neurologic deficit and death following hemorrhage is 50%. Microsurgical resection, endovascular embolization, and stereotactic radiosurgery are used separately or in combination as treatments of AVMs. The efficacy of radiosurgery in the management of small AVMs (3-cm diameter) is well documented. Indeed, AVMs represent the most accepted indication for stereotactic radiosurgery.

The literature supports a cure rate of 70% to 95% for small AVMs treated with radiosurgery (27–32). Complete obliteration of the AVM nidus and normalization of the vascular anatomy are regarded as the defining points of AVM cure (29–32). A number of factors are associated with radiosurgical failure (29,32–34). Imprecise delineation of the lesion by two-dimensional stereotactic angiography accounts for a significant percentage of these errors (33). Some practitioners argue that two-dimensional imaging fails to demarcate the complexity of AVM architecture and that this failure is magnified as the size of the AVM increases. Previous embolization may further complicate the marginal structure of the AVM, again decreasing the likelihood of precisely defining the lesion. Studies comparing stereotactic angiography to magnetic resonance angiography (MRA) demonstrate that the former is more likely to accurately define small AVMs (less than 1 cm) but is equivalent or slightly worse than the latter in delineating medium-size and large lesions. These results suggest that the optimal treatment protocol should employ both angiographic and magnetic resonance techniques as the basis of therapeutic planning. Finally, incomplete angiography, specifically failure to perform external carotid injections, can also account for imprecision in AVM definition (33).

Perhaps the most salient complication of radiosurgery in the treatment of AVMs is rupture during the latency period of obliteration (30–32,34–36). Resolution of the nidus and normalization of the angiographic architecture typically evolves over a 2- to 3-year period following treatment (30,31,34,36) (Fig. 30-4). Controversy exists as to whether the risk of AVM rupture during the latency period is lower than the rate defined by the natural history of AVMs (2–4% per year) (31,34,35). While early studies supported a protective effect of radiosurgery during the latency period, more recent analyses have documented equivalence to the natural rate of AVM rupture. Microsurgery offers the advantage of immediate cure if complete resection is achieved. This option may be untenable, however, in cases of deep-seated or eloquently located malformations. Other advantages of radiosurgery include no risk of mortality and a significantly lower risk of acute morbidity than microsurgery. These advantages, however, must be weighed against the possibility of AVM rupture during the latency period after radiosurgery, a risk that apparently does not differ from the lesion's natural history (31–33,35).

A number of technical considerations affect the success of radiosurgery in the treatment of AVMs (27,28,30,31). An AVM nidus may persist if treatment is based on the earliest phase of arterial filling as delineated by angiography. Later-filling components of the lesion may not be irradiated during treatment. Similarly, an incompletely resolved hematoma may compress portions of the nidus, preventing irradiation of the entire lesion. The marginal radiation dose is another factor determining AVM obliteration. A minimum dose of 15 Gy to the periphery of the lesion is required, although reports currently suggest that doses of 22 to 25 Gy are optimal (29,30,32). Higher doses, however, are associated with an increased likelihood of edema surrounding the AVM (27–30,37). This complication typically ensues over a 5- to 18-month period following radiosurgery in up to a third of patients (27,30,37). Symptoms are those of mass effect and typically resolve with corticosteroid therapy.

MENINGIOMAS

Microsurgical resection remains the treatment of choice for meningiomas. Complete excision results in cure and is

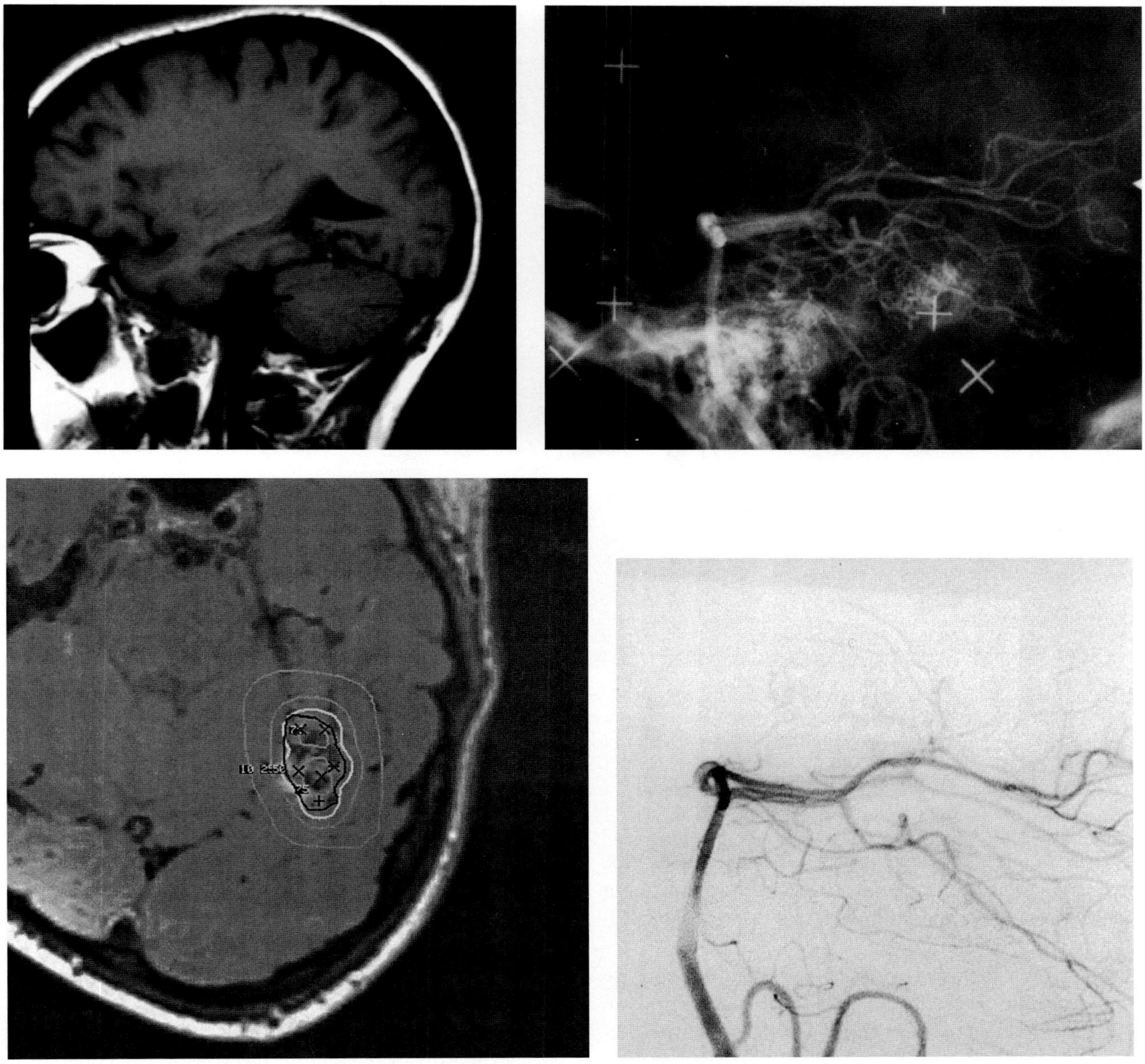

A B C D

FIG. 30-4. Sagittal MRI **(A)** and lateral stereotactic angiography **(B)** demonstrate a 2-cm arteriovenous malformation (AVM) below the region of the left trigone in a 37-year-old woman. Seventy-five percent of the maximum dose is delivered to the AVM nidus **(C)**. Three years later, lateral angiography **(D)** demonstrates resolution of the AVM and normalization of the arterial anatomy.

most easily achieved in lesions located over the convexities. Resection of skull base tumors, however, is more cumbersome. The surgical mortality rate averages from 5% to 9%, while the risk of permanent morbidity ranges from 24% to 43% (38–40). Moreover, the rates of incomplete resection and recurrence are high for this subgroup. Based on these factors, radiosurgery has emerged as a standard adjunct in the treatment of skull base residual and recurrent tumors and as a primary therapeutic modality in patients with risk factors for a poor surgical outcome.

As a group, skull base lesions account for 35% to 50% of all intracranial meningiomas (38–42) (Figs. 30-5 and 30-6). A number of factors determine the likely outcome of surgery. The patient's current health, tumor location and size, and involvement of critical neurovascular structures are perhaps the most important considerations. Sites of occurrence include the CPA, petrous ridge, sphenoid wing, cavernous sinus, and olfactory groove (38–43).

Radiosurgery is typically reserved for small (less than 3.5 cm diameter) residual or recurrent lesions and in those cases in which the patient's overall health dictates a noninvasive therapy (39,40). Tumor control rates are excellent, typically ranging from 85% to 100% (38,40–43). Complications occur in up to 6% of cases and include delayed cranial nerve

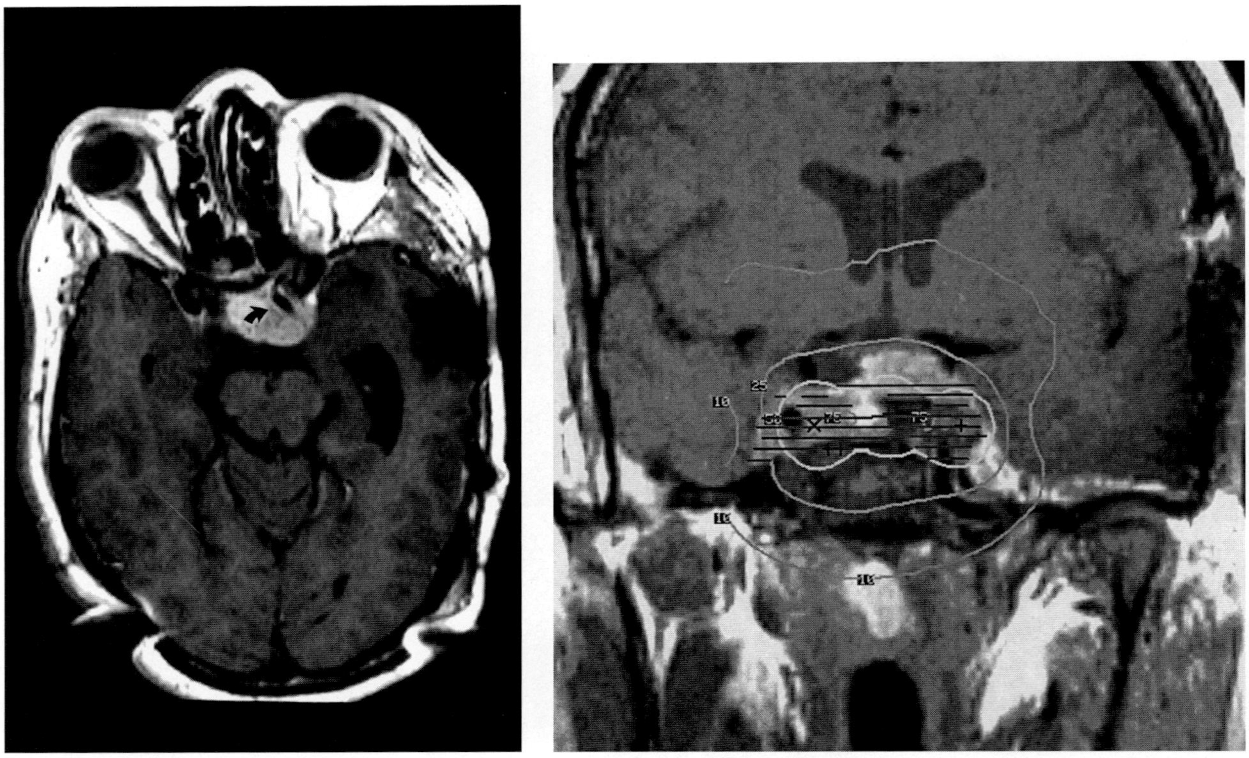

A B

FIG. 30-5. This 39-year-old woman presented with headache. MRI **(A)** reveals a meningioma in the region of the left cavernous sinus. The carotid artery (*arrow*) is encased by tumor, thus increasing the risks of microsurgical resection. Treatment planning **(B)** must account for the optic apparatus and pituitary gland.

injury, cerebral necrosis with secondary neurologic deficits, symptomatic peritumoral edema, and uncontrolled tumor growth. Symptomatic deterioration is an indication for surgical extirpation (38,41–43).

Technical considerations in the treatment of skull base meningiomas must account for the irregular contour of these neoplasms as well as their proximity to vital structures. Lesions smaller than 3.5 cm in diameter and situated at least 5 mm from critical structures are ideal (38–43). Radiosurgery of larger lesions is associated with a significantly higher rate of complications (up to 40%). Because of the irregular architecture of skull base meningiomas, multiple isocenters are often employed. Marginal radiation doses typically vary from 15 to 20 Gy (38–40,42,43). The slow-growing nature of meningiomas allows an adequate period for the vascular and cytotoxic effects of radiation to develop. Finally, the treatment region may be extended to include the dural blood supply of these lesions, thus increasing the likelihood of a tumoricidal effect (38–42).

In summary, radiosurgery is a potent adjunct to microsurgery in the treatment of skull base and convexity meningiomas. The availability of radiosurgical techniques dictates a conservative surgical approach in the management of skull base lesions, which are more likely to involve critical structures and are associated with a high operative risk. The use of radiosurgery as a primary therapy is unusual for convexity meningiomas as these are often curable via surgery. However, in patients with skull base neoplasms and coexistent morbidity, primary radiosurgical therapy is often the only alternative.

TUMORS OF THE ANTERIOR SKULL BASE

Neoplasms of the anterior skull base are unique in their ability to encroach upon neurovascular structures. This tendency accounts for the relatively high morbidity and mortality of microsurgical resection. These complications primarily include injury to cranial nerves and the carotid artery, as well as CSF leak (44,45). Nevertheless, microsurgery remains the primary therapy in most cases because of the proportionally higher morbidity of unchecked tumor growth and mass effect. Endocrinopathies and visual compromise are specific examples attributable to sellar lesions (44,45). Radiosurgery is generally reserved for recurrent and residual tumors, although its use as a primary therapy may be applicable in medically unfit or elderly patients. Those patients with neoplastic involvement of the carotid artery who also fail test occlusion of the vessel are other potential candidates for primary radiosurgical treatment.

Tumors of this region vary in their histology and malignancy. Meningiomas, pituitary adenomas, craniopharyngiomas, and metastases are the most common neoplasms to

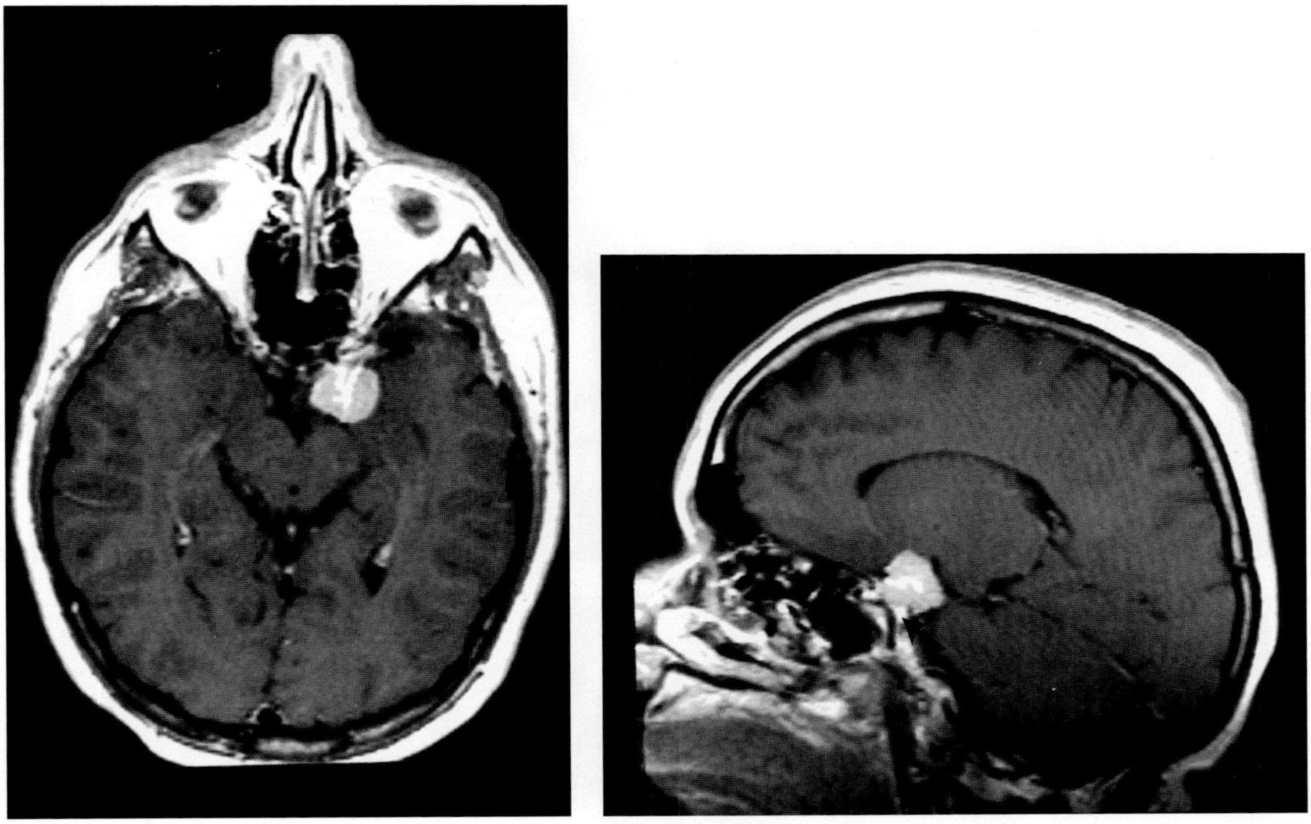

A B

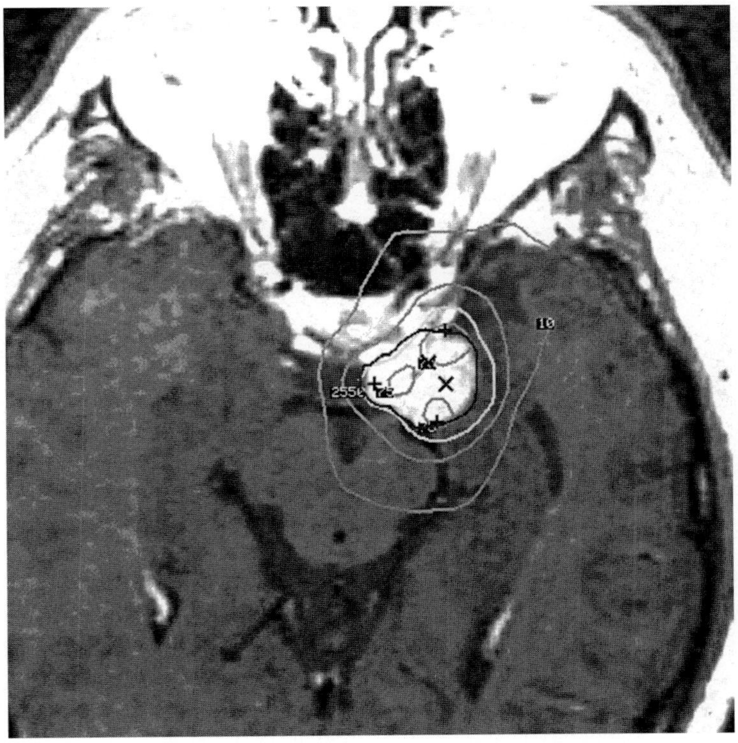

C

FIG. 30-6. This 29-year-old woman demonstrates a left cavernous meningioma on axial **(A)** and sagittal MRI **(B)**. Proximity to the carotid artery (*arrow*) is noted on the sagittal image. Treatment planning **(C)** reveals that the left cerebral peduncle receives only 10% of the maximum radiation dose.

occur in the anterior skull base (44,45). Pituitary tumors may become symptomatic either through the functional production of pituitary hormones or releasing factors, or through the generation of mass effect, which may disrupt the hypothalamic-pituitary axis or compress the optic chiasm and pathways (44,45) (Fig. 30-7). Meningiomas arising from the paraclinoid region, sphenoid wing, cavernous sinus, and olfactory groove may produce similar compromise of the optic

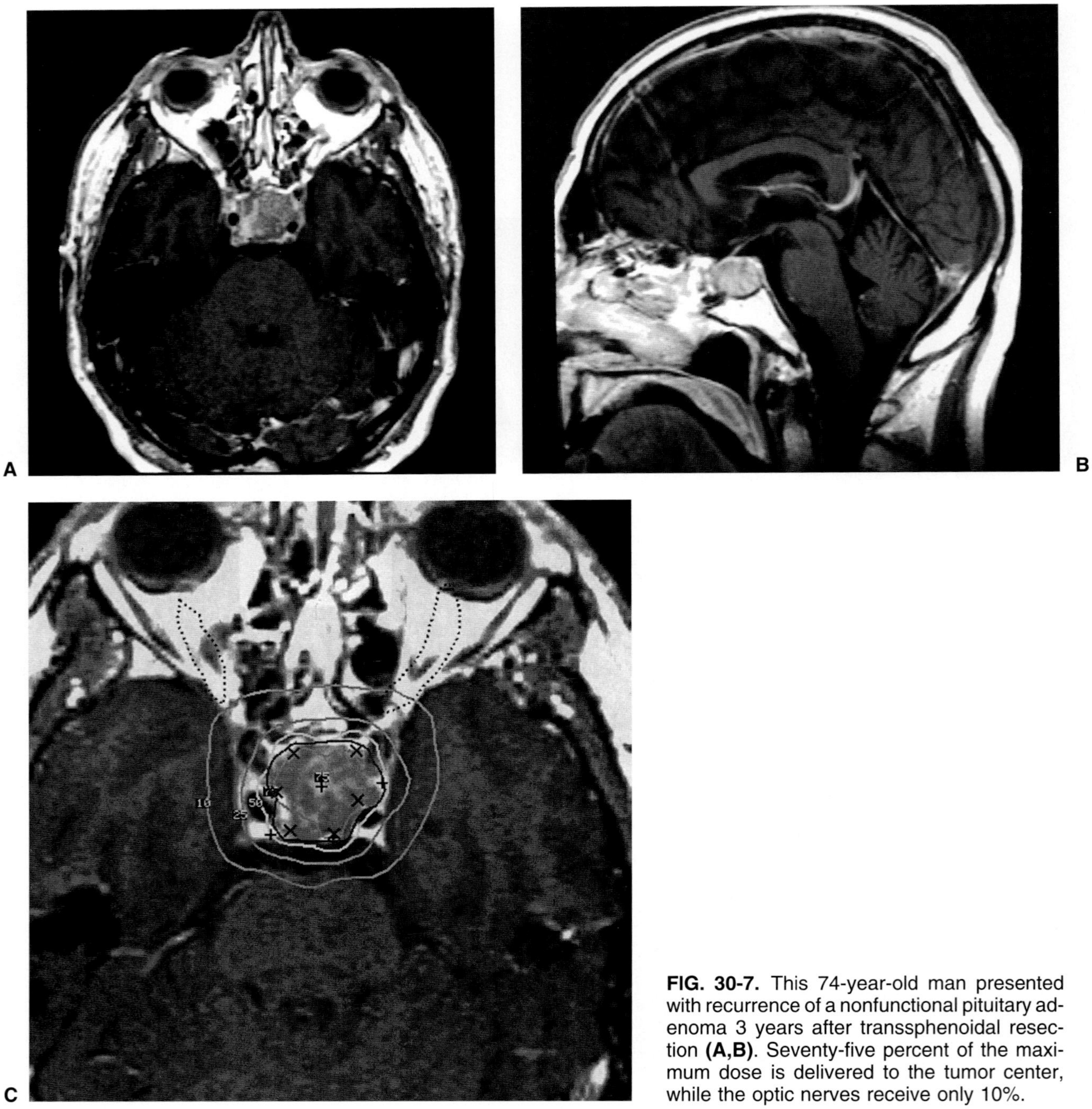

FIG. 30-7. This 74-year-old man presented with recurrence of a nonfunctional pituitary adenoma 3 years after transsphenoidal resection **(A,B)**. Seventy-five percent of the maximum dose is delivered to the tumor center, while the optic nerves receive only 10%.

pathways, as well as cranial neuropathy, carotid stenosis, and disruption of higher cortical function such as that which occurs with large, subfrontal tumors. Craniopharyngiomas produce symptoms through their generation of hypothalamic-pituitary dysfunction, optic pathway compromise, and mass effect. Metastases include a variety of head and neck tumors such as adenoid cystic carcinoma, mucoepidermoid carcinoma, squamous cell carcinoma, and melanoma, as well as spread from renal cell and colon carcinomas (45). Symptoms of these neoplasms are site specific, although they can mimic the behavior of primary tumors in this region.

In light of the significant morbidity of visual pathway compromise and endocrine dysfunction, microsurgery remains the treatment of choice for sellar lesions (44,45). Microsurgical excision allows decompression of vital structures and the potential for rapid reversal of endocrinopathy. Those patients with residual or recurrent tumors of this region are potential candidates for radiosurgery. Pituitary tumor control rates range from 90% to 95% following radiosurgery, while the likelihood of normalization of endocrine status varies according to tumor histology from 60% to 100% (44,45). The effects of tumor volume reduction and endocrine improvement are delayed and, therefore, of little benefit to the acutely ill patient. Meningiomas demonstrate similar response patterns following radiosurgery (45). The likelihood of cranial nerve or vascular injury often relegates these lesions to partial microsurgical resection, with radiosurgery serving as an effective and safe means of controlling residual or recurrent lesions (45). The efficacy of radiosurgery in the control of metastatic disease and head and neck tumors is discussed in other sections of this chapter. The effects of systemic metastases and aggressive primary disease accounts for the relatively poor prognosis of this subset of neoplasms. Craniopharyngiomas are less responsive than pituitary lesions to radiosurgery, although large series with adequate follow-up have yet to be reported (45). Nonetheless, the high attendant morbidity and mortality of aggressive surgical resection of craniopharyngiomas warrants consideration of other treatment options such as stereotactic radiosurgery (45). Tumor control rates of 75% and higher have been reported, although the follow-up periods are too short to derive an accurate estimate of the efficacy of radiosurgical treatment (45).

Technical considerations in the radiosurgical treatment of anterior skull base lesions are critical in the prevention of complications (see below). A minimum distance from lesion to optic apparatus of 5 mm is generally regarded as the gold standard requirement that must be met prior to treatment (43,45). At this minimum distance and with doses to the optic apparatus of no more than 9 Gy, the likelihood of visual compromise is less than 5% (43,45). The likelihood of injury to the motor nerves of the cavernous sinus is even lower, while no documented cases of delayed injury to the carotid artery have been reported (43,45). The use of multiple isocenters and beam-blocking techniques are other means of reducing the potential for morbidity after radiosurgery in this region.

METASTATIC TUMORS

Intracranial metastasis is the most frequent neurologic complication of cancer, affecting nearly 50% of patients and accounting for 13% to 42% of all intracranial tumors (46–49). In addition, metastases are one of the most common causes of death in this patient population. The goals of radiosurgery in such cases include control of intracranial tumor growth, minimization of treatment-related side effects, preservation of an adequate quality of life, and prolongation of survival.

The results of radiosurgery for this diverse group of lesions have steadily improved. Commonly treated tumors include metastases from breast, lung, renal, and thyroid tumors, as well as malignant melanoma (46–49). Tumor histology plays a variable role in treatment success (Fig. 30-8). Breast metastases are associated with a longer survival than tumors of other histology, while melanoma and renal cell lesions demonstrate superior local growth control.

Retrospective studies document a 1-year local control rate of 80% to 90% (46–49). New metastases occur in 5% to 20% of cases (46–49). Mean survival rates typically range from 30 to 50 weeks, while Karnofsky performance scores are improved or stable for the majority of the survival period (46–48). Data are similar for patients with solitary and multiple lesions except for the 2-year survival rate, which falls to less than 10% in the latter group. Progression of the primary neoplastic disease is the most common cause of death in this population, occurring in more than 60% of cases (46–49). With improved survival after radiosurgery, the likelihood of progression of the primary disease increases. This finding supports aggressive management of the patient's underlying disease both prior to and after stereotactic radiosurgery of the metastatic lesion.

Radiation-induced, peritumoral edema is the most frequent complication of radiosurgery for metastases (27,46–49). Pharmacologic therapy generally suffices to resolve those neurologic deficits produced by peritumoral edema. Surgical extirpation of the offending lesion may be required in rare cases in which edema produces intractable symptoms. Permanent deficits from radiation injury are typically delayed and occur in a small minority of patients (<5%) (46–48). Intra- or peritumoral hemorrhage may complicate the treatment of melanomas, renal cell tumors, and thyroid metastases, all of which show a proclivity for bleeding even without stereotactic irradiation. The sequelae of such hemorrhages include death and permanent neurologic deficit.

TRIGEMINAL NEURALGIA

Stereotactic radiosurgery is an effective treatment for medically or surgically refractory trigeminal neuralgia (50–52). Primary radiosurgical therapy may be appropriate for elderly patients, as well as those with concomitant medical problems. Patients taking anticoagulant medication are also potential candidates for primary treatment. Radiosurgery effects good to excellent pain control in 80% to 94% of patients, with the remainder suffering therapeutic failures (50–52). The latency until pain relief ranges from 1 to 8 weeks. Symptomatic improvement is durable in the majority of patients. Those with severe pain associated with eating and drinking may not tolerate a delay in symptom relief, and therefore are best managed through a medical or surgical regimen (50–52).

A number of technical considerations guide the use of radiosurgery in the treatment of trigeminal neuralgia. The root entry zone is the preferred target because of its sensitivity to radiation and its ease of identification by MRI (50–52). Doses of 70 to 90 Gy are typically delivered to a single 4-mm isocenter at this site (50–52). The heightened sensitivity to radiation at the root entry zone is likely the result of its pattern of myelination. Oligodendrocytes, which are more prone to radiation-induced injury, myelinate this region, while Schwann cells myelinate the gasserian ganglian and distal nerve branches.

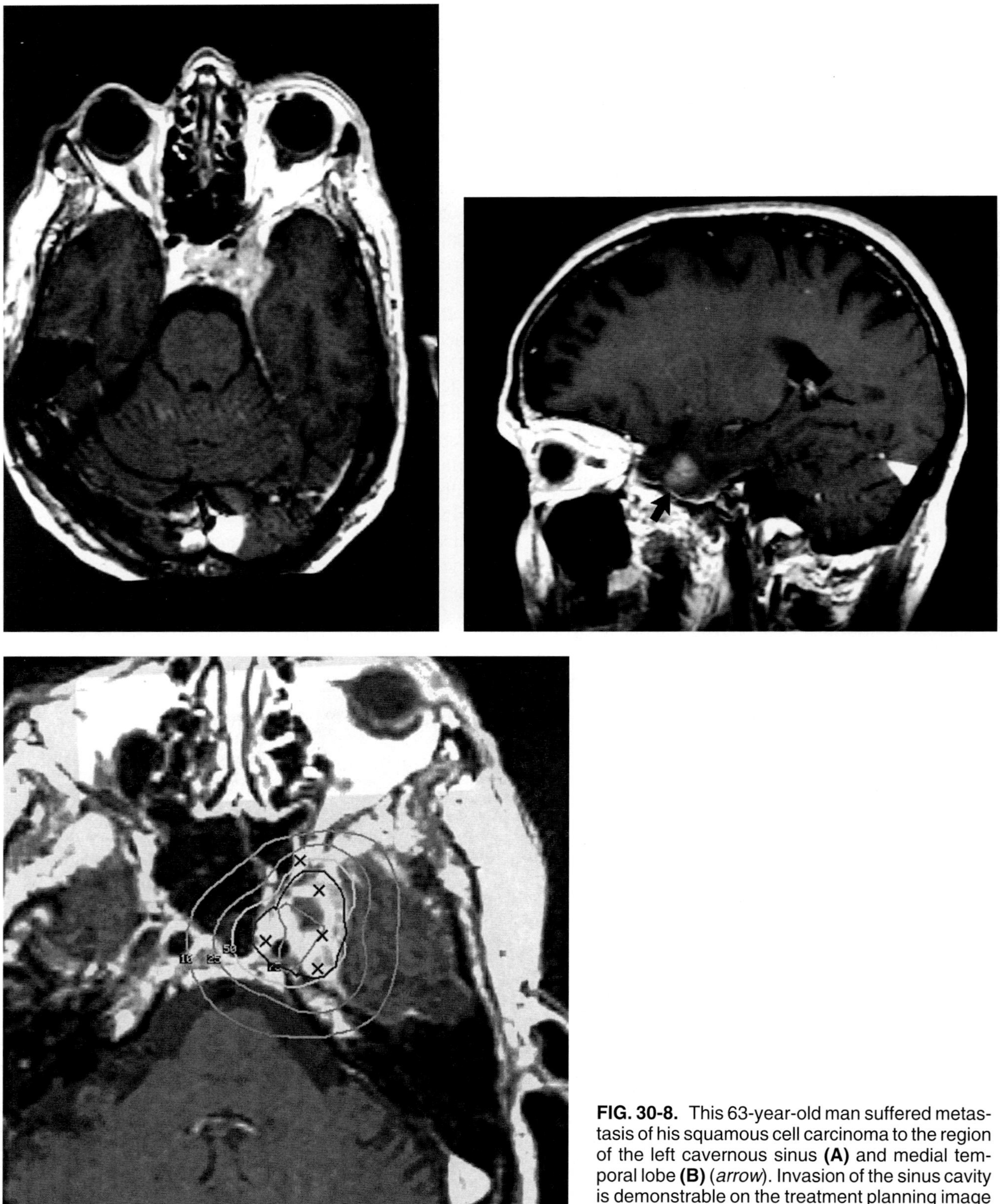

FIG. 30-8. This 63-year-old man suffered metastasis of his squamous cell carcinoma to the region of the left cavernous sinus **(A)** and medial temporal lobe **(B)** (*arrow*). Invasion of the sinus cavity is demonstrable on the treatment planning image **(C)**.

RADIATION-INDUCED COMPLICATIONS OF RADIOSURGERY

Despite the frequency of its application, the complications attendant to conventional external beam irradiation and to stereotactic interstitial brachytherapy have only rarely been reported following gamma radiosurgery (53). This fact may result from methodologic constraints in detecting such complications rather than from the special protection that gamma radiosurgery confers against iatrogenic insults when compared with other forms of radiotherapy. For instance, biopsies and autopsies are not commonly performed after gamma knife treatment, making neuropathologic confirmation of the complications problematic. The latency for developing these complications often exceeds the life expectancy of patients harboring the types of lesions currently treated by radiosurgery. Finally, it is often difficult to verify that the pathologic changes reflect complications of the radiation treatment, rather than the natural history of the disease process itself.

In addition to the dose, dose rate, and treatment volume, the risks of radiation-induced brain injury following radiosurgery are dependent on the location of the target and the nature of the pathologic condition being treated (54–56). Radiation necrosis of adjacent brain has been reported following gamma radiosurgery of numerous intraaxial targets, including AVMs, metastatic tumors, gliomas, and thalamic nuclei for intractable pain (57–63). In each of these conditions, the risk of significant brain necrosis is typically in the range 2% to 5%. By contrast, large series have suggested that more than 40% of patients undergoing interstitial brachytherapy have required further surgery to manage radiation-induced edema and necrosis (64).

The risk of brain necrosis following gamma radiosurgery of skull base lesions is expected to be even lower, since many of these conditions remain extraaxial and can be targeted with sufficient precision to minimize the radiation dose to surrounding neural tissue. The combination of multiple isocenters with various beam diameters (using different collimator sizes) and selective plug patterns should permit isodose configurations that deliver conformal radiotherapy to irregularly shaped tumor volumes while sparing the adjacent brainstem (65–69). Thus, while many series of radiosurgical treatment of acoustic neuromas have reported injury to the fifth, seventh, and eighth cranial nerves, accounts of persistent brainstem injury are sparse (66,68,70). Approximately 5% to 9% of such patients may develop edema of the cerebellum, brainstem, or middle cerebral peduncle 6 to 12 months after treatment, but this reaction is almost always transient and only rarely causes disturbing vertigo or ataxia (68,69,71,72). Although brainstem edema following radiosurgery is frequently asymptomatic, Kondziolka et al. (68,73) observed temporary neurologic symptoms (trigeminal hypesthesia and contralateral hemiparesis) in one patient with a petrous apex meningioma who developed edema in the adjacent pons. This process is characterized by increased signal intensity on T2-weighted MRI and by gadolinium-enhancement from blood–brain barrier disruption in the peritumoral region on T1-weighted scans (68,69). The possible causes of edema or blood–brain barrier breakdown after radiosurgery include demyelination, axonal swelling, and disruption of vascular endothelial integrity, which have been reported to occur in a delayed fashion after fractionated radiotherapy (68,73). Because these MRI signal changes resolve over time, however, they are not likely to represent true radiation necrosis (68).

Morikawa et al. (57) reported a patient with probable radiation necrosis of the pons developing 26 months after gamma knife treatment of a CPA AVM. The radiation dose prescribed to that region of the pons was not specified. The necrosis was recognized as a persistent, ring-enhancing area encircling the site of the previous nidus (57). Thallium 201 SPECT has also been reported to be an accurate test to detect radiation necrosis after gamma knife radiosurgery (62).

Acutely, up to 10% to 20% of patients undergoing gamma knife treatment of acoustic neuromas or cavernous sinus meningiomas may experience nausea and vomiting lasting less than a day (54,65). The risk of this reaction appears to be related to incidental irradiation of the area postrema in the medulla and may be mitigated by premedication with corticosteroids (54).

For radiosurgery of sellar, suprasellar, and parasellar tumors, radiation injury to the hypothalamus, pituitary gland, and optic pathways are probably more salient considerations than effects on the brainstem. Thus, following gamma knife treatment of pituitary adenomas, hypopituitarism may develop in 10% to 50% of patients, while neuronal complications such as temporal lobe injury or brain necrosis occur in less than 1% of cases (54,74).

The cranial nerves at the skull base show marked variation in their susceptibility to radiation-induced injury, with the sensory nerves being less tolerant than motor nerves. It is postulated that this variation in radiosensitivity is related to the type of myelin involved, since sensory nerves carry central rather than peripherally derived myelin (68). The optic nerve and chiasm appear to be the most radiosensitive (68), and it is recommended that the radiation dose to the optic pathways not exceed 9 Gy, although doses as high as 15 Gy have been tolerated in some cases (75). A 5-mm margin between the tumor and optic apparatus has been proposed as a selection criterion among patients being considered for radiosurgical treatment (65,68).

After the optic nerve, the cochlear nerve and the trigeminal nerve appear to be the most radiosensitive (68). Thus, following gamma knife treatment of acoustic neuromas, the actuarial risk of clinically significant auditory neuropathy is approximately 66%, while that of trigeminal neuropathy is 33% (66,68). In contrast, the purely motor nerves of the cavernous sinus have sustained doses as high as 40 Gy with impunity (71). For instance, in Duma et al.'s (65) series of 34 patients with cavernous sinus meningiomas, no patient developed a new extraocular muscle paresis, and the incidence of delayed cranial nerve complications was only 6%. In addition to the nature of the cranial nerve and the dose it receives, the length of nerve irradiated is an important determinant of the risk for subsequent neuropathy (68,71).

Numerous in vitro experiments have confirmed the carcinogenic potential of ionizing gamma radiation and have clarified the molecular mechanisms of radiation-induced transformation from cobalt 60 sources (76–79). In clinical practice, however, the risk of malignant degeneration of benign skull base tumors following gamma radiosurgery is impossible to quantify. Neuropathologic confirmation of the malignant change is only rarely sought. Furthermore, even in the absence of irradiation, spontaneous malignant transformation may occur as part of the natural history of many cranial base lesions, including schwannomas of the frontoethmoid sinus complex (80) and benign enchondromas of the skull (81).

Although postradiation vasculopathy predominantly affects smaller caliber vessels, conventional radiotherapy has been implicated in occlusion of the major intracranial arteries as well (82,83). Several large series have reported a 5% to 10% incidence of this latter complication following radiotherapy of pituitary tumors and other skull base lesions (74). However, animal models of gamma knife irradiation have found no changes in the basilar or middle cerebral arteries up to 2 years after treatment with doses as high as 100 Gy (71). In Lindquist and Steiner's (71) clinical experience of several hundred patients whose major cerebral vessels have been exposed to radiosurgical doses of 15 to 25 Gy, stenosis or occlusion has been seen in less than 1% and has caused clinical deficit in only one case. Likewise, MRI studies performed after gamma knife treatment of skull base chondrosarcomas, clival chordomas, and cavernous sinus meningiomas have demonstrated preservation of flow-void signals from major vessels within the radiosurgical treatment volume (65,67). Thus, in clinical practice, the major vessels never limit the radiation dose prescribed for skull base lesions, since it is assumed that endothelial damage sustained by vessels with large lumina is quickly repaired and does not lead to persistent thrombosis (71).

CONCLUSION

Stereotactic radiosurgery is an effective treatment for a number of diseases that come to the attention of both the neurosurgeon and otolaryngologist. Factors that limit the morbidity of this technique include patient selection and the adherence to specific technical considerations. Its future use as a primary or adjuvant therapy in the treatment of neoplastic, vascular, and functional disorders is predicated on a review of its long-term results, although initial data support a broad utility.

REFERENCES

1. Larson DA, Bova F, Eisert D. Current radiosurgery practice: results of an astrosurvey. *Int J Radiat Oncol Biol Phys* 1993;28:523–526.
2. Yu C, Luxton G, Apuzzo MLJ, MacPherson DM, Petrovich Z. Extracranial radiation doses in patients undergoing gamma knife radiosurgery. *Neurosurgery* 1997;41:553–560.
3. Albuquerque FC, Giannotta SL. Cranial nerve preservation in surgery of the cerebellopontine angle. *Neurosurg Q* 1996;6(1):31–50.
4. Foote RL, Coffey RJ, Swanson JW. Stereotactic radiosurgery using the gamma knife for acoustic neuromas. *Int J Radiat Oncol Biol Phys* 1995;32:1153–1160.
5. Hirato M, Inoue H, Zama A, Ohye C, Shibazaki T, Andou Y. Gamma knife radiosurgery for acoustic schwannoma: effects of low radiation dose and functional prognosis. *Stereotact Funct Neurosurg* 1996; 66(suppl 1):134–141.
6. Ito K, Kurita H, Sugasawa K, Okuno T, Mizuno M, Sasaki T. Neuro-otological findings after radiosurgery for acoustic neurinomas. *Arch Otolaryngol Head Neck Surg* 1996;122:1229–1233.
7. Kondziolka D, Lunsford LD, Flickinger JC. Stereotactic radiosurgery for acoustic tumors: technique and results. *Tech Neurosurg* 1997;3: 154–161.
8. Mendenhall WM, Friedman WA, Bova FJ. Linear accelerator-based stereotactic radiosurgery for acoustic schwannomas. *Int J Radiat Oncol Biol Phys* 1994;28:803–810.
9. Noren G, Arndt J, Hindmarsh T, Hirsch A. Stereotactic radiosurgical treatment of acoustic neurinomas. In: Lunsford LD, ed. *Modern stereotactic neurosurgery*. Boston: Martinus Nijhoff, 1988:481–489.
10. Ogunrinde OK, Lunsford LD, Flickinger JC, Kondziolka DS. Cranial nerve preservation after stereotactic radiosurgery for small acoustic tumors. *Arch Neurol* 1995;52:73–79.
11. Ogunrinde OK, Lunsford LD, Kondziolka DS, Bissonette DJ, Flickinger JC. Cranial nerve preservation after stereotactic radiosurgery of intracanalicular acoustic tumors. *Stereotact Funct Neurosurg* 1995;64: 87–97.
12. Pama H, Kobayashi T, Kida Y, et al. Early changes in volume and non-enhanced volume of acoustic neurinoma after stereotactic gamma-radiosurgery. *Neurol Med Chir* 1994;34:607–611.
13. Seo Y, Fukuoka S, Nakagawara J, et al. Effect of gamma knife radiosurgery on acoustic neurinomas. *Stereotact Funct Neurosurg* 1995; 66(suppl 1):93–102.
14. Hudgins WR. Patients attitude about outcomes and the role of gamma knife radiosurgery in the treatment of vestibular schwannomas. *Neurosurgery* 1994;34:459–465.
15. Pollock BE, Lunsford LD, Kondziolka D, et al. Outcome analysis of acoustic neuroma management: a comparison of microsurgery and stereotactic radiosurgery. *Neurosurgery* 1995;36:215–224.
16. Flickinger JC, Kondziolka D, Lunsford LD. Dose and diameter relationships for facial, trigeminal, and acoustic neuropathies following acoustic neuroma radiosurgery. *Radiother Oncol* 1996;41:215–219.
17. Ito K, Kurita H, Sugasawa K, Mizuno M, Sasaki T. Analyses of neuro-otological complications after radiosurgery for acoustic neurinomas. *Int J Radiat Oncol Biol Phys* 1997;39:983–988.
18. Linskey ME, Flickinger JC, Lunsford LD. Cranial nerve length predicts the risk of delayed facial and trigeminal neuropathies after acoustic stereotactic radiosurgery. *Int J Radiat Oncol Biol Phys* 1993;25: 227–233.
19. Pendl G, Ganz JC, Kitz K, Eustacchio S. Acoustic neurinomas with macrocysts treated with gamma knife radiosurgery. *Stereotact Funct Neurosurg* 1995;66(suppl 1):103–111.
20. Bajada C, Selch M, De Salles A, et al. Application of stereotactic radiosurgery to the head and neck region. *Acta Neurochir* 1994;62: 114–117.
21. Dong RH, Gao ZW, Hu ZQ, Xu WM, Pan L. Preliminary application of gamma knife in the treatment of nasopharyngeal carcinoma. *Stereotact Funct Neurosurg* 1995;66(suppl 1):201–207.
22. Firlik KS, Kondziolka D, Lunsford LD, Janecka IP, Flickinger JC. Radiosurgery for recurrent cranial base cancer arising from the head and neck. *Head Neck* 1996;18:160–166.
23. Kaplan ID, Adler JR, Hicks WL, Fee WE, Goffinet DR. Radiosurgery for palliation of base of skull recurrences from head and neck cancers. *Cancer* 1992;70:1980–1984.
24. Kocher M, Voges J, Staar S, Treuer H, Sturm V, Mueller RP. Linear accelerator radiosurgery for recurrent malignant tumors of the skull base. *Am J Clin Oncol* 1998;21:18–22.
25. Kondziolka D, Lunsford LD. Stereotactic radiosurgery for squamous cell carcinoma of the nasopharynx. *Laryngoscope* 1991;101:519–522.
26. Solberg TD, Holly FE, De Salles AAF, Wallace RE, Smathers JB.

Implications of tissue heterogeneity for radiosurgery in head and neck tumors. *Int J Radiat Oncol Biol Phys* 1995;32:235–239.
27. Hall EJ, Brenner DJ. The radiobiology of radiosurgery: rationale for different treatment regimes for AVMs and malignancies. *Int J Radiat Oncol Biol Phys* 1993;25:381–385.
28. Karlsson B, Lax I, Soderman M, Kihlstrom L, Lindquist C. Prediction of results following gamma knife surgery for brain stem and other centrally located arteriovenous malformations: relation to natural course. *Stereotact Funct Neurosurg* 1995;66(suppl 1):260–268.
29. Lunsford LD, Kondziolka D, Bissonette DJ, Maitz AH, Flickinger JC. Stereotactic radiosurgery of brain vascular malformations. *Neurosurg Clin North Am* 1992;3:79–98.
30. Lunsford LD, Kondziolka D, Flickinger JC, et al. Stereotactic radiosurgery for arteriovenous malformations of the brain. *J Neurosurg* 75: 512–524.
31. Pollock BE, Lunsford LD, Kondziolka D, Maitz A, Flickinger JC. Patient outcomes after stereotactic radiosurgery for operable arteriovenous malformations. *Neurosurgery* 1994;35:1–7.
32. Yamamoto M, Jimbo M, Ide M, Lindquist C, Steiner L. Gamma knife radiosurgery in cerebral arteriovenous malformations: postobliteration nidus changes observed on neurodiagnostic imaging. *Stereotact Funct Neurosurg* 1995;64(suppl 1):126–133.
33. Gallina P, Merienne L, Meder JF, Schlienger M, Lefkopoulos D, Merland JJ. Failure in radiosurgery treatment of cerebral arteriovenous malformations. *Neurosurgery* 1998;42:996–1004.
34. Porter PJ, Shin AY, Detsky AS, Lefaive L, Wallace MC. Surgery versus stereotactic radiosurgery for small operable cerebral arteriovenous malformations: a clinical and cost comparison. *Neurosurgery* 1997;41: 757–766.
35. Flickinger JC, Kondziolka D, Pollock BE, Maitz AH, Lunsford LD. Complications from arteriovenous malformation radiosurgery: multivariate analysis and risk modelling. *Int J Radiat Oncol Biol Phys* 1997; 38:485–490.
36. Karlsson B, Kihlstrom L, Lindquist C, Steiner L. Gamma knife surgery for previously irradiated arteriovenous malformations. *Neurosurgery* 1998;42:1–6.
37. Flickinger JC, Lunsford LD, Kondziolka D, et al. Radiosurgery and brain tolerance: an analysis of neurodiagnostic imaging changes after gamma knife radiosurgery for arteriovenous malformations. *Int J Radiat Oncol Biol Phys* 1992;23:19–26.
38. Chang SD, Adler JR. Treatment of cranial base meningiomas with linear accelerator radiosurgery. *Neurosurgery* 1997;41:1019–1027.
39. Nicolato A, Ferraresi P, Foroni R, et al. Gamma knife radiosurgery in skull base meningiomas. *Stereotact Funct Neurosurg* 1995;66(suppl 1):112–120.
40. Pendl G, Schrottner O, Friehs GM, Feichtinger H. Stereotactic radiosurgery of skull base meningiomas: stereotactic radiosurgery of skull base meningiomas. *Stereotact Funct Neurosurg* 1994;64(suppl 1):11–18.
41. Hakim R, Alexander E, Loeffler JS, et al. Results of linear accelerator-based radiosurgery for intracranial meningiomas. *Neurosurgery* 1998; 42:446–454.
42. Hudgins WR, Barker JL, Schwartz DE, Nichols TD. Gamma knife treatment of 100 consecutive meningiomas. *Stereotact Funct Neurosurg* 1995;66(suppl 1):121–128.
43. Leber KA, Bergloff J, Pendl G. Dose-response tolerance of the visual pathways and cranial nerves of the cavernous sinus to stereotactic radiosurgery. *J Neurosurg* 1998;88:43–50.
44. Ganz JC. Gamma knife treatment of pituitary adenomas. *Stereotact Funct Neurosurg* 1994;64(suppl 1):3–10.
45. Lunsford LD, Witt TC, Kondziolka D, Flickinger JC. Stereotactic radiosurgery of anterior skull base tumors. *Clin Neurosurgery* 1994;23: 99–119.
46. Fukuoka S, Seo Y, Takanashi M, Takahashi S, Suematsu K, Nakamura J. Radiosurgery of brain metastases with the gamma knife. *Stereotact Funct Neurosurg* 1995;66(suppl 1):193–200.
47. Gerosa M, Nicolato A, Berlucchi S, et al. Gamma knife radiosurgery of primary and metastatic malignant brain tumors: a preliminary report. *Stereotact Funct Neurosurg* 1994;64(suppl 1):56–66.
48. Gerosa M, Nicolato A, Severi F, et al. Gamma knife radiosurgery for intracranial metastases: from local tumor control to increased survival. *Stereotact Funct Neurosurg* 1995;66(suppl 1):184–192.
49. Tago M, Aoki Y, Terahara A, et al. Gamma knife radiosurgery for brain stem metastases: two autopsy cases. *Stereotact Funct Neurosurg* 1995;66(suppl 1):225–230.
50. Kondziolka D, Flickinger JC, Lunsford LD, Habeck M. Trigeminal neuralgia radiosurgery: the University of Pittsburgh Experience. *Stereotact Funct Neurosurg* 1996;66(suppl 1):343–348.
51. Kondziolka D, Lunsford LD, Flickinger JC, et al. Stereotactic radiosurgery for trigeminal neuralgia: a multiinstitutional study using the gamma unit. *J Neurosurg* 1996;84:940–945.
52. Regis J, Manera L, Dufour H, Porcheron D, Sedan R, Peragut JC. Effect of the gamma knife on trigeminal neuralgia. *Stereotact Funct Neurosurg* 1994;64(suppl 1):182–192.
53. Flickinger JC. An integrated logistic formula for prediction of complications from radiosurgery. *Int J Radiat Oncol Biol Phys* 1989;17: 879–885.
54. Anscher MS, Swift PS, Gaspar LE, Marks LB. Radiation injury of the brain and spinal cord. In: Wilkins RH, Rengachary SS, eds. *Neurosurgery*. New York: McGraw-Hill, 1996:1928–1933.
55. Kondziolka D, Somaza S, Martinez AJ, et al. Radioprotective effects of the 21-aminosteroid U-74389G for stereotactic radiosurgery. *Neurosurgery* 1997;41:203–208.
56. Wiet RJ, Micco AG, Bauer GP. Complications of the gamma knife. *Arch Otolaryngol Head Neck Surg* 1996;122:414–416.
57. Morikawa M, Numaguchi Y, Rigamonti D, et al. Radiosurgery for cerebral arteriovenous malformations: assessment of early phase magnetic resonance imaging and significance of gadolinium-DTPA enhancement. *Int J Radiat Oncol Biol Phys* 1996;34:663–675.
58. Steiner L, Lindquist C, Adler JR, Torner JC, Alves W, Steiner M. Clinical outcome of radiosurgery for cerebral arteriovenous malformations. *J Neurosurg* 1992;77:1–8.
59. Tanaka T, Kobayashi T, Kida Y, Oyama H, Niwa M. Comparison between adult and pediatric arteriovenous malformations treated by gamma knife radiosurgery. *Stereotact Funct Neurosurg* 1996;66(suppl 1):288–295.
60. Yamamoto M, Ban S, Mitsunobu I, Jimbo M. A diffuse white matter ischemic lesion appearing 7 years after stereotactic radiosurgery for cerebral arteriovenous malformations: case report. *Neurosurgery* 1997; 41:1405–1409.
61. Flickinger JC, Kondziolka D, Lunsford LD, et al. A multi-institutional experience with stereotactic radiosurgery for solitary brain metastasis. *Int J Radiat Oncol Biol Phys* 1994;28:797–802.
62. Kline JL, Noto RB, Glantz M. Single-photon emission CT in the evaluation of recurrent brain tumor in patients treated with gamma knife radiosurgery or conventional radiation therapy. *Am J Neuroradiol* 1996; 17:1681–1686.
63. Young RF, Vermeulen SS, Grimm P, et al. Gamma knife thalamotomy for the treatment of persistent pain. *Stereotact Funct Neurosurg* 1995; 64(suppl 1):172–181.
64. Tada E, Matsumoto K, Kinoshita K, Furuta T, Ohmoto T. The protective effect of dexamethasone against radiation damage induced by interstitial irradiation in normal monkey brain. *Neurosurgery* 1997;41: 209–219.
65. Duma CM, Lunsford LD, Kondziolka D, Harsh GR, Flickinger JC. Stereotactic radiosurgery of cavernous sinus meningiomas as an addition or alternative to microsurgery. *Neurosurgery* 1993;32:699–705.
66. Flickinger JC, Lunsford LD, Linskey ME, Duma CM, Kondziolka D. Gamma knife radiosurgery for acoustic tumors: multivariate analysis of four year results. *Radiother Oncol* 1993;27:91–98.
67. Kondziolka D, Lunsford LD, Flickinger JC. The role of radiosurgery in the management of chordoma and chondrosarcoma of the cranial base. *Neurosurgery* 1991;29:38–46.
68. Kondziolka D, Lunsford LD, Linskey ME, Flickinger JC. Skull base radiosurgery. In: Alexander E, Loeffler JS, Lunsford LD, eds. *Stereotactic radiosurgery*. New York: McGraw-Hill, 1993:175–188.
69. Lunsford LD, Kondziolka D, Flickinger JC. Stereotactic radiosurgery for benign intracranial tumors. *Clin Neurosurg* 1993;40:475–497.
70. Kobayashi T, Tanaka T, Kida Y. The early effects of gamma knife on 40 cases of acoustic neurinoma. *Acta Neurochir* 1994;62(suppl):93–97.
71. Lindquist C, Steiner L. Radiosurgery for tumors. In: Wilkins RH, Rengachary SS, eds. *Neurosurgery*. New York: McGraw-Hill, 1996: 1887–1907.
72. Oyama H, Kobayashi T, Kida Y, et al. Early changes in volume and non-enhanced volume of acoustic neurinoma after stereotactic gamma-radiosurgery. *Neurol Med Chir* 1994;34:607–611.
73. Kondziolka D, Lunsford LD, Coffey RJ, Flickinger JC. Stereotactic radiosurgery of meningiomas. *J Neurosurg* 1991;74:552–559.

74. Larson DA. Radiation therapy of pituitary tumors. In: Youmans JR, ed. *Neurological surgery*. Philadelphia: WB Saunders, 1996:2970–2979.
75. Kobayashi T, Tanaka T, Kida Y. Stereotactic gamma radiosurgery of craniopharyngiomas. *Pediatr Neurosurg* 1994;21(suppl 1):69–74.
76. Iijima M, Mihara K, Kondo T, Tsuji T, Ishioka C, Namba M. Mutation in p53 and de-regulation of p53-related gene expression in three human cell lines immortalized with 4-nitroquinoline 1-oxide or 60Co gamma rays. *Int J Cancer* 1996;66:698–702.
77. Kasid U, Suy S, Dent P, Ray S, Whiteside TL, Sturgill TW. Activation of Raf by ionizing radiation. *Nature* 1996;382:813–816.
78. Reinhold DS, Walicka M, Elkassaby M, et al. Malignant transformation of human fibroblasts by ionizing radiation. *Int J Radiat Biol* 1996;69: 707–715.
79. Sugihara S, Mihara K, Marunouchi T, Inoue H, Namba M. Telomere elongation observed in immortalized human fibroblasts by treatment with 60Co gamma rays or 4-nitroquinoline-1-oxide. *Hum Genet* 1996; 97:1–6.
80. Kautzky M, Sailer H, Franz P, Susani M. Malignant transformation of a peripheral nerve sheath tumor in the area of the paranasal sinuses. *Laryngorhinootologie* 1996;75:691–696.
81. Maleux G, Demaerel P, Vanslambrouk K, Aerts P, Brijs S, Tanghe W. [Chondrosarcoma of the skull base: CT, MR, and pathological features.] *Rofo Fortschr Geb Rontgenstr Neuen Bildgeb Verfahr* 1996;165: 599–601.
82. Hirata Y, Matsukado Y, Mihara Y, Kochi M, Sonoda H, Fukumura A. Occlusion of the internal carotid artery after radiation therapy for the chiasmal lesion. *Acta Neurochir (Wien)* 1985;74:141–147.
83. Murros KE, Toole JF. The effect of radiation on carotid arteries: a review article. *Arch Neurol* 1989;46:449–455.

Neurosurgical Issues in Otolaryngology: Principles and Practice of Collaboration,
edited by Moisés A. Arriaga and J. Diaz Day.
Lippincott Williams & Wilkins, Philadelphia © 1999.

CHAPTER 31

Anterior Skull Base: Otolaryngology—Head and Neck Surgery Perspective

Richard E. Hayden and Scott E. Strome

Surgery of the anterior skull base has undergone revolutionary change in the past two decades. The foundation for this growth is based on two fundamental features: (a) technological advances, which have enabled more accurate preoperative diagnosis and intraoperative patient monitoring; and (b) the development of a team approach. The otolaryngologist–head and neck surgeon is an integral member of the skull base team, lending a dynamic appreciation of the anatomy of the mid-face, the orbits, and the lateral nasal wall/frontoethmoid complex, the understanding of which can be utilized to design approaches to the anterior skull base. Additionally, the otolaryngologist provides a working knowledge of sinonasal disease, which represents a significant percentage of anterior skull base pathology. From a technologic perspective, recent advances in endoscopic sinus surgery have allowed the design of minimally invasive approaches to this region. Finally, the evolving role of head and neck reconstruction as a subspecialty of otolaryngology has reduced the morbidity of tumor ablation by decreasing associated complications with secondary improvement of function and cosmesis in this patient population.

SURGICAL APPROACHES

Craniofacial Resection

Surgical approaches to the anterior skull base have traditionally relied upon combined intracranial/extracranial resections, which afford the skull base team the ability to approach a particular lesion under direct visualization. While the techniques employed are dependent on the nature of the disease process, they are historically based on the classic craniofacial resection and the en bloc orbitectomy/craniectomy with the potential inclusion of the maxilla. Craniofacial resection was first described by Dandy (1) for the treatment of orbital neoplasms with intracranial extension. This approach was adapted for the exenteration of sinonasal tumors by Smith et al. (2) in 1954, and later popularized by Ketcham et al. (3) in a report detailing the resection of 17 malignant sinonasal tumors.

The technique for craniofacial resection is extensively described in the literature. Briefly, a bicoronal incision is performed and elevated in a subpericranial fashion to the level of the supraorbital rims. Leaving the pericranium attached to the flap helps to ensure that it remains moist during the procedure. If necessary, the entire bony nasal dorsum may be exposed to the level of the upper lateral cartilages. Laterally, the bicoronal flap can be elevated over the body of the zygoma, but care must be taken to dissect in the fat inferior to the temporal line of fusion to protect the frontal branch of the facial nerve. The flap can also be carried down over the supraorbital rims as required, but the supraorbital pedicle must be maintained to preserve sensation to the forehead and the blood supply to the pericranial flap. Because the orbital roof curves sharply posterior and superior, the surgeon must maintain the correct angle of dissection to prevent inadvertent penetration through the periorbita (4).

Following flap elevation, a standard bifrontal craniotomy/craniectomy is performed with bone, dura, and brain parenchyma resected as dictated by the underlying disease process. The midface is generally approached via a Weber-Ferguson, Lynch, or Sewell incision. When performing these incisions, a Webster modification is often useful in the medial canthus region to prevent postoperative hooding. Price et al. (5) have described a sublabial transnasal degloving approach, which affords the same access to the frontoethmoid region but avoids the cosmetic issues associated with facial incisions.

R. E. Hayden and S. E. Strome: Department of Otolaryngology, Allegheny University of the Health Sciences, Philadelphia, Pennsylvania 19103.

Following flap elevation the disease process is approached from below, via exenteration of the frontoethmoid complex. The orbital contents and the maxilla are incorporated into the dissection as required by the underlying disease. The intra/extracranial resections are then connected by intracranial elevation of the olfactory tracts and resection of the cribriform plate with en bloc specimen removal. Reconstruction of this defect is detailed later in the chapter; it can generally be accomplished with a pericranial flap if the dura remains intact.

Craniofacial resection is useful for large sinonasal tumors with intracranial involvement and is less commonly employed for infectious and traumatic disease processes. A realistic assessment of the morbidity and mortality associated with this approach is confounded by the large variety of benign and malignant disease processes that occur in this region. A series by Shah et al. (6) of 71 patients who had undergone anterior craniofacial resection for a variety of anterior skull base tumors documented an overall survival of 56% and a mean survival of 4.2 years. A similar series by Jackson et al. (7) evaluating 79 patients revealed only one operative mortality and two deaths secondary to recurrent tumor. Significant morbidity can be associated with cerebrospinal fluid (CSF) leak, pneumoencephalus, or local infection leading to meningitis, encephalitis, or brain abscess. Infection or loss of the nonvascularized frontal craniotomy bone flap can produce significant long-term problems. Risk of orbital complications are more common with diplopia, enophthalmos, and telecanthus occurring most frequently. With careful planning and execution, the classic craniofacial resection should produce rare and minimal negative side effects.

Despite the relative success of this procedure, there are several potential disadvantages. Complete anosmia is expected postoperatively. Because of the need to expose the floor of the anterior cranial fossa, significant prolonged retraction is often required on the frontal lobes. This can delay return of normal brain function, especially in the frontal lobes. Additionally, the use of transfacial incisions can result in significant cosmetic deformity, particularly in patients prone to keloid formation. Thus, while this procedure still has a role for the treatment of massive sinonasal tumors, its utility has largely been supplanted by procedures that provide a more refined approach to the anterior cranial base.

Subcranial Approach

The subcranial approach to the anterior cranial fossa was introduced by Raveh (8) in 1979 for the treatment of congenital craniofacial anomalies. This has rapidly evolved to become the procedure of choice for a variety of disease processes involving the anterior skull base. The essential features of this technique involve the removal of the frontal nasal glabellar complex, providing exposure to the cribriform region, planum sphenoidale, clivus, paranasal sinuses, and the orbits. Because the procedure is performed entirely through a bicoronal incision, cosmetic deformity is minimized. Additionally, removal of the glabellar complex provides direct visualization of the anterior cranial fossa floor without necessitating brain retraction.

The procedure, like the classic operation, is initiated by the placement of a lumbar drain. Following this a bicoronal flap is elevated, taking care to preserve the pericranial flap for later use. The flap must be elevated to a sufficient extent to expose the entire bony dorsum, superior orbit, and the zygoma. The anterior ethmoid arteries are identified and ligated. As discussed in the previous section, care must be taken to preserve the supraorbital neurovascular pedicle and the frontal branch of the facial nerve. A limited bifrontal craniotomy is then performed, with the frontal sinus included. The nasal glabellar complex is then removed while protecting the intracranial and orbital contents. Subsequent tumor ablation is dependent on tumor histology and location. Following tumor extirpation, closure of the defect can generally be accomplished using the pericranial flap. This flap is positioned in the bone kerf between the frontal and the nasal glabellar bone flaps. Prior to replacement of the frontal bone flap, the frontal sinus is cranialized. Care must be taken to accurately attach the medial and lateral canthal tendons. Additionally, it is important to reattach the temporal line of fusion to prevent excess facial laxity. At the conclusion of the procedure, either a tracheotomy is performed or bilateral nasal trumpets are placed and sutured into position to prevent postoperative pneumocephalus.

There are several advantages to the subcranial approach relative to classic craniofacial resection. The absence of dural retraction minimizes postoperative frontal lobe sequelae. Additionally, cosmesis is excellent as the entire procedure is performed through a bicoronal flap. Finally, the procedure can be adapted for the treatment of inflammatory, traumatic, and congenital disease, with more limited procedures employed for processes such as localized CSF leaks or encephaloceles.

From a disease standpoint, this approach has documented efficacy in the therapy of a variety of skull base neoplasms. In an initial study by Raveh (9), 48 patients with benign and 38 patients with malignant tumors of the anterior skull base were treated via subcranial resection. The patients with benign disease enjoyed a 91% survival, while patients with malignant tumors had a 57% survival at time intervals ranging from 6 to 63 months (9). This has been substantiated in other series (10,11). Perhaps more importantly, patients undergoing subcranial resection had a reduced number of complications compared to those reported in large series of craniofacial resections (6). In the initial series reported by Raveh et al. (10), complications included CSF leak in two patients, epidural infection in two patients, frontal lobe contusion (one), tension pneumocephalus (one), frontal sinus dysfunction (one), pneumonia (one), and pulmonary embolism (one). Although tumor variability precludes direct comparison of these with the large craniofacial series, these statistics appear favorable. This minimal postoperative morbidity in combination with reduced frontal lobe retraction and improved cosmesis makes the subcranial approach a particularly attractive technique for treating a variety of anterior skull base diseases.

Endoscopic Approaches

The advent of functional endoscopic sinus surgery, popularized in Europe by Wigand and Stammberger and championed in the United States by Kennedy, has allowed the design of minimally invasive approaches to the anterior skull base (12–14). Endoscopic approaches are premised on a dynamic appreciation of the anatomy of the lateral nasal wall/ ethmoid complex. This anatomy is extensively reviewed in the literature, and must be studied in a supervised setting prior to attempting any of these techniques on patients.

The advantages of endoscopic sinus approaches to the anterior cranial base are minimal morbidity and improved visualization. Thus, these approaches lend themselves to the therapy of a variety of inflammatory, traumatic, and neoplastic disease processes. For example, endoscopic techniques are particularly well suited to the therapy of traumatic/iatrogenic CSF leaks and other benign skull base neoplasms such as inverted papilloma. Moreover, the improved visualization of the nasal contents provided by the endoscopes makes these techniques a valuable adjunct to both the classic craniofacial resection and subcranial approaches. Optimistically, innovative new tracking systems for the endoscopes will broaden the utility of these techniques in the treatment of anterior skull base disease (15).

RECONSTRUCTION OF ANTERIOR SKULL BASE DEFECTS

The techniques used for the reconstruction of anterior skull base largely depend on the location of the defect, the integrity of the dura, and the degree of cosmetic deformity. The variety of disease processes occurring in this region mandates that reconstructive efforts be premised on a stepladder approach in which patient safety is the primary goal, with functional and cosmetic considerations playing important but secondary roles. Thus, the initial goals of the reconstructive surgeon are to provide an adequate barrier between the brain and the nasal contents, in hopes of preventing secondary CSF contamination. External bone support is often necessary to avoid subsequent brain trauma. Functional considerations include accurate reconstruction of the lacrimal system to reduce chances of postoperative epiphora or dacryocystitis, creation of a barrier between the dura and the orbital contents to prevent pulsatile exophthalmos, and the provision of an adequate nasal airway. Cosmetic concerns are centered on achieving an image that will allow patient integration into society. It is important to counsel the patient that the requirements of the ablative procedure may eliminate the potential for maintaining preoperative appearance, yet an excellent cosmetic result is often attainable.

As with all reconstructive efforts, the first and most important component is elimination of the primary disease process. Meticulous dissection in the ablative portion of the procedure, e.g., preserving one olfactory tract in unilateral cribriform involvement, will maximize the overall result. Following eradication of the primary disease process, the reconstructive team has several options for defect repair that can be broadly categorized into pedicled fascial flaps, pedicled myocutaneous flaps, free tissue transfer techniques, and autologous/synthetic bone replacement. The choice of techniques depends on the surgical defect and the experience of the reconstructive surgeon.

Pedicled Fascial Flaps

There are essentially two pedicled fascial flaps commonly employed for anterior skull base reconstruction: (a) the pericranial flap, and (b) the temporoparietal fascial flap (TPFF). These flaps are similar in that each provides a thin pliable layer for dural support or repair. The advantages of these flaps include their excellent vascular supply and their proximity to the anterior skull base. Even in the ablation of large sinonasal tumors, meticulous dissection often allows preservation of the blood supply to these flaps.

The pericranial flap is perhaps the most common type of reconstructive procedure employed for defects of the anterior skull base. This flap can be used in isolation or as an adjuvant to pedicled or free tissue transfer. Because the elevation of this flap is discussed in the earlier part of this chapter, only the key points will be highlighted.

The pericranial flap receives its primary blood supply from the supraorbital neurovascular bundle with secondary contributions from the superficial temporal system. The flap can be based on a unilateral supraorbital pedicle, allowing its utilization after unilateral orbital roof resection. If this flap is considered for use, it is important to design the bicoronal flap far enough posterior to ensure adequate pericranial length. Alternative methods to augment length include posterior reflection of the scalp in a supraperiosteal plane, allowing more posterior pericranial elevation, or the creation of a hockey stick-shaped flap. As mentioned previously, it is the authors' preference to elevate the bicoronal flap in a subperiosteal plane, with flap elevation from the scalp at the time when it is required for use. This prevents flap desiccation and helps to reduce the incidence of inadvertent periosteal injury during bicoronal flap elevation. The flap is elevated by incision through the periosteal layer followed by blunt dissection with a dry sponge. During the resection, the bicoronal/pericranial flap is kept moist with a sponge, which an assistant irrigates at regular intervals. At the conclusion of the ablative portion of the procedure, the flap is dissected under direct visualization away from the scalp. It is then used to reinforce the dura, by suturing it to the floor of the anterior cranial fossa. This can often be facilitated by the placement of microscrews in bony remnants at the anterior skull base, which are used to anchor the flap. Following flap insertion, it is important to pack the nasal cavity, providing additional support to the flap from below.

The TPFF, like the pericranial flap, provides a pliable layer of vascularized tissue for dural coverage or repair. The temporoparietal fascia, or superficial temporal fascia, is a continuation of the superficial musculoaponeurotic system (SMAS), and is found just deep to the subcutaneous fat. It is a layer distinct from the temporalis muscular fascia. The flap is 2 to 3 mm thick and receives its blood supply from the superficial temporal artery and vein (16).

Because the temporoparietal fascia is transected during standard elevation of a bicoronal flap, preoperative planning is critical. The flap is elevated in a plane just deep to the hair follicles, taking care to prevent injury. The temporal vessels penetrate the parotid fascia at the level of the tragus, with inferior and anterior flap dissection restricted by the frontal branch of the facial nerve. The TPFF can be elevated in conjunction with either the muscular fascia of the temporalis or the temporalis muscle itself, providing a potential second layer for defect closure (16).

The TPFF has been used extensively for the reconstruction of anterior skull base and mastoid defects (16,17). It is particularly useful in filling orbital defects. The utility of the TPFF is enhanced by its potential for use as a free flap. Disadvantages of the TPFF are the need for a preoperative decision regarding flap use. The thin nature of the flap prevents its utilization for large-volume defects and entails the risk of alopecia along the parietal scalp wound secondary to ischemia of hair follicles. Despite these concerns, the TPFF provides an extremely well-vascularized tissue supply, which is excellent for reinforcing dural dehiscences and useful for the augmentation of smaller defects.

Pedicled Muscle/Myocutaneous Flaps

Pedicled muscle/myocutaneous flaps (PMMFs) have a distinct role in the reconstruction of anterior skull base defects because they provide a well-vascularized muscle bulk, which is useful in the ablation of large defects. In fact, prior to the advent of free flaps, PMMFs were the standard second-level option for anterior skull base reconstruction. They can be divided into two categories: local flaps and regional flaps. Because these flaps are well described in the literature, techniques for individual flap elevation are not reviewed here. Rather, this section focuses on features unique to this type of reconstruction.

The predominant local PMMF used for reconstruction of the anterior skull base is the temporalis muscle flap. This muscle is supplied by deep temporal branches of the internal maxillary artery, which run deep to the zygoma on the undersurface of the muscle. Following reflection of the temporalis fascia, the flap can be elevated from its bed and rotated into a variety of anterior and lateral defects. The advantage of this flap is the relative ease of flap dissection and its local availability. The primary disadvantage is the limited arc of rotation, which often prevents adequate midline coverage. Moreover, repositioning of the temporalis muscle results in a considerable cosmetic deformity. Although cosmesis may be improved with synthetic bone replacement or autologous fat, this issue must be considered when employing the temporalis muscle flap.

There are several regional pedicled flaps available for anterior skull base reconstruction. Most commonly employed are the pectoralis major myocutaneous flap, the latissimus dorsi flap, and the lower island trapezius flap (18–21). These flaps are advantageous in that they provide a significant amount of muscle bulk and have a cutaneous portion useful for the reconstruction of skin defects. The primary disadvantage to using regional PMMFs for anterior skull base reconstruction is the fixed vascular pedicle length, which limits their ability to fill the distal portion of large defects. Specifically, the critical distal portion required for dural coverage is at the greatest risk for vascular compromise based on either a random pattern of perfusion or tension on the pedicle. While there are several potential means to combat the problem of distal flap compromise, e.g., removing a portion of the clavicle to increase the range of a pectoralis major myocutaneous flap or delay of the random portion of the skin paddle, tenuous viability of the distal flap remains of paramount concern when considering the utilization of a regional PMMF. By far, the regional flap with the greatest arc of rotation is the latissimus dorsi flap.

Free Tissue Transfer Techniques

Free tissue transfer techniques have revolutionized the field of anterior skull base surgery, providing coverage for extensive defects, which were previously not amenable to surgical therapy. These flaps offer all of the advantages of the PMMF, but are not restricted by a fixed pedicle. Additionally, the many flap alternatives provide choice of flap thickness and surface area, and of tissue utilized, such as skin, fat, fascia mucosa, or vascularized bone, useful for midface or anterior cranial base reconstruction. While a variety of free flaps can be employed for reconstruction of the anterior cranial base, those most commonly utilized include the rectus abdominis, latissimus dorsi, scapula radial forearm, and external iliac flaps (22,23). Because of the number of potential donor sites available for free flap reconstruction of the anterior cranial base, the general advantages of free flap reconstruction will be discussed without focusing on any particular flap.

The primary advantage of free flap reconstruction for anterior skull base defects is the ability to transfer a reliable source of vascularized tissue without the limitations imposed by a fixed vascular pedicle. Because free tissue transfer, by definition, relies on a microvascular anastomosis to provide blood supply to the flap, this tissue can usually be utilized with no regions of random blood supply. As these flaps are often harvested from distant sites, they allow a two-team approach, with simultaneous flap harvest and tumor ablation minimizing operative tissue. Utilization of a distant site also provides for nonirradiated donor tissue in cases of secondary reconstruction after radiotherapy. Finally, the use of certain osseous free flaps from the scapula and iliac crest regions permits the transfer of vascularized bone, enhancing the ability to reconstruct defects requiring bone resection.

The disadvantages of free flap reconstruction are relatively few. Because of the need for specialized harvesting and microvascular surgical skill, additional training is required for the reconstructive surgeon. As with all types of head and neck reconstruction, there is the potential for donor site morbidity, but this can be minimized with meticulous surgical planning and technique. Perhaps the greatest risk of free flap reconstruction is flap failure. This is of critical importance in the anterior skull base, where this tissue provides the primary barrier between the brain and the nasal contents. The rate of free flap failure varies, but is usually substantially less than failure rates with PMMFs and ranges between 1.2% and 5% in several large series (24,25). The primary determinant of flap viability is surgical experience. Additional factors are continuous flap monitoring, either by direct visualization or Doppler studies to ensure the integrity of the vascular anastomosis. Early recognition of a compromised pedicle can result in a high rate of flap salvage with rapid return to the operating theater and revision of the vascular anastomosis.

Autologous/Synthetic Bone Replacement

Free tissue transfer techniques have the ability to provide vascularized bone to large defects of the anterior cranial base. Smaller ablative procedures, with minimal or no soft tissue loss, often lend themselves to reconstruction with nonvascularized sources of bone, either autologous or synthetic. Free bone grafts receive their blood supply from the surrounding tissue, making them unsuitable for contaminated or infected sites or areas with decreased oxygen supply, e.g., the irradiated field. Additionally, because they require vascular ingrowth for survival, adequate fixation with a limited potential for rotational stress is critical to their survival. Two types of nonvascularized bone replacement are currently available: (a) autologous/allogenic and (b) synthetic.

Autologous vascular bone can be harvested from several sites including iliac crest, rib, and calvarium. Iliac crest and rib grafts offer viable sources of endochondral bone; however, their utility is limited by the need for a second surgical field and the potential for significant donor site morbidity (26). Specifically, split rib graft harvest may be complicated by pneumothorax with additional concerns of postoperative respiratory splinting and associated atelectasis. Maintaining an intact posterior periosteal layer at the time of graft harvest reduces the risk of pneumothorax. Similarly, iliac crest grafts are associated with significant postoperative pain, often resulting in delayed ambulation and an increased potential for deep venous thrombosis. Despite these drawbacks, both the iliac crest and split rib graft offer a significant amount of endochondral bone stock for the reconstruction of anterior skull base defects or cranioplasty.

Unlike iliac crest and split rib grafts, split calvarial grafts are locally harvested with minimal donor site morbidity, assuming the use of appropriate surgical technique. Specifically, grafts should be elevated posterior to the coronal suture over the parietal region to garner adequate bone stock, and computed tomography (CT) scans with bone windows must be studied preoperatively to ensure the presence of an adequate diploic layer. The grafts should be harvested at least 1 cm lateral to midline to prevent inadvertent injury to the sagittal sinus in the event of intracranial penetration. Following graft elevation, the edges of the donor site should be beveled to prevent a palpable bony step-off or an overt cosmetic deformity (26).

Utilizing these techniques, split calvarial grafts can adequately fill osseus defects of the anterior skull base. The donor site can be chosen so that a graft can be designed to fit the size and contour of a specific defect. Additionally, several grafts may be spliced together with miniplates or wires for complex three-dimensional reconstruction. This is especially relevant for combined defects of the orbital floor and rim. Finally, the ability to wrap these grafts in vascularized soft tissue like the temporoparietal fascial flap both enhances vascularity and offers the potential for improved cosmesis by eliminating bony contact with subcutaneous scalp fat.

Recently, bone replacement in the anterior skull base has been revolutionized with the development of synthetic bone sources such as hydroxyapatite cement (HAC). The ideal synthetic bone source would be pliable, biologically inert, allow vascular ingrowth, and be relatively inexpensive. Hydroxyapatite (HA), which forms the principal mineral component of bone, has been available in the synthetic implant form since the early 1970s. Early forms of this material were available only in porous or dense ceramic forms. While both compounds are relatively inert, the dense ceramic form is relatively nonpliable and resistant to fibro-osseus tissue integration. The porous form permits fibro-osseus integration, yet remains difficult to shape and subject to fracture, limiting its utility for reconstruction of stress-bearing regions (27).

Newer forms of HAC are produced as a nonceramic material. When this dry compound is mixed with appropriate quantities of nonpyrogenic water, a paste is formed that can be molded into a particular defect. This sets in approximately 15 minutes and is converted to HA within 4 hours. Perhaps more importantly, this form of HAC is gradually resorbed over a period of months to years and replaced with physiologically normal bone. Because this form of HAC has limited shear resistance it is currently approved only for non–stress-bearing regions.

Nonceramic HAC has been utilized for reconstruction of a variety of anterior skull base defects including CSF leaks, cranioplasty, and orbital/malar fractures/augmentation (28–31). Implantation of 45 patients over a 13-month period produced no toxic reactions and an infection rate of 5% with the majority of implants exposed to paranasal sinus mucosa (27). In the authors' experience, there are three keys to successful use of this material: (a) use of appropriate amounts of nonpyrogenic water, (b) maintenance of an extremely dry field when the implant is hardening, and (c) prevention of implant migration. Nonceramic HAC is extremely sensitive to overhydration, making the paste too liquid for clinical utility. This problem can be avoided by adding exact amounts of water in appropriate quantities with a tuberculin syringe. The field is kept dry by covering the implant with Surgicel during the initial drying period and covering the Surgicel with neurosurgical pledgets that are replaced every 5 minutes. Implant migration is avoided by placing several miniscrews or mesh in the surrounding bone, providing a latticework to maintain implant position.

Nonceramic HAC is a relatively safe alternative when compared with autologous bone grafts. The long history of human use with a low infection rate and minimal toxicity attests to the biologic inertness of this compound. Additionally, there is no associated donor site morbidity, and the substance can be adapted to fill a variety of defects. Despite such advantages, newer forms of HAC are extremely costly, are inappropriate for use in stress-bearing areas, and have a slightly higher rate of infection than that associated with autologous bone use. These factors must be considered when choosing between autologous and synthetic reconstructive options.

CONCLUSION

The otolaryngologist–head and neck surgeon serves as an integral member of the skull base team. His unique appreciation of the anatomy of the lateral nasal wall and paranasal sinuses has facilitated the creation of novel approaches to the anterior skull base with improved cosmesis and reduced morbidity. Perhaps more importantly, the integration of state-of-the-art reconstructive techniques into the field of anterior skull base surgery has enhanced the ability to resect more advanced disease. Perhaps this increased surgical aggression will afford prolonged survival to individuals with advanced cancer. In any case, the current predictability and relative safety of anterior cranial base surgery has been provided by those reconstructive techniques that provide reliable separation of the CSF and the contaminated sinonasal cavities.

REFERENCES

1. Dandy WE. *Orbital tumors: results following the transcranial operative attack.* New York: Oskar Priest, 1941:1154.
2. Smith RR, Klopp CT, Williams JM. Surgical treatment of cancer of the frontal sinus and adjacent areas. *J Cancer* 1954;7:991–994.
3. Ketcham AS, Wilkins RH, Van Buren JM, Smith RR. A combined intracranial approach to the paranasal sinuses. *Am J Surg* 1963;106: 698–703.
4. Kellman RM, Marentette LJ. *Atlas of craniomaxillofacial fixation.* New York: Raven Press, 1995.
5. Price JC, Holliday MJ, Johns ME, Kennedy DW, Richtsmeier WJ, Mattox DE. The versatile midface degloving approach. *Laryngoscope* 1988;98:291–295.
6. Shah JP, Krauss DH, Arbit E, Galicich JH, Strong EW. Craniofacial resection for tumors involving the anterior skull base. *Otolaryngol Head Neck Surg* 1992;106(4):387–393.
7. Jackson IT, Marsh R, Hide TAH. Treatment of tumors involving the anterior cranial fossa. *Head Neck Surg* 1984;6:901–913.
8. Raveh J. Schwere gesichtsschadelverletzungen: eigene erfahrungen und modifkationen. *Aktuel Probl ORL* 1979;3:145.
9. Raveh J. The extended frontal approach. *J Neurosurg* 1992;77: 655–656.
10. Raveh J, Laedrach K, Speiser M, et al. The subcranial approach for fronto-orbital and anteroposterior skull-base tumors. *Arch Otolaryngol Head Neck Surg* 1993;119:385–393.
11. Jung TM, TerKonda RP, Haines SJ, Strome SE, Marentette LJ. Outcome analysis of the transglabellar/subcranial approach for lesions of the anterior cranial fossa.
12. Mattox DE, Kennedy DW. Endoscopic management of cerebrospinal fluid leaks and encephaloceles. *Laryngoscope* 1990;100:857.
13. Kennedy DW, Zinreich SJ, Johns ME. Functional endoscopic sinus surgery. *The principles and practice of rhinology.* New York: Wiley, 1987.
14. Lanza DC, O'Brien DA, Kennedy DW. Endoscopic repair of cerebrospinal fluid fistulas and encephaloceles. *Laryngoscope* 1996;106: 1119–1125.
15. Senior BA, Lanza DC, Kennedy DW, Weinstein GS. Computer-assisted resection of benign sinonasal tumors with skull base and orbital extension. *Arch Otolaryngol Head Neck Surg* 1997;123:706–711.
16. Cheney ML, Varvares MA, Nadol JB. The temporoparietal fascial flap in head and neck reconstruction. *Arch Otolaryngol Head Neck Surg* 1993;119:618–623.
17. Cheney ML, Megarian CA, Brown MT, McKenna MJ, Nadol JB. The use of the temporoparietal fascial flap in temporal bone reconstruction. *AJO* 1996;17(1):137–142.
18. Baek S, Lawson W, Biller HF. An analysis of 133 pectoralis major myocutaneous flaps. *Plast Reconstr Surg* 1982;69(3):460–467.
19. Maves MD, Panje WR, Shagets FW. Extended latissimus dorsi myocutaneous reconstruction of major head and neck defects. *Otolaryngol Head Neck Surg* 1984;92(5):551–557.
20. Urken ML, Naidu RK, Lawson W, Biller HF. The lower island trapezius flap revisited. *Arch Otolaryngol Head Neck Surg* 1991;117:502–511.
21. Netterville JL, Panje WR, Maves MD. The trapezius myocutaneous flap: dependability and limitations. *Arch Otolaryngol Head Neck Surg* 1987;113:271–281.
22. Urken ML, Turk JB, Weinberg H, Vickery C, Biller HF. The rectus abdominis free flap in head and neck reconstruction. *Arch Otolaryngol Head Neck Surg* 1991;117:857–866.
23. Taylor GI, Corlett RJ, Boyd JB. The versatile deep inferior epigastric (inferior rectus abdominis) flap. *Br J Plast Surg* 1984;37:330–350.
24. Shaw WW. Microvascular free flaps: the first decade. *Clin Plast Surg* 1983;10:3–20.
25. Khouri RK. Avoiding free flap failure. *Clin Plast Surg* 1992;19: 773–781.
26. Frodel JL, Marentette LJ, Quatela VC, Weinstein GS. Calvarial bone graft harvest: techniques, considerations, and morbidity. *Arch Otolaryngol Head Neck Surg* 1993;119:17.
27. Constantino PD, Friedman CD, Lane A. Synthetic biomaterials in facial plastic and reconstructive surgery. *Facial Plast Surg* 1993;9(1):1–15.
28. Ducic Y. Midface reconstruction with titanium mesh and hydroxyapatite cement: a case report. *J Cranio Max Trauma* 1997;3(2):35–39.
29. Constantino PD, Friedman CD, Jones K, Chow LC, Sisson GA. Experimental hydroxyapatite cement cranioplasty. *Plast Reconstr Surg* 1992; 90(2):174–185.
30. Stelnicki EJ, Hoffman WY, Ousterhout DG. A method for repairing zygomatic arch fractures using hydroxyapatite cement paste (bone source). *J Craniofac Surg* 1997;8(3):236–239.
31. Shindo ML, Constantino PD, Friedman CD, Chow LC. Facial skeletal augmentation using hydroxyapatite cement. *Arch Otolaryngol Head Neck Surg* 1993;119:185–190.

Subject Index